Advances in Biomaterials, 7

Biomaterials and Clinical Applications

EUROPEAN SOCIETY FOR BIOMATERIALS

ADVANCES IN BIOMATERIALS

Previous volumes (1–4) published by Wiley, New York.

Volume 5.	Biomaterials and Biomechanics 1983 (edited by P. Ducheyne, G. Van der Perre and A.E. Aubert)
Volume 6.	Biological and Biomechanical Performance of Biomaterials (edited by P. Christel, A. Meunier and A.J.C. Lee)
Volume 7.	Biomaterials and Clinical Applications (edited by A. Pizzoferrato, P.G. Marchetti, A. Ravaglioli and A.J.C. Lee)

Advances in Biomaterials, 7

Biomaterials and Clinical Applications

Proceedings of the Sixth European Conference on Biomaterials,
Bologna, Italy, September 14–17, 1986

edited by

A. Pizzoferrato
Centro di Ricerca per la Biocompatibilità dei Materiali da Impianto, Istituto Ortopedico Rizzoli, Università di Bologna, Bologna, Italy

P.G. Marchetti
Clinica Ortopedica, Università di Bologna, Bologna, Italy

A. Ravaglioli
Istituto di Ricerca Technologica per la Ceramica, CNR, Faenza, Italy

and

A.J.C. Lee
Department of Engineering Science, University of Exeter, Exeter, England

with the assistance of

G. Ciapetti and S. Stea
Istituto Ortopedico Rizzoli, Bologna, Italy

ELSEVIER
Amsterdam — Oxford — New York — Tokyo 1987

ELSEVIER SCIENCE PUBLISHERS B.V.
Sara Burgerhartstraat 25
P.O. Box 211, 1000 AE Amsterdam, The Netherlands

Distributors for the United States and Canada:

ELSEVIER SCIENCE PUBLISHING COMPANY INC.
52, Vanderbilt Avenue
New York, NY 10017, U.S.A.

Library of Congress Cataloging-in-Publication Data

European Conference on Biomaterials (6th : 1986 :
Bologna, Italy)
Biomaterials and clinical applications.

(Advances in biomaterials ; v. 7)
Includes bibliographies and indexes.
1. Biomedical materials--Congresses. 2. Bio-
compatibility--Congresses. I. Pizzoferrato, A.
II. European Society for Biomaterials. III. Title.
IV. Series. [DNLM: 1. Biocompatible Materials--
therapeutic use--congresses. 2. Implants, Artificial--
congresses. W3 AD23 v.7 / QT 34 E882 1986b]
R857.M3E87 1986 610.28 87-24566
ISBN 0-444-42883-6 (U.S.)

ISBN 0-444-42883-6 (Vol. 7)
ISBN 0-444-42353-2 (Series)

Printed in The Netherlands

SERIES FOREWORD

Biomaterials is that branch of biomedical engineering that is concerned with the materials aspects of medical devices. Any material, metal, ceramic, plastic or organic, brought into contact with the fluids, cells and tissues of the living body comes within the domain of biomaterials science. Included are surgical implant and dental materials, dressings orthotics, prosthetic materials, and those used in extracorporeal circulation devices. Biomaterials scientists are concerned with the physical and chemical properties of materials and their suitability for a particular device. They are concerned with how these properties are altered by the biological environment and how the materials may affect the body. The subject spans the physical and life sciences.

Biomaterials science has expanded rapidly in the last years, nurtured by enthusiasts in the medical profession, in universities, commerce, and government agencies. Many universities now offer undergraduate and postgraduate teaching courses. Among the societies that exist to promote the safe and efficient use of biomaterials and to encourage the development of a sound rational basis for this discipline are: the Society for Biomaterials (U.S.A.) founded in 1974, the Biological Engineering Society (U.K.) founded in 1960 and which established a specialist topic group in biomaterials in 1974, and the European Society for Biomaterials founded in 1976. Japanese and Canadian societies were inaugurated in 1979. These societies play a major part in the development of our subject by organising international meetings which provide a forum for the exchange of ideas in clinical and basic research.

It was to complement the valuable activities of these societies that the idea for this series on "Advances in Biomaterials" was born. It is intended to provide a vehicle for the publication of the proceedings of meetings on biomaterials which will grow into a valuable reference library. Volumes dealing with special topics may be commissioned as appropriate. The first four volumes in the series were published by John Wiley and Sons. The fifth and sixth volumes were published in 1984 and 1986 by Elsevier Science Publishers and were sponsored by the European Society for Biomaterials. With this, the seventh volume in the series, we continue the collaboration between Elsevier and the ESB and hope that these volumes will continue to fulfil the stated purpose of the series: to build a coherent body of knowledge for the use of students and practitioners in biomaterials, for the ultimate benefit of patients.

June 1987

A.J.C. LEE
President of the European Society
for Biomaterials

PREFACE

The present volume contains the Proceedings of the European Congress on Biomaterials organized through the joint collaboration of the Rizzoli Orthopaedic Institute in Bologna and the ESB, and held in Bologna (Italy) from September 14–17, 1986 in celebration of the tenth anniversary of the founding of the European Society for Biomaterials.

The well-known lecture, "The potential use of ceramics in orthopaedic implants," given by Prof. Samuel Hulbert (then at Clemson University, South Carolina) on March 3, 1973 at the Rizzoli Institute, served to stimulate the existing interest in the study of biomaterials. Following an initial meeting on October 3, 1975 in the Anatomical Drawing Room at the Rizzoli Institute, the European Society for Biomaterials was officially founded on March 12, 1976, by a group of European scientists with the goal of furthering the study of biomaterials used for implants in the human organism. The Executive Board was elected on that date: President, G.D. Winter (Great Britain); Secretary, S. Sandrolini Cortesi (Italy); Treasurer, A. Pizzoferrato (Italy) and Members of the Board, J.L. Leray (France), F.L. Burny (Belgium), G. Heimke (West Germany) and K. De Groot (Holland).

The Congress held in Bologna was divided into three scientific days during which 26 speakers were asked to give keynote and invited lectures on current issues, while the 21 sessions included 295 scientific papers by authors from all over the world. It was the main purpose of the Congress to verify the state of the art in the use of biomaterials and to allow for the participation of surgeons in the topics discussed. Problems specific to each field of application were included. In orthopaedic surgery, for example, cementless prostheses, the replacement of knee ligaments, fracture and spinal fixation devices were dealt with; in maxillo-facial surgery and dental implantology, maxillary reconstruction, dental implants and new dental materials, as well as materials for plastic surgery; in vascular surgery, the problems of small-bore vascular prostheses and the use of reabsorbable materials; in ocular surgery, polymers utilized for contact lenses and possible materials for retinal detachment or lens replaement. Particular emphasis was given to current materials such as composites and porous surface materials.

The round table discussion on the standardization of biomaterials covered several minimal requirements for biomaterial use and went into methods used in defining these requirements. The large variety of topics included in the Congress is proof of the multifaceted and interdisciplinary nature of the science of biomaterials.

The scientific papers collected in this volume constitute the final result of the Congress. They represent a vast amount of work by each author and by the scientists who assumed the task of acting as referees during the various stages of the Congress. We wish to thank all involved for their intense collaboration, which made it possible to maintain the high scientific level which characterizes the activities of the ESB.

Bologna, June 1987

The Editors

G. Agrifoglio
P. Bartolozzi
A. Bertoluzza
W. Bonfield
J. Breme
M. Campanacci
R. Caramazza
C. Cavina
M. D'Addato
K. De Groot
P. Ducheyne
J.O. Galante
P.E. Gallenga
G. Galletti
K.L. Gerlach
P. Giusti
R.M. Greenhalg
A.G. Gristina
U. Gross
G. Hastings
G. Heimke
A. Hensten-Pettersen
J. Kopecek
M. La Placa
D.L. Leake
A.J.C. Lee
P.G. Marchetti
G. Marotti
P.L. Melanotte
K. Merritt
C. Migliaresi
I. Oh
J.P. Paul
N.A. Peppas
A. Pizzoferrato
H. Plenk
T. Rae
B.A. Rahn
A. Ravaglioli
E. Rinonapoli
A. Ruggeri
R. Savini
G. Stea
P. Tranquilli-Leali
P.J. van Mullem
A.M. Weinstein
D.F. Williams

Contents

Section 3. Biomaterials for soft tissues and cardiovascular devices

Section 4. Structural, chemico - physical and biocompatibility characterization of biomaterials

Section 5. Drug delivery, infections and immunological aspects of biomaterials

Section 6. Experimental applications of prosthetic materials

Section 7. Standards and assessment of biomaterials

Biomaterials and Clinical Applications,
edited by A. Pizzoferrato, P.G. Marchetti, A. Ravaglioli and A.J.C. Lee
Elsevier Science Publishers B.V., Amsterdam, 1987 — Printed in The Netherlands

BIOMATERIALS AND INFECTION: CLINICAL EXPERIENCE

A.PIZZOFERRATO
Centro di Ricerca per la Biocompatibilità dei Materiali da Impianto, Istituto Ortopedico Rizzoli, Via Codivilla 9 - 40136, Bologna (Italy)

SUMMARY

Infections are one of the major complications in the use of prosthetic devices. The mechanisms by which the implantation of foreign objects increase susceptibility to infections are not completely understood, nevertheless clinical studies from many fields of surgery clearly demonstrate an association between the implantation of foreign materials and an increased incidence of infections. As reported by many Authors, the incidence of many types of prosthesis associated infection has decreased over recent years, and this finding is confirmed by our experience in the field of orthopedics.

INTRODUCTION

Prosthesis associated infection is one of the most feared complications in the use of prosthetic devices.

It is characterised by its persistency, even in the face of antimicrobial therapy and the defenses of the host.

In most cases the only possible cure is the removal of the prosthesis (Ref. 1).

A patient undergoing prosthetic surgery runs a high risk of infection, since nosocomial infections, which are acquired during the patients stay in hospital, are more common in this kind of surgery.

There are various causes that favour the high incidence of infection during prosthetic surgery:

- Insufficient cleanliness in the operating theatres
- Alteration of the immunological response
- Special features of the local response
- Emergence of antibiotic-resistant micro-organisms
- Intrinsic properties of the biomaterials
- Inaccurate sterilisation of the biomaterials

The degree of bacterial contamination within the operating room environment plays an important part in favouring the onset of the prosthesis associated infection.

It is however obvious that it is not only the air in the operating theatre and the type of clothing worn that influence the onset of infection. Other factors are associated with it, such as asepsis of the medical or nursing staff, the accuracy of the disinfection of the patient and post-operative care.

Alteration in the general host response constitutes another cause for the increase in the incidence of prosthesis associated infection.

This alteration may be due to poor nutrition, extreme old age and obesity, to pre-existing diseases such as rheumatoid arthritis, mellitus diabetes or other concurrent infectious diseases.

Therapeutic care, such as corticosteroid or anti-tumour treatments may modify the overall response capacity.

Another cause for the increased frequency of prosthesis associated infection is the alteration of host tissue response. The damage to the tissues caused by the surgery leads to the formation of an ideal ground for the trapping and development of bacteria.

In addition the surgical technique, and thus the time of exposure of the wound to the environment, increases the possibility of bacterial contamination.

The emergence of multiple antibiotic resistant organisms, which limits the use of treatment with antibiotics, may be one of the reasons for the increase in surgical infection; however, only some causes apply specifically to prosthesis associated infections.

One of these causes is the intrinsic properties of the biomaterials; particulate debris of metals such as cobalt and nickel and of the cobalt-chrome alloy or the PMMA cement, used for fixing the prosthesis, damage the host defense mechanisms. In particular, it has been shown "in vitro" that particles of these materials hinder chemotaxis and phagocytosis (Ref. 2).

Moreover, some biomaterials represent a foreign body to which bacteria, supplied by a polysaccharidic glycocalyx, adhere and increase rapidly in "protected" colonies (Ref. 3).

The unsuitable sterilisation of the biomaterials is another cause of increased incidence of the infection.

Sterilisation procedures, such as irradiation, may modify the properties of the material and lead to the formation of residues of liquid or gas that alter the host's response.

The diagnosis of the infection is based on the clinical evaluation, on the laboratory tests and on standard radiographs as well as on specialised diagnostic techniques (Ref. 4). A sure diagnosis of prosthesis associated infection is given by the examination of culture and by a histological examination of tissue samples collected at the removal or at the revision of the prosthesis.

The bacteriological examination should be carried out for both the aerobic and the anaerobic micro-organisms. The tissue samples should be obtained from more than one site around the prosthesis, so it is possible to establish the etiology of the sepsis and whether the infection is monomicrobial or polymicrobial.

The histological examination of frozen sections is mandatory before proceeding to immediate re-implantation of the prosthesis. An examination of paraffin-embedded slices makes it possible to ascertain the type and grade of infection.

It should be remembered that false negative or positive results may be obtained at the histological examination as well as at the bacteriological examination.

CLINICAL EXPERIENCE

Infections represent a serious complication in all the fields of application of surgical prostheses.

Infections associated with arterial and heart valve prostheses.

In vascular grafts for arterial reconstruction such complications may even be fatal.

The true incidence of infection following reconstructive arterial surgery is difficult to ascertain because the infections may remain dormant for years before becoming clinically evident (Ref. 5).

Some percentages of infection reported by various Authors are listed in table 1.

Most of these infections are due to Staphylococcus aureus, Staphylococcus epidermidis and enterobacteria.

TABLE 1
Incidence of synthetic vascular graft infections

N° Cases	N° Infections	%	Author
201	12	6	Hoffert et al 1965
890	12	1.3	Lindenaner et al 1967
435	22	5	Conn et al 1970
3397	40	1.9	Szilagyi et al 1972
566	27	2.5	Goldstone et al 1974
664	15	2.5	Jamieson et al 1975
859	22	2.5	Liekweg et al 1977
590	32	2.5	Yashar et al 1978
671	16	2.4	Martin-Paradero 1983

The number of infections due to Gram-negative bacteria or to polymicrobial association of aerobic and anaerobic germs is steadily increasing (Ref. 6).

The same Author also claims that early infections are mainly caused by Pseudomonas aeruginosa, E. coli and S. aureus whereas late infections are often caused by Staphylococcus epidermidis.

The anatomical site of the implant may affect the sepsis rate: the aorta-femoral area is the one most at risk.

The infections may be due to hematogenous contamination of the prosthesis or to direct contamination from a pre-existing infection of the arterial wall, by micro-organisms present in the adjacent lymph nodes, or arising from the surgery itself.

The infections, at least those due to direct contamination, should now be on the decrease thanks to the improvement in surgical techniques and in the sterilisation of the biomaterials, as well as improvements in the operating theatre.

Both early and late infections are associated with the implant of prosthetic heart valves. The early infections arise at the time of the implantation and are due to various types of germs.

Late endocarditis, the frequency of which varies from 0.9% to 3.9% as reported in table 2, is most commonly caused by streptococcus of the oral cavity.

TABLE 2
Incidence of prosthetic valve endocarditis

N° patients	N°infections	%	Author
1235	48	3.9	Slaughter 1973
1671	37	2.2	Dismukes 1973
4586	45	0.9	Wilson 1975
2184	50	2.3	Rossiter 1978
1282	46	3.6	Masur 1980

The bacteriemia of such germs may lead to seeding of the endothelialized surface of the prosthetic valves (Ref. 7).

Infections associated with ocular prosthetic devices

Infections associated with ocular prosthetic devices present different incidence rates and are due to different germs, depending on the site of their application.

Hard contact lenses are made of a material (PMMA) that does not support the growth of micro-organisms.

Soft contact lenses (pHEMA), may, on the contrary, provide a receptacle for micro-organisms and may easily lead to conjunctivitis unless decontaminated.

Even gas permeable lenses do not produce significant alterations to the endogenous ocular flora, but these too must be conserved and decontaminated with cleansing solutions.

Bacterial conjunctivitis, which may be associated with the use of contact lenses, are generally caused by Staphylococcus or Streptococcus, but infection has also been reported from Proteus species, Escherichia coli and Pseudomonas contaminating cleansing solutions (Ref. 8).

The incidence of cornea infections due to contact lenses is low, but may even reach 6% when there is extended wear of soft lenses (Ref. 9).

Numerous micro-organisms, such as Staphylococcus aureus, Pseudomonas, Streptococcus, Serratia, Enterobacter, Escherichia coli and Acinetobacter, may cause infectious keratitis.

Intraocular lenses implanted at removal of crystalline lenses affected by cataracts do not give rise to a high percentage of infection, however severe endophthalmitis may occur (Ref. 10).

Late infections are more common than acute infections in the surgical treatment of retinal detachment requiring the use of a biomaterial.

The most frequently isolated micro-organisms in treatment with silicon buckles are reported in table 3 (Ref. 11).
The infections are most frequently due to Staphylococcus epidermidis.

The incidence of clinical infections varies from 1.3 to 18%.

TABLE 3
Micro-organisms isolated from infected scleral buckles
(From Cobo et al, 1984)

	Lincoff (1970)	Hitchings (1974)	Ulrich (1974)	Hahn (1979)
Staphylococcus aureus	11	1	14	29
S. epidermidis	14	5	9	2
Proteus sp.	2		3	4
Klebsiella sp.			1	1
Enterobacter sp.			1	1
Alpha-hemolytic Strep.				1
No growth		4		11
	27	10	28	49

Infections associated with intrauterine devices

The mechanism by which an infection develops in the genital tract in relation to an IUD may vary. It is possible for bacteria to be introduced when the device is inserted, but it is also possible that the uterus becomes infected by the ascending contamination along the "tail" of the IUD, especially if this is made of a polyfilament (Ref. 12).

The erosion of the uterine wall, caused by IUD may favour the growth of bacteria (Ref. 13).

The infections can spread widely and may lead to pelvic inflammatory disease and ovarian abscesses.

Infections associated with oral and dental implants

In the field of oral and dental prostheses, implant associated infection is a complication to be feared.

The bacterial plaque that collects around the neck of the implant does not only cause gum infection but frequently determines a periodontal disease due to the lack of a seal between the implant and the mucosa (Ref. 14).

Deep infection leads to the resorption of the alveolar bone and to loosening of the implant.

The germs that determine such an infection are mainly anaerobic (Ref. 15).

Those most frequently involved are Bacteroid, Fusobacterium, Peptococcus and Actinomyces.

These infections may, albeit in extremely rare cases, spread to the neck and head with very serious complications (Ref. 16).

Infections associated with orthopedic devices

The percentages of infection associated with orthopedic devices reported in literature concern total joint prostheses. These percentages vary according to the Author and according to the site of the implant of the artificial joint under consideration (Table 4).

TABLE 4
Incidence of infection in total arthroplasties

N° Prostheses	N° infections	%	Author
5800 (hip)	85	1.6	Charnley 1972
298 (hip)	0	0	Colles et al. 1976
3120 (hip)	42	1.3	Fitzgerald et al. 1977
1065 (hip)	73	6.8	Carlsonn 1977
16054 (hip)	198	1.23	Rand et al. 1984
1000 (hip)	22	2.2	Ainscow 1984
2012 (hip)	18	0.89	Poss et al. 1984
1957 (knee)	11	0.57	Poss et al. 1984
821 (knee)	14	1.7	Gorgan 1986
471 (knee)	25	5.3	Johnson 1986

The percentage for hip arthroprostheses goes from the 0% reported by Colles in 1976 to the 6.8% of Carlsonn in 1977 and for knee arthroprostheses from 0.57 found by Poss (1984) to the 5.3% of Johnson in 1986.

It is however difficult to collect adequate data for the evaluation of the incidence of infection, as well as the variations in this incidence depending on the period of time and the type of implant.

This is because in many case-reports the cases are followed only for a period of 2 or 3 years; it is known that implants may have to be removed many years after their implantation, because of infection.

In order to establish the incidence of early infections due to prostheses it could be useful to evaluate the ratio between the rate of infected post-operative wounds with prosthetic devices versus the rate of infected surgical wounds without prosthesis, such as joint resections, arthrodesis and osteotomy.

In order to establish the incidence of late infections we consider that a bacteriological examination of the periprosthetic bioptic material should be carried out (Ref. 17). Specimens should be collected from different sites, as Fig. 1 shows.

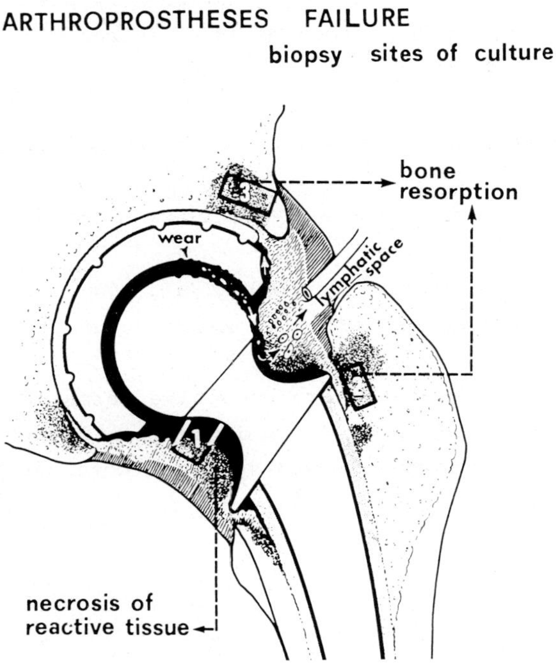

FIGURE 1

Table 5 reports the data collected in 403 cases of hip arthoprosthesis removed more than 2 years after implantation at the Istituto Rizzoli from 1977 to the present time.

The annual percentage enables us to follow the trend of late infection.

TABLE 5
Examined cases of hip prosthesis failure

YEARS	NUMBER OF CASES	POSITIVE CULTURE No.	%
1977-78-79	161	79	49.1
1980	53	26	49.1
1981	36	10	27.8
1982	37	11	29.7
1983	24	7	29.2
1984	27	9	33.3
1985	43	8	18.6
1986 (Jan.-July)	22	2	9

The percentage of positive results, from 49.1% in the first 3 years, drops to 27.8% in 1981.

A more noticeable drop occurred in 1985 and in the first six months of 1986.

In agreement with other Authors (Refs. 18,19), we attribute the drop mainly to improvements in prophylactic measures adopted before, during and after surgery, both as regards the patient and the medical and nursing staff present in the operating and after-care areas.

Many types of micro-organisms were identified as reported in table 6.

In each of the three-year periods there was a predominance of gram-positive germs over gram-negative.

Of the gram-positive germs those most commonly arising are Staphylococcus aureus, Staphylococcus epidermidis, Micrococcus and Streptococcus faecalis.

The Enterobacteria account for 75% of the gram-negative germs in the first three-year period, but this percentage decreases in the subsequent periods (approx. 57%) and Pseudomonas species increases (from 13% to 33%).

The isolation of anaerobic bacteria is rare.

TABLE 6
Micro-organisms isolated from 403 removed hip prostheses

Strains	'77-'79	'80-'82	'83-'85	1986 (Jan-July)
Staphylococcus epidermidis	18	23	6	1
Micrococcus	10	6	2	
Staphylococcus aureus	11	3	6	
Alpha-haemolytic Streptococcus		3	1	
Non-haemolytic Streptococcus	9			
Group A beta-haemolytic Streptococcus	1			
Group B beta-haemolytic Streptococcus	4	1		
Streptococcus faecalis	11	6	3	1
Diphteroid bacilli	6	1		
Propionibacterium acnes			1	
Proteus mirabilis			1	
Proteus vulgaris	2	1		
Proteus rettgeri	7			
Proteus morganii	4	1		
Serratia marcescens	9	2		
Enterobacter agglomerans	3			
Enterobacter cloacae	1	3	1	
Escherichia coli	1		3	
Klebsiella pneumoniae	4			
Citrobacter freundii	3			
Pseudomonas aeruginosa	4	1	3	
Pseudomonas fluorescens	1	1		
Pseudomonas species	1	2		
Acinetobacter calcoaceticus var. Lwoffi	4	1		
Acinetobacter calcoaceticus var. anitratus			1	
Bacteroides fragilis ss. fragilis	1			

The polymicrobial associations are reported in table 7.

TABLE 7
Polymicrobial associations in infected hip endo-artroprostheses (1980-1986)

1) Serratia marcescens + Pseudomonas species
2) Proteus mirabilis + Enterobacter cloacae
3) Streptococcus faecalis + Serratia marcescens
4) Streptococcus faecalis + Escherichia coli
5) Streptococcus faecalis + Enterobacter cloacae
6) Strept. faecalis+Proteus morganii+Proteus vulgaris+Staph. aureus
7) Staphylococcus epidermidis + micrococcus
8) Staphylococcus epidermidis + alpha-haemolytic streptococcus
9) Staphylococcus epidermidis + Pseudomonas species
10) Staphylococcus epidermidis + acinetobacter calcoaceticus var.lwoffi

The types of association are various, this means that the source of the infection is also variable.

CONCLUSIONS

The problem of prosthesis associated infections may be related to the more general problem of post-operative nosocomial infections.

However, biological phenomena related directly to the characteristics of the biomaterials themselves determine the greater incidence and seriousness of prosthesis associated infections, when compared to other post-operative infections.

The immediate damage to tissue, due to the insertion of the prosthesis, or the subsequent damage to tissue, caused by wear or corrosion of the implanted material, lead to the formation of an area around the prosthesis that is more prone to infection.

The action that favours the collection of bacteria or that inhibits the phagocytosis of some biomaterials enhances bacterial growth.

The result is the persistence of any bacterial contamination arising at the time of surgery or subsequently by hematogenous routes.

A rapid colonisation of the bacteria may follow, leading to the development of a severe infection, which is certainly more serious than infections that are not prosthesis associated.

Treatment with antibiotics is often ineffective and the only possible solution is the removal of the implant.

However, the incidence of many types of prosthesis associated infection has considerably decreased over recent years, as confirmed by our experience in the field of orthopedics.

This decrease is due not so much to a specific prophylaxis for the prosthetic implantation, as to the rigorous measures of hygiene adopted in the last few years aimed at containing all nosocomial infections (Ref. 20).

However, the implants that are positioned through the mucosa, and which therefore communicate with the outside, have not had the same good results.

In cases such as dental implants, in which there is a lack of sealing between the mucosa and the material, micro-organisms are more likely to adhere. In this respect the shape of the implant plays an important role.

A solution to the problem can not be reached with only a better understanding of the pathogenesis of the infections and their treatment with antibiotics. An increase in our knowledge of the biomaterials and the prosthetic models is also required.

REFERENCES

1 G.C. Canner, M.E. Steinberg, R.B. Heppenstall, R. Balderston, The infected hip after total hip arthroplasty, J. Bone Joint Surg. 66A(9) (1984) 1393-1399.
2 T. Rae, A study on the effects of particulate metals of orthopaedic interest on murine macrophages in vitro, J. Bone Joint Surg., 57B (1975) 444-456.
3 A.G. Gristina, J. Kolkin, Current Concepts Review. Total joint replacement and sepsis, J. Bone Joint Surg., 65A(1) (1983) 128-134.
4 J.A. Rand, B.F. Morrey, Management of the infected total joint arthroplasty, Orthop. Clin. of North Am., 15 (3) (1984) 491-505.
5 W.J. Liekweg, L.J. Greenfield, Vascular prosthetic infections: collected experience and results of treatment, Surg., 81 (3) (1977) 335-342.
6 J. Goldstone, Infections in vascular grafting: pathogenesis prevention and treatment in: S.H. Skotnicki (Ed.), Proc. Symposium on Recent Advances in Vascular Grafting, Nijmegen, The Netherlands, April 26-28, 1984, pp. 207-215.
7 W.R. Wilson, G.K. Danielson, E.R. Giuliani, J.E. Geraci, Prosthetic valve endocarditis, Mayo Clin. Proc., 57 (1982) 155-166.
8 J.F. Morgan, Complications associated with contact lens solutions, Ophthalmology, 86 (1979) 1107-1120.
9 D.A. Snyder, S.M. Litensky, H. Gelender, Hypopyon iridocyclitis associated with extended wear soft contact lenses, Am. J. Ophthalmol., 93 (1982) 519-527.
10 R.K. Forster, R.L. Abbot, H.Gelender, Management of infectious endophthalmitis, Ophthalmology, 87 (1980) 313-318.
11 L.M. Cobo, G.N. Foulks, J. Tiedman, Infections associated with ocular devices, in: B. Sugarman, E.J. Young (Eds.), Infections associated with prosthetic devices, CRC Press, Boca Raton, 1984, pp. 43-59.
12 L.J. van Bogaert, A clinicopathological study of IUD users with special reference to endometrial patterns in endometritis, Gynecol. Obstet. Invest., 126 (1983) 129-135.
13 W.Jr. Cates, H.W. Ory, IUD complications: infection, death and ectopic pregnancy, in: K.S. Moghissi (Ed.), Controversies in contraception, Williams and Wilkins, Baltimore, 1979, pp. 187-202.
14 S.Michieli, D. Leake, A. Pizzoferrato, F. Gasparini, L. Cini, S.Sandrolini , Design comparison of alumina coated dental implants, J. Clin. Engineering, 4 (3) (1979) 269-274.
15 M.G.Newman, The role of Bacteroides Melaninogenicus and other anaerobes in periodontal infections, Rev. Infect. Dis., 1 (1979) 313-320.
16 Ch. A. Babbush, Infections associated with oral and dental implants, in: B. Sugarman, E.J. Young (Eds.), Infections associated with prosthetic devices, CRC Press, Boca Raton, 1984, pp. 61-71.
17 A. Pizzoferrato, F. Fiori, L. Savarino, Microbiological investigation on 161 cases of hip endo-arthroprosthesis failure, Chir. Org. Mov., 66 (3), (1981) 297-307. e and outcome of infection following total joint arthroplasty, Clin. Orthop., 182 (1984) 117-126.
18 J.Charnley, Post-operative infection after total hip replacement with special reference to air contamination in the operating room, Clin. Orthop., 87 (1972) 167-187.

19 R.Poss, T.S.Thornhill, F.C.Ewald, W.H.Thomas, N.J.Batte, C.B.Sledge, Factors influencing the incidence and outcome of infection following total joint arthroplasty, Clin. Orthop., 182 (1984) 117-126.
20 A. Pizzoferrato, F. Fiori, E. Cenni, Controllo delle infezioni nosocomiali, Min. Med., 76 (1985) 1473-1486.

Biomaterials and Clinical Applications, 13
edited by A. Pizzoferrato, P.G. Marchetti, A. Ravaglioli and A.J.C. Lee
Elsevier Science Publishers B.V., Amsterdam, 1987 — Printed in The Netherlands

NEW TRENDS IN IMPLANT MATERIALS

W. Bonfield

Department of Materials, Queen Mary College, London. El 4NS, England.

SUMMARY

The application of synthetic materials for bone and joint replacement is now well established. In general, metallic alloys from one of three major types, namely austenitic stainless steel, cobalt-chromium and Ti 6 wt% Al 4 wt% V, are used in the majority of major load bearing applications. Such alloys exhibit a range of mechanical properties, which depend sensitively on the microstructure developed by prior metallurgical conditioning. The development of optimised properties in these alloys for application as implant materials is reviewed, with particular reference to the comparative properties of the cortical bone being replaced. It is suggested that mechanical - as well as bio-compatibility is of importance if stress shielding and consequent bone resorption is to be avoided at areas of fixation. The development of analogous materials to the natural tissue for longer term applications is also considered.

INTRODUCTION

A prerequisite for any synthetic material implanted in the body is that it should be biocompatible in the sense of not producing an inflammatory tissue reaction. In addition, the implanted material is expected to withstand applied physiological forces without substantial dimensional change, catastrophic brittle fracture, or fracture in the longer term from creep, fatigue or stress corrosion. Within this context the application of synthetic materials for bone and joint replacement is now well-established. Each of the implant materials currently used has different mechanical properties and hence has particular advantages or disadvantages for a particular clinical situation. The paper is concerned with a comparison of the metallic alloys currently favoured in orthopaedic surgery with a forward look at some novel non-metallic materials. The corresponding properties for normal adult weight bearing cortical bone are also considered as it is recognised that mechanical compatibility between the implant and the natural tissue is of particular importance if stress shielding, and consequent bone resorption, is to be avoided at areas of fixation. Thermodynamic stability is only achieved in the ideal situation of an equivalent replacement material in an identical structure to that of the natural tissue. Any departure from this situation will create a different stress state in the remaining tissue and hence the potential for bone resorption and implant loosening. Whether this thermodynamic instability is significant in practice depends on the kinetics of the bone remodelling, but is well illustrated by the relative "success" of total hip replacement in elderly patients (i.e. ~ 90% achieve a lifetime > 10 years) as compared with the relative "failure" of identical procedures for more active, middle aged patients (with lifetimes < 2 years). In either group the major cause of failure (apart from infection) is implant loosening. Hence the bone-implant "circuit" deserved serious consideration if current orthopaedic implant procedures are to be optimised to produce longer "in vivo" lifetimes.

Cortical bone

Cortical bone from the major support bones has anisotropic mechanical properties with a maximum parallel to, and a minimum perpendicular to, the long axis (Ref.1). The stiffness of cortical bone, as represented by the Young's modulus varies between ~ 10-25 GPa. In fact bone is only linear elastic in behaviour at relatively low applied stresses, as a small viscoelastic component of deformation is also noted within the range of physiological stressing. Bone fracture, in tension, the weakest mode, requires an applied stress of ~ 50-150 MPa, although a statement of fracture in terms of a stress alone is misleading, given that bone is notch sensitive with a limited elongation to fracture (~ 0.5-3%). Hence, a measure of the fracture toughness of bone, requiring both a stress and a characterised crack, is required and values have been established (Ref.2) for the critical stress intensity factor, K_C (~ 2-12 $MNm^{-3/2}$) and the critical strain energy release rate, G_C (~ 600-5000 Jm^{-2}). Such fracture data for cortical bone defines the baseline which must be exceeded by an implant material in an equivalent structural design.

Metallic alloys

The vast majority of implants for bone and joint replacement are based on three major alloy types, namely austenitic stainless steel, cobalt-chromium and titanium 6 wt% Al 4 wt% V. Each alloy has a characteristic Young's modulus which increases from titanium (106 GPa) to stainless steel (200 GPa) to cobalt chromium (230 GPa), i.e. all three alloys are considerably stiffer than cortical bone. While Young's modulus is approximately independent of metallurgical condition for all three alloy types, the values of yield stress (which defines the limit of elastic behaviour and hence, divisible by a safety factor, determines the useable stress range for the implant), as well as of ultimate tensile strength, K_C and G_C, all depend sensitively on grain size, porosity, and the size and distribution of the individual phases. In general, optimum properties correspond to a minimum grain size and, obviously, a minimum porosity, while uniform properties necessitate a uniform grain size distribution. In addition, austenitic stainless steel is ductile in the annealed condition and shows a strong response to cold working, which increases the yield stress and ultimate tensile strength at the expense of the elongation to fracture. Hence a range of yield stress values can be obtained, which, depending on the particular composition and metallurgical processing, are approximately 207-1160 MPa and 430-1028 MPa for stainless steel and cobalt-chromium respectively (Ref.3). For implant purposes, the upper end of this range is used, with corresponding elongations to fracture of ~ 10%.

The titanium alloy is not sufficiently ductile in the annealed condition to permit cold working, but comparable values of yield stress and elongation to fracture to those near the upper end of the ranges for stainless steel and cobalt chromium are obtained, namely 780-1050 MPa and ~ 10%, respectively (Ref.3). Hence, it is important to appreciate that each alloy type does not have single values of yield stress. In general the yield stress values for all three alloys comfortably exceed the ultimate tensile strength of cortical bone (50-150 MPa), while the limiting fracture toughness values are also considerably enhanced (Table 1). Consequently, given that the applied stress is defined by the applied force divided by the cross sectional area, a comparison of the relative areas of cortical bone and implant would indicate that all three alloys will qualify as candidates for bone replacement on a strength basis.

An allowance should also be made for the fatigue process occurring with time under cyclic loading. Indeed, as this process initiates at the surface, it is essential that the implant surface is carefully polished and free from defects. Reducing the effective yield stresses by a maximum factor of ~ 0.5 to allow for fatigue (Ref.3), still leaves an appreciable safety margin with respect to cortical bone. However a major consequence of the current trend to produce porous implant surfaces, as a means of encouraging bone ingrowth, is to accelerate the fatigue process by facilitating crack nucleation. Indeed the stress level to produce fatigue fracture at 10^7 cycles can be reduced to potentially critical levels, as shown in Table 2. Such a situation requires careful control as the natural hard tissue can effectively resist fatigue crack propagation at a relatively high proportion of its ultimate tensile strength by "self repair" bone remodelling. Certainly the variations in yield stress values between the three alloys with polished, non-porous surfaces are of small consequence as compared to the large difference of all three with the natural tissue. All three alloy types are accepted as biocompatible, although there is a growing awareness of the accumulation of metal ions (particularly of nickel) in tissues in the longer term, which would suggest that stainless steel is less suitable than cobalt-chromium and titanium for applications with an expected lifetime greater than one year.

One distinction between the three alloy types in mechanical behaviour, is with respect to their Young's modulus. None match cortical bone, but titanium is certainly a factor two less stiff than stainless steel and cobalt-chromium, and consequently, for a similar cross section produces less stress shielding, and hence is intrinsically more desirable in a bone-implant contact position.

An alternative approach to the difference in invariant alloy properties such as Young's modulus is to reduce the structural stiffness for a given alloy through a reduction in the implant cross section. Such a procedure would be counter to the current trend to "fill" the medullary cavity, but could become feasible in future macro-composites designs, as discussed in the following section, and would require an enhancement in the alloy mechanical properties. From this standpoint, the Co-Cr alloy still has considerable potential for development, given the large grain size and compositional heterogeneity ("coring") present in the as cast structure, which, as shown in Figure 1, is only partially homogenised by a subsequent annealing heat treatment (Ref.3). While this non-optimised microstructure provides adequate mechanical properties for present implant design, various metallurgical processing routes could effectively improve the strength and ductility. It has been demonstrated on related alloys (Ref.4) as well as on Co-Cr (Ref.5), that a reduction in carbon content produces an increased room temperature ductility. Hence the pronounced response of the matrix austenite phase to work hardening can be utilised, with the subsequent formation of fcc deformation twins and hcp ϵ-martensite platelets providing an effective strengthening mechanism (Ref.4). In contrast, the Ti 6% Al 4% V implant is already effectively optimised in terms of its metallurgical structure (Ref.3), with a relatively fine grain size (~ 10 μm) and a homogeneous two phase α-β microstructure (Figure 2). Consequently future improvements in fatigue and ultimate strength characteristics may depend on the utilisation of potentially higher strength, lower modulus alloys such as Ti 15% V 3% Cr 3% Sn 3% Al and Ti 6% Al 5% Zr 0.5% Mo 0.25% Si.

Analogue materials

An alternative approach to bone replacement is to develop new composite materials with analogous properties to bone and one such composite, hydroxyapatite reinforced polyethylene, is now entering clinical trials (Ref.6). Such composites can only be used in an equivalent structural position to that of the natural tissue and for example, a medullary spike, with maximum surface stresses of 145-575 MPa (Ref.3), would not prove adequate if manufactured from either cortical bone or a synthetic equivalent. One advantage of the hydroxyapatite-polyethylene composite is that a range of mechanical properties can be producing depending on the particular volume fraction of hydroyapatite selected. Consequently an appropriate balance between stiffness and fracture toughness can be achieved, so as to obtain approximate modulus matching, with a superior fracture toughness as compared with cortical bone. In particular, the incorporation of the hydroxyapatite phase in a polymer matrix produces a significantly higher fracture toughness than would be obtained for hydroxyapatite by itself. As the favourable bone bioactivity created by hydroxyapatite is retained in high volume fraction composites, then bone appositional growth can be encouraged (Ref.7). Hence the considerable potential for such materials is to allow cementless fixation to bone without any major stress shielding. Indeed, a major materials prospect for the future is the development of multi component systems, involving a combination of one or more of the conventional alloys with analogous composites to provide a spectrum of mechanical behaviour for the orthopaedic surgeon to exploit in various clinical situations.

ACKNOWLEDGEMENTS

The author gratefully acknowledges the contribution of the Biomaterials Group at Queen Mary College and the continuing major support of the Science and Engineering Research Council.

REFERENCES

1 W. Bonfield, Elasticity and viscoelasticity of bone in Natural and Living Biomaterials, CRC Press, Boca Raton, FL., 1984, 43-60.

2. W. Bonfield, Biomechanical compatibility of composites analogous to bone. Biocompatibility of tissue analogs, CRC Press, Boca Raton, FL., 1985, 89-102.

3 R.M. Pilliar and G.C. Weatherly, Developments in implant alloys in CRC Critical Reviews in Biocompatibility, CRC Press, Boca Raton, FL., 1985, 371-403.

4 M. Assefpour-Dezfuly and W. Bonfield, Strengthening mechanisms in Elgiloy, J. Mater. Sci., 19, 1984, 2815-2836.

5 K. Rajan and J.B. Van der Sande, Room temperature strengthening mechanisms in a Co-Cr-Mo-C alloy, J. Mater. Sci., 17, 1982, 769-778.

6 W. Bonfield, Composites for bone replacement, Shell Polymers, 9, 1985, 79-85.

7 W. Bonfield, C. Doyle and K.E. Tanner, In vivo evaluation of hydroxyapatite reinforced polyethylene composites, Biological and Biomechanical Performance of Biomaterials, ed. P. Christel, A. Meunier and A.J.C. Lee, Elsevier Science Publishers BV, Amsterdam, 1986, 153-158.

TABLE 1

A comparison of some mechanical properties of current implant materials with those of cortical bone

Material	E/GPa	UTS/MPa	$K_{IC}/MNm^{-3/2}$	G_{IC}/Jm^{-2}
Cobalt-chromium alloys	230	430-1,028	~ 100	~ 50,000
Austenitic stainless steel	200	207-1,160	~ 100	~ 50,000
Ti 6 wt% Al 4 wt% V	105	780-1,050	~ 80	~ 10,000
Cortical bone	7-30	50-150	2-12	~ 600-5,000
PMMA (bone cement)	3.5	70	1.5	~ 400
Polyethylene	1	30	-	~ 8,000

E - Youngs modulus
UTS - Ultimate tensile strength
K_{IC} - Critical stress intensity factor
G_{IC} - Critical strain energy release rate

TABLE 2

A comparison of 10^7 cycles fatigue fracture

<u>Fatigue stresses</u> (10^7 cycles)/MPa	
Stainless steel	190-700
Co-Cr	250-670
Co-Cr (porous coat)	(150)
Ti-6 Al-4V	500-625
Ti-6 Al-4V (porous coat)	(200)

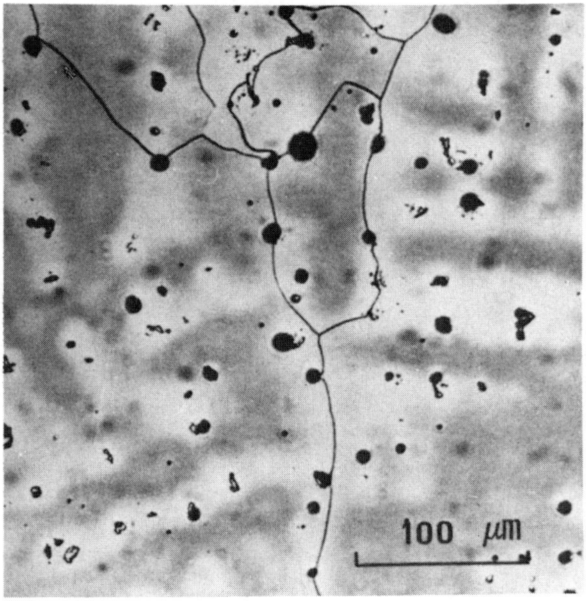

Fig.1. A heterogeneous microstructure in Co-Cr remaining after a solution anneal at 1230°C/1 hr (Ref.3).

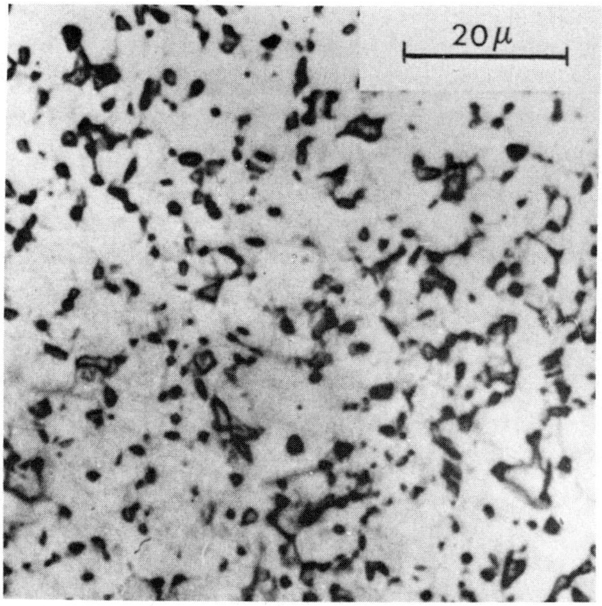

Fig. 2. A homogeneous microstructure in Ti 6% Al 4% V (Ref.3).

Biomaterials and Clinical Applications,
edited by A. Pizzoferrato, P.G. Marchetti, A. Ravaglioli and A.J.C. Lee
Elsevier Science Publishers B.V., Amsterdam, 1987 — Printed in The Netherlands

CEMENTLESS FIXATION

LARRY L. HENCH[1]

[1]Graduate Research Professor of Materials Science and Engineering and Director Bioglass Research Center and Co-Director Advanced Materials Research Center, University of Florida, Gainesville, Florida 32611

INTRODUCTION

Use of alloplastic prostheses in joint reconstruction has been one of the most significant and successful advances in orthopaedic surgery. Figure 1, prepared from Hori et al (ref. 1) and Rutkow (ref. 2) shows the large continuing increase in repair and plastic operations on joint structures in the United States during 1976-1983. Similar increases have occurred in Europe and Japan. The cumulative number of joint operations in the U.S. during the 1976-1986 decade is nearly 6,000,000, an approximately 6 fold increase over the previous decade. A substantial fraction of these operations involve implants, either in primary or revision cases.

This enormous growth in total joint surgical procedures is due to a very low morbidity (<1%) and high rate (>95%) of

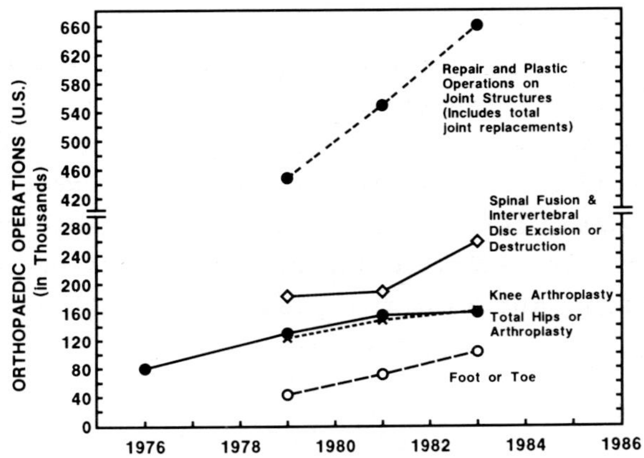

Figure 1. Orthopaedic operations (U.S.) from 1976-83 (refs. 1,2).

immediate post-operative success for patients with cemented orthopaedic prostheses. The immediate relief from pain and increased mobility results in a dramatic improvement in the patients' quality of life (ref. 3).

THE PROBLEM

However, from the late 70's to the present there has become a growing awareness of the complications associated with long term (>5 years) use of implants (refs. 4,5,6,7,8,9,10,11,12). Loosening, fracture, wear, and late infection all contribute to loss of prostheses. Concerns regarding long term systemic effects, such as metal ion toxicity or carcinogenicity are also beginning to emerge, (refs. 13,14,15,16,17). The probability of failure from each of these factors increases with time, each factor is additive, and in many cases the complications are synergistic. A consequence of synergistic, additive failure modes is an ever growing rate of revision operations which could reach epidemic proportions by the end of this century (ref.12), (ref. 18).

The reported results of 30-50% loosening of cemented femoral components by 10 years and 30-50% of cemented acetabular components by 15 years, multiplied by the nearly 6,000,000 joint operations in the last decade, assuming the same rates of long term loosening for all cemented prostheses, could result in 1,800,000 to 3,000,000 revisions between now and 1996. This is an annual rate of revision as large as present primary surgery (see Fig. 1). Use of cemented prostheses in younger patients (<45 yrs) will almost surely result in revision and therefore often cannot be justified.

Many circumstances affect the balance between stability of an implant and loosening. Lee and Ling (ref. 19), have summarized the interrelationship between biological and bio-mechanical factors that can lead to loosening (Fig. 2). The problem of loosening, of course, is focused at the bone-implant interface. It is the progressive deterioration of this interface that results in loosening and mechanical failure of either the bone or the device.

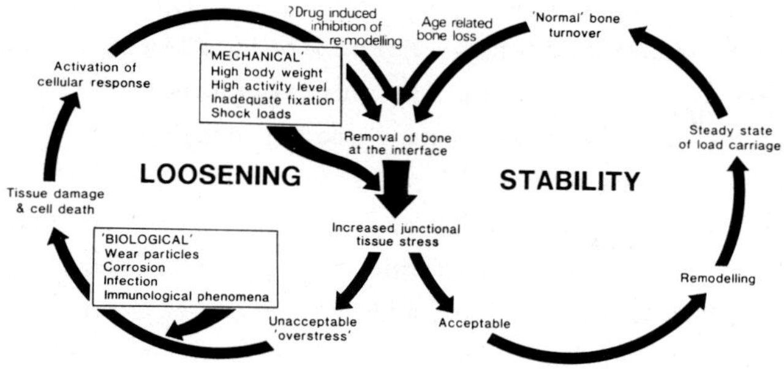

Figure 2. Biomechanical factors affecting loosening or stability of implants. (from Lee and Ling, ref. 19)

The presence of PMMA bone cement at the viable bone-implant interface has been implicated in most studies of loosening (refs. 19,20,21). Consequently, there is a rapidly growing interest in alternative, cement-free methods for anchoring prostheses in bone. Three primary approaches to cementless fixation have evolved: 1) "Morphologic fixation", by mechanical interlocking, 2)Porous ingrowth of bone or "Biological fixation" and 3) "Bioactive fixation" or surface-active interfacial bonding. The objective of this paper is to review the concepts and the relative advantages and disadvantages of these three alternatives.

However, it is important to keep in mind that for any fixation method to be judged superior to cement, the prognosis for failure should be less than 5% at 5 years, and the prognosis for success should be greater than 70% at 10 years. This is a difficult mark to meet. It is fortunate indeed for the millions of patients with cemented devices that this goal is so high.

MORPHOLOGIC FIXATION

The primary advantages of cemented prostheses lie in 1)

spreading the load over a wider area of bone and, 2) achieving load bearing soon after surgery. Morphologic fixation attempts to spread the load by increasing the surface area of the implant. Many designs of both acetabular and femoral components or knee prostheses have been advocated to achieve "physiologic" loading of non-cemented prostheses (see Morscher, ref. 11 for examples of these devices). Various combinations of grooves, ribs, holes, indendations, etc on a variety of materials have been investigated. For success, great attention must be paid to adapting the bone and the design of the morphologic prosthesis since the interfacial strength is very low compared to cemented devices (Fig. 3).

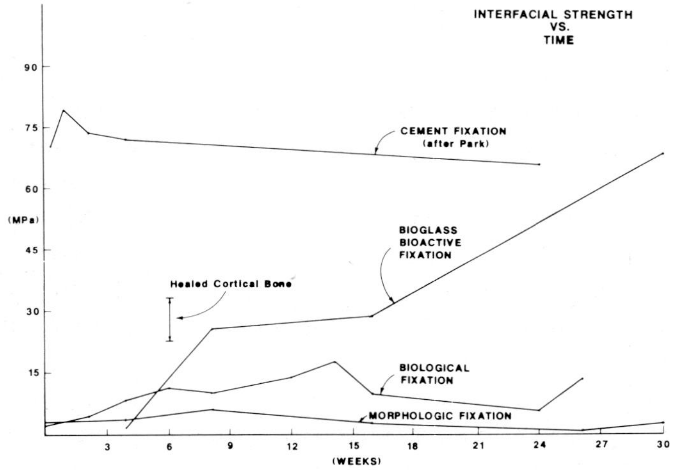

Figure 3. Interfacial bond strength (MPa) of various types of implants as a function of post-implantation time.

Although there is for morphologic prostheses relatively little follow-up data longer than 5 years, the clinical results appear to be at least as good as cemented hip arthroplasty, and loosening has not been a major problem (ref. 11). A potential advantage clinically for morphologically fixed devices is the absence of cement damage to bone stock should revision be necessary. However, revision techniques are complicated by bony ingrowth into indentations and surface irregularities. The surgical technique required to achieve perfect adaptation of the prosthesis and bone is reported to be precise and demanding and the incidence of intraoperative complications greater (ref. 11). Even so, there is a growing indication that morphologic fixation should be the system of choice for younger, active persons. However, until substantial 10 year follow-up data is available, such a conclusion must be one of guarded optimism.

BIOLOGICAL FIXATION

Ingrowth of bony tissue into porous implants or porous implant surfaces with a large surface area is the basis for "biological fixation". This concept should distribute the loads transmitted from the prosthesis to bone over a large interfacial area and thereby minimize localized stress gradients. Ideally, such a "living bone-implant interface" should remodel in response to stress variations over an indefinite period of time, unlike the dormant cement-prosthesis interface, and interfacial loosening should be delayed or prevented altogether.

Bone ingrowth into porous metal implants (refs. 22,23,24,25), porous ceramics (ref. 26) and porous polymers (refs. 27,28,29), has been well documented in animals. (See Chapters 3,4 and 5 in ref. 16 for a general review of this subject.) A pore size of 100 to 400 micrometers has been shown to be optimum. An optimum depth of ingrowth is also required, i.e. at least 3 layers of beads, to achieve maximum shear strength of the interface, (ref. 30).

In experimental animals, uniform ingrowth of bone has been demonstrated in both non-cemented polymers and porous metals (refs. 24,27,30). A compilation of results from a large number of animal studies show that the interfacial strength of porous implants changes with time, requiring 2 to 3 months to reach a maximum of 15-20 MPa (Fig 3). However, there is a tendency for interfacial strength to decrease at longer times. These values of interfacial strength are less than those for repaired cortical bone, tested with a similar push out model but are certainly sufficient to anchor prostheses even with a small area of the device coated with porous material.

There are several areas of concern regarding biological fixation, especially if the method is expected to be used for young patients with 20-40 years of post-operative lifetime. These include: 1) Reduced strength and/or fatique resistance of Co-Cr metal prostheses due to sintering of porous coatings, (ref. 31); 2) Increased notch sensitivity of Ti implants due to porous coatings (ref. 32); 3) Subsidence of implants and bone resorption due to stress shielding;(refs. 11,33,34); 4) Loss of surface beads and bead migration (refs. 35,36); 5) Enhanced corrosion and metal ion release due to the large metal surface area when fretting-corrosion occurs at the implant-tissue interface (ref. 37); 6) Potential for immune hypersensitivity and malignant neoplasms due to increased local levels of Co, Cr, or Ni (refs. 13,14,15,16,17); 7) Careful selection of sizes and precise technique to ensure post operative fixation and a sensation of stability (refs. 11,33,34); 8) Controlled post-operative loading regimen to ensure progressive bone ingrowth and stabilization (ref. 33); 9) Difficult revision procedures (refs. 11,33); and 10) Lack of uniform bone growth into porous implants, especially for elderly or arthritic patients or young patients with poor bone quality. For example, soft tissue has always been found at some parts of the interface between bone and non-cemented polyethylene tibial prostheses (ref. 39). In contrast, the same team (ref. 40), using the same type of device in animals achieved excellent bone ingrowth. These differences show that there is a need for long term animal studies of the interfacial stability of porous prostheses with arthritic and osteoporotic bone before wide spread clinical use can be justified.

Obviously, these concerns are not always realized, especially in the short term. Results reported by Engh and Bobyn for example (refs. 33,34), indicate clinical results in primary cases using biological fixation that are very encouraging and compare favorably with the results of cemented arthroplasty. They have seen relatively minor early subsidence in only 5% of femoral stems and only one case of symptomatic acute subsidence. They observe a high percentage of perfect scores for pain and walking for younger patients with biological fixation which is consistent with Lord and Mittlemeier's observations using morphologic fixation in younger patients.

These results suggest that biological fixation may some day

replace cement fixation. However, the documented concerns listed above necessitate continuation of cautious, careful clinical trials in a few centers with detailed 10 year follow up periods before biological fixation should be recommended for general use in orthopaedics.

BIOACTIVE FIXATION

The concept of direct chemical bonding of implants to tissues was first proposed by the author in 1967, demonstrated in animal tests in 1969 and published in 1971 (ref. 41). The bioactive material was one of a special composition range of SiO_2-Na_2O-CaO-P_2O_5 glasses, termed Bioglasses®, which are summarized in Fig. 4. Subsequent studies established details of the Bioglass® bond bonding boundary, shown as region A in Fig. 4, the mechanisms of bone bonding (refs. 41,45), absence of toxicity (ref. 46), preclinical functional tests for fixation of orthopaedic prostheses in monkeys (ref. 47) and tooth rooth implants in baboons (ref. 48). After extensive comparative biomaterials studies in the mouse middle ear (ref. 49), FDA approvals were granted for sales of Bioglass® middle ear prostheses in 1984. FDA approval of endosseus ridge maintenance implants (ref. 50) and maxillofacial augmentation implants (ref. 51) using bulk 45S5 Bioglass® are expected in early 1987.

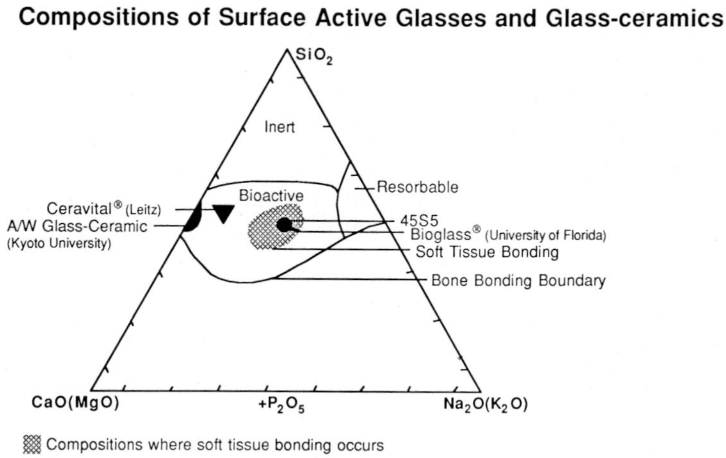

Figure 4. Compositional ranges of bioactive glasses and glass-ceramics.

A less reactive bioactive glass-ceramic (Ceravital®) was developed in the mid 70's (refs. 52,53) and shown by Gross and Strunz (ref. 54), to bond to bone. (See Fig. 4) Clinical use as an ossicular chain prosthesis (ref. 55) and in maxillofacial repair (ref. 56), soon followed. A higher strength bioactive glass-ceramic composed of apatite and wollastonite, termed A/W glass-ceramic (See Fig. 4), was developed in Japan by Kokubo et al (ref. 57) and is now in clinical use as vertebral prostheses by Yamamuro (ref. 58). Höhland and associates have recently developed a bioactive glass-ceramic that is machineable (ref. 59).

There has also been extensive use of dense hydroxylapatite as a bioactive implant in various clinical applications, such as periodontal treatment (ref. 60), alveolar ridge augmentation (ref. 61) and tooth root implants (refs. 62,63).

The major limitation of this broad range of bioactive materials is their weak tensile strength and low fatique resistance. Consequently, bioactive fixation of load bearing prostheses, such as total joints, require use of the bioactive material as a coating on a high strength substrate. Coatings of bioactive glasses and glass-ceramics on surgical alloys have been tested (refs. 47,64,65,66) and found to bond to bone. The major advantage of such a fixation system is that the interfacial bonding strength is very high (Fig. 3) and in fact is stronger than bone. When the bond forms, the interface does not fail in tension or torsion.

The major limitation of bioactive fixation is the long term stability of the metal-glass interface. Bioactive glasses easily lose bioactivity if metal ion impurities are incorporated in the glass during processing (refs. 42,56). Adhesion of glass to metal requires forming a diffusional zone of oxidized metal. If this zone becomes too thick or metal ions, such as Cr, Co, Fe, Ni, migrate through the glass it will no longer be bioactive. In other words, the bone-bonding boundary of Fig. 4 shrinks as the concentration of $M^{+3,+4}$ ions increases. Only a few % are required to eliminate the formation of the bioactive hydroxylapatite film on the glass coating surface. When this happens the coating becomes inert and will not bond.

Conversely, if the metal-glass bonding zone is not sufficiently developed the glass will flake or spall off the metal. The metal-glass interface is especially susceptible to attack by water or body fluids. Consequently, the fatique resistance of bioactive coatings is often very poor.

Clinical orthopedic applications of bioactive fixation systems cannot be justified until the coatings have passed long term in-vitro fatique studies. As yet, there are no such studies reported to the author's knowledge.

An intermediate, alternative use for bioactive materials may be as bioactive cements (refs. 67,68), or in conjunction with biological fixation devices to accelerate the rate of bone ingrowth, as shown by Ducheyne, et al (ref. 69).

CONCLUSIONS

1) No cementless fixation system yet reported shows long term (>10 years) results superior to cemented prostheses. Therefore, only careful, limited clinical trials in selected centers are justified until >70% results at 10 years are proven.
2) Considerable more research on the biomechanics of interfacial failure modes is needed. 3) Improved prostheses designs to eliminate or minimize stress shielding is required. 4) Long term in- vitro fatigue studies on bioactive coatings and composites are necessary. 5) Development of improved bioactive cements may be the best solution. 6) Methods for joint resurfacing for young patients should be developed to save bone stock. 7) Research on biomaterials responses to aged, arthiritic and osteoporotic bone is needed.

REFERENCES

1. R.Y. Hori, J.L. Lewis, J.R. Zimmerman, C.I. Compere, "The Number of Total Joint Replacements in the United States" Clinical Orthopaedics and Related Research (1978) Vol. 132, pp. 46.
2. I.M. Rutkow, "Orthopaedic Operations in the United States 1979 through 1983", J. Bone and Joint Surgery, Vol. 68-A, No. 5 June 1986 (pp. 716-719).
3. J. Charnley, "Acrylic Cement in Orthopaedic Surgery" Edinburgh, London, Livingstone. (1970).
4. J. Charnley, "The Long Term Results of Low Friction Arthoplasty of the Hip Performed as a Primary Intevention", J. Bone and Joint Surg. 54B: (1972) p. 61
5. J. Charnley, and F. Cupic, "The 9-10 Year Results of Low Friction Arthroplasty of the Hip", Clin. Orthop. 111:105 (1973).

6. H.C. Amstutz, K.L. Markolf, G.M. McNiece, "Loosening of Total Hip Components: Cause and Prevention", in the Hip Society, Hip Proceedings of the Fourth Open Meeting of the Hip Society. St. Louis, CV Mosby (1978).
7. T.A. Gruen, G.M. McNiece, H.C. Amstutz, "Modes of Failure of Cemented Type Femoral Components: A Radiographic Analysis of Loosening", Clin. Orthop. 141:17 (1979).
8. H.R. Chandler,F.T. Reineck, R.I. Wixon, T.C. McCarthy, "Total Hip Replacement of Patients Younger than 30 years Old". J. Bone Joint Surg. 63A:1426 (1981).
9. C.J. Sutherland, H. Wilde, L.S. Borden, K.E. Marks, "A Ten Year Followup of One Hundred Consecutive Mueller Curved Stem Total Hip Replacement Arthroplasties", J. Bone Joint Surg. 64A:970 (1982).
10. R.N. Stauffer, "Ten Year Followup Study of Total Hip Replacement", J. Bone Joint Surg. 64A:983 (1982).
11. E.W. Morscher, "Cementless Total Hip Orthoplasty" Clin. Orthop., 181:76-91, (1983).
12. R.S.M. Ling, ed. Complications of Total Hip Replacement, Churchill-Livingstone (NY,NY) (1984).
13. J.H. Dumbleton, and J. Black, "Chapter 13, Some Long-Term Complications" ibid. (1984).
14. J.C. Heath, M.A.R. Freeman, and S.A.V. Swanson, "Carcinogenic Properties of Wear Particles from Prostheses Made in Cobalt-Chromium Alloy", Lancet i:564 (1971).
15. V.A. Memoli, J.C. Woodman, R.M. Urban, J.O. Galante, "Malignant Neoplasmo Associated with Orthopaedic Implant Materials", Orthop. Trans. 6:264 (1982).
16. D.F. Williams, Biocompatibility of Orthopedic Implants, Vol. 11, D.F. Williams, ed. CRC Press, Boca Raton, FL (1982).
17. J.L. Woodman, J. Black, and S.A. Jiminez, "Isolation of Serum Protein Organometallic Corrosion Products from 316LSS and HS-21 in vitro and in-vivo", J. Biomed. Mater. Res. 18: (1984) pp. 99-114.
18. L.L. Hench, Guest editorial, J. Biomed. Mat. Res. 15:iii-vii (1981).
19. A.J.C. Lee, and R.S.M. Ling, "Loosening" (Chapter 9) in Complications of Total Hip Replacement, ed. R.S.M. Ling, Churchill-Livingstone (NY, NY) (1984) pp. 110-145.
20. H.G. Willert, and M. Semlitsch, "Problems Associated with the Cement Anchorage of Artificial Joints" in Advances in Artificial Hip and Knee Joint Technology (1st Ed) Berlin, Heidelberg, NY, Springer Verlog (1976).
21. L. Linder, "The Tissue Response to Bone Cement" in Biocompatibility of Orthopedic Implants, Vol. 11, D.F. Williams, ed. CRC Press, Boca Raton, FL (1982).
22. J. Galante, W. Rostoker, R. Luech, R.D. Ray, "Sintered Fiber Metal Composites as a Basis for Attachment of Implants to Bone", J. Bone and Joint Surg. 53A:101 (1971).
23. R.M. Pilliar, H.U. Cameron, I. McNab, "Porous-Surface Layered Prosthetic Devices", J. Biomed. Eng. 10:126 (1975)
24. H.U. Cameron, R.M. Pilliar, and I. Macnab, "The Rate of Bone Ingrowth into Porous Metal", J. Biomed. Mater. Res. 10: (1976) pp. 295-302.
25. I.D. Bobyn, R.M. Pilliar, H.U. Cameron, and G.C. Weatherly "The Optimum Pre Size for the Fixation of Porous-Surfaced Metal Implants by the Growth of Bone, Clin. Orthop., 150 (1980) pp. 263-270,
26. J.J. Klawitter, and S. Hulbert, "Application of Porous Ceramics for the Attachment of Load Bearing Internal

Orthopedic Application", J. Biomed Mater Res Symp. 2:161 (1971)
27. R.P. Welsh, R.M. Pilliar, and I. Macnab, "Surgical Implants. The Role of Surface Porosity in Fixation to Bone and Acrylic". J. Bone and Joint Surg. 53-A: July (1971) pp. 963-977.
28. J.J. Klawitter, J.G. Bagwell, A.M. Weinstein, B.W. Sauer, and J.R. Pruitt, "An Evaluation of Bone Growth into Porous High Density Polyethylene", J. Biomed. Mater. Res. 10: (1976) pp. 311-323,
29. C.A. Homsy, T.E. Cain, F.B. Kessler, M.S. Anderson, J.W. King, "Porous Implant Systems for Prosthesis Stabilization", Clin. Orthop. 89:220 (1972).
30. S.D. Cook, K.A. Walsh, and R.J. Haddad, Jr., "Interface Mechanics and Bone Growth into Porous Co-Cr-Mo Alloy Implants", Clin. Orthop. 193: (1985) pp. 271-280.
31. R.M. Pilliar, "Powder Metal Made Orthopaedic Implants with Porous Surface for Fixation by Tissue Ingrowth", Clin. Orthop. 126: (1983) pp.42-46.
32. G. Miller, "Personal Communication"
33. C.A. Engh, and J.D. Bobyn, Biological Fixation in Total Hip Arthroplasty, Slack, Inc. N.J. (1985).
34. J.D. Bobyn, and C.A. Engh, "Biologic Fixation of Hip Prostheses: Review of the Clinical Status and Current Concepts", Adv. Orthop. Surg. 7:137-150 (1983).
35. R. Rosenquist, B. Bylander, K. Knutson, U. Rydholm, B. Rooser, N. Egund, and L. Lindgren, "Loosening of the Porous Coating of Bicompartmental Prostheses in Patients with Rheumatoid Arthritis", J. Bone and Joint Surgery Vol. 68-A, No. 4, April 1986 pp. 538-542.
36. L. Ryd, "Micromotion in Knee Arthroplasty Thesis", Dept. of Orthopedic Surgery, University Hospital, Lund, Sweden, (1985).
37. P.K. Buchert, B.K. Vaughn, T.H. Mallory, C.A. Engh, and J.D. Bobyn, "Excessive Metal Release due to Loosening and Fretting of Sintered Particles on Porous Coated Hip Prostheses", J. Bone and Joint Surgery, Vol. 68-A, No. 4, April 1986 pp. 606-609.
38. H.G. Willert, and M. Semlitsch, "Reactions of the Articular Capsule to Wear Products of Artificial Joint Prostheses", J. Biomed. Mater. Res. 11:157, (1977).
39. M.A.R. Freeman, J.D. Blaha, G. Brown, W. Day, H.P. Insler, and P.A. Revell, "Cementless Fixation of a Tibial Component for the Knee". Trans. Orthop. Res. Soc. 6: (1981) p. 157.
40. J.D. Blaha, H.P. Insler, M.A.R. Freeman, P.A. Revell, and R.C. Todd, "The Fixation of a Proximal Tibial Polyethylene Prostheses without Cement", J. Bone and Joint Surg. 64-B: (1982) pp. 326-335.
41. L.L. Hench, R.J.M. Splinter, W.C. Allen, T.K. Greenlee, Bonding Mechanisms at the Interface of Ceramic Prosthetic Materials. J. Biomed Mater Res Biomed Mater Symp 2: (1971) pp. 117-141.
42. L.L. Hench, J. Wilson, Surface Active Biomaterials. Science (Wash. D.C.) 226: (1984) pp. 630-636.
43. L.L. Hench, E.C. Ethridge, Biomaterials-An Interfacial Approach. Academic Press, New York (1982).
44. L.L. Hench, A.E. Clark, Adhesion to Bone. In: Williams D.F. (Ed.), Biocompatibility of Orthopaedic Implants. CRC Press, Boca Raton, FL, Vol. 2, Ch. 6 (1982).
45. L.L. Hench, H.C. Paschall, Direct Chemical Bonding Between

Bio-active Glass-ceramic Materials and Bone. J. Biomed. Mater. Res. Biomed. Mater. Symp. 4: (1973) pp.25-42.
46. J. Wilson, G.H. Pigott, F.J. Schoen, L.L. Hench, Toxicology and Biocompatibility of Bioglass®. J. Biomed. Mater. Res. 15: (1981) pp. 805-811.
47. G. Piotrowski, L.L. Hench, W.C. Allen, and G.J. Miller, J. Biomed. Mater. Res., 9(6), (1975) pp. 47-61.
48. H.R. Stanley, L.L. Hench, R. Going, C. Bennett, S.J. Chellemi, C. King, N. Ingersoll, E. Ethridge, and K. Kreutziger, Oral Surg., Oral Med., Oral Pathology, 42: (1976) pp. 339-356.
49. G.E. Merwin, J.S. Atkins, J. Wilson, L.L. Hench, Otolaryngol Head Neck Surg. 90:(1982) pp. 461-469.
50. H.R. Stanley, A.E. Clark, M.B. Hall, C. King, F. Colaizzi, D. Spilman and Hench, paper presented at 12th Annual Meeting of the Society for Bio-materials (1986).
51. G.E. Merwin, L. Rogers, J. Wilson, and R. Martin, Arch. of Otolaryngol. (Head and Neck Surgery) 112: March, 1980 pp. 280-284.
52. H. Bromer, E. Pfeil, and H.H. Kas, German Patent No. 2, (1973) pp. 326,100.
53. B.A. Blenke, H. Bromer, and K.K. Deutscher, J. Biomed. Mater. Res. 12: (1978) pp. 307-316.
54. U.M. Gross, and V. Strunz, J. Biomed. Mater. Res. 14: (1980) pp.607-618. 55. R. Reck, Clin. Otolaryngol., 6:63-65 (1981).
56. U. Gross, and V. Strunz, Clinical Applications of Biomaterials (1982) pp. 237-244.
57. T. Kokubo, M. Shigematsu, Y. Nagashima, M. Tashiro, T. Nakamura, T.Yamamuro, and S. Higashi, Bull. Inst. Chem. Res., Kyoto Univ., 60: (1982) pp. 260-268.
58. T. Yamamuro, "Private Communication"
59. W. Höhland, J. Naumann, W. Vogel, J. Gummel, Z. Wiss, Freidrich Schiller Univ. Jena Math. Naturwiss, Reihe 32:571 (1983).
60. P.J. Boyne, and B.A. Shapton, Trans. 4th Ann. Meet. Soc. Biomater. 115 (1978).
61. J. Kent. R. James, I. Finger, M. Jarcho, J. Taggart, and S. Cook, First World Biomat. Cong. 3.8.2 (abstract) (1980)
62. H.W. Denissen, K. deGroot, P. Kakkes, A. ven den Hooff, and P.J. Klopper, First World Biomat. Cong. 3.8.1. (abstract) (1980).
63. Ogiso, et al, Trans. Soc. for Biomat., Vol. IV, 52 (1981).
64. E. Barth, Bioactive Glass Ceramic on Titanium Substrate: The Effect of Molybdenum as an Intermediate Bond Coating. Biomaterials 7, 4 July 1986 pp. 273-276.
65. S. Contoli, A. Krajewski, and A. Ravaglioli, Histocompatibility and Bio-Physico-Chemistry of Doped Bioglass®. Ceramics in Surgery, (Ed.), P. Vincenzini, Elsevier Scientific Publishing Company Amsterdam (1983) pp. 187-197.
66. M. Ogino, "Personal Communication"
67. W. Hennig, B.A. Blencke, H. Bromer, K.K. Deutscher, A. Gross, and W. Ege, J. Biomed. Mater. Res. 13: (1983) pp. 89-99.
68. J. Raveh, H. Stich, P. Schawalder, C. Ruchti, and H. Cottier, Biocement - A New Material, Acta Otolaryngol 94: (1982) pp. 371-384.
69. P. Ducheyne, L.L. Hench, A. Kagan, M. Martens, A. Bursens, and J.C. Mulier, J. Biomed. Mater. Res. 14:225 (1980).

Biomaterials and Clinical Applications,
edited by A. Pizzoferrato, P.G. Marchetti, A. Ravaglioli and A.J.C. Lee
Elsevier Science Publishers B.V., Amsterdam, 1987 — Printed in The Netherlands

CLINICAL APPLICATIONS OF BIOMATERIALS IN MAXILLOFACIAL, PLASTIC AND RECONSTRUCTIVE SURGERY

Donald Leake, D.M.D., M.D., F.A.C.S.

Harbor-UCLA Medical Center
1000 West Carson Street
Torrance, California 90509

INTRODUCTION

Surgeons have been more successful in reconstructing or replacing hard tissues, i. e., bone and teeth, than soft tissue. Metals, ceramics, polymers and composites are commonly used in reconstructive surgery of bones of the cranial and maxillofacial regions. Metals most often are used for fixation devices in the form of rods, pins, screws, sutures and bone plates. The ceramic hydroxylapatite has been extensively used for alveolar ridge augmentation in atrophic mandibles and maxillae and/or small contour defects of facial bones, for example, the malar bone and the chin. New bioactive materials such as Bioglass also promise to be useful in the restoration of facial contour defects. Collagen, polymers and polymer composites, such as polyurethanes, silicone rubbers, PMMA and polytetrafluoroethylene may be useful in certain non-stress bearing bony contour defects, but large curvilinear defects that characterize cranial and facial bone defects including the mandible, are now reconstructed with anatomic precision using computer assisted technology. Three dimensional computed tomography scans are reformatted and used to direct a computer assisted lathe in the fabrication of a model of the deformity as well as the mirror image of the normal side. When the defect is small, the choice of polymer or ceramic depends on the anatomic site and the surgeon. Where possible, however, large bony defects are best reconstructed using autogenous material. Because it is difficult to achieve an aesthetic result that is lasting, bone by itself is not very satisfactory. Remodelling favoring resorption for the long term, and unevenness of the surface, initially, are drawbacks of using bone alone. An implant to impose form in combination with bone graft material provides the optimum aesthetic outcome.

A biomaterial whose potential is yet to be achieved in reconstructive surgery is collagen. Particularly promising is collagen in combination with hydroxylapatite or Bioglass® for small bony defects of the facial skeleton.

Metals

The use of metals in the reconstruction of facial bones has now largely been superceded by other materials. The use of perforated stainless steel or titanium metallic trays for the reconstruction of bony contour defects of the jaws was popular for a number of years but because of stress shielding, and the resultant resorptive loss of bone with time, the popularity of metallic trays for mandibular reconstruction has decreased. Metallic plates used in the reconstruction of defects of the neurocranium were superceded by the use of acrylic. Acrylic is now giving way to the use of better materials, particularly those used in combination with bone grafting, for the reconstruction of large defects of the neurocranium. Metal mini-plates, however, are enjoying an upsurge in the use of fixation of facial fractures. The merits of compression versus non-compression plates are widely discussed. The principle advantage of the use of metal plates for fracture fixation involving the mandible or maxilla, or in the fixation of bone after orthognathic surgery, is that intermaxillary fixation can be avoided thus allowing the patient to lead a more nearly normal life. It is particularly advantageous for the surgeon because the patient can eat a reasonable, albeit soft, diet shortly after surgery. Bone plates for the fixation of mandibular fractures are not without complications, however. Bone plates used to stabilize mandibular fractures fail if the surgeon is not attentive to detail or if the patient is non-compliant by excessively loading the mandible by eating a normal diet too soon. Titanium compared to other metals is particularly attractive as a bone plate material because of its high strength and low rate of corrosion. Its light weight and lower modulus of elasticity than other metals in use, which reduces the stresses around the implant by flexing with the bone, suggest better acceptance by patients due to decreased awareness of the implant.

Ceramics

Hydroxylapatite in granular form or block form, Bioglass, HTR (porous methacrylates) and aluminum oxides are materials used either for reconstruction of facial bones or as coatings for materials to enhance their biocompatibility. An interesting combination is the use of hydroxylapatite in granular form placed under an implant made of OsteoMesh™. Hydroxylapatite in block form, carved freehand to conform to the defect, works well in treating small contour defects of facial bones such as the malar bone. HTR has also been used for facial contour reconstruction. A major application of hydroxylapatite to date has been the granular material for alveolar ridge augmentation to restore the atrophic mandible to a suitable clinical shape in order to support the denture. The extreme fragility due to brittleness of block hydroxylapatite is a shortcoming in its application for facial contour reconstruction and makes it unsuitable unless there is adequate underlying bone to support it.

HTR™ (hard tissue replacement) is a material developed by Bruins and Ashman made by adding a leachable substance such as sodium chloride to a mixture of powdered polymethylmethacrylate. This is placed in a mold and heat polymerized. On removal from the mold, the material is abraded enough to remove the impervious skin surface and the salt is leached out to provide porosity. By controlling the particulate size of the salt, the pore size can be predetermined. Pore size of 200-400 microns allows bone ingrowth. This material was modified by the addition of 2-hydroxylethylmethacrylate (HEMA) to enhance its hydrophylic characteristics. HEMA added to PMMA makes the surface tacky. The beads, wetted with HEMA, are pressed into a mold and heated in a dielectic oven which converts approximately 90 percent of the HEMA to polymer. The contact surface of the beads becomes attached to one another. The POLYHEMA that fails to crosslink is dissolved in boiling water. This material has been proposed for use as dental replicas to replace teeth following dental extraction. Our experience is limited to correcting an inadequate chin by placing HTR subperiosteally for chin augmentation, and to use it in patients with severely atrophic mandibles where precise fitting implants were made to fit on the superior border of the mandible. By using CAD/CAM technology, a 3-D scan of the mandible is used to create a model of the mandible with a computer driven lathe. Custom fabrication of the HTR implants to fit on the superior border of the mandible with anatomic precision is possible based on the precise model of the mandible. The surgical technique requires a flap elevated in the buccal mucosa so that the implant is remote from the suture line. When the tunneling technique was used in one side in one patient, the suture line dehisced over the implant. This gradually exposed an area of approximately one square centimeter of implant. Several weeks after implantation, the exposed area of the implant was reduced using a large round burr in a Hall air driven drill. The implant had become well vascularized in the inferior portion near the bone. This suggests that the application of HTR for contour defects of bone has great promise.

Bioglass® is a bioactive, nonporous, transparent material proposed for use in facial augmentation. Composed of oxides of silicon, calcium, sodium and phosphorous, bioreactivity can be varied from virtual inertness to dissolution in-vivo. When the material is only slightly reactive, a series of events take place wherein hydrogen ions from the biologic host exchanges with alkali ions from the Bioglass resulting in adherence at the interface. When Bioglass has been placed in a bone defect, loading of the bone has lead to some bone-Bioglass bonding. When placed passively on bone, better bonding occurs if the implant is placed under the periosteum and is stabilized securely. Failure to immobilize the implant may result in an inferior degree of bonding and loss of the implant. Successful application of Bioglass for facial augmentation requires an adequate means of immobilization of the implant during the time required for bonding. The Bioglass can be contoured intraoperatively by using diamond burrs, however, its greatest use in facial augmentation will occur, I predict, when 3-D scanning and model making using the mirror image are employed to provide an anatomically precise model for the reconstructed defect. With the model of the defect available, the implant can be prepared preoperatively.

Polymer and Polymer Composites

Silastic^R, a silicone rubber, when used to improve facial contours is highly successful for the short term. In the course of time, however the underlying bone almost invariably responds to the overlying implant's pressure by resorbing. Chin implants have been reported to erode through the entire thickness of the mandible and extrude into the floor of the mouth. Malar implants may erode into the maxillary antrum. Large sections of the mandible have been replaced with solid Silastic custom molded implants, but the host bone-Silastic implant interface could not withstand the forces placed on it by the mandible in function and the implant invariably extruded through the mucosa at the interface. When the implant overlapped bone, the bone resorbed. Silastic has also been used to hold bone grafts much as the various perforated metallic tray devices, but the bone resorbs in a Silastic tray presumably due to the lack of adequate vascular ingrowth. Although Silastic can be molded with anatomic precision and can impose form, it lacks the internal strength required to support cancellous bone grafts in stress bearing areas, and the obstruction of vascular ingrowth prevents its use in supporting bone grafts in non-stress bearing or passive areas.

Finger joints and breast prostheses continue to be popular clinical biomaterial applications of Silastic.

Proplast^R

The use of a PTFE carbon composite was advocated for alveolar ridge augmentation, but this has not proved successful due to extrusion and infection. As a filler for facial contour defects, however, the material has been more successful. It may migrate in spite of its porous nature unless it is securely fastened by suturing. It has also proved to be quite susceptible to infection. Numerous studies evaluating its uses as a coating for metals have been undertaken. As a passive bone contour filler, its applications include the nose for saddle nose deformity, the malar bone, for chins and small defects of the forehead.

Silastic[R] and Proplast[R] are commonly used materials to replace the meniscus after meniscectomy of the temporomandibular joint. In a recent study using rabbits, Timmis placed 2 mm Dacron reinforced Silastic implants in the glenoid fossa adapted to allow articulation with the condyle after meniscectomy. In another group, 1.3 mm Proplast sheeting laminated to non-porous Teflon was trimmed and stabilized using 4-0 sutures just as the Silicone elastomer had been treated. The animals were sacrificed at 2, 4, 8, and 20 weeks after surgery. Histologically, the silicone group showed increasing fragmentation of the implant material and the formation of foreign body giant cells which reached the peak at the eighth week. Resorption of the condyle and articular eminence were noted in this group. Implant fracture was noted in one-fifth of the animals. In the Proplast group, osteoclastic activity with resorption and severe degenerative changes in both condyle and glenoid fossa were noted. Foreign body giant cell reaction was severe throughout all time intervals and increased with time. The implant fractured in nearly half of the Proplast treated cases. In our clinical practice, we have the Proplast meniscus replacements from two patients and histologically have observed foreign body giant cell reactions.

The Mandible

The best material for replacing large sections of the mandible is bone. Whenever possible, it is best to reconstruct the defect primarily, i. e., in the same surgical operation as the resection. This is true even when the resection is for cancer. Historically, a Kirschner wire was used to help maintain the position of the bone fragments after resection of several centimeters to hemimandibulectomies and to try to reposition the attachment of the muscles and soft tissues in as normal a way as possible. Elaborations of the K-wire have included plates with joints connected with screws or bolts. Perforated stainless steel, Vitalium[R], tantalum and titanium trays were the next elaboration to hold bone grafts taken as particulate marrow from the iliac crest region. OsteoMesh[TM], a porous Dacron cloth stiffened with urethane has a number of advantages over metal trays: easier to adapt in surgery, radiolucent, bone will not resorb because of stress shielding as in metal trays, and there is no radiation interface effect leading to radiation dosage increase on the near side of the beam. The head of the condyle of the mandible can be fashioned out of solid urethane attached to the OsteoMesh[TM] tray for reconstruction of total hemimandibles.

The Temporomandibular Joint

The replacement of the head of the condyle with metal prostheses has been a standard for some years. Polymers may prove superior when an adequate means of attachment of the head of the condyle to the ascending ramus has been developed. Acrylic or Silastic condylar head replacements have been used but they tend to become loose or in the case of acrylic, to fracture after a while at the interface with bone.

The meniscus has been replaced routinely with Silastic sheet placed in the glenoid fossa of the skull. Recently, Proplast has been sold for this purpose but both Proplast and Silastic may result in foreign body giant cell reactions in this application. Some surgeons now advocate removing these implants after three or four months and leaving the fibrous capsule that has formed around the implant to serve as the new pseudo-disk or meniscus. Tanned collagen may provide the solution to this problem by being slowly resorbed leaving behind a tough fibrous capsule to serve as pseudomeniscus.

Maxilla

Defects of the maxilla have been restored with removable prostheses made of denture acrylic although bone grafting for some defects seems to be increasingly advocated. Dental implants, which deserve a special chapter, are now commonly placed in the maxilla to stabilize removable dentures or in some cases a dentition of cast bridgework attached to the implants.

Orbit

Orbital blowout fractures resulting in the loss of the orbital floor due to comminution and the frequently resultant entrapment of the orbital musculature, the inferior rectus and inferior oblique muscles, require surgical exploration to release the muscles and to repair the orbital floor with alloplastic materials. Silastic and Supramid sheets are commonly used today. Large defects are not easily restored with these materials, however, and even with thicker than usual sheeting, the results may be unsatisfactory. The use of OsteoMesh™ for orbital floor repair has the advantages of being contoured to fit the shape of the orbit and of porosity so that it will be stabilized by connective tissue ingrowth. Prudent surgeons may wish to wire orbital implants to the orbital rim to assure accurate positioning.

Eyelid

When there is loss of function in the orbicularis oculi, ectropion of the lower lid with epiphora, and exposure of the cornea, may occur. The upper lid generally moves about a centimeter in closing the eyes and the lower lid may rise only a barely measureable amount. Thus, paralysis of the muscles used to close the eyes is treated by placing an implant subcutaneously in the upper lid. This adds weight to the lid and allows it to close while the patient is upright. Small gold plates seem to be well tolerated.

The Skull

Cranioplasty is essential when there is a bony defect in the skull after resection for tumor, traumatic loss of bone or infection, both to protect the brain and to restore appearance. It is generally agreed that autogenous bone is the best material to restore the integrity of the skull but it is technically difficult to provide an aesthetically acceptable smooth contour with the use of bone grafts alone. The pressure of the scalp on bone grafts also may contribute to uneven healing, either flattening the contour or when ribs are used resulting in a washboard effect. Thus, the invention of OsteoMesh^{TM} has provided an ideal solution to this vexing problem. The defect is exposed through the previous incision, or through a bicoronal flap in the case of a frontal defect, and the bone margins are freshened. Either split and contoured ribs or bone from the iliac crest may be used. The OsteoMesh^{TM} implant is then placed over the bone graft in the skull defect overlapping by a centimeter or more of the margins of the defect. This imposes form to the healing bone and protects it from the pressure of the scalp during the healing phase. With the advent of CAD/CAM technology, an anatomically precise implant can be fabricated.

The Zygoma

The zygoma may be deficient secondary to traumatic defects, congenital hypoplasia, as in Treacher-Collins Syndrome, or because of tumor resection. Anatomically precise reconstruction is now possible with the use of CAD/CAM technology where 3-D scanning provides the basis for the model of the defect as well as the mirror image of the normal side to restore symmetry. For small defects, block hydroxylapatite can be carved, HTR (porous methacrylate) can be molded or for larger defects, OsteoMesh^{TM} can be made over the model of the mirror image of the normal side and either filled with bone or the synthetic materials mentioned above. Carved Silastic block or molded implants of Silastic fail after time because of resorption of the underlying bone.

The Nose

Where possible, bone or cartilage should be used to replace or restore form to nasal defects. Many synthetic materials have been used but in the course of time most have been abandoned. Whether natural or synthetic material is used, the implants are placed in a subcutaneous pocket on the bridge of the nose approached through the columella, the nasal vestibule or the upper buccal sulcus. The typical design is an L-shaped strut with the long arm used to support the bridge of the nose and short arm to support the tip of the nose as the vertical component of the columella. Failure usually results from pressure necrosis of the skin at the tip of the nose. Where there is adequate intrinsic support at the tip of the nose, a boat-shaped implant may be used to restore saddle deformities. Proplast is a currently useful material for this application.

The Ear

The construction of the external ear is a challenge because of lack of soft tissue and because of inadequate materials to form the cartilaginous framework. One advance has occurred through the use of inflatable silicone bags to expand the tissue thus creating adequate soft tissue for coverage. The Silastic bag can be filled progressively with sterile saline. Over the course of several weeks, there will be adequate skin to encompass the implant or autogenous graft.

Cartilage is excellent material but it is difficult to obtain and a particular challenge to carve to the required shape. With time, however absorption may occur and the delicate contours may become distorted. Soft silicone rubber appears to be the most popular of the synthetic materials for reconstruction of the pinna of the ear.

The Trachea

A reconstructive problem as yet unsolved but within reach, given world enough and time as the poet said, is that of tracheal replacement. Mesh materials allowing connective tissue and vascular ingrowth have resulted in mucosal regeneration throughout large areas of the tracheal lumen in the area restored, but all samples studied have had varying but significant degrees of stenosis.

Prostheses with adequate porosity, lightweight in design, but rigid enough to maintain patency of the airway, yet flexible enough to allow some movement of the vital contiguous structures and not dehisce at the suture line, become infected, develop chronic leakage or stenosis, will solve the need.

The Future

The history of the clinical application of biomaterials is one of trial and error. Happily, the empirical method is giving way to scientific principle. Technology, too, continues to advance bringing insights and solutions to reconstructive surgical problems that were only dreams two decades ago. The host-implant interface response can be predicted with a multitude of materials. Controlled bioactive surfaces and computer aided custom fabrication will revolutionize the reconstruction of contour defects of the facial and cranial bones as well as the mandible.

Biomaterials and Clinical Applications,
edited by A. Pizzoferrato, P.G. Marchetti, A. Ravaglioli and A.J.C. Lee
Elsevier Science Publishers B.V., Amsterdam, 1987 — Printed in The Netherlands

POLYMERS AND COMPOSITE MATERIALS IN BIOMEDICAL APPLICATIONS

Paolo Giusti

Dipartimento di Ingegneria Chimica Laboratorio di Bioingegneria
Via Diotisalvi 2, 56100 Pisa, Italy

SUMMARY

After having examined the definition of biomaterial and the main medical area where polymers and composites have found a wide use, a modern approach to the realization of new polymeric biomaterials is considered.

Four different routes for the substitution of biological polymers and composites are suggested.
Namely: 1) the re-use of materials of human or animal origin, 2) the production of polymers and composites structurally identic to the natural ones, 3) the production of synthetic polymers and composites purposely designed in order to imitate natural biomaterials, 4) the regeneration of natural tissue through a natural pathway using synthetic polymers as a support.

= = = =

At the Consensus Development Conference on the Clinical Applications of Biomaterials held at the National Institute of Health on November 1-3, 1982 in the USA a biomaterial was defined as any substance (other than a drug) or combination of substances, synthetic or natural in origin, which can be used for any period of time, as a whole or as a part of a system which treats, augments or replaces any tissue, organ or function of the body.

Successively in Chester on March 3-5, 1986 a Consensus Conference on Definitions in Biomaterials proposed the following: a biomaterial is a non-viable material used in a medical device intended to interact with biological systems.

Whatever will be the most generally accepted definition by people working in this field, there are no doubts that polymers and polymeric composites make up by far the broadest and most diverse class of biomaterials. The main medical area where polymer and composites have found a wide use are: artificial organs, the cardiovascular system, orthopaedics, dentistry, ophtalmology, drugs and drug delivery systems.

Polymers for artificial organs are mainly thermoplastic elastomers for the artificial heart, and polymers easily formable in hollow fibres (cuprophan, acrylic, polycarbonate etc.) for artificial kidney, hybrid artificial pancreas and liver.

Polymers for cardiovascular applications are mainly thermoplastic elastomers (polyurethanes), Dacron fabrics and pliant composite with fibres imbedded in a rubbery matrix as well as PTFE.

Fairly traditional polymers, like PMMA as bone cement or UHMWPE as bearing part, have found applications in orthopaedics until now.

Quite recently new composite materials have been successfully used both for bone replacement and in plates for fracture fixation as well as for artificial tendons.

Dentistry applications mainly involve the use of acrylic polymers and composites, although new classes of monomers and new composites are now being developed particularly in restorative dentistry.

The main polymer still used for contact lenses is PHEMA.

The application of polymers in delivering medications is a relatively new development, either for use as drug delivery systems or as polymeric drugs. For the first application, bioresorbable materials appear very promising, while for the second, very special polymers are used depending on the pharmacological effect desired.

The large use of polymers and composites as biomaterials, as shown previously, is due to the fact that synthetic polymers are available with a wide variety of compositions, properties and forms and also because they may be fabricated readily into complex shapes and structures. Until quite recently commercial polymers were used as biomaterials almost without any attempt to design new and more suitable performance characteristics.

The biomaterial science has grown very quickly during the last few years, so we are now able to project new polymers and composites for biomedical applications.

I will describe in the following a modern approach to the realization of new polymeric biomaterials.

When something which is no longer working in the right way must be replaced, the best approach is certainly to use a "spare part" which is the same as the natural one. Transplantation is obviously an application of such an approach for replacing ill organs and tissues and it has had a great success in these recent years.

However, the problems connected to transplantation are well-known, the main being the lack of donors.

A second solution is represented by the use of different materials, either synthetic or natural, designed to imitate in the best way the biological materials the ill part is made up of.

The more we know about the chemical nature, the structure and properties of the natural components of tissues and organs, the more such a solution is likely to be successful.

An interesting aspect is, at least for those working in the field of polymers and of macromolecular composites, that pratically all materials in the animal world are made up of macromolecules, which are rarely of one kind but more often are intercombined with others or with non-macromolecular materials in composites.

The macromolecular aspect of the biological matter, even though encouraging, must not lead to false enthusiasm, for biological polymers (or biopolymers) are very complex. Nevertheless, it is evident that the best starting point for a correct approach to the production of biomaterials is to know the structure, properties and function of biopolymers very well, as well as to know how they intercombine or interact with different materials in the formation of composites.

The main biopolymers synthesized by cells are: polynucleotides (DNA or RNA), polysaccharides and proteins. Only the last two are important as biomaterials because they constitute fundamental parts of tissues and organs. From this point of view some of the most important proteins are: silk, keratin, collagen, elastin.

The structure of silk, keratin and collagen are well known, while the structure of elastin is not yet well-known, even though we know that it has properties similar to those of vulcanized elastomers.

Among polysaccharides with well known structure let us mention cellulose, kitin and kitosan and glycosaminoglycans.

Less clearly defined are the interactions among biopolymers, as well as those between biopolymers and low molecular weight substances in composite structures constituting tissues and other structural biomaterials. Examples of such composite biological materials are: skin, blood vessels, tendons and bones.

All these tissues are mainly made up of connective tissue.

The term connective tissue describes the extracellular matrix plus the cells found in it, such as fibroblasts, macrophages, and mast cells.

Two of the main classes of the extra-cellular macromolecules that make up the matrix are the collagenes and the polysaccharides glycosaminoglycans, which are usually covalently linked to proteins to form proteoglycans.

The glycosaminoglycan and proteoglycan macromolecules constitute a gel like, highly hydrated substance where the collagen fibers are embedded.

In many tissues elastin fibers are also present as well as fibronectin and laminin which has been found only in basal lamina until now.

The mechanical properties of soft connective tissues depend mainly on the properties and architecture of the collagen and elastin fibers interacting with each other.

As an example of how the interactions among different proteins are important in determining the properties of a tissue let us consider the blood vessel wall.

The blood vessel wall has to distend in response to a pulse wave and subsequently to recoil actively in order to contribute to the propulsion of blood. This function is achieved by a complicated interaction between collagen and elastin fibers; the smooth muscle cells present mainly regulate the tone (and consequently the diameter) of the vessel wall. The interaction between collagen and elastin have been investigated by removing collagen and elastin from alternate specimens from the same tissue (ref. 1). Results from such experiments have shown that the removal of collagen markedly lowers the stress-strain curve but does not affect the initial part of it.

The removal of elastin, on the other hand, results in marked increase in extensibility and lowering of strength.

This is contrary to the current opinion that collagen is responsible for the main part of the tensile strength of elastic arteries.

An interaction between collagen and elastin elements is thus responsible for the mechanical properties of elastic arteries as the aorta and the strength of the tissue is not derived from its collagen fibers per se (ref. 2).

Which is then the best approach to replace these complicated natural structures? Two ideas stem directly from the solution given in the past to the need of producing substitutes of the natural products cotton fibers and natural rubber. Once the structure of cellulose, which is the main constituent of cotton, was understood, and once it was discovered that the same polymer can be found in wood in large quantities, wood was used as a raw material for the production of fibers similar to cotton.

All this was achieved through the viscose and cuprammonium processes which allow the production of artificial fibers (the well-known rayons) of the same chemical structure as cotton and with similar properties. At the same time similar fibers were also produced from petroleum derivatives: the success of such fibers, known as· nylon, terital, meraklon has discouraged any further attempt to exactly reproduce exactly the complex structure of natural cellulose starting from low molecular weight petroleum derived substances.

Things have evolved in a different way for natural rubber, a polyisoprene 1-4 cis, since a natural alternative source of this material is not available at a low cost. The research was concentrated on the direct synthesis starting from low molecular weight molecules.

Up to the 60's it was not possible to reproduce the exact structure of rubber because of its high structural regularity.

Nonetheless a great number of polymeric materials imitating its properties were synthesized. Such products are still in use today as synthetic elastomers. The exact reproduction of the structure of rubber was achieved thanks to discovery of stereospecific catalytic systems due to Prof. Natta who was awarded the Nobel Prize in 1964.

We can now suggest four different routes for the substitution of biological polymers and composites, bearing in mind what has been said in the case of cotton and natural rubber.

The first route is the re-use of materials of animal or human origin which are either already structurally organized or in molecules.

This route has already led to interesting results in the case of human or bovine fibrin and collagen which have been used successfully in different medical fields. The same can be said about the use of bovine dura mater and pericardium in the construction of cardiac valves and finally, let us mention porcine cardiac valves used for the valvular substitution in humans.

The second route is the production of polymers and composites structurally identic to the natural ones.

This is a very complicated approach if carried out through

synthetic pathways. However, it may be achievable with the aid of biotechnology (enzyme catalysis or DNA recombinant technique).

The third route is represented by the use of synthetic polymers and composites industrially available or purposely designed in order to imitate both mechanical properties and, possibly, the biological behaviour of natural biomaterials.

All the synthetic polymers mentioned above may be used, eventually modified by grafting biologically active molecules on their backbone.

New polymers may be synthesised in order to obtain some peculiar biomedical properties. New composites with peculiar properties may be produced through a correct choice of materials in combination with micromechanics and lamination theories.

A fourth route is the regeneration of natural tissue through a natural pathway using synthetic polymers (eventually biodegradable and bioresorbable) as a support.

This idea was suggested by the observation of spontaneous neointima formation in prosthetic blood vessels of large internal diameter, and has already been applied for the construction of nerve guide channels, artificial skin and some other few applications.

We now wish to describe an example of the reconstruction of a natural tissue such as the skin, through a process involving almost all the routes described above.

Skin is made up of epidermis and derma. Epidermis includes a superficial layer of keratinized squames, a central layer of germinal cells and a basal cells layer adhering to the underlying basal lamina which separates the epidermis from the derma.

An artificial skin made up of a suturable membrane comprising a top layer of silicon elastomer and a bottom layer of a biodegradable porous collagen-glycosaminoglycans covalently crosslinked network, was studies in Cambridge at the MIT" (ref. 3).

During application, the collagen-GAG layer undergoes

biodegradation at a controlled rate and is replaced by neodermal tissue while the silicon layer is spontaneously ejected following formation of a neoepidermal compliant layer under it. Successively the technique was improved by seeding autologous epidermal basal cells into the membranes before grafting.

Finally I would like to mention the solution given in our laboratories to the problem of substituting damaged natural vessels of small diameter. This is still an unsolved problem since commercially available synthetic polymeric prostheses frequently fail when the internal diameter is less than 5 mm.

In order to contribute to the solution of this problem we studied a new "biolized" polymeric material obtained by mixing synthetic polyurethanes with the plasma protein fibrinogen of human origin. Once that the tube was constructed the blend was submitted to the enzymatic treatment with thrombin to convert the fibrinogen into fibrin, and with factor XIIIa and calcium ions to covalently cross-link fibrin (ref. 4).

This new composite material has been used successfully in animal experiments and its success is mainly due, in our opinion, to the fact that the synthetic polymer confers the mechanical properties while the fibrin increase the blood compatibility of the prostheses, since the tissue ingrowth and the neointima formation are favoured by the biodegradation of the natural protein.

REFERENCES

1 F. Missirilis, Use of enzymolysis techniques in studying the mechanical properties of connective tissue components. J. Bioengineering, 1 (1977) 215-222.

2 A. Vüdik, C.C. Danielsen and H. Oxlund. On fundamental and phenomenological models, structure and mechanical properties of collagen, elastin and glycosaminoglycan complexes. Biorheology, 19 (1982) 437-451.

3 I.V. Yannas, J.F. Burke, E. Chen, D.P. Orgill and E.M. Skrabut Stage 2 Artificial skin: a polymeric template for regeneration of new skin. Proceedings IUPAC MACRO 82, July 1982, pag. 336.

4 P. Giusti, G. Soldani, M. Palla, M. Paci, New Fibrin containing thermoplastic elastomers for cardiovascular applications. Proceedings of the 5th European Conference on Biomaterials, Paris, September 4-6, 1985, Published in Advances in Biomaterials, Elsevier, Amsterdam, 6, 1986, pp. 221-226.

Biomaterials and Clinical Applications,
edited by A. Pizzoferrato, P.G. Marchetti, A. Ravaglioli and A.J.C. Lee
Elsevier Science Publishers B.V., Amsterdam, 1987 — Printed in The Netherlands

THE ROLE OF PORE SIZE ON BONE INGROWTH AND IMPLANT SUBSTITUTION IN HYDROXYAPATITE AND TRICALCIUM PHOSPHATE CERAMICS; A HISTOLOGIC AND MORPHOMETRIC STUDY IN RABBITS.

P.S. EGGLI[1], W. MUELLER[2] and R.K. SCHENK[1]
[1]Institute of Anatomy, University of Bern, Postfach 139, 3000 Bern (Switzerland)
[2]Mathys Co, 2544 Bettlach (Switzerland)

SUMMARY

Hydroxyapatite and tricalcium phosphate cylinders with the same porosity but a different range of pore size were implanted in the metaphysis of the distal femur and proximal tibia of 15 NZW rabbits for up to six months. The hydroxyapatite ceramic was practically not substituted, whereas up to 85% of the tricalcium phosphate material had been degraded after six months. The rate of implant substitution (for tricalcium phosphate) and bone ingrowth (for tricalcium phosphate and hydroxyapatite) depended upon pore size. The implants with the smaller pore size range of 50-100µm showed a significantely higher rate of implant degradation and bony ingrowth than the implants with a larger pore size range of 200-400µm. An explanation of this rather surprising result are preexisting pore interconnections of up to 20µm diameter between the smaller pores. They allow rapid ingrowth of vessels and cells involved in implant resorption and bone formation.

INTRODUCTION

Besides the use of porous calcium phosphate ceramics as bone substitutes, their application as delivery systems for antibiotics, osteogenic substances or other drugs will be of major future interest. Especially for the latter purpose ceramics with regularly distributed pores are needed, allowing bone ingrowth and implant substitution at predictable rates. The aim of this study was to present quantitative data concerning the influence of chemical composition and pore geometry on these processes.

MATERIALS AND METHODS

Hydroxyapatite and tricalcium phosphate ceramics with a homogeneous pore distribution, a porosity of 60% and two different pore size ranges of either 50-100µm or 200-400µm were prepared by MATHYS Co, Bettlach, Switzerland. Cylinders of 3mm diameter were implanted in the metaphysis of the distal femur and proximal tibia of 15 NZW rabbits for up to six months. From the plastic embedded material saw cuts were made and first used for microradiography. They then were mounted on opalescent glass plates, milled down to approximately 60µm and superficially stained for histologic evaluation (for details see ref. 1). Morphometric methods were applied to measure bony ingrowth and implant substitution.

RESULTS AND DISCUSSION

Biodegradability of hydroxyapatite is still under discussion. In our material we could not detect any implant degradation for the smaller porous hydroxyapatite (HAPS) after four months (Fig.1a), whereas a loss of 5% was observed in the larger porous hydroxyapatite (HAPL) (Figs.1a,2a). This loss reflects probably not an actual implant resorption, but is rather due to mechanical detachment of superficially located ceramic particles.

Biodegradation of tricalcium phosphate is documented by several authors and quantitative data are given in literature (refs.2-4). Our most remarkable observation is the faster substitution of the tricalcium phosphate with the smaller pores (TCPS) compared to the modification with a larger pore size (TCPL). Already after two weeks 23% of the TCPS had disappeared (Fig.1a), whereas the reduction of TCPL was only 7%. The respective values after four weeks are 41% and 9% implant resorption. This difference established after four weeks is then approximately maintained during the entire period of six months with a final implant resorption of 85% for TCPS and 62% for TCPL (Figs.1a,2b,c).

There is also a major difference in the rate of bone ingrowth into the tricalcium phosphate ceramics. 40% of the total implant area of the TCPS cylinders are occupied by bone after four weeks, compared to 17% of the TCPL cylinders (Fig.1b). After four weeks and six months the amount of bone within the implant area of TCPS is the same with a decrease after four months, whereas the part of TCPL cylinders filled by bone is increasing during the entire period of implantation.

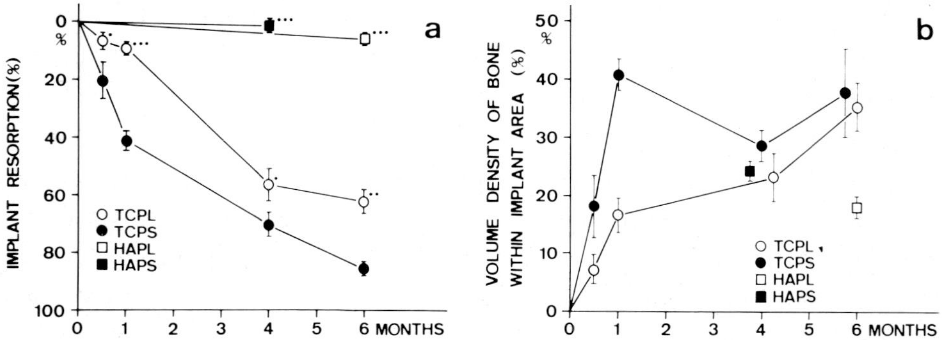

Fig. 1.(a) Implant resorption as a function of time. Means ± SEM. Significances are given in relation to the data obtained for TCPS: *$p < 0.05$, **$p < 0.005$, ***$p < 0.0005$. (b) Volume density of bone within the implant area. Means ± SEM. Abbreviations see text.

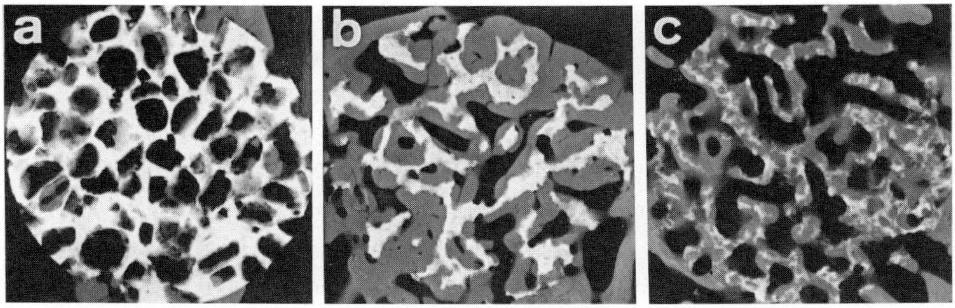

Fig.2. Microradiographs of cross-sections of ceramic cylinders after six months of implantation. Bone (dark gray) and implant material (light gray) can be discerned. x 13. (a) HAPL, (b) TCPL, (c) TCPS.

The preponderance of the smaller pore size may be partially explained by a surface enlargement, exposing a larger part of the material for resorption and bone deposition. But the main reason are numerous preexisting interconnections between the smaller pores. Scanning electron microscopy shows, that the walls of the larger pores are relatively thick and interconnections occur only occasionally (Fig.3a). The smaller pores are separated by very thin walls and multiple gaps of up to 20µm can be observed (Figs.3b,c). These interconnections favour rapid ingrowth of bone and implant resorbing cells, whereas in the larger porous material the majority of the septa have to be perforated by resorption before tissue ingrowth and implant degradation can proceed. This view is supported by

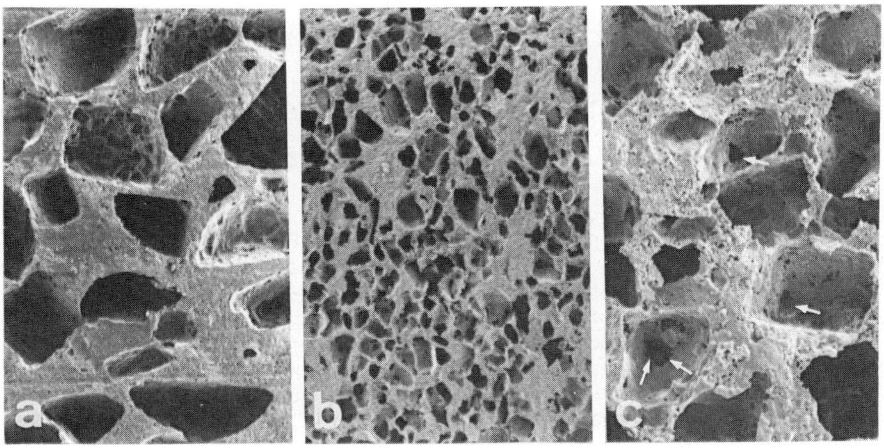

Fig. 3. Scanning electron microscopy of implant cylinders. TCPL (a) and TCPS (b) at the same magnification. x 45. Higher magnification of the TCPS (c), arrows indicating pore interconnections. x 166.

the fact, that after four months the smaller porous hydroxyapatite is penetrated by bone to a similar degree as the tricalcium phosphate ceramics, though no implant resorption has taken place, whereas bone ingrowth into the larger porous hydroxyapatite stays significantly lower ($p < 0.005$) even after six months (Figs.1b,2a).

It is a kind of dogma, that a pore size of over 100μm is required for sufficient bone ingrowth (ref. 5). We could show, that a pore size of 50-100μm with pore interconnections of 20μm allows bony ingrowth over a distance of at least 1.5mm, even when pores and pore interconnections can not be widened by resorption. The pore size per se, however, is not responsible for the better tissue ingrowth and implant substitution. The essential factor lies in the texture resulting from the production of smaller pores, i.e. rarefication of the septa and formation of pore interconnections, which favour vascular and cellular invasion (ref. 4).

CONCLUSIONS

Two major conclusions can be drawn from the presented data: 1.) Rather the existence of pore interconnections than pore size determines the rate of bone ingrowth and in the case of tricalcium phosphate the rate of implant resorption. 2.) Tricalcium phosphate is biodegradable, whereas practically no degradation occurs in the hydroxyapatite material.

Bearing in mind these facts one can choose the adequate ceramic material for the application as bone substitute or drug delivery system. Especially the smaller porous ceramics might be of future interest, because rapid tissue ingrowth is in most situations an important advantage.

REFERENCES

1 R.K. Schenk, A.J. Olah and W. Herrmann, Preparation of calcified tissues for light microscopy. In: G.R. Dickson (ed.), Methods of calcified tissue preparation, Elsevier, Amsterdam, 1984, pp1-56.

2 C.P.A.T. Klein, A.A. Driessen, K. de Groot and A. van den Hooff, Biodegradation behaviour of various calcium phosphate materials in bone tissue, J. Biomed. Mater. Res., 1983, 769-784.

3 W. Renooij, H.A. Hoogendoorn, W.J. Visser, R.H.F. Lentferink, M.G.J. Schmitz, H.V. Ieperen, S.J. Oldenburg, W.M. Janssen, L.M.A. Akkermans and P. Wittebol, Bioresorption of ceramic strontium-85-labeled calcium phosphate implants in dog femora, Clin. Orthop. Rel. Res., 197, 1985, 272-285.

4 K. Shimazaki and V. Mooney, Comparative study of porous hydroxyapatite and tricalcium phosphate as bone substitute, J. Orthop. Res., 3, 1985, 301-310.

5 J.J. Klawitter and S. Hulbert, Application of porous ceramics for the attachement of load bearing internal orthopedic applications, J. Biomed. Mater. Res., 1971, 161-229.

Biomaterials and Clinical Applications,
edited by A. Pizzoferrato, P.G. Marchetti, A. Ravaglioli and A.J.C. Lee
Elsevier Science Publishers B.V., Amsterdam, 1987 — Printed in The Netherlands

EXPERIMENTAL BONE INGROWTH STUDY OF 3-D POROUS CERAMIC COATING (PORAL°) FOR CEMENTLESS HIP PROSTHESIS.

A. TONI[1], A. PIZZOFERRATO[2], A. VENTURINI[3], A. SUDANESE[1], N. BALDINI[1], G. CIAPETTI[2] and S. STEA[2]

[1]Clinica Ortopedica 1, Istituto Rizzoli, Università di Bologna, Italy

[2]Centro di Ricerca per la Biocompatibilità dei Materiali da Impianto, Istituto Rizzoli, Bologna, Italy

[3]Istituto di Patologia Chirurgica Veterinaria, Università di Bologna, Italy

SUMMARY

A ceramic alumina-bioglass composite is presented as new porous coating for prosthetic devices. The porous alumina (PORAL°) utilized for implant samples briefly characterized. The bone ingrowth study was performed implanting the PORAL° samples in rabbit distal femur metaphysis. Retrievals were done at 2,4 and 6 weeks. Specimens were embedded in methylmethacrylate and stained with paragon. At 2 weeks bone ingrowth is still poor, while at 4 weeks the ceramic pores are quite filled with new trabeculae. At 45 days, the bone ingrowth into the ceramic porosity is impressive, with initial bone remodeling already taking place.

INTRODUCTION

Cementless prosthetic replacement presents increasing popularity among orthopaedic surgeons. The bone-ingrowth fixation requires a porous surface. To reach a valid bone-implant interlocking, such porosity should be around 25-45%, with a medium pore size ranging between 200 and 500 microns. Our aim was to make a porous alumina-bioglass ceramic composite to couple the advantages of the ceramic-ceramic bearing surfaces with the improved biocompatibility of the porosity totally made by ceramics versus metal alloys.

This experimental study of bone-ingrowth into a three dimensional macroporosity obtained with a new ceramic coating composite was performed in order to test this original solution for cementless articular prosthesis.

Before presenting the biological results, we will briefly overview a few morphological, chemical and mechanical characteristics of this ceramic composite.

MATERIAL AND METHODS

Porous alumina (PORAL°): composition

This material, called PORAL° for porous alumina, is made by two or three layers of alumina beads bonded with an high temperature bioglass to an alumina core, for instance the outer surface of hip prosthetic socket.

The alumina utilized is a 99.7% pure aluminim oxide, which presents fairly common properties for this kind of ceramic. The bioglass is based on alumina silicates with low alkali and alkaline earth contents. The binding process is performed at 1400 °C.

PORAL° morphological and chemical characterization

The bead diameter varies from 500 to 750 microns. The porous alumina mesh obtained bonding these beads give a 27% average porosity, while the pore size ranges between 290 and 510 microns, averaging 400 microns. The average interconnecting pore size is 350 microns. These porous character istics are well included among the ranges commonly considered as an optimal for bone ingrowth biology.

The bioglass cumulative release was also studied to evaluate the leaking property of the glass into biological solutions. The test was performed with PORAL° samples left in a daily stirred Ronger solution for 5000 hours. The sample weight losses were considered as the bioglass release and were measured every 500 hours. The cumulative bioglass resorption at 5000 hours is only 1.8 mg, with a trend that is decreasing with time. The bioglass resorption rate (Fig.1) gives an even clearer view such a trend, which enables us to evaluate the time necessary to reach the 10% of bioglass weight loss in 21 years.

PORAL° mechanical characterization

The alumina-bioglass bonding strengh was evaluated by testing the shear strength at the beads-core interface. A loading jig applied to an Instrom measured the force required to remove the outer poral ring from an alumina cylindric core. The strength ranged from 18 to 46 MPa, averaging 32 MPa. Such a variability is commonly seen in composite structures. The average value of 32 MPa is considered to be safe enough for the application of this porous alumina into human bone.

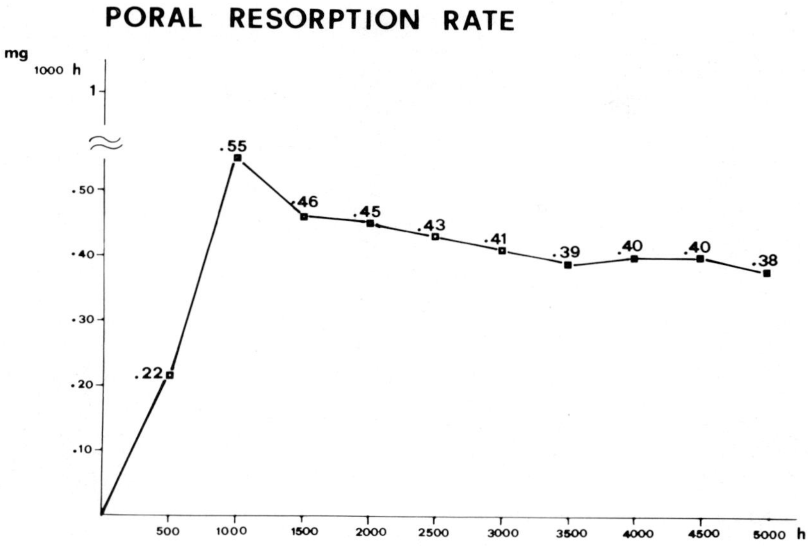

Fig. 1.

Bone-ingrowth study

The experimental study of the bone ingrowth into porous alumina was performed implanting 4 mm PORAL cylinders in general anesthetized rabbit distal femoral metaphyses. Animals were then sacrified at 2, 4, 6 weeks intervals. During the tests, tetracycline was administered. The specimens retrieved were embedded in methylmethacrylate, cut with a diamond blade saw and stained with Paragon. In almost all cases the ceramic composite was lost during the slice preparation, due to its brittleness when thinned to 80 microns. In pictures the ceramics must then be seen as void spaces.

RESULTS

Two weeks after surgery, connective reparative tissue is mainly present around the ceramic beads as you can see in Fig. 2, were the bony structure is emphasized by the polarized light. In fact, the bony trabeculae are still highly disorganized and adapting trabecular system seldom develops.

After 4 weeks bone ingrowth is more evident (Fig.3). It it then possible to evaluate the relevance of the pore sizing for the tissue ingrowth rate. Two pores are represented in Fig. 3: the narrow (a) one is 290 microns, while the larger one (b) is 390 microns. It is evident how the bone ingrowth

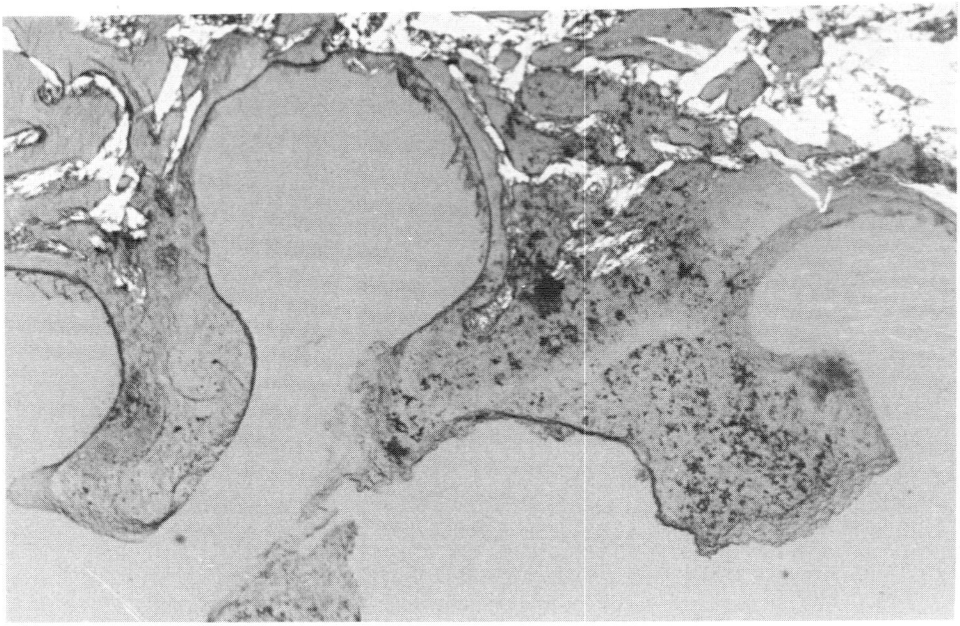

Fig. 2. Seven days after surgery the porous volume is filled up mainly with fibrous tissue (polarized light; 2.5 X).

Fig. 3. Four weeks after surgery; a: pore size 270 microns; b: pore size 390 microns (4 X).

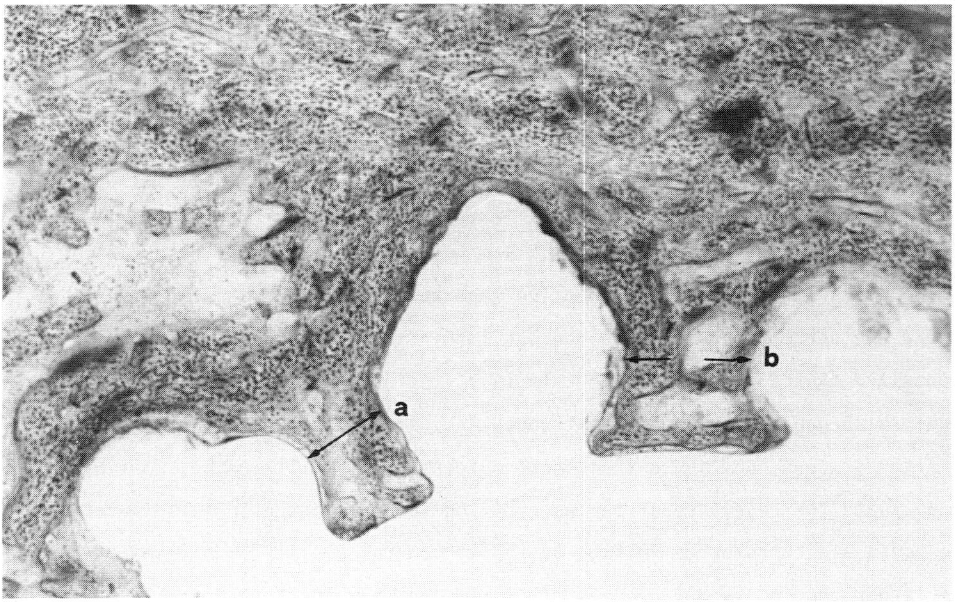

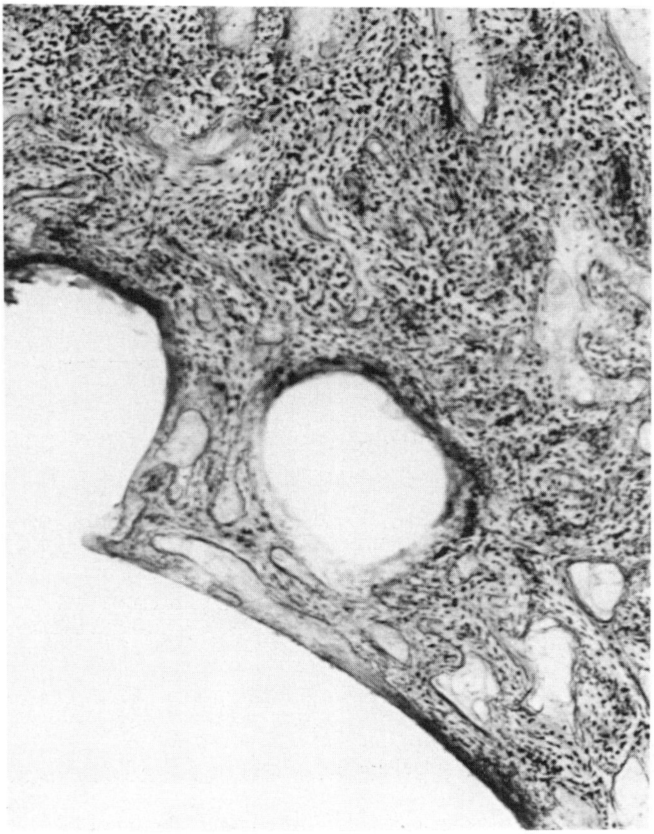

Fig. 4. Fourty-five days after surgery. The bone ingrowth is completely filling the ceramic porosity, reaching a close contact with the ceramic surfaces (void spaces) (4 X).

actually progresses quicker in the larger pore than in the narrower one.

After 45 days bone ingrowth into the porous alumina is impressive (Fig. 4). The trabeculae show an intimate contact with the beads, even at the bottom of the pore, where the bone shows already an initial adaptive remodeling to the porosity shape, though the bony structure is not yet well organized. Almost no connective tissue is interposed between bone and ceramic.

CONCLUSIONS

The porous alumina (PORAL) is a chemically stable composite, with a good mechanical strength, as confirmed by the 32 MPa average alumina-beads-bioglass shear modulus.

The ceramic porosity of PORAL shows a good bone biocompatibility, as confirmed by the quick and intimate bone ingrowth.

Biomaterials and Clinical Applications,
edited by A. Pizzoferrato, P.G. Marchetti, A. Ravaglioli and A.J.C. Lee
Elsevier Science Publishers B.V., Amsterdam, 1987 — Printed in The Netherlands

HISTOLOGICAL EXAMINATION OF THE BONE/METAL INTERFACE IN REMOVED POROUS COATED HUMAN PROSTHESES USING A NEW PROCESSING METHOD

J. F. DICHIARA AND P. A. HIGHAM

Howmedica, 309 Veterans Blvd., Rutherford, New Jersey 07070 (USA)

ABSTRACT

A recently developed method for the production of thin sections permits the preparation of 20 to 30 micron sections of the tissue/metal interface of retrieved prostheses. Examination of all three components of a total knee prosthesis removed at autopsy 13 months after implantation show excellent bone apposition and ingrowth into the porous coating. A thin (50 to 100 micron) oriented fibrous tissue layer surrounds the core of the prosthesis as well as many of the beads. Examination of a porous coated hip removed at autopsy, two months after implantation, shows complete tissue ingrowth into the coating, good apposition of calcified bone and a few distinct areas of bony spicules within the porous coated area. A fibrous membrane was also found around the core of this prosthesis.

INTRODUCTION

The increased use of biologically fixed prostheses has created a need for a more detailed examination of the histology of the tissue/implant interface. This type of detailed examination is necessary to determine the viability of porous ingrowth surfaces and to provide a correlation between the clinical results and histology.

A number of problems exist with performing this type of examination. The acquisition of samples that will provide the most reliable scientific data is difficult. Many researchers have only conducted animal studies; however, this does not provide an accurate evaluation of the human clinical case(1, 2). Others have examined human prostheses removed for revision(3, 4, 5). These samples are interesting for histological correlation to clinical history, but do not represent the results obtained in a clinically successful case.

In this study two autopsy samples were examined: 1) all three components (tibial, patellar and femoral) from a total knee arthoplasty implanted for thirteen months, and 2) a hip stem implanted for two months.

MATERIALS & METHODS

All samples were fixed in 10% Millonig's Buffered Formalin for one to three weeks depending on sample size. During this period excess bone around the prosthesis was removed using a diamond wire saw. After fixation the samples were transferred to 70% ethanol for storage to await further processing.

Sections of approximately 3 mm were cut through the hip, tibial component and patella. The knee femoral component had first to be cut in such a manner as to separate each of the condyles and the anterior portion of the sample. Each of these pieces could then be cut into 3 mm sections.

The sections were dehydrated through graded ethanol solutions, to absolute ethanol for a total dehydration time of 24 to 36 hours, and then infiltrated with a methylmethacrylate solution for 12 to 24 hours. The methyl methacrylate contained 0.1% of the initiator bis (4-tert-butylcyclohexyl)per- oxydicarbonate (BBPD) and 10% Plastoid-N to aid in penetration of the solution into the bone (6). The infiltration required four to five changes of the above solution and the entire procedure was performed under vacuum pulsed in 30 minute cycles.

The samples were polymerized for 24 to 48 hours in a 37°C water bath. After polymerization, the embedded samples were cut and thinned to approximately 0.5 mm on a metallurgical grinding wheel, and then mounted on plexiglass slides using an epoxy adhesive and flattened on one side using a Logitech Thin Section Lapping Machine. (The Logitech system uses a rotary lapping plate with a constant flow of 3 or 9 micron alumina to slowly thin the sample while maintaining control over flatness to within 2 microns over the length of the sample). A microradiograph was made of the sample. Each sample and a flattened glass slide were cleaned with freon and bonded together with an epoxy adhesive. After curing, sections were thinned to approximately 100 to 200 microns on a grinding wheel before being transferred to the Logitech machine for thinning to the final thickness of 20 to 30 microns. Sections were then polished on a felt polishing wheel with 0.05 micron alumina.

The sections were stained with hematoxylin for twenty to thirty minutes at 50°C and eosin for approximately 20 minutes at the same temperature. The staining was monitored to achieve the desired results. Staining of the sections can be done with most commonly used histological stains; however, penetration of the plastic requires a longer time and heating. After staining the sections were allowed to dry before coverslipping with permount. The sections were examined using a Leitz Orthoplan microscope under both plain and polarized light.

RESULTS AND DISCUSSION

Case 1

A seventy-five-year-old male with a history of osteoarthritis underwent a PCA™ total knee replacement. The joint was clinically successful with the patient experiencing no pain. The patient died thirteen months post operatively of unrelated causes. All three components of the knee were removed post mortem and deep frozen prior to examination. At examination the samples were removed from the freezer and excess bone removed. The samples were then immediately transferred to a 10% buffered formalin solution. Processing was carried out as outlined above.

Histological examination of the tibial component showed a morphology that can be divided into four zones. The first zone, closest to the substrate of the tibial tray, shows a dense fibrous tissue layer which surrounds the core of the implant and some of the beads. This layer is composed of lenticular collagen fibres orientated parallel to the substrate. The fibrous layer has a uniform thickness of 50 to 100 microns when apposing the prosthesis core and approximately 10 to 30 microns when around the beads.

The second zone, described as the area within the porous coating, has a more varied histology. It consists of a well vascularized loose fibrous tissue and bone with some globules of fat. Polarized light microscopy shows distinct tissue elements similar to Sharpey's Fibres. These fibres appear to be attached to calcified bone growing into the porous coating (Fig. 1, 2).

The second zone has extensive ingrowth of woven bone. Most bone ingrowth is found posterior to the fixation pegs and in some areas this bone can be seen close to the core of the prosthesis. Although there are some areas that appear to have bone directly apposing the metal prosthesis, examination of a number of sections suggests that there is always a thin fibrous membrane separating the calcified bone from the metal prosthesis.

The third zone, from the periphery of the porous coating to the edge of the original normal appearing bone and marrow, consists of bone apposing the porous coating and a fatty marrow with areas of hematopoesis (Fig. 3). This zone consists of both woven and lamellar bone. Areas of new woven bone can be seen directly on spicules of lamellar bone that previously existed. There are other areas in which new bone formation appears to be derived directly from the underlying marrow. Bone appositon to the porous coating is seen throughout most of the prosthesis. The extent of the hematopoesis in the marrow of this zone is not as great as that seen in the original marrow but appears to increase with increasing distance from the prosthesis. Zone four consists of a normal appearing marrow and bone.

The femoral component demonstrates a morphology similar to that described in the tibial plateau. The amount of bone ingrowth is somewhat less than that seen in the tibia with the most extensive ingrowth seen on the condylar areas parallel to the tibial plateau.

In zone two, the fibrous tissue on the posterior portion of the femoral component is denser than on the remainder of the sample and some hematopoetic fatty marrow is observed.

The tissue morphology seen in the patellar component is similar to that of the other two components. One difference is in the amount of bone ingrowth in zone two. The patella shows bone ingrowth into more than 50% of the sample with some local areas of higher concentration (Fig. 5).

Case 2

A seventy year old female with a history of osteoarthritis underwent a PCA™ total hip replacement. The femoral component, implanted for 2 months, was received post mortem upon the patients death of unrelated causes. It was removed from the bone by the surgeon prior to formalin fixation.

Histological examination of the femoral component shows a dense fibrous layer surrounding the core of the prosthesis and many of the beads; the thickness was similar to that seen in the tibial tray.

In some areas a histiocytic region can be observed between the prosthesis and the fibrous tissue layer (Fig. 4). Occasional giant cells can be seen in this region along with a mild inflammatory response.

Within the porous coating is a zone of loose connective tissue. Tissue histiocytes and mononuclear cells are seen throughout this highly vascularized area. The sample shows evidence of new bone formation with occasional calcified bone spicules within the porous coating.

In the zone immediately adjacent to the prosthesis good apposition of woven bone to the porous coating is seen. This zone is characterized by fatty tissue and bone with varying amounts of hematopoesis. It resembles a fatty marrow in some areas and normal bone and marrow in others.

In general the histology of this sample, implanted for two months, is similar to that seen in the early stages of fracture repair.

SUMMARY

Our examination, based on the limited number of suitable samples available, shows a very consistent morphology to the pattern of tissue ingrowth in these clinically successful surgeries. The histology of these samples can be conveniently divided into four distinct zones: Zone 1, a dense fibrous membrane surrounding the core of the prosthesis and many of the beads; Zone 2, a well vascularized loose fibrous tissue similar to Sharpey's Fibres and areas of calcified bone ingrowth; Zone 3, a fatty marrow with areas of normal hematopoesis, and Zone 4, a normal appearing marrow and bone.

The pattern of bone ingrowth in these samples appears to be progressing in a manner similar to that of fracture healing. The only difference is that no cartilage formation was noted in these prostheses as would be expected in a fracture callus formation.

This paper provides a look at two clinical cases consisting of four components. Considerably more work on autopsy samples implanted for varying times must be performed to develop a complete picture of the time course involved in ingrowth into porous coatings in clinical cases and the amount of calcified bone versus soft tissue that is required for stable fixation. This work combined with examination of samples received from revision surgeries will help to provide a more accurate evaluation of the histological results associated with varying clinical cases.

REFERENCES

1 J.D. Bobyn, R.M. Pilliar, H.U. Cameron and G.C. Weatherly, The optimum pore size for the fixation of porous-surfaced metal implants by the ingrowth of bone, Clin. Orthop. 150: 263 (1980).
2 R.M. Pilliar, H.U. Cameron and I. Macnab, Porous-surfaced layered prosthetic devices, J. Biomed. Eng. 10: 126 (1975).
3 J.D. Bobyn and C.A. Engh, Human histology of the bone-porous metal interface, Orthopedics 7(9) (1984) pp. 1410-1421.
4 M.B. Mayor, C.O. Townley, J.B. Fenning and F.F. Buechel, Histology of Retrieved Porous-Coated Knee Prosthesis, AAOS, New Orleans (1986) No. 14.
5 R.J. Haddad and J.O. Edmunds, Histologic and Microradiographic Analysis of Noncemented Retrieved PCA Knee Components, AAOS, New Orleans (1986) No. 15.
6 R. Buijs and A.A. Dogterom, An improved method for embedding hard tissue in polymethyl methacrylate, Stain Technol. 58(3) (1983) pp. 135-141.

ACKNOWLEDGEMENTS

Professor Fernandez-Fairen and Dr. Hungerford for supplying the samples and Dr. V. Vigorita for reviewing the histology.

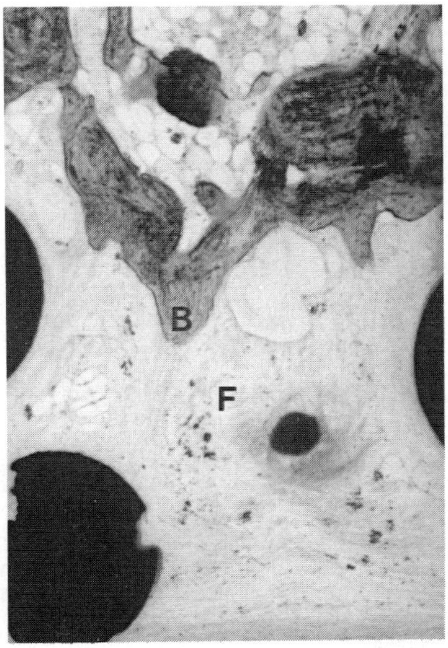

Fig. 1. Loose Fibrous Tissue (F) in the porous coating of the Femoral knee component. Calcified Bone (B).

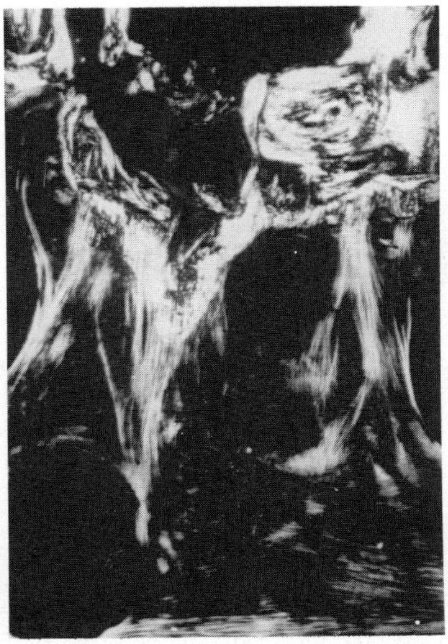

Fig. 2. Polarized light view of Figure 1. Note the fibres attached to the bone (Sharpey's Fibres).

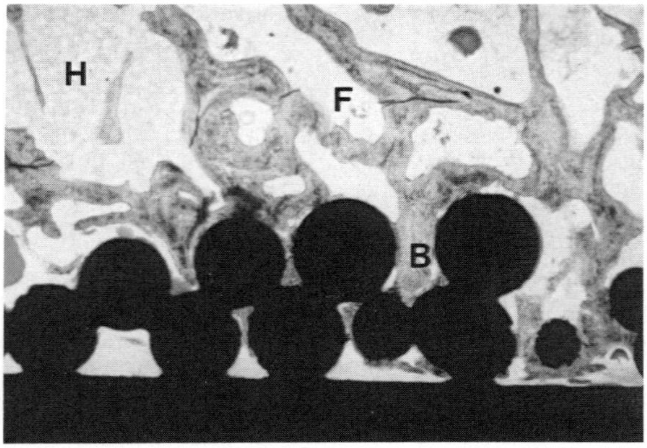

Fig. 3. Bone (B) Ingrowth into the porous coating of the tibial tray. Areas of hematopoesis (H) and fatty marrow (F).

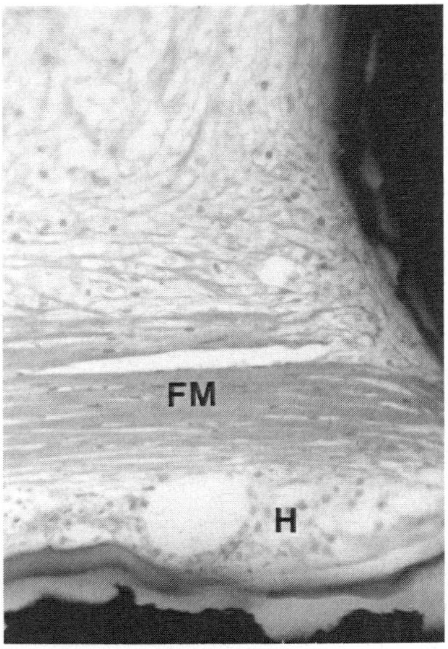

Fig. 4. Dense Fibrous Membrane (FM) surrounding the core of the hip. Histiocytic region (H) below the membrane.

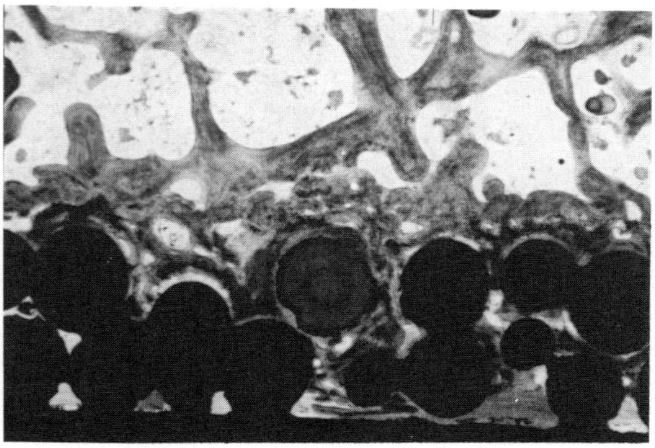

Fig. 5. Extensive ingrowth of woven bone into the patellar component.

Biomaterials and Clinical Applications,
edited by A. Pizzoferrato, P.G. Marchetti, A. Ravaglioli and A.J.C. Lee
Elsevier Science Publishers B.V., Amsterdam, 1987 — Printed in The Netherlands

HYDROXYLAPATITE COATING ON Ti AND Al_2O_3 —— STUDIES ON THE BIOLOGICAL FIXATION

H. OONISHI M.D.[1], S. MIYAMOTO Ph.D.[2], A. KOHDA M.D.[2], H. ISHIMARU Ph.D.[2] and E. TSUJI Ph. D.[3]

[1]Department of Orthopaedic Surgery, Artificial Joint Section and Biomaterial Research Laboratory, Osaka-Minami National Hospital, 677-6, Kido-Cho, Kawachinagano-Shi, Osaka 586, JAPAN

[2]Sumitomo Chemical Co.

[3]Osaka Prefectural Industrial Research Institute

ABSTRACT

Fundamental studies have been made on materials which are obtained by coating HAP on alumina or metal surfaces by means of the spatter method and plasma spray. After two weeks, spaces between the bone and the plasma spray coated HAP were filled with homogeneous bony substances and bone salts. Four weeks later, the bone completely bonded with HAP. As time elapsed to 4, 6 and 13 weeks, there occurred a difference in bonding strength between the material [A] coated with 100% HAP, [B] coated with a mixture of 80% HAP and 20% alumina and [C] with only shot blasting as a control. The adhering strength of material [B] was 80% material [A], but no histological difference was found. In the case of alumina coated with HAP by means of spatter method, the bone directly contacted to the materials even after HAP disappeared, and alumina coated with HAP had adhering force more than about five times stronger than that of alumina.

INTRODUCTION

Apatite coating is available as one way of obtaining cementless fixation which is intended for obtaining reliable fixation relatively early by means of chemical bonding. Latterly, the porous metal has come to be used to allow early, strong fixation with the bone. On the other hand, for earlier, stronger fixation, apatite coating on the porous metal surface was considered more useful. Thus, fundamental studies for applications to orthopedic surgery have been made on materials which are obtained by coating hydroxylapatite (HAP) on alumina or metal surfaces by means of the spattering method and plasma spray.

HYDROXYLAPATITE COATING ON Ti BY MEANS OF PLASMA SPRAY

1) Method

A) Preparations of materials and samples

Ti cylinders of 5mm in diameter and 15mm in height as well as wedge-like Ti plates with a height of 12mm were prepared by cutting. Then the surfaces of these were processed with shot blasting.

Hydroxylapatite was produced by wet synthesis and made into dry spheres by spray drying. Mixed with alumina of 99.99% in purity, it was again made into spheres. Those spheres were used as raw materials for plasma spray.

They were plasma-sprayed to the Ti surfaces which had been made uneven by shot blasting, by using a plasma jet sprayer.

The experimental samples consisted of (A) materials sprayed with 100% HAP, (B) those sprayed with mixture of 80% HAP and 20% alumina, respectively, and (C) pure Ti applied with only shot blasting as a control. X-ray diffraction analyses were made on the HAP phases and crystal structure which had been created due to mixture with alumina and also to spraying. In addition, measurements were made on changes in the strength of the membrane depending on the mixing ratio of alumina.

B) Animal experiment

In the animal experiment, tibiae and greater trochanters of 20 mature beagles were used. On the right and left tibial shafts, three holes each with a diameter larger by 0.2mm to 0.3mm than that of the cylinders to be implanted were made. Each piece of the experimental samples (A), (B) and (C) was implanted to the respective tibiae. Similarly, on the greater trochanters, three holes each with a thickness greater by 0.2mm than the thickness of the wedge were made. Then, the wedges were driven into the respective holes just as in the case with the tibiae. After 2, 3, 4, 6, 12 and 24 weeks, a total of 12 beagles were sacrificed and hard preparations were made after embedding with resin. Observations were made on them by light microscope, tetracycline labeling, CMR, SEM and COMPO pictures.

C) Adhering strength to the bone

In order to measure the adhering strength to the bone, four each of the same cylindrical samples (A), (B) and (C) as used for the previous observations of histological pictures, were implanted to the tibiae. After 2, 4, 6 and 12 weeks, a total of 8 beagles were sacrificed and immediately the pushing-in test was made using Instron Universal Tester at a head rate of 0.1mm/min.

2) Results and discussion

A) Materials and samples

The titanium surfaces processed by shot blasting was several μm to several hudred μm in roughness and the HAP surface several ten μm to several hundred μm. Thus, HAP membrane with a thickness of several μm to several hundred μm was formed. No change and resolution due to spraying were found on the phase of HAP (Fig. 1). As the mixing ratio of alumina increased, the strength of the membrane became greater.

B) Animal experiment

After two weeks, from the COMPO pictures, the space between the bone and

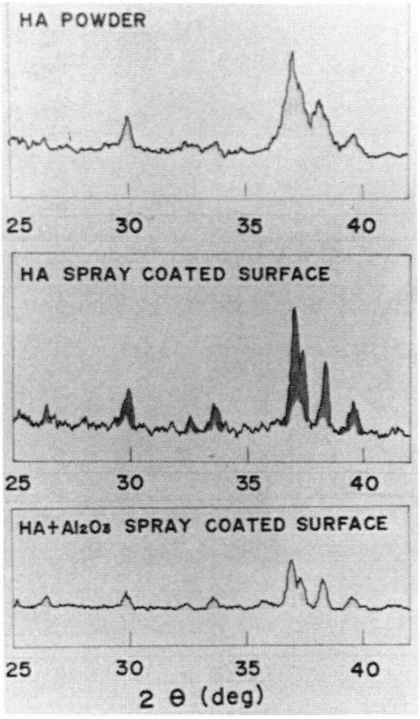

Fig. 1. X-ray diffraction analyses at the HA and HA + Al_2O_3 spray coated surface.

HAP was seen to be filled with homogeneous substance and with the HAP powder particles that were produced when they were inserted into bone (Fig. 2 (a)). By the HE-stained preparations, elemental analyses and CMR, that space was also seen to be filled with bone salt. There was no soft tissue observed. In the control group, bone invasion into the rough surfaces had already started, but existence of soft tissues was found without fail. Four weeks later, in the histological pictures, the bone extensively and completely bonded with HAP, and this was same six weeks later (Fig. 3). In the COMPO pictures, as 2, 4 and 6 weeks passed, bone tissues which appeared to be homogeneous gradually changed into apparent bone tissues (Fig. 2 (a, b)). Comparisons were made between 100% HAP and mixture of 80% HAP and 20% Al_2O_3. Throughout the course of time, no histological difference was found. In the control group, bone invasion into the rough surfaces gradually increased, but no difference was noticed after 4 weeks and after 6 weeks. With respect to the histological pictures taken 12 and 24 weeks after implantation, SEM, COMPO pictures and stained preparations showed that HAP directly bonded with bone, that homogeneous tissues disappeared, that bone tissues in the interface were completely ossified, and that the interface became clear (Fig. 4 (a, b, c)).

C) Adhering strength to the bone

Two weeks after implantation, the material (A) coated with 100% HAP was

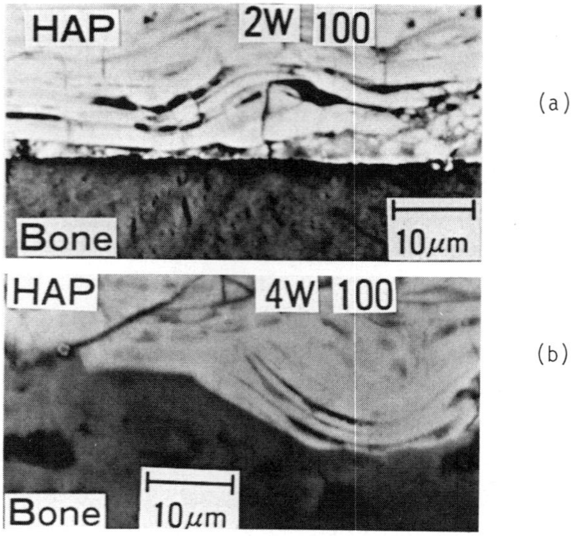

Fig. 2 (a, b). COMPO pictures.
(a) Two weeks after the implantation
(b) Four weeks after the implantation

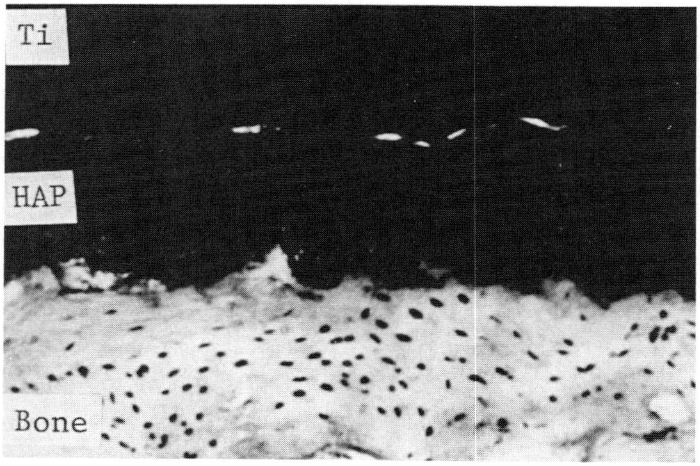

Fig. 3. HE stained preparations. Four weeks after the implantation.

slightly superior in adhering strength to the material (C) with no coating, but there was no substantial difference between the two. At this stage, the interface had not sufficient strength since only homogeneous substance existed there. As time elapsed to 4, 6 and 13 weeks, there occurred a difference in bonding strength between the material (A), (B) and (C). The adhering strength

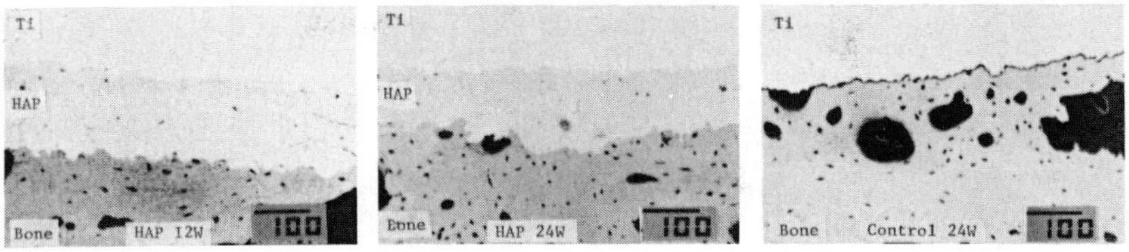

(a) (b) (c)

Fig. 4 (a, b, c) COMPO pictures. (a) 12 weeks after the implantation, (b) 24 weeks after the implantation and (c) 24 weeks after the implantation (control)

of sample (B) with a mixture of 80% HAP and 20% alumina was 80% sample (A) with 100% HAP. Namely, these adhering strength ratios were almost coincident with the mixing ratio of HAP to alumina. Bone tissues invaded the material (C) and mechanical bonding was obtained. The SUS 316L with smooth surfaces, as a control, was very low in adhering strength even after long implantation. In any of the materials (A), (B) and (C), as the implanted period became longer, the adhering strength with bone increased (Fig. 5). In any case, about 80% adhering strength was acquired six weeks after implantation. In our experiment on porous metal, there was the same tendency. Thus, all the above factors were closely related to bone growth and formation. Therefore, six weeks after surgery can be an index for postoperative exercise and loading clinically.

When the sample surfaces were observed with SEM after the pushing-in test, samples (A) and (B) were broken at the HAP layers. Sample (C) was broken at the layer of bone and connective tissues. In the control SUS 316L sample with smooth surfaces, connective tissue membrane was exfoliated off the sample.

HYDROXYLAPATITE COATING ON ALUMINA BY MEANS OF THE SPATTER METHOD

1) Method

The following implant test pieces were prepared: (1) a column of Fe-Cr-Al alloy (4mm in diameter and 12mm in height) the surface of which had α-Al_2O_3 dispersed by heat treatment (Fe-Cr-Al + Al_2O_3), (2) the same implant test piece over which HAP was coated by the spatter method (Fe-Cr-Al + Al_2O_3 + HAP) and (3) a column of SUS 316L. The tibial cortical bone of a goat was drilled with the same diameter as that of the test pieces, and each set of four test pieces were implanted into both tibiae. After three months, the goat was sacrificed and the following tests and observations were carried out.

a) Pushing-in test of each implanted test piece: When the pushing-in test of the test pieces was conducted, a fixing base was prepared by using MMA so that the cylindrical test pieces might be positioned vertically.

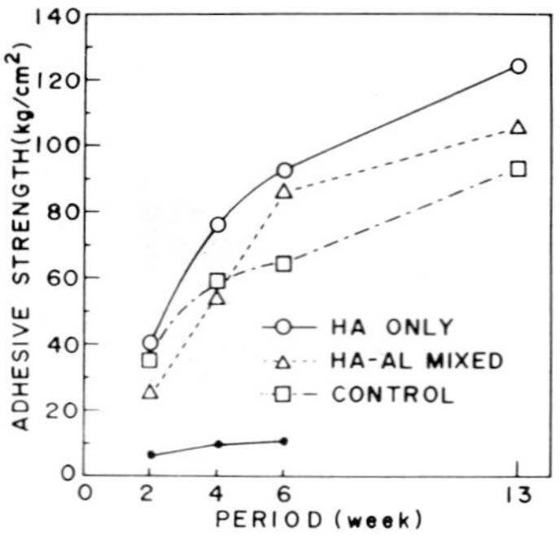

Fig. 5. Results of pushing-in test. In order to compare the adhering strength to the bone, the following materials were used: (A) materials sprayed with 100% HAP, (B) those sprayed with mixture of 80% HAP and 20% alumina, (C) pure Ti applied with only shot blasting as a control and (D) SUS 316L with smooth surface as a control.

b) Observation on the interface between an implanted test piece and a bone by means of SEM, COMPO and X-ray microanalyzer.

2) Results and discussion

a) The results of the pushing-in test indicated that the adhering force of (1) the alloy with α-alumina (Fe-Cr-Al + Al_2O_3), (2) the alloy with α-alumina coated with HAP (Fe-Cr-Al + Al_2O_3 + HAP) and (3) SUS 316L to the bone was, on an average, about 9 kg/cm^2, about 50 kg/cm^2 and about 3 kg/cm^2, respectively.

b) When the interfacial sections between the implanted test pieces and the bones were observed by SEM and element analyses, there were almost no differences between (1) and (2). However, very thin fibrous membrane was seen in same areas in the case of (1). From this fact, it was presumed that bone tissues directly touched to the test pieces even after HAP disappeared.

CONCLUSION

Metals, polymeric materials, alumina and apatite have their own characteristics as biomaterials and cannot be always used individually. Therefore, in order to utilize the excellent characteristics of each material, the composite use of several kinds of materials is desirable.

REFERENCES

1 Okabe, H., Tsuji, E., Ike, H. and OOnishi, H.: A study on the Fe-Cr-Al alloy as a biomaterial — Mechanical properties corrosion resistance and Al_2O_3 formation —, J. of Jap. Soc. for Biomat., 3, 1, 55-63, 1985.
2 Oonishi, H., Okabe, H., Ike, T. and Tsuji, E.: Development of Fe-Cr-Al alloy with α-alumina layer diffused on the surface — Studies on biocompatibilities — , J. of Jap. Soc. for Biomat. In print.
3 Oonishi, H., Tsuji, E., Kohda, H., Ishimaru, H. and Sugimoto, T.: Studies on Ti-6A-4V beads coated with HAP, 6th Orthopaedic Ceramic Implant, 1986.

Biomaterials and Clinical Applications,
edited by A. Pizzoferrato, P.G. Marchetti, A. Ravaglioli and A.J.C. Lee
Elsevier Science Publishers B.V., Amsterdam, 1987 — Printed in The Netherlands

STRENGTH OF BONDING BETWEEN A-W GLASS CERAMIC AND THE SURFACE OF BONE CORTEX

SATORU YOSHII[1], YOSHIAKI KAKUTANI[1], TAKAO YAMAMURO[1] AND TADASHI KOKUBO[2]

[1]Department of Orthopaedic Surgery, Faculty of Medicine, Kyoto University. Kyoto 606 (Japan)

[2]Laboratory of Ceramic Chemistry, Institute for Chemical Research, Kyoto University, Uji, 611 (Japan)

SUMMARY

We examined the bonding strength of apatite- and wollastonite-containing glass-ceramics (A-W glass-ceramic) to the surface of bone cortex. A semi-column-shaped block of A-W glass-ceramic was fixed with a screw on the surface of the tibia of a rabbit.

The load required to detach the implant from the surface of the bone was measured at 2, 4, 8 and 25 weeks after implantation.

The bonding strength of the ceramics increased with time reaching a maximum of 18 kg/cm2.

From these studies, we conclude that A-W glass-ceramic has good bonding capability to the surface of bone.

INTRODUCTION

In the field of bone and joint replacement, one of the most important problems is fixing the implant to bone. The implant fixed to bone by mechanical interlocking is liable to loosen with time. Glass and glass-ceramics containing CaO and P_2O_5 as well as hydroxyapatite ceramics are reported to bind chemically with bone (refs. 1-3).

However, the mechanical strength of these materials are inadequate to be used as orthopedic implants (ref. 4). We have developed glass-ceramics by the method of precipitating a second crystalline. These new glass-ceramics contain oxyapatite and wollastonite as major components. In this report, these glass-ceramics are referred to as A-W glass-ceramic. The mechanical strength of the A-W glass-ceramic is superior to the mechanical strength of cortical bone (ref. 5). Nakamura has reported its excellent bonding strength to bone when A-W glass-ceramic is implanted in the bone (ref. 6).

For the clinical application, especially in maxillo-facial

surgery, it is important that the implant binds firmly to the surface of cortical bone. In these studies, we examined the bonding strength of A-W glass-ceramic to the surface of bone cortex.

MATERIALS AND METHODS

1. Preparation of materials

The chemical composition of our A-W glass-ceramic is as follows: MgO,4.6, CaO,44.6, SiO_2,34.2, P_2O_5,16.3, CaF_2,0.5 in weight ratio.

Glass powders of the composition were compacted and heated up to 1050°C at a rate of 5°C/min and held at 1050°C for 2 h to be sintered and crystallized. The resultant glass-ceramics showed high bending and compressive strengths of 157 and 1060 MPa, respectively (ref. 5). X-ray diffraction analysis showed that these glass-ceramics were composed mostly of oxyapatite and wollastonite crystals. Alumina-ceramics were used for control.

A-W glass-ceramic and alumina-ceramics were shaped into semi-column blocks, 4 x 10 x 8 mm, with holes of 2 mm-diameter at their centers (see Fig. 1). The flat base of the block was 70 mm^2. Their surfaces were polished with No. 1500 SiC paper. The blocks were heat-sterilized in the conventional manner.

2. Implantation of materials

Mature male rabbits weighing 3.0 to 3.5 kg were anesthetized with pentobarbital (50 mg/kg). The operations were performed under aseptic conditions. A 2-cm skin incision was made on the antero-medial portion of the tibial metaphyses of the rabbit. The cortex of tibia was exposed subperiosteally about 10 x 10 mm. A 2-mm diameter hole was made by a drill at the center of the exposed cortex through the bone. The ceramic block was placed on the flat surface of the bone cortex and fixed with a stainless steel screw through the hole in the block. The wound was closed in layers.

The blocks of A-W glass-ceramic were implanted in tibiae of 12 rabbits. The blocks of alumina-ceramics were implanted in tibiae of 6 rabbits.

The rabbits were housed in temperature- and humidity-controled room with a 12-h light cycle. They were fed food and water freely.

3. Evaluation of bonding strength

The rabbits implanted with the A-W glass-ceramic were sacrificed 2, 4, 8 and 25 weeks after implantation with a lethal dose of pentobarbital solution. The rabbits implanted with the alumina-ceramics were sacrificed 4 and 8 weeks after implantation.

The tibia was excised with the ceramic block, and cut transversely at 3 mm proximal and distal to the block. The bone tissue covering the block was removed completely and the block was placed in contact with the bone only at its flat surface. The screw was carefully removed. The block and the piece of bone were held by hooks. The hooks were connected to an Instron-type tensile load tester (Autograph S-500, Shimadzu Seisakujo,Kyoto,Japan).

The block was pulled perpendicularly to the surface contacting the bone. The load required to detach the implant from the bone or to break the bone was measured.

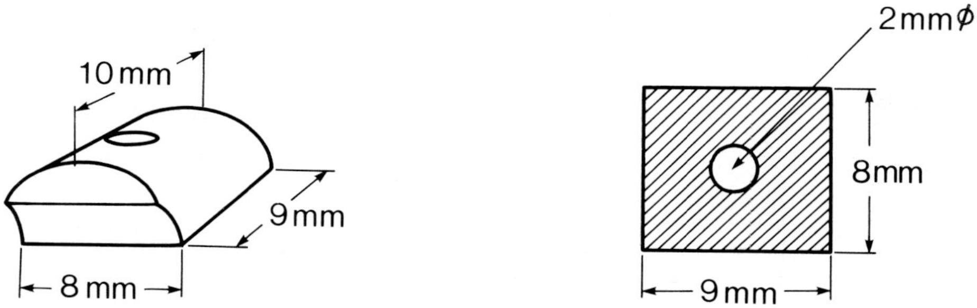

Fig. 1. Illustrations showing the form of ceramic implant.
The right-sided one shows the base of the block.

RESULTS

Table 1 summarizes the detaching load of both ceramics. Two weeks after implantation, the detaching load of A-W glass-ceramic was 0 kg. Four weeks after implantation, it became 8.4±1.1 kg/cm^2 and increased to 14.6±3.1 kg/cm^2 8 weeks after implantation.

The detaching load was 18.5±7.3 kg/cm^2 25 weeks after implantation. The detaching load of alumina-ceramics was 0.5±0.6 kg/cm^2 8 weeks after implantation.

Fig. 2 shows that the bonding strength of A-W glass-ceramic increased rapidly 4 weeks after implantation. Its bonding strength was 80% of the maximum bonding strength 8 weeks after implantation.

DISCUSSION

From the present results, it is apparent that A-W glass-ceramic makes strong chemical bonding with the surface of bone cortex.

TABLE 1

Detaching loads of ceramic implants

Time after Implantation	Means ± SD kg/cm² ( ): No. of Samples	
	Alumina-ceramics	A-W glass-ceramics
2W		0 ± 0 (6)
4W	0 ± 0 (6)	8.4 ± 1.1 (6)
8W	0.5 ± 0.6 (5)	14.6 ± 3.2 (5)
25W		18.5 ± 7.3 (3)

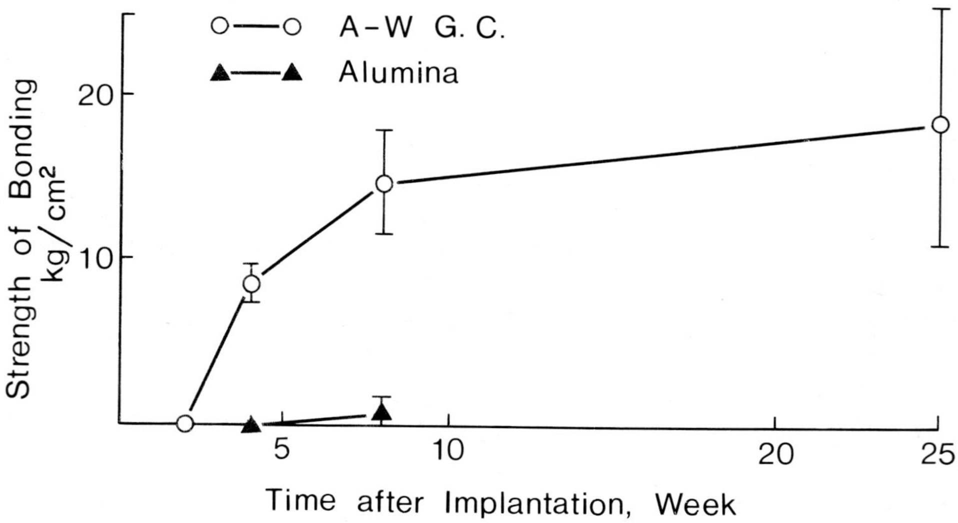

Fig. 2. Diagram showing the relationship between the strength of bonding of ceramic implants and the time after implantation.

The finding that 1 cm^2 contacting surface supports a detaching load of 18 kg indicates that a contacting surface of only 2.5 x 2.5 cm supports a load over 100 kg.

With sufficient mechanical strength superior to that of cortical bone and with this excellent bonding capability, A-W glass-ceramic is regarded as a leading implant material to cover defects of bone or to build up a new bony structure in orthopedic surgery, maxillo-facial surgery and neurosurgery.

REFERENCES

1 L.L. Hench, R.J. Splinter, W.C. Allen and T.K. Greenlee, Bonding mechanisms at the interface of ceramic prosthetic materials, J. Biomed. Mater. Res. Symp., 2, (1971) 117-141.
2 B.A.Blencke, E. Pfeil and H.H. Kas, Implant aus Glass-keramik in der Knochenchirurgie (Tier-experimentelle Untersuchungen), Langenbechs Arch. Chir. Suppl. Forum, 1973 (1973) 107-110.
3 M. Jarcho, J.F. Kay, K.I.Gumaer, R.H. Doremus and H.P. Drobeck, Tissue, cellular and subcellular events at a bone-ceramic hydroxyapatite interface, J. Bioeng., 1 (1977) 79-92.
4 D.T. Reilly and A.H. Burstein, The mechanical properties of cortical bone, J. Bone Jt. Surg., 56-A, (1974) 1001-1022.
5 T. Kokubo, M. Shigematsu, Y. Nagashima, M. Tashiro, T. Nakamura, T. Yamamuro and S. Higashi, Apatite- and wollastonite-containing glass-ceramics for prosthetic application, Bull. Inst. Chem. Res. Kyoto Univ., 60 (1982) 260-268.
6 T. Nakamura, T. Yamamuro and S. Higashi, A new glass-ceramic for bone replacement: evaluation of its bonding to bone tissue, J. Biomed. Mater. Res., 19 (1985) 685-698.

Biomaterials and Clinical Applications,
edited by A. Pizzoferrato, P.G. Marchetti, A. Ravaglioli and A.J.C. Lee
Elsevier Science Publishers B.V., Amsterdam, 1987 — Printed in The Netherlands

CALCIUM PHOSPHATE CERAMICS FOR BONE IMPLANTS: BIORESORPTION OF POROUS CERAMICS OF STRONTIUM-85 LABELED HYDROXYAPATITE AND TRICALCIUM ORTHOPHOSPHATE IMPLANTED IN DOG FEMORA

H.A. HOOGENDOORN [1], W.J. VISSER [2], S.J. OLDENBURG [3], L.M.A. AKKERMANS [1], P. WITTEBOL[1] and W. RENOOIJ[1]

Departments of [1]Surgery, [2]Internal Medicine, and [3]Nuclear Medicine, Utrecht University Hospital, Catharijnesingel 101, 3511 GV UTRECHT (The Netherlands)

SUMMARY

Blocks of sintered macroporous hydroxyapatite and tricalcium orthophosphate (dimensions 2.5 x 1.25 x 0.5 cm) were implanted into surgically created defects in dog femora. Bioresorption was evaluated from histologic preparations, and was quantitated by labeling implants with radioactive strontium-85 apatite or tristrontium-85 orthophosphate. Hydroxyapatite implants were not affected by bioresorption processes during 3.5 years of observation. Tricalcium orthophosphate implants were subject to extensive cell-mediated biodegradation. The radioactivity over the implant sites showed a decrease of 25%-30% in 22 weeks. Resorption debris from these implants was found in mononuclear phagocytes.

INTRODUCTION

In the fields of medicine and biomechanical engineering, much effort has been directed to the development of bone implant materials, which can be used as a scaffold for bone growth in defects resulting from disease or trauma. In particular, calcium phosphate compounds -- hydroxyapatite ($Ca_{10}(PO_4)_6(OH)_2$) and tricalcium orthophosphate ($Ca_3(PO_4)_2$) -- have recieved wide attention.

It has been unambiguously demonstrated that ceramic tricalcium orthophosphate implants are subject to biodegradation processes (see ref. 1, for an extensive review; ref. 2). Hydroxyapatite implants do not show signs of bioresorption (refs. 1,2), although some reports suggest that hydroxyapatite implants are affected by bioresorption processes (refs. 3,4).

In most reports, time-dependent resorption of implants in vivo was studied by estimating the decrease in radiolucency of roentgenograms. In this study a novel method is presented to quantitate resorption of calcium phosphate ceramic implants. The authors developed a procedure to prepare strontium-85 labeled porous ceramic implants of hydroxyapatite and tricalcium orthophosphate. Bioresorption of the implants was quantitated by measuring the radioactivity over the implant sites. Strontium-85 was selected because it fulfills the following requirements: strontium is chemically and biologically related to calcium; the

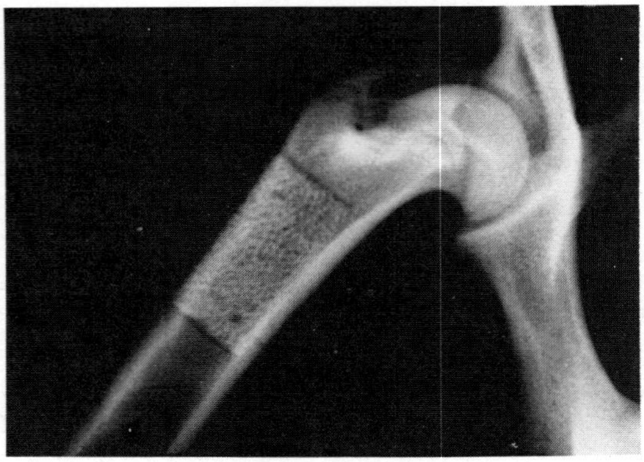

Fig. 1. Roentgenogram of an implant in a dog's femur immediately after surgery.

half-life of the isotope is 64.7 days, which permits relatively long-term studies; and the isotope is a gamma emitter (energy, 514keV), which allows detection outside the body.

METHODS

The preparation of labeled ceramic implants, and the surgical and analytical procedures were extensively described elsewhere (refs. 5,6). Therefore, these methods will only be outlined briefly.

Labeled strontium hydroxyapatite was chemically synthesized from dibasic ammonium phosphate and (^{85}Sr)strontium nitrate. Labeled tristrontium orthophosphate was synthesized from (^{85}Sr)strontium nitrate and dibasic sodium phosphate. The reaction products were taken up in slurries of a 1000-fold excess of calcium hydroxyapatite or tricalcium orthophosphate in 1.5% or 2.5% hydrogen peroxide. The slurries were baked at 80 °C forming porous bodies, which were subsequently sintered at 1300 °C (hydroxyapatite) or 1150 °C (tricalcium orthophosphate). After cooling, the bodies were cut into blocks of 2.5 x 1.25 x 0.5 cm. The blocks were heat-sterilized. The porosity of the implants was 50%-56%. The average pore size was 0.18-0.26 mm^2.

Under general anesthesia, a window of cortical bone of the size of the implants was removed from the proximal third of the left femoral shaft just distal to the trochanter major. The implant was placed in that window and secured in position with two sutures.

Unlabeled hydroxyapatite implants were placed in the left femur of 14 dogs (beagles, 10-15 kg). The dogs were killed at intervals of 1.5-2 months up to two years after the implantation date. Two dogs were killed after about 3.5 years. Labeled blocks of either hydroxyapatite or tricalcium orthophosphate were implanted in the left femur of four dogs, two dogs for each type of

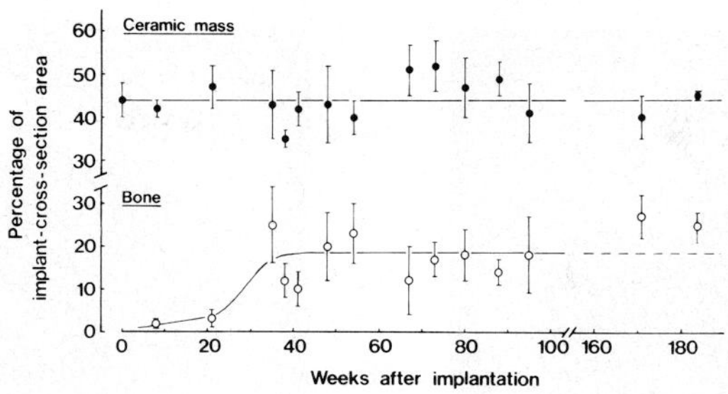

Fig. 2. Relative surface areas of bone and ceramic mass in cross sections of hydroxyapatite implants. The data presented are the averages ± S.D. of the data obtained from three histologic slides per implant.

compound. These four dogs were killed one year after the implantation date.

Periodically, the areas over the implant sites were scanned with a radioactivity detector-scanner for precise localization of the implants. Subsequently, the radioactivity was measured with a counter for thyroid-function analysis.

Femora were retrieved after the animals were killed. Bone segments were processed for histology and microradiography.

RESULTS

Figure 1 is a typical roentgenogram showing the position of a ceramic implant in a femur immediately after surgery. Healing occurred uneventful. No adverse tissue reactions could be observed.

Figure 2 shows the relative surface areas of bone and ceramic mass of hydroxyapatite implants in histologic sections. Apposition of bone in the pores became evident after 20 weeks and reached a maximum level after 35 weeks. No significant change in bone mass occurred afterward. Figure 3 is a microradiogram of a 184-week-old hydroxyapatite implant. It illustrates that the implant remained intact. New bone enveloped the implant, while the original medullary cavity seems to extend into the implant pores.

In contrast, Figure 4 shows a microradiogram of a 50-week-old tricalcium orthophosphate implant, where extensive resorption of the implant occurred.

Figure 5 shows the results of radioactivity measurements over the implant sites. The radioactivity of the hydroxyapatite implants did not change, while the radioactivity of the tricalcium orthophosphate implants showed a gradual decrease of 25%-30% in 22 weeks.

Figure 6 illustrates that contact between hydroxyapatite and newly formed bone at the surface of the implant pores is extensive. Osteoblasts can be seen lining the surface of the pores and depositing seams of osteoid directly against the hydroxyapatite surface (Fig. 7). Figure 8 shows that contact

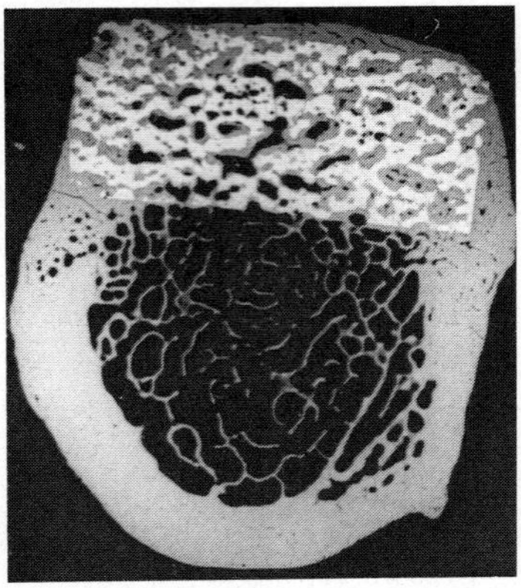 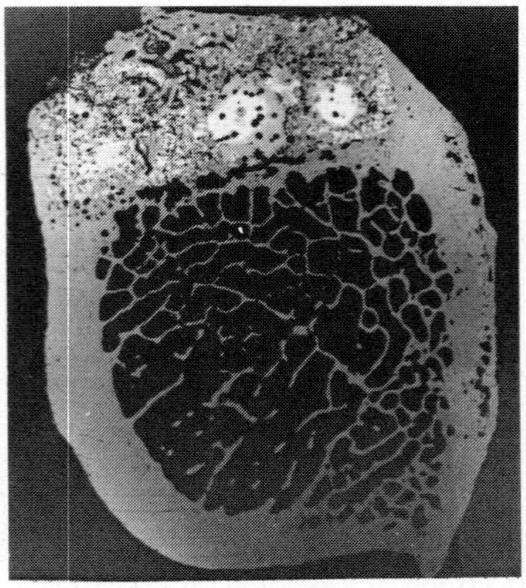

Fig. 3. Microradiogram of bone and hydroxyapatite implant at 184 weeks.
Fig. 4. Microradiogram of bone and tricalcium orthophosphate implant at 50 weeks.

between bone and tricalcium orthophosphate ceramic is made over short distances only.

Bioresorption of tricalcium orthophosphate implants occurs, at least partly, via a cell-mediated process. Figure 9 shows mononuclear phagocytes loaded with debris from tricalcium orthophosphate ceramic inside the cell interior.

DISCUSSION

The results clearly demonstrate that hydroxyapatite implants are not affected by bioresorption processes. In Figure 7 osteoblasts are lining the ceramic surface suggesting that these cells do not discriminate between mineralized bone and a synthetic-hydroxyapatite surface. However, the implants

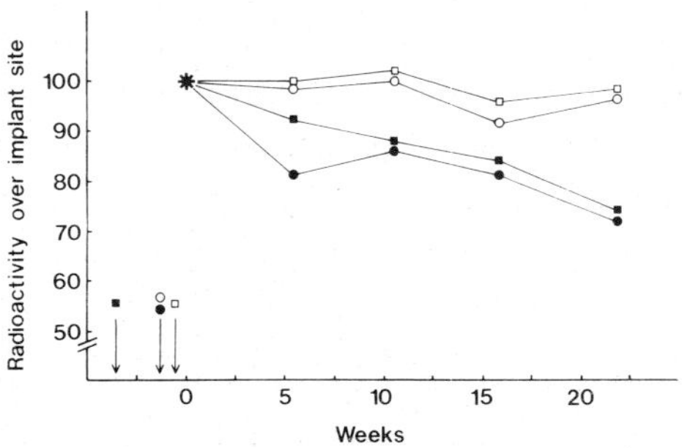

Fig. 5. Radioactivity measured over the implant sites. The radioactivity, corrected for physical decay, is expressed as percentage of the radioactivity at time zero. The vertical arrows indicate the time between implantation date and zero-time for radioactivity measurements. ○,□ -^{85}Sr-labeled hydroxyapatite; ●,■ -^{85}Sr-labeled tricalcium orthophosphate.

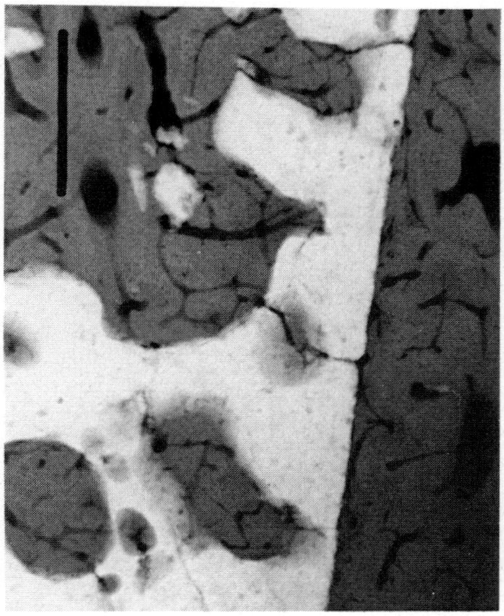

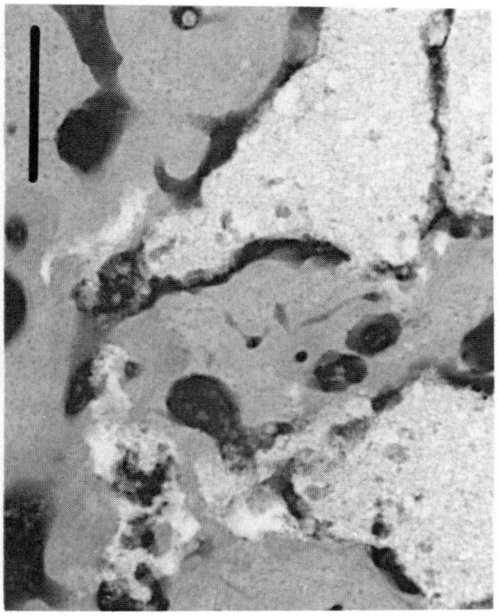

Fig. 6. Microradiogram of a hydroxyapatite implant. Scale = 0.5 mm.
Fig. 8. Microradiogram of a tricalcium orthophosphate implant. Scale = 0.5 mm.

serve only as a scaffold for bone growth without inducing osteogenesis, because defects that were left open were practically healed within 16 weeks, when bone growth into the implant pores had only just started (see Fig. 2).

Tricalcium orthophosphate implants are subject to extensive bioresorption during which process the implants are replaced by newly formed bone. This would make the material ideally suited for temporary bridging of a bone defect.

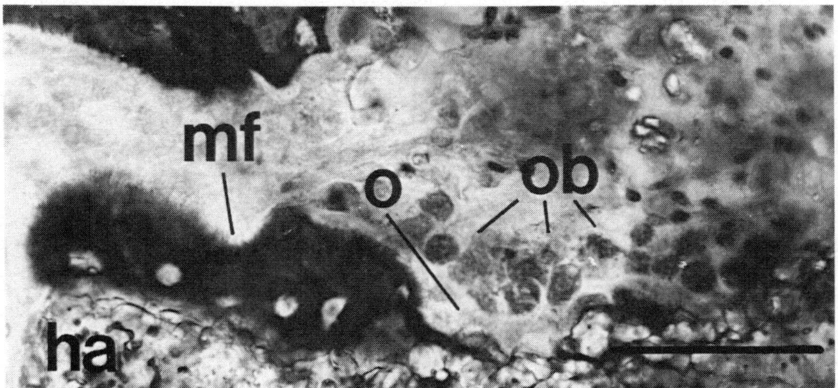

Fig. 7. Histology of a 21-week-old hydroxyapatite implant. ha = hydroxyapatite implant; ob = osteoblasts; o = osteoid; mf = mineralization front. Scale = 50 μm.

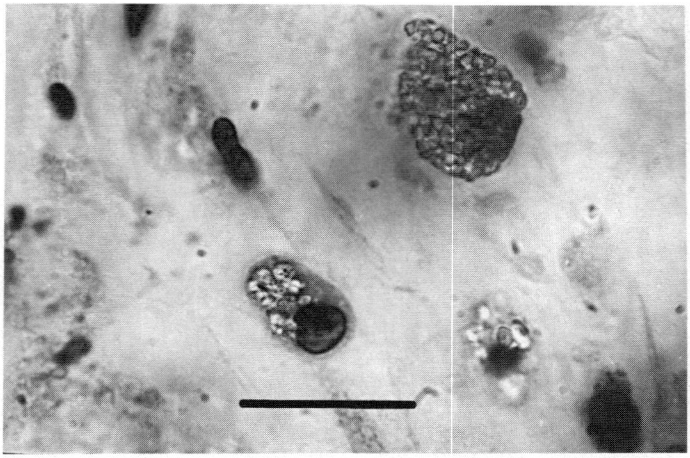

Fig. 9. Mononuclear phagocytes carrying ceramic debris from a tricalcium orthophosphate implant in their cytoplasm. Scale = 20 μm.

Figure 5 illustrates that the extent of resorption can be adequately quantitated in vivo by labeling the implants with strontium-85 analogs of the calcium phosphate compounds, which might provide a valid improvement in the methodology of implantation research.

REFERENCES

1 M. Jarcho, Calcium phosphate ceramics as hard tissue prosthetics, Clin. Orthop., 157 (1981) 259-278.
2 C.P.A.T. Klein, A.A. Driessen, K. de Groot and A. van den Hooff, Biodegradation behaviour of various calcium phosphate materials in bone tissue, J. Biomed. Mater. Res., 17 (1982) 769-784.
3 J.G.J. Peelen, B.V. Rejda, J.P.W. Vermeiden and K. de Groot, Sintered tricalcium phosphate as bioceramic, Sci. Ceramics, 9 (1977) 226-236.
4 B.V. Rejda, J.G.J. Peelen and K. de Groot, Tri-calcium phosphate as a bone substitute, J. Bioeng., 1 (1977) 93-97.
5 H.A. Hoogendoorn, W. Renooij, L.M.A. Akkermans, W.J. Visser and P. Wittebol, Long-term study of large ceramic implants (porous hydroxyapatite) in dog femora, Clin. Orthop., 187 (1984) 281-288.
6 W. Renooij, H.A. Hoogendoorn, W.J. Visser, R.H.F. Lentferink, M.G.J. Schmitz, H. van Ieperen, S.J. Oldenburg, W.M. Janssen, L.M.A. Akkermans and P. Wittebol, Bioresorption of ceramic strontium-85-labeled calcium phosphate implants in dog femora. A pilot study to quantitate bioresorption of ceramic implants of hydroxyapatite and tricalcium orthophosphate in vivo, Clin. Orthop., 197 (1985) 272-285.

Acknowledgement

The Figures 1-3, 7-9 are reproduced with permission of CLINICAL ORTHOPAEDICS AND RELATED RESEARCH.

Biomaterials and Clinical Applications,
edited by A. Pizzoferrato, P.G. Marchetti, A. Ravaglioli and A.J.C. Lee
Elsevier Science Publishers B.V., Amsterdam, 1987 — Printed in The Netherlands

MORPHOLOGICAL STUDIES ON TITANIUM IMPLANTS INSERTED IN RABBIT KNEE-JOINTS

P. Thomsen, A.S. Eriksson, R. Olsson, L.M. Bjursten, P.-I. Brånemark and L.E. Ericson

Department of Anatomy, University of Göteborg, P.O. Box 33031, S-400 33 Gothenburg (Sweden)

SUMMARY

Long-term clinical studies with jaw-bone anchored threaded titanium fixtures indicate that titanium could be used also for reconstructive joint surgery. In the present experimental study the subchondral bone, cartilage and synovial tissue adjacent to non-alloyed titanium screws were morphologically evaluated 2, 4 and 6 weeks after insertion in rabbit knee-joints. A transient inflammatory reaction, due to the surgical trauma, was present. The amount of bone within the screw threads increased with time and a direct contact, without an intervening fibrous tissue layer, between the surface of the implant and surrounding bone was evident. Depending on implant insertion site, articular cartilage or synovial tissue regenerated and covered the titanium screw.

Observations in this study, together with recent findings in studies of titanium implants in soft tissues, indicate that titanium provides an inert surface supporting the proliferation and differentiation of tissues in vivo. This study indicates that non-alloyed titanium implants can be used for several purposes in the joint.

INTRODUCTION

A prerequisite for a successful joint reconstruction with prostheses is a firm anchorage with good load-bearing capacity. In the jaw-bone a direct contact is established between screws of pure titanium and bone, without an intervening soft tissue layer (ref. 1). This indicates that non-alloyed titanium might be used also for the purpose of reconstructive joint surgery. In order to further develop the use of titanium in different clinical situations much more has to be learnt about tissue reactions around implants inserted in or close to joints.

Using experimentally inserted implants, as well as implants from patients, we are currently studying the interaction between implant and surrounding soft and hard tissues. In this first study in a series of experiments focussing on the healing-in of titanium in normal and arthritic knee-joints of the rabbit we now report that non-alloyed titanium implants heal in normal joints with a direct contact between the fixture and bone and that cartilage and synovial tissue regenerate and cover the fixture.

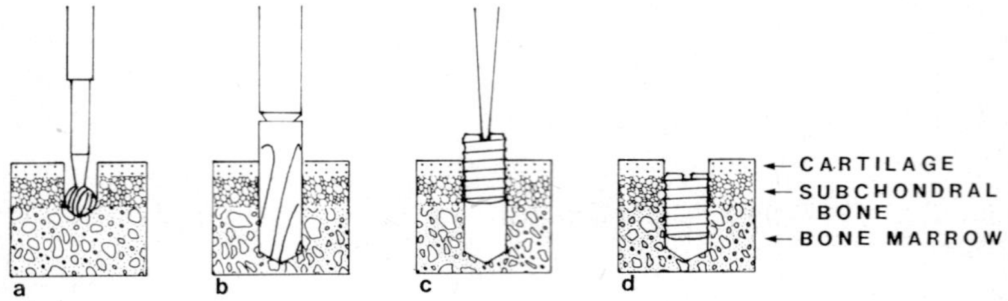

Fig. 1. Schematic presentation of the implantation procedure. a. Spherical drill. b. Cylindrical drill. c. Insertion of screw. d. Final position of screw with upper surface at the bone-cartilage junction.

MATERIAL AND METHODS

Titanium implants

Surgery was performed under sterile conditions using a dissecting microscope. After skin incision and opening of fascia layers the joint capsule was opened. The titanium screws were inserted through the cartilage in the femoro-patellar groove or through the synovial tissue on the medial femoral condyle in altogether 30 knee-joints.

The hole through the cartilage and bone into the bone marrow was drilled under cold saline irrigation using a dentist drill at low speed. The screws inserted through the cartilage had their upper surface at the bone-cartilage junction (Fig. 1).

The joint cavity was washed with saline before the joint capsule and skin was closed by sutures. The rabbits were allowed free motion postoperatively.

Two, 4 and 6 weeks after surgery the animals were sacrificed by an overdose of pentobarbital i.v. and the joints opened and examined.

Specimen processing and evaluation

The titanium screw and surrounding tissue were excised under profuse saline irrigation using a dental drill with a diamond saw blade. The specimens were fixed in 3% glutaraldehyde in 0.1 M sodium cacodylate (pH 7.4). After fixation the specimens were divided along the axis of the screw and the tissue was demineralized for ten days in 10% EDTA. After careful removal from the screw the tissue was postfixed in 2% osmium tetroxide, dehydrated in alcohol and embedded in epoxy resin. One μm thick sections for light microscopy were stained with 0.5% Azur 11 and 0.5% methylene blue in 0.1% disodium tetraborate. In addition synovial tissue biopsies were obtained from all joints. They were fixed in 3% glutaraldehyde in 0.1 M sodium cacodylate, postfixed, dehydrated and embedded essentially as described above.

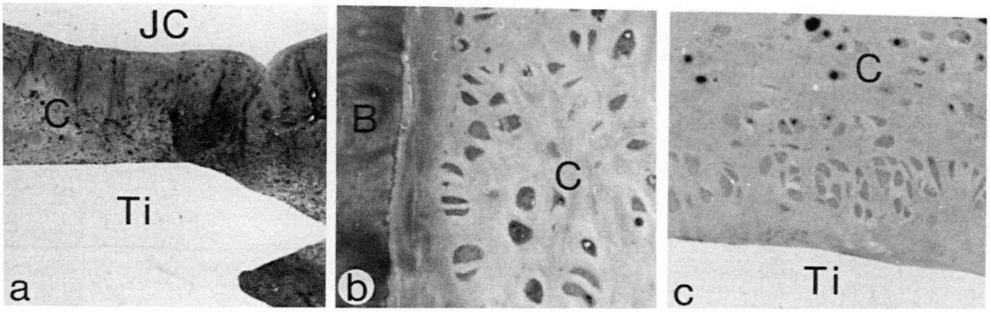

Fig. 2. Micrographs of newly formed cartilage tissue covering intraarticular titanium screw. a. Survey. b. Clustered chondrocytes close to bone-cartilage junction. c. Clustered chondrocytes close to the titanium surface. B = bone; C = cartilage; JC = joint cavity; Ti = (removed) titanium screw.

RESULTS

Morphology of tissue close to titanium implants inserted through cartilage

In rabbits sacrificed 2 weeks after surgery, macroscopic observations showed that the titanium screws were covered by a whitish tissue which partly filled the hole in the cartilage. After 4 and 6 weeks the whitish repair tissue had filled the entire hole. No hyperemia, bleeding or increased capsule thickness were detected at any observation time.

The repair tissue which covered the screws had a morphology similar to the surrounding hyaline cartilage (Fig. 2a). The chondrocytes were often distributed in clusters, most notably at the border between cartilage and bone (Fig. 2b) and close to the titanium surface (Fig. 2c).

Light microscopy of the bone close to the implant surface at 2 weeks revealed a pronounced bone-forming and bone-resorptive activity. Macrophages and osteoclasts were located on the surface of old bone and also surrounded displaced fragments of old bone present between the threads. A striking feature at 2 weeks was the finding of newly formed bone between the threads mainly present at the implant surface and with the largest amounts detected in the inner corner between the threads (Fig. 3). Four and 6 weeks after surgery signs of inflammation or bone resorption were rare. The amount of newly formed bone between the threads had increased (Fig. 4). At these time intervals a layer of newly formed bone covered the distal threads and the distal surface of the screw which protruded into the bone marrow cavity.

Morphology of tissue close to titanium implants inserted through synovial tissue

A direct contact was observed between bone and implant surface, similar to that observed when implants were inserted through the cartilage. The defect

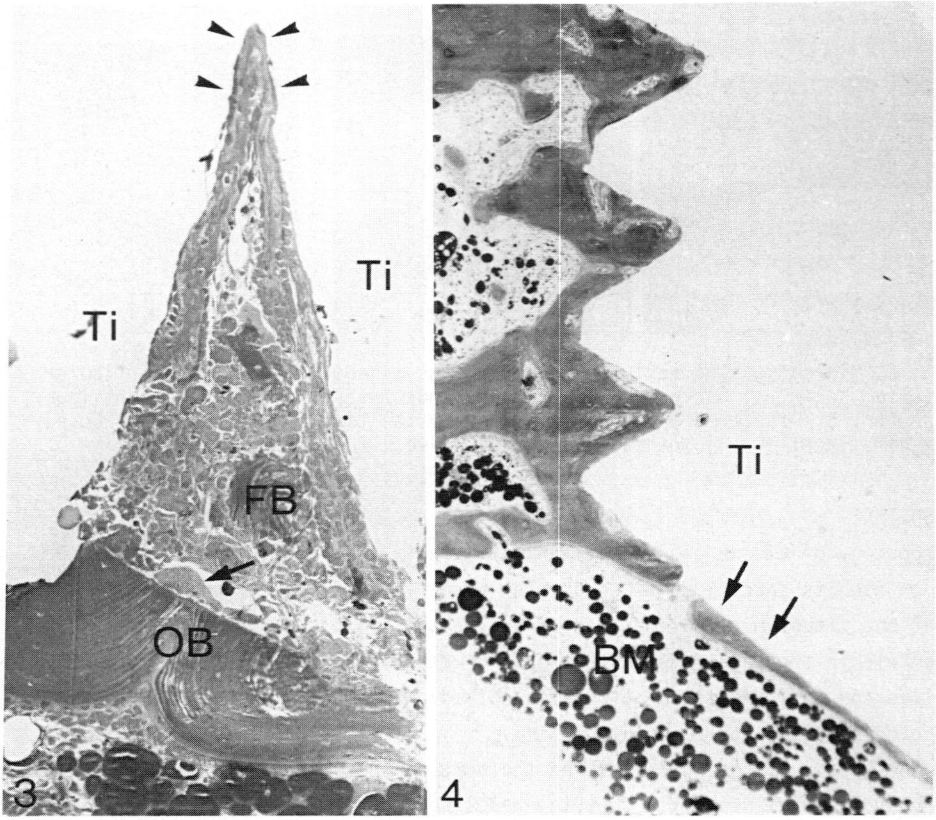

Fig. 3. Tissue between threads 2 weeks after implantation. Newly formed bone (arrow-heads) is located at the titanium surface in the inner corner between the threads. FB = fragment of old bone; OB = old bone. Arrow = osteoclast at the surface of old bone. Ti = (removed) titanium screw.

Fig. 4. Four weeks after implantation. The space between the threads is filled with newly formed bone. Bone (arrows) also covers the distal end of the screw projecting into the bone-marrow (BM). Ti = (removed) titanium screw.

in the synovial membrane was filled by connective tissue and covered by a normal synovial lining layer.

Morphology of synovial tissue

Biopsies obtained at the time of sacrifice were examined with respect to possible inflammatory changes induced by the presence of the intra-articular implant. No adverse effects were found in any of the biopsies examined.

DISCUSSION

The present study shows that intra-articularly inserted titanium implants become anchored in the subchondral bone without any intervening fibrous tissue. This important finding was evident regardless of access route to the bone, via drilling through the cartilage or the synovial tissue.

Formation of new bone was observed at 2 weeks. At this time an inflammatory response, with resorption of old bone by phagocytic cells was evident. This inflammation was probably due to the injury caused by the implant insertion and was not caused by the implant per se. This conclusion is supported by the finding that phagocytic cells were preferentially located at injured bone tissue and not at the surface of the implant and also by the transient nature of the inflammatory reaction. Furthermore, recent experimental studies in soft tissues showing a rapid disappearance of the initial inflammation close to titanium implants (ref. 2) support this conclusion. Taken together, these experimental studies indicate the importance of the early material surface-cell interaction for the interfacial tissue composition and long-term fate of an implant.

Although this study mainly concerned the qualitative morphological changes it was found that the amount of newly formed bone between the threads increased with time. Our preliminary observations indicate that the amount of newly formed bone between the threads can be quantified by morphometry. Thus, a quantitative comparison of the bone tissue response to e.g. different types of implant materials can be made using this implant design and surgical procedure.

Non-alloyed titanium might serve as a supporting surface of "substrate surface" for the proliferation of bone cells. This is supported by the following findings (1) osteoblasts were located at the implant surface, (2) initially new bone formation was most evident in the inner corner between the threads and (3) newly formed bone appeared also on the distal part of the implant projecting into the bone marrow cavity.

The capacity to repair defects in cartilage is controversial (ref. 3). In the present study the upper surface of the screw was covered by cartilage. Although further studies are needed to establish the role played by titanium for the proliferation of cartilage our findings suggest that titanium can serve as a supporting surface for the formation of new cartilage, replacing the subchondral plate otherwise considered to be required for the healing of an articular cartilage defect.

The present study in the rabbit knee-joint shows that

1) no inflammation is observed in the synovial tissue of joints with implanted titanium screws,
2) new synovial tissue is rapidly formed over titanium implants inserted in non-cartilaginous areas,

3) intra-articularly inserted titanium screws become integrated in subchondral bone, and
4) cartilage has the capacity to regenerate on the upper surface of titanium screws integrated in subchondral bone.

REFERENCES

1 R. Adell, U. Lekholm. B. Rockler and P.-I. Brånemark, A 15 year study of osseointegrated implants in the treatment of the edentulous jaw. Int. J. Oral Surg. 10 (1981) 387-416.
2. P. Thomsen, L.M. Bjursten and L.E. Ericson, Implants in the abdominal wall. Scand. J. Plast. Reconstr. Surg. In press (1986).
3. E.L. Radin and D.B. Burr, Hypothesis: Joints can heal. Seminars in Arthritis and Rheumatism, 13, 3 (1984) 293-302.

This study was supported by grants from Swedish National Association against Rheumatism; Gothenburg Medical Society; King Gustav V 80-years Fund; Medical Faculty, University of Göteborg.

Biomaterials and Clinical Applications,
edited by A. Pizzoferrato, P.G. Marchetti, A. Ravaglioli and A.J.C. Lee
Elsevier Science Publishers B.V., Amsterdam, 1987 — Printed in The Netherlands

CERAMICS IN DENTAL IMPLANTOLOGY

G. HEIMKE[1], B. D'HOEDT[2], and W. SCHULTE[2]

[1]Friedrichsfeld GmbH, Steinzeugstr. 50, 6800 Mannheim 71 (Germany)

[2]Zentrum für ZMK und Sonderforschungsbereich "Implantologie", Universität Tübingen, Osianderstr. 2 - 8, 7400 Tübingen (Germany)

ABSTRACT

Ceramics suitable for medical applications can be subdivided into two groups for which the terms "bioinert" and "bioactive" have been coined. The main representative of the bioinert materials is the dense, pure Al_2O_3-ceramic. The term bioactive has been used to describe a particular type of interface reaction of bony tissue along some Ca-phosphate ceramics and Ca-phosphate containing glasses and glass ceramics.

It was found that the bioinert ceramics allow for an interface remodelling as in fracture healing if the same precautions of relative rest along the interface are taken. This remodelling is mainly controlled by the stress and strain field created by the insertion of the implant. Thus, correctly designed implants can become and remain well osseo-integrated under full load application. More than ten years of clinical experience have fully confirmed this concept in different fields of surgery. For dental implants this motionless fixation also avoids any mechanical irritation of the gingiva/implant interface. The reactive materials have been shown to allow for an adhesion of bony tissue in the sense of a glueing effect. All attempts to use this ability for the fixation of really loaded implants failed because of the severe fatigue these materials suffer in body environment.

INTRODUCTION

In material science the term "ceramics" comprises all none metallic, inorganic materials. From this large group of materials some have been found to have a combination of properties from which improvements of implants could be expected. Amongst these "bioceramics" two subgroups can be distinguished: the "bioinert ceramics" do not influence the surrounding tissue biochemically, the so-called reactive or "bioactive ceramics" have the fascinating ability to stimulate a deposition of calcified tissue along their surface if inserted in a bony environment, resulting in a strong adhesion between the implant and the living tissue.

MATERIALS

Bioinert ceramics

The main representative of the bioinert ceramics is the dense, high purity Al_2O_3-ceramic. Its use as an implant material was commenced in 1964 (ref. 1) and some of its modifications were studied experimentally in the late sixties (ref. 2). In the early seventies the dense, more pure versions were tested in cell cultures (ref. 3), in rodents under nearly load free conditions (ref. 4) and as fully loaded hip replacements in sheep and dogs (ref. 5, 6, 7). From one series of these experiments (ref. 8, 9,) and experiments with dental implants the following conclusions could be drawn:

1. The dense, high purity Al_2O_3-ceramic does not influence the adjacent tissue biochemically (ref. 3, 4).
2. This material does not stimulate immune reactions (ref. 4, 10).
3. No material induced sarcomas could be detected (ref. 11).
4. The remodelling processes of bony tissue adjacent to an Al_2O_3-ceramic implant are the same as in fracture healing if the same precautions of relative rest along the interface are observed (ref. 8, 12).
5. This direct contact of well proliferating bony tissue can be maintained during functional loading at all those interfaces along which relative movements can be excluded (ref. 12).
6. A sufficiently dense arrangement of surface undulations can prevent relative movements even along tangentially loaded interfaces by interlocking (ref. 13, 14).

The correlations between the biomechanically controlled tissue reaction and the shape of an implant of a bioinert material are summarized schematically in Fig. 1.

Besides the Al_2O_3-ceramic some modifications of carbon (ref. 15) had been shown to reach the same level of biocompatibility and had, therefore, also been considered for dental implants. More recently, some ZrO_2-, Si_3N_4-, and SiC-ceramics have been tested biologically (ref. 16, 17). The results are not yet completely conclusive.

Bioactive ceramics

The strong adhesion of a calcium and phosphate containing SiO_2 based glass-ceramic to bony tissue was first observed in the late sixties (ref. 18). The details of this "glueing" effect, its dependence on the degree of devitrification and on composition has been studied in many details since (ref. 19, 20).

A similar adhesion to bony tissue was found for some calcium and phosphate containing ceramics in the early seventies (ref. 21). The influences of the chemical and phase composition, crystal structure, and ceramic processing on the tissue responses have been evaluated by several groups (ref. 22, 23, 24). Dense hydroxylapatite ceramics (HA) were found to be relatively stable in body environment, for porous tricalciumphosphate ceramics (TCP) different resorption rates had been described (ref. 25).

The results obtained by all these efforts for these two kinds of bioactive materials can be summarized in a few sentences:

1. The static (initial) mechanical strength remains low (for practical applications not more than about 100 N/mm^2 or one quarter of the strength required for Al_2O_3-ceramics according to international standards (ref. 26)).
2. In body environment the mechanical strength is further reduced considerably by fatigue.
3. The adhesion of dense HA to bony tissue can withstand several years of funtional loading by shear forces (ref. 27).

Therefore, at present, uses of these materials are confined to mainly none load bearing applications. The research efforts are concentrated on reinforcing these materials. Attempts to solve this problem for dense HA by prestressing have not been successful (ref. 28). The probability of success of this prestressing concept or of coating hydroxylapatite on metal substrates mainly depends on the kind of the fatigue process. If the disintegration of the grain boundaries (ref. 29) turns out to be an inherent material property of this kind of ceramic and is not caused by contaminations accumulated along the grain boundaries, the ability of such coatings to withstand functional loading for long periods of time appears doubtful.

CLINICAL APPLICATIONS

From all ceramic materials mentioned above Al_2O_3-ceramics only have found large scale applications for load bearing dental implants. Carbon and the bioactive ceramics are presently not or no longer used for directly supporting superstructures. The reasons, of course, are mechanical problems as mentioned above previously. The bioactive materials are mainly used for defect fillings or alveolar ridge augmentation or some segmental replacements or corrections in maxillo facial surgery in which the implants are, if at all, mainly pressure loaded.

Dental implants

The implant systems using Al_2O_3 ceramics are mainly based on two widely different design principles. One group more or less duplicate implant shapes which had been used previously with metals, the basic features of which are expressed in Fig. 1a, left side. In a smaller group the implants had been designed to strictly account for the remodelling ability of the bony tissue under the influence of the stress and strain distribution created by the implant in the surrounding bone. These implants can, therefore, result in a direct bony anchorage as shown

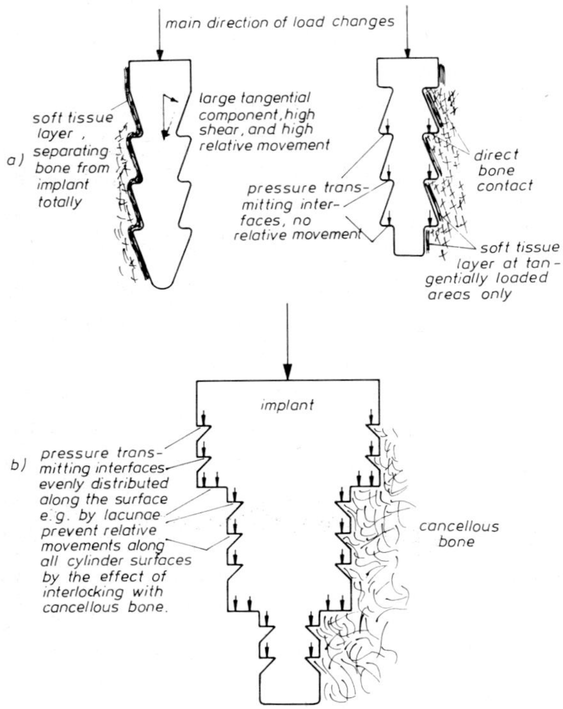

Fig. 1. The influence of the shape of the implant on the kind of interfacial load transfer and on the remodelling of the surrounding bony tissue. (a) Stepped (and screw shaped) design: left: no interfaces with perpendicular load transfer (forces perpendicular to interface = pressure), soft tissue interlayers along all tangentially loaded surfaces (shear forces); right: stepped (or screw) design with pressure transmitting interfaces along which direct bone contact can be maintained. (b) Correctly oriented surface undulations like lacunae result in an interlocking with the ingrown cancellous bone preventing relative movements even along surfaces oriented tangentially to the forces.

schematically in Fig. 1b. For such a direct bony fixation the term osseo-integration was coined. The idea to try to achieve this osseo-integration resulted from the well established correlation between the thickness of a soft tissue interlayer, the degree of implant mobility, and implant failures (ref. 30).

The Al_2O_3-ceramic implants of the first group are either screw type implants with cross sections of the threads mainly following the shape shown in Fig. 1a, left side (ref. 31, 32, 33) or they duplicate more or less directly previous metal blade implants (ref. 33, 34, 35). These two design groups do not offer sufficiently large pressure transmitting interfaces. Most of these implants are, therefore, encapsulated by a soft tissue interlayer which, on its outer side, is separated from the cancellous bone by some kind of a lamella of cortical bone. There is no follow-up study available for these systems which would come close to the requirements of the Havard Consensus Conference of 1978.

Transdental fixation pins of Al_2O_3-ceramics or corundum single crystals have been in clinical application since the late seventies (ref. 36). As these pins are rigidly cemented into the remainder of the teeth which are still suspended in their desmodontal ligaments the apical portions of these pins maintain some freedom of movement in the surrounding bone. They are, therefore, soft tissue encapsulated (ref. 36).

Dental implant systems of Al_2O_3-ceramic of the second group closely following the ideas expressed in Fig. 1a, right side, had been tested clinically around the mid seventies, but did not reach large scale applications (ref. 37, 38).

The design features necessary for the full osseo-integration of a dental implant as expressed in Fig. 1b have been realised with the FRIALIT Tübingen dental implant (ref. 39)(Fig. 2). The implant body includes a circular groove into which the marginal gingival border and its internal epithelial seam can be placed. In order to account for the requirements of fracture healing an unloading period of three months was observed.

Up to 3 years animal studies were performed in dogs. Histologically, normally proliferating and well load bearing bony tissue along nearly all interfaces could be demonstrated (Fig. 3) (ref. 40).

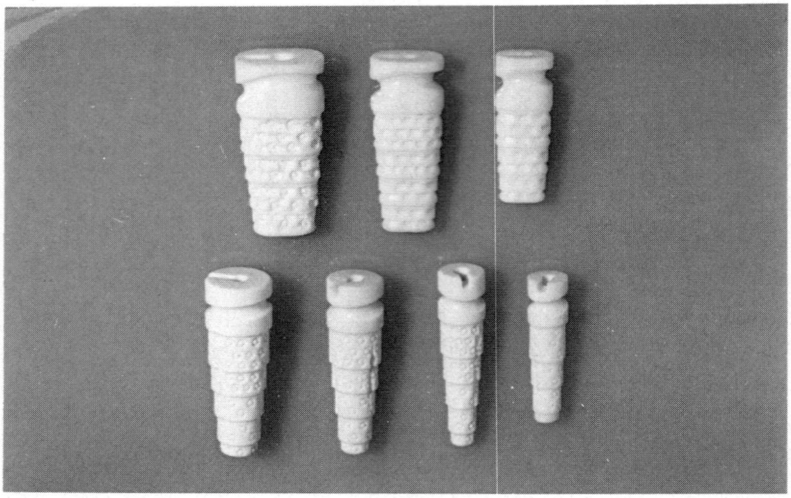

Fig. 2. The Tübingen implants made of FRIALIT Al_2O_3-ceramic. There are four round implants with diameters of 4, 5, 6, and 7 mm and three oval ones with short axis of cross section of 4, 5, and 6 mm.

Histology of bony tissue adhering to parts of human implants which became available after an implant fracture due to trauma completely confirmed the results of animal experiments (ref. 41). However, none invasive methods were developed to test the state of bony contact clinically. By measuring the intrusion paths of implants and natural teeth a sinking-in difference could be detected. Whilst natural teeth sink into their alveola by about 0,1 mm under a load of 10 to 20 N due to the deformation of the desmodontal ligament, the implants of this kind do not move for more than 8 to 10 μm, a movement completely controlled by the elastic properties of the cancellous bone (ref. 42). A similar result was obtained by measuring the recoil movement of teeth and implants (ref. 43). In daily clinical routine the frequency level of the percussation sound allows to distinction between osseo-integration and soft tissue encapsulation.

These studies were supplemented by measurements about the integration of the implants into the neurophysiological feedback system (ref. 44). It was found that the sensitivity thresholds are greater by the factor of 10 for implants than for natural teeth until one year after insertion. After that time this threshold decreases slowly until after 3 to 4 years it approaches the values for natural teeth. Thus, implants are at risk to traumatic or parafunctional stresses in particular during the first year after implantation.

Parameters describing the state of the gingival attachment like the pocket depth, bleeding index, and the sulcus fluid flow rate were also determined and recorded (ref. 40).

The patients who received FRIALIT implants in the Tübingen clinic have been kept in a strict recall system. All data are computerised. Fig. 4 is a black and white reproduction of the survival board containing all implants. Nearly all of the implants inserted during the first year (1975/76) are still functioning well. In the second year some variations of implant shape, surface properties and of the unloading (healing-in) period had been tested clinically. After a high failure rate became evident, the clinic returned to the original design and procedure. This original technique was subsequently called "standard treatment". Most of the problems observed in the next years could be traced back to their origins and, thus, be used to further improve the standard treatment. The results of this learning process can be seen in Table 1:

TABLE 1
Summary of the 10 years' follow-up evaluation of all FRIALIT Tübingen implants inserted according to the standard treatment.

all standard treatments 1975 - 1985			treatments commenced after reaching final routine 1982 - 1985	
	610	total number of treatments commenced	352	
	18	disappeared in follow-up	5	
(100 %)	592	treatments remaining in follow-up	347	(100 %)
(15,5 %)	92	failed treatments	26	(7,5 %)
	14	attempts of reimplantation contained in these failures	5	
(84,5 %)	500	successful treatments	321	(92,5 %)
	28	reimplantations contained in the successful treatments	10	

The term "treatment" is used to describe any commenced implantation procedure according to the standards mentioned above, eventually including reimplantation.

The comparison of the two different follow-up periods (10 years in the left and 3 years in the right column) is justified by the fact that implant losses of this system are confined nearly completely to the healing-in and early loading period, so, at any rate to the

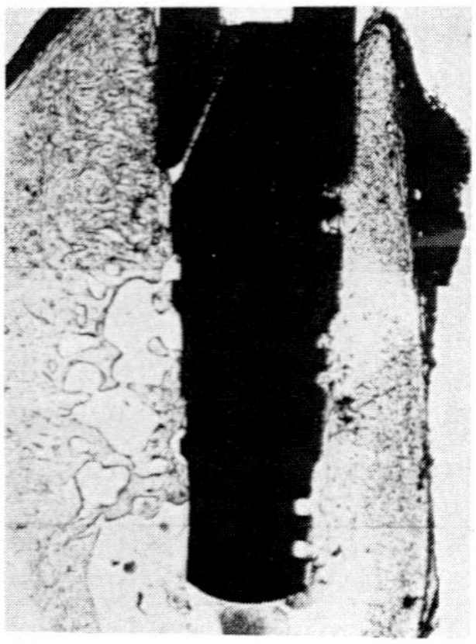

Fig. 3. Histological section of Tübingen implant after 2 years in a beagle dog.

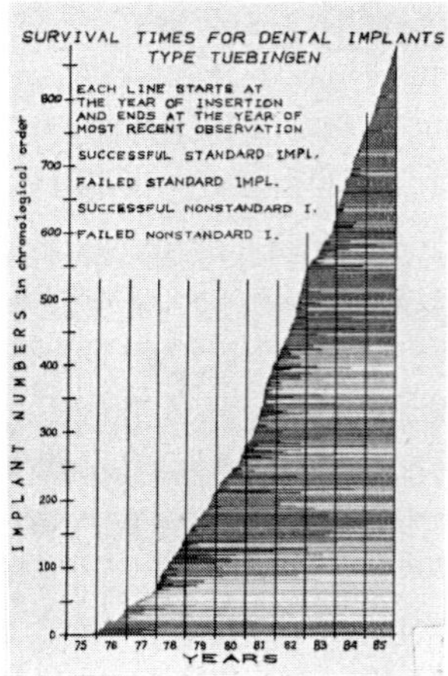

Fig. 4. Survival board of all FRIALIT implants inserted in the Tübingen clinic from 1975-1985.

first year. This had already been shown in the 5 years statistical evaluation (ref. 41) and is clearly confirmed by the 10 years' statistic. From our more detailed evaluations (ref. 41, 45) of all the data including those treatments which deviated from the standard, the following additional results are worth mentioning:

1. The success rate does not depend on the location of the implant.
2. The success rate is reduced considerably for any deviation from the standard procedure, in particular if no initial press-fit can be achieved or the implants are loaded before 3 months p.o.
3. The sulcus fluid flow rates are identical with those measured for teeth of the same patients, and they are constant over time as are the pocket depths.
4. There are indications of a markedly reduced plaque adhesion to Al_2O_3-ceramic as compared to metal implants or teeth.
5. The observations indicate that the shape of the alveola ridge is maintained around these implants as around natural teeth.

In this abbreviated version of the statistical evaluation the only criteria of failure was the removal of an implant. This simplification. as compared e. g. with rules given by the Harvard Consensus Conference of 1978, is justified by the properties inherent to this implant system: Because of the complete lack of any undercut any osteolysis resulting in considerable degrees of mobilities for other implant systems would immediately result in the extrusion of these implants. Thus, mobilities which are still allowed according to the Consensus Conference standards do not occur at all with the FRIALIT Tübingen implant system.

There is an additional point of view which follows from the data given in Table 1. The loss of an implant with extended undercuts also always involves severe bone destruction. In contrast to this situtation 18 and 10 treatments could be carried on successfully by supplying the implant bed with another implant. This is another indication for the absence of bone distruction in the failure cases. It also clearly demonstrates that the simple comparison of implant losses does not fully express the advantages of undercut free implants.

If implants are inserted in the front area, cosmetic problems must be considered. Here implants with diameters coming close to those of the natural teeth and which allow for a shaping using normal grinding procedures are of considerable advantage.

The results reported here clearly indicate the advantages of the direct fixation of implants in the bony tissue without soft tissue interlayers and confirm the validity of the design principles from which they had been derived. The considerable improvement of the success rate due to the learning effect as shown in Table 1 also demonstrates the necessity of a thorough and careful clinical follow-up study before any new or modified implant system should be made available to the general practitioner.

<u>Cavity fillings and augmentations</u>

The clinical applications of the bioactive ceramics have mainly remained confined to cavity fillings and augmentations. For cavity fillings TCP- and HA-ceramics are used, mostly in the shape of granules with diameters between 0,1 to several millimeters. More or less dense granules of HA have found large scale application in alveolar ridge augmentations and fillings of periodontal pockets (ref. 46).

In these augmentations and pocket fillings the implant material is in contact with bony tissue along a small fraction of its surface only. As the formation of bony tissue along these materials needs a close contact to well proliferating bony tissue, and because this bone formation is a slower process than the invasion of soft tissue, the granules of these fillings are mostly embedded into a granulation tissue. The follow-up studies on such treatments indicate that a sufficient gain in the height of the ridge remains and is maintained for the time of these studies (ref. 47).

FINAL REMARK

During the last decade ceramics have made considerable contributions to dentistry which can be looked at from different points of view:

1. Because of the availability of a really bioinert material, the reactions of bony tissue to new stress and strain fields, created by the insertion of implants, could be studied with the strict exclusion of biochemical influences.
2. Other basic problems could be dealt with, like the neurophsiological response and the maintenance of the alveolar ridge after the insertion of adequately designed implants.
3. The results of the follow-up studies on the FRIALIT Tübingen implant system and on the alveolar ridge augmentations with HA ceramic document the creation of new, reliable possibilities for dental rehabilitation.

REFERENCES

1 S. Sandhaus, Bone implants and drills and tapes for bone surgery, British Patent 1083769, 1967.

2 S.F. Hulbert, F.A. Young, R.S. Mathews, J.J. Klawitter, C.D. Talbert and F.H. Stelling, Potential of ceramic materials as permanently implantable skeletal prostheses, J. Biomed. Mater. Res., (4) (1970) 433-456.

3 G. Heimke, P. Griss, G. Jentschura, B. Krempien, E. Gugel, I. Petzenhauser, H.W. Hennicke, Keramische und keramikbeschichtete Knochenersatzwerkstoffe, Forschungsberichte des Bundesministers für Forschung und Technlogie, BMFT-FBT 77 - 70, 1977.

4 P. Griss, H. von Andrian-Werburg, B. Krempien, G. Heimke, Biological activity and histocompatibility of dense Al_2O_3/MgO ceramic implants in rats. J. Biomed. Mat. Res. Symposium, (4) (1973) 453-462.

5 R.L. Hentrich, G.A. Graves, H.G. Stein and P.K. Baipai, An evaluation of inert and resorbable ceramics for future clinical orthopaedic applications. J. Biomed. Mat. Res., (5) (1971) 25.

6 P. Griss, B. Krempien, H. von Andrian-Werburg, G. Heimke, R. Fleiner, Th. Diehm, Experimental analysis of ceramic tissue interactions: a morphologic, fluorescense-optic, and radiographic study of dense alumina oxide ceramic in various animals, J. Biomed. Mater. Res. Symposium, (5) (1974) 39-48.

7 P. Boutin, Arthroplastie totale de la hanche par prothèse en alumine frittée. Revue de chirurgie orthopédique et réparatrice de l'appareil moteur, Paris, (58) (1972) 229-246.

8 P. Griss, G. Heimke, H. von Andrian-Werburg, B. Krempien, S. Reipa, H.J. Lauterbach and H.J Hartung, Morphological and bio-

biomechanical aspects of Al_2O_3 ceramic joint replacement: experimental results and design considerations for human endoprostheses, J. Biomed. Mater. Res. Symposium, (6) (1975) 177-188.

9 P. Griss, R. Silber, B. Merkle and K. Haehner, Biomechanically induced tissue reactions after Al_2O_3 ceramic hip joint replacement: experimental and early clinical results. J. Biomed. Mater. Res. Symposium, (7) (1976) 519-528.

10 P. Griss, B. Krempien, H. von Andrian-Werburg, G. Heimke and R. Fleiner, Experimentelle Untersuchung zur Gewebeverträglichkeit oxidkeramischer (Al_2O_3) Abriebteilchen., Arch. Orthop. Unfall-Chir., (76) (1973) 270-279.

11 P. Griss, E. Werner, R. Buchinger, C.M. Büsing and G. Heimke, Zur Frage der unspezifischen Sarkomentstehung um Al_2O_3-keramische Implantate. Arch Orthop. Unfall-Chir.,(90) (1977) 29-40.

12 G. Heimke, P. Griss, W. Werner, G. Jentschura, The effects of mechanical factors on bio-compatibility tests, J. Biomed. Engng., (3) (1981) 209-213.

13 C.M. Büsing, G. Heimke, W. Schulte and W. Linn, Gibt es ein Lastschattenphänomen? Biomechanische Aspekte bei Zahnimplantaten aus Al_2O_3-Keramik, Der Pathologe, (1) (1979) 61

14 G. Heimke, W. Schulte, B. d'Hoedt, P. Griss, C.M. Büsing, D. Stock, The influence of fine surface structures on the osseointegration of implants, The International Journal of Artificial Organs, 3(5) (1982) 207-212.

15 J.C. Bokros, V.L. Gott, L.D. a Grange, A.M. Fudali and M.D. Ramos, Heparin sorptivity and blood compatibility of carbon surfaces, J. Biomed. Mater. Res., (4) (1970) 145.

16 R.C. Garvie, C. Urbani, D.R. Kennedy and J.C. McNeuer, Biocompatibility of magnesia partially stabilized zirconia (Mg-PSZ) ceramics, J. Mater. Sci., (19) (1984) 3224-3228.

17 P. Griss, E. Werner and G. Heimke, Alumina ceramic, bioglass, and silicon nitride: a comparitive biocompatibility study, in: G.W. Hastings and D.F. Williams (Eds.), Mechanical Properties of Biomaterials, John Wiley and Sons, New York, 1980, pp. 217-226.

18 L.L. Hench, R.J. Splinter, W.C. Allen and T.K. Greenlee, Bonding mechanisms at the interface of ceramic prosthetic material, J. Biomed. Mater. Res. Symposium, (2)(1971) 117

19 L.L. Hench, R.W. Petty and G. Piotrowski, An investigation of bonding mechanisms at the interface of a Prosthetic Material, Rep. 9, U.S. Army R & D Command, Contract No. DADA 17-70-C-0001, Washington, D. C. 1978.

20 B.A. Blencke, H Brömer and E. Pfeil, Rasterelektronemikroskopische Untersuchungen der Reaktion des Knochens auf glaskeramische Implantate, Z. Orthop. Ihre Grenzgeb.,(112) (1974) 978.

21 T.D. Driskell, C.R. Hassler, V.J. Tennery, I.R. McCoy and W.J. Clarke, Calcium phosphate resorbable ceramics: a potential alternative to bone grafting, J. Dent. Res., (52) (1973), 123

22 K. de Groot, Bioceramics consisting of calcium phosphate salts, Biomaterials, (1) (1980) 47.

23 M. Jarcho, Calcium phosphate as hard tissue prosthetics, Clin. Orthop., (157) (1981) 259.

24 K. Köster, H., Heide and R. König, Resorbierbare Calciumphosphatkeramik im Tierexperiment unter Belastung, Langenbecks Arch. Chir., (343) (1977) 173-181.

25 K. de Groot, Degradable ceramics, in: Biocompatibility of Clinical Implant Materials, D.F. Williams (Ed.), Vol. 1, CRC Press, Boca Raton, Fla., 1981, 199.

26 ISO 6474, DIN 58 835.

27 C. de Putter, K. de Groot, P.A.E. Sillevis Smitt, Implants of Dense Hydroxyapatite in Prosthetic Dentistry, in: A.J. Lee, T. Albrektsson and P.-I. Branemark (Eds.), Clinical Application of Biomaterials, John Wiley & Sons Ltd., 1982, p. 125.
28 C. de Putter, G.L. de Lange and K. de Groot, Permudosal dental implants of dense hydroxylapatite in prosthetic dentistry, paper presented at Symposium "Ceramics in Clinical Applications", Milan, Italy, June 26-28, 1986. To be printed in conference procedures.
29 J.F. Osborn, Implantatwerkstoff Hydroxylapatitkeramik/ Grundlagen und klinische Anwendung, Quintessenz-Verlags GmbH, Berlin, 1985.
30 H. Spiekermann, Clinical and animal experiences with enosseous metal implants, in : G. Heimke (Ed.), Dental Implants, Hanser Verlag, München, 1980, pp. 49-54.
31 S. Sandhaus, Neue Aspekte der Implantologie, Medica Verlag Dr. Walter Schmid, Stuttgart, 1975.
32 H. Kawahara, M. Hirayashi and T. Shikita, Single crystal alumina for dental implants and bone screws, J. Biomed. Mater. Res., (14) (1980) 597-605.
33 E. Brinkmann, Indikation und Anwendung keramischer Implantate aus Aluminiumoxid (Biolox), Swiss Dent, (4) (1983) 23-36.
34 E. Mutschelknauss and E. Dörre, Enossale Stiftimplantate aus Aluminiumoxidkeramik, Zahnärztl. Prax., (29) (1978) 3.
35 H. Kawahara, Cellular responses to implant materials: biological, physical, and chemical factors, International Dental Journal, 33 (4) (1983) 350-375.
36 H. Kirschner, U. Bolz, K.W. Hüttemann and J. Sturm, Autoplastic tooth reimplantation with partial ceramic roots made of Al_2O_3, in: G. Heimke (Ed.), Dental Implants, Hanser Verlag, München, 1980, 55-62.
37 R. Fritz, G. Killius and G. Heimke, Experiences with an Al_2O_3-dental implant in a dental office, in: G. Heimke (Ed.), Dental Implants, Hanser Verlag, München, 1980, 89-95.
38 T.D. Driskell and A.L. Heller, Clinical use of aluminum oxide enosseous oral implants, J. Oral Implantol, (7) (1977) 53-76.
39 W. Schulte and G. Heimke, Das Tübinger Sofortimplantat, Quintess. Zahnärztl., Lit 27 (1976) 5456
40 Issue no. 5 of Dtsch. Zahnärztl. Z. 33 (1978), complete issue.
41 W. Schulte, C.M. Büsing, B. d'Hoedt and G. Heimke, Enosseous implants of aluminum oxide ceramics - A 5-years' study in humans, in: H. Kawahara (Ed.) Proceedings of International Congress of Implantology and Biomaterials in Stomatology, Kyoto, Japan, 1980, pp. 157-167.
42 W. Schulte, The intra-osseous Al_2O_3 (Frialit) Tuebingen Implant. Developmental Status after Eight Years (1 - 3), Quintessence International, (15) (1984) 1-39.
43 F. Scholz, Bewegungsverhalten bei Stoßanregung des Tübinger Implantates im Vergleich zum natürlichen Zahn, Dtsch. Zahn. Z., (36) (1981) 567-570.
44 L. Mühlbradt, J. Meyle, D. Lukas, W. Schulte, Die Tastsensibilität Tübinger Sofortimplantate, Dtsch. Zahnärztl. Z., (35) (1980) 334-338.
45 B. d'Hoedt, 10 Jahre Tübinger Implantat aus Frialit, Z. f. Zahnärztl. Implantologie, 2 (1986) Special Issue July 6-10.
46 J.N. Kent, H.J. Quinn and M. Jarcho, Augmentation of deficient alveolar ridges with nonresorbable hydroxylapatite alone or with autogenous cancellous bone, J. Oral Maxillofac. Surg., (41) (1983) 629-642.
47 H. Dielert, personal communication.

Biomaterials and Clinical Applications,
edited by A. Pizzoferrato, P.G. Marchetti, A. Ravaglioli and A.J.C. Lee
Elsevier Science Publishers B.V., Amsterdam, 1987 — Printed in The Netherlands

EVALUATION OF SUBMERGED BULK AND FIBRE REINFORCED BIOGLASS DENTAL IMPLANTS.

E.SCHEPERS[1], M.DE CLERCQ[2], P.DUCHEYNE[3]

[1]Dept. of Prosthet. Dent., Cath. Univ. Leuven, Belgium
[2]Dept. of Bioeng., Univ. of Pennsylvania, Philadelphia, U.S.A.

SUMMARY

In this study the bone bonding capacity of bulk and fibre reinforced bioglass dental root implants is investigated by microchemical, histological and histomorphometrical analysis. Microchemically, three types of interface can be detected. In the first type a smooth transition of the CaP profile can be seen when the implant-bone interface is scanned. This implies histologically a connection between bone tissue and the bioglass surface. In the second type the sudden interruption of the CaP profile stands for a fibrous tissue encapsulation of the implant. The third type is probably time depending, since it is only seen after 16 months. Here a gradual decrease of the CaP profile can be seen towards the surrounding tissues. This implies a certain degree of calcification of the fibrous tissue at the implant interface. Histomorphometrical analysis shows the influence of detrimental factors such as some material's aspects, some surgical trauma and some biomechanical factors which can impede the osteogenesis.

INTRODUCTION

The clinical success of dental implants seams to be very much related to the interfacial response elicited by the root part of that implant. When this root part shows a direct bone apposition, favourable results can be expected(ref.1,2) When such a direct bone contact can be transformed into an effective bond, those positive results will not decrease.

Bioglass is a material able to bond with bone (ref. 3,6),but due to it's poor mechanical properties it can not be used as a dental implant material. By reinforcing it with ductile stainless steel fibres, a material suitable for load bearing devices is reached (ref. 7,8).

The aim of this study is to evaluate microchemically, histologically and histomorphometrically the interfacial response of those bioglass composite dental root implants.

MATERIALS AND METHODS

Preformed sintered networks of stainless steel fibres are dipped in molten bioglass according to the method described by Ducheyne (ref. 7-9). The dipped samples are ground and polished until the final dimensions are reached. After gassterilization those implants are subgingivally installed in the partial edentulous jaws of 4 Beagle dogs. At least one year prior to the implantation the premolars of the dogs were extracted. After 4 and 16 months the jaws are resected and processed for analysis with the implants in situ. Sections are made with a sawing microtome (Leitz, Wetzlar, Germany) and further treated for microchemical analysis (Jeol Superprobe 733) and histological analysis in microscopes using transmitting and reflecting light. A histomorphometrical method is applied to quantify the amount of bone connection and fibrous tissue at the implant surface. This technique gives also the opportunity to quantify the influence of detrimental factors such as some material's aspects, the surgical technique and the biomechanical factors.

RESULTS AND DISCUSSION

The formation of a Si-rich layer covered by a CaP-rich layer on the bioglass surface can be detected by microprobe analysis. The formation of these layers is essential for the connection between bioglass and bone, as demonstrated in other studies (ref. 3,4,8-11).

Microchemically, three types of interface can be observed (ref. 11,13,16). In the first type a smooth transition of the CaP profile across the implant-bone interface is found (fig. 1). This means that the CaP content of the outer glass surface is similar to that of bone. Histologically, this type of interface corresponds to a bone connection (fig. 2) and is preferentially found at the level of the cortical bone.

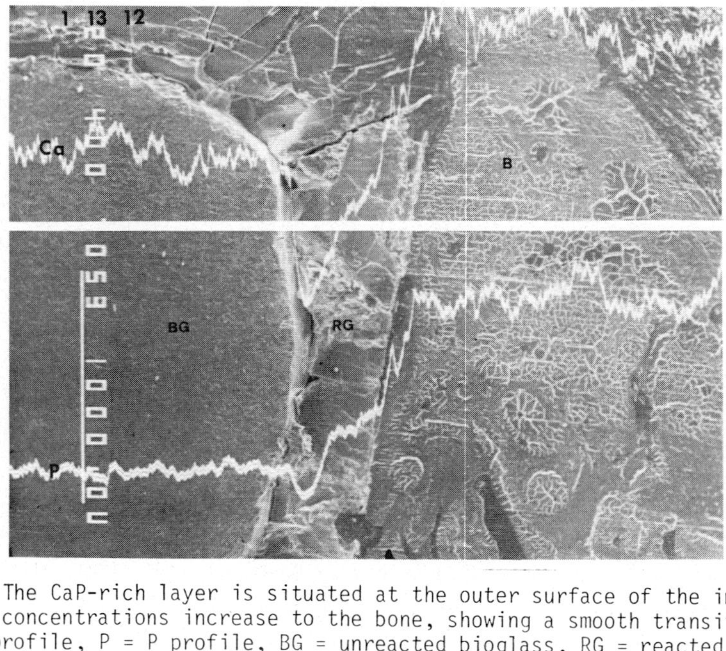

Fig. 1 : The CaP-rich layer is situated at the outer surface of the implant. The Ca and P concentrations increase to the bone, showing a smooth transition.
Ca = Ca profile, P = P profile, BG = unreacted bioglass, RG = reacted glass layer, B = bone.

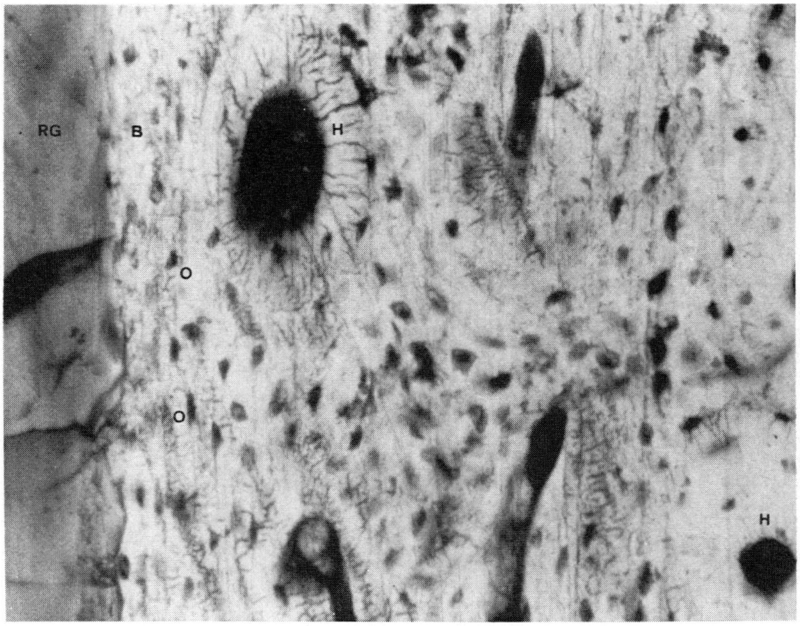

Fig. 2 : Bone is in direct connection with the bioglass surface. O = osteocyt, H = Haversian system, B = bone, RG = reacted glass layer (x 250).

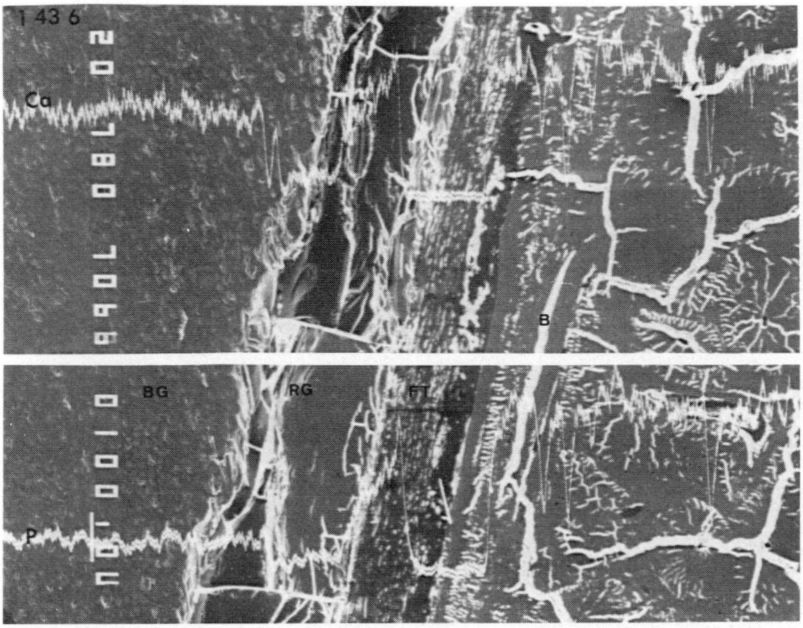

Fig. 3 : Across a fibrous interface a sudden interruption of the CaP profile can be detected. Ca = Ca profile, P = P profile, BG = unreacted bioglass, RG = reacted glass layer, FT = fibrous tissue, B = bone.

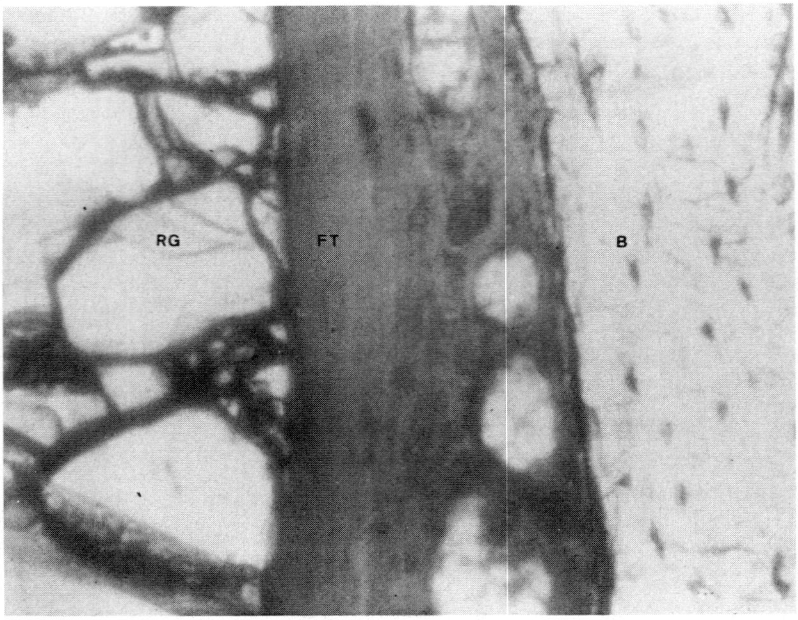

Fig. 4 : Bone is separated from the bioglass by fibrous tissue. The fibres in this tissue are running parallel to the surface. RG = reacted glass layer, FT = fibrous tissue, B = bone (x 125).

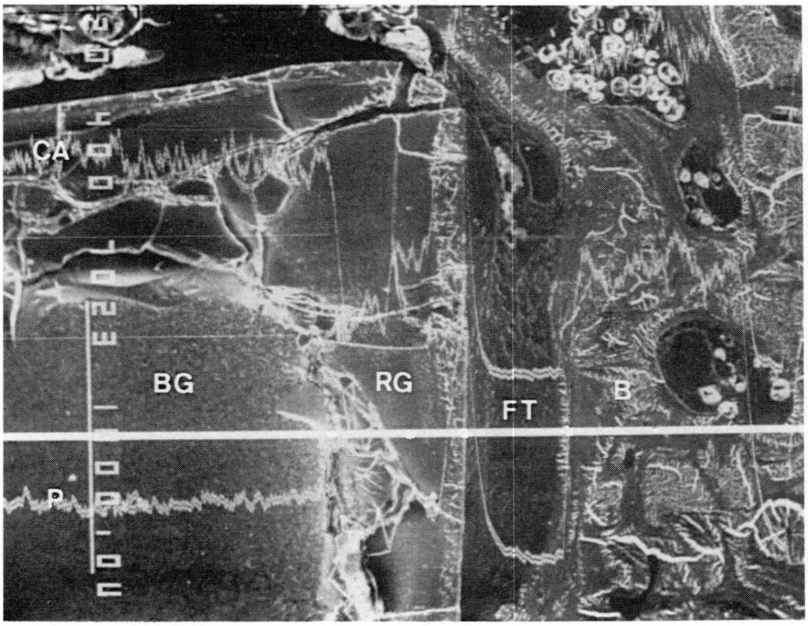

Fig. 5 : With microprobe analysis a gradual decrease of the Ca and P concentrations can be seen when the fibrous tissue is analyzed. Ca = Ca profile, P = P profile, BG = unreated glass, RG = reacted glass layer, FT = fibrous tissue, B = bone.

The second type of interface shows a sudden decrease in the CaP profile (fig. 3). Here the implant is separated from the bone tissue by a fibrous tissue layer (fig. 4). The third type of interface shows a gradual decrease of the CaP profile (fig. 5). This means that Ca and P ions are present in the surrounding fibrous tissue. Point analyses confirm the presence of these ions up to a depth of 70 µm. Since this type of interface is only seen after 16 months, the CaP enrichment of the surrounding tissues is probably time dependant.

The bone connection can be impeded by factors such as surgical trauma, lack of bone tissue to submerge and stabilize the implant and a poor fitting of the implant (ref. 10, 12, 14-16). Also, damage of the implant, establishing a direct contact with the stainless steel fibres, can inhibit locally the osteogenesis. In the cracks of the outer glass rim, microprobe analysis reveals the presence of metal ions. Those metal ions are, probably by a synergistical effect with glass ions, responsible for the lack of osteogenesis (fig.6).

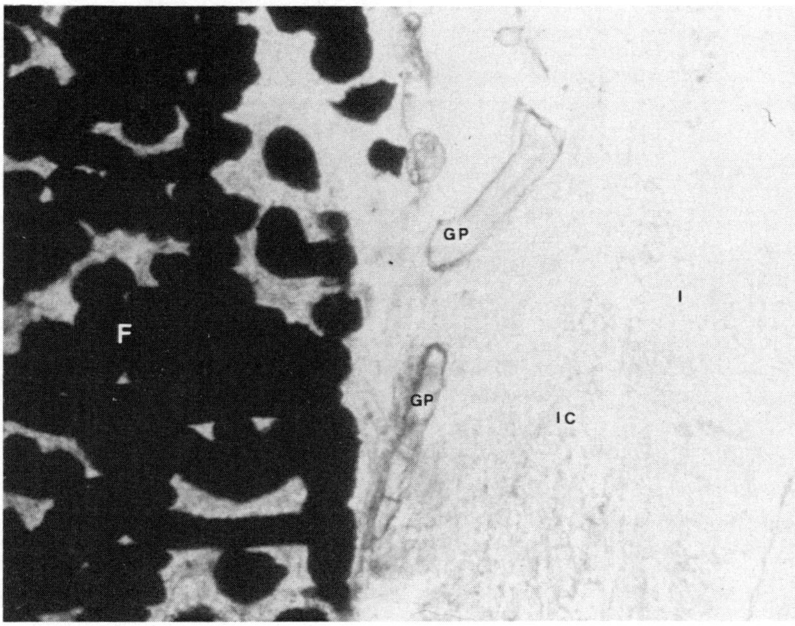

Fig. 6 : A direct contact with the stainless steel fibres inhibits locally the osteogenesis and can eventually elicit an inflammation reaction. F = metal fibre GP = glass particle, IC = inflammatory cell, (x 62,5)

The influence of those detrimental factors can be demonstrated by histomorphometrical analysis. If those factors are perfectly controlled, more than 100 % bone connection can be expected when compared to the initial contact area of the implant with bone tissue. This means that new bone is formed by osteoconductivity and can eventually encapsulate totally the implant (fig. 7). The bone can grow out along the implant surface in the apical direction as well as in the cervical direction, starting from the contact area with cortical bone. Such · an outgrowth of bone can also occur in the spongious bone, starting from the contact areas with bone trabeculae (ref. 15,16).

No diferences can be seen between the interfacial behaviour of bulk and intact fibre reinforced bioglass implants.

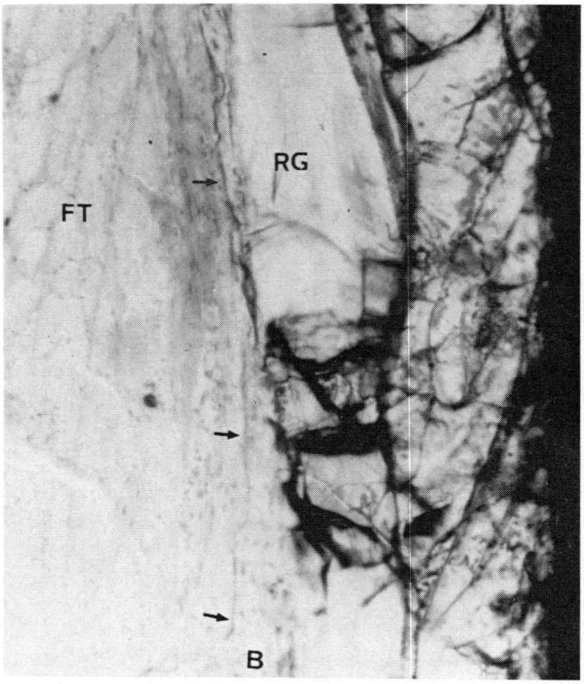

Fig. 7 : Outgrowth of bone (➚) from the cortical bone border in the cervical direction over a distance of 1850 μm. B = bone, RG = reacted glass layer, FT = fibrous tissue.

CONCLUSIONS

Three types of microchemical interface can be detected. The first type shows a smooth transition of the CaP profile, the second an abrupt interruption in this profile and the third a gradual decrease. These types correspond histologically with a bone connection, a fibrous tissue encapsulation and a calcification of the fibrous tissue in contact with the implant surface. The latter is probably time dependent since it is only seen after 16 months of implantation. No differences can be detected between the interfacial behaviour of bulk and fibre reinforced bioglass dental implants.

Histomorphometrical analysis reveals the noxious influence of some aspects of the material, the surgical technique and some biomechanical factors. This study not only demonstrates the bone bonding capacity of bioglass but also the fact that bone growth can be stimulated by osteoconductivity.

REFERENCES

1 R.Adell, U.Lekholm, B.Rockler, P.I.Bränemark, A 15 year study of osseointegrated implants in the treatment of the edentulous jaw, Int. J. Oral Surg., 10 (1981) 387 - 416.

2 A.Kirsch, Titan-spritzbeschichtete Zahnwurzelimplantaten unter physiologischer Belastung beim Menschen, Dtsch. Zahnärtzl. Z., 35 (1980) 112 - 115.

3 L.L.Hench, R.J.Splinter, W.C.Allen, T.K.Greenlee, Bonding mechanisms at the interface of ceramic prosthetic materials, J. Biomed. Mater. Res. 2 (1971) 117 - 141.

4 L.L.Hench, H.A.Paschall, Direct chemical bond of bio-active glass-ceramic implants to bone and muscle, J. Biomed. Mater. Res. 4 (1973) 25 - 42.

5 U.M.Gross, V.Strunz, The anchoring of glass-ceramics of different solubility in the femur of the rat, J. Biomed. Mater. Res. 14 (1980) 607 - 618.

6 U.M.Gross, V.Strunz, The interface of various glasses and glass-ceramics with a bony implantation bed, J. Biomed. Mater. Res. 19 (1985) 251 - 271.

7 P.Ducheyne, L.L.Hench, Metal fibre reinforced bioglass composites. Biomaterials 1 (1980) 21 - 26.

8 P.Ducheyne, L.L.Hench, The processing and static mechanical properties of metal fibre reinforced bioglass. J. Biomed. Mater. Res. 15 (1981) 441 - 445.

9 P.Ducheyne, Bioglass coatings and bioglass composites as implant materials, J. Biomed. Mater. Res., 19 (1985) 273 - 291.

10 P.Ducheyne, M.Martens, A.Burssens, Materials, clinical and morphological evaluation of custom-made bioreactive-glass-coated canine hip prostheses. J. Biomed. Mater. Res., 18 (1984) 1017 - 1030.

11 M.DeClercq, E.Schepers, P.Ducheyne, Microchemical analysis of bulk and fibre reinforced bioglass submerged dental root implants in dogs, In : van Steenberghe D. (Ed.) Tissue integration in oral and maxillo-facial reconstruction, Exerpta Medica, Amsterdam, 1986,pp. 138 -143.

12 E.Schepers, M.De Clercq, P.Ducheyne, Histological evaluation of bulk and fibre reinforced bioglass submerged dental root implants in dogs. In: D. van Steenberghe (Ed.) Tissue integration in oral and maxillo-facial reconstruction, Exerpta Medica, Amsterdam, 1986, pp. 144 - 149 .

13 M.De Clercq, E.Schepers, P.Ducheyne, Microchemical analysis of bulk and fibre reinforced bioglass dental implants. J. Dent. Res., 65 (4) (1985) 540.

14 E.Schepers, M.De Clercq, P.Ducheyne, Histological evaluation of bulk and fibre reinforced bioglass dental implants. J. Dent. Res., 65 (4) (1985) 544.

15 E.Schepers, M.Declercq, P.Ducheyne, Histomorphometrical evaluation of bulk and fibre reinforced bioglass dental implants. J Dent. Res., 65 (1986) 751.

16 E.Schepers, Vezelversterkt bioglas als een potentieel tandheelkundig implantaatmateriaal. Thesis, Cath. Univ. Leuven, Belgium, 1986.

Biomaterials and Clinical Applications,
edited by A. Pizzoferrato, P.G. Marchetti, A. Ravaglioli and A.J.C. Lee
Elsevier Science Publishers B.V., Amsterdam, 1987 — Printed in The Netherlands

HOW TO MEASURE STRENGTH OF DENTAL FILLING MATERIALS

U. SOLTESZ[1], B. KLAIBER[2] and J. SANDER[2]

[1] Fraunhofer-Institut für Werkstoffmechanik, Wöhlerstr. 11, D 7800 Freiburg

[2] ZMK-Klinik der Universität, Hugstetter-Straße 55, D 7800 Freiburg, FRG

SUMMARY

The strength behaviour of different types of dental filling materials was studied in order to find out the most informative and the most convenient testing procedure. Several common compression, tensile and bending tests were utilized. Additionally, size and shape of the specimens or the surface treatment were varied in some series. The results not only show the well known large differences in the strength values depending on the testing method but also contradictory evaluation when comparing materials. From these findings it is concluded that pure compression tests are not useful. Furthermore, taking into account the practicability of the different procedures it is proposed to perform diametral tensile tests in order to determine volume strengths, or 4-point-bending-tests if surface influences are of interest.

INTRODUCTION

For the characterization of the strength properties of dental filling materials several test methods are used at present. These tests differ greatly in specimen size, shape and loading conditions. An axial compression test is generally performed for amalgams, as recommended by DIN and ISO. On the other hand, for polymers and composite materials DIN and ISO require a 3-point-bending arrangement. The ADA, however, demands a diametral tensile test for composites. In the literature some authors propose 4-point-bending or pure uniaxial tensile tests as being correct from the theoretical point of view. All these procedures result in quite different strength values even for the same material and frequently produce contradictory results when comparing various materials.

In order to investigate the differences between the test methods and to check their usefulness and practicability, representatives of the different types of filling materials were examined under the mentioned loading conditions.

MATERIALS AND METHODS

Eight commercial materials were chosen for this investigation. They are listed in Table 1.

For the determination of the strengths five principally different arrangements were used. They are shortly described in Table 2. Some of them correspond to standard tests, the other ones are adapted to those.

TABLE 1 Materials investigated

Type	Trade name	Filler Material	Filler Vol.%	Filler mean size [μm]
Conventional Composites	Adaptic	quartz	58	15
	Classecond	quartz	66	2
	Nimetic	quartz	60	30
Hybrid Comp.	Coltène Brilliant	glass/SiO_2	54	2/.05
Microfilled Composites	Estic Microfill	pyr. SiO_2	35	.05
	Nimetic Dispers	pyr. SiO_2	40	.05
Pure Polymer	Sevriton			
Amalgam	Amalcap	non-γ-2		

TABLE 2 Materials investigated

Loading device	Specimen's shape	Specimen's dimensions [mm]	Standard
Axial Compression	cylinder	diameter x height 4 x 8 4 x 4; 4 x 12; 8 x 8	DIN 13904
Uniaxial tension	flat tapered	length x thickn. x width 25 x 2 x 2 (free 16)	
Diametral tension	cylinder	diameter x depth 6 x 3 4 x 2; 4 x 4; 4 x 8	ADA Spec. 27
3-point bending	square bar	length x thickn. x height 25 x 2 x 2 (support 20)	DIN 13922 ISO 4049 (DP)
4-point bending	square bar	as 3-point-bending (loading roller dist. 10)	

Additionally, to find out possible influences of sample volume, specimens of different size were tested under axial compression and diametral tension.

Finally, for the demonstration of the effect of preparation, specimens with differently treated surfaces were studied in 3- and 4-point-bending. For this purpose the composite bars were ground with finishing strips, whereas the amalgam specimens were polished. (Further details regarding materials and testing procedures may be taken from [1]).

RESULTS

The most evident result of the measurements is, at first, the strong difference in the strength values obtained by different testing methods. This well-known effect is illustrated in Fig. 1 in which only the three standard arrange-

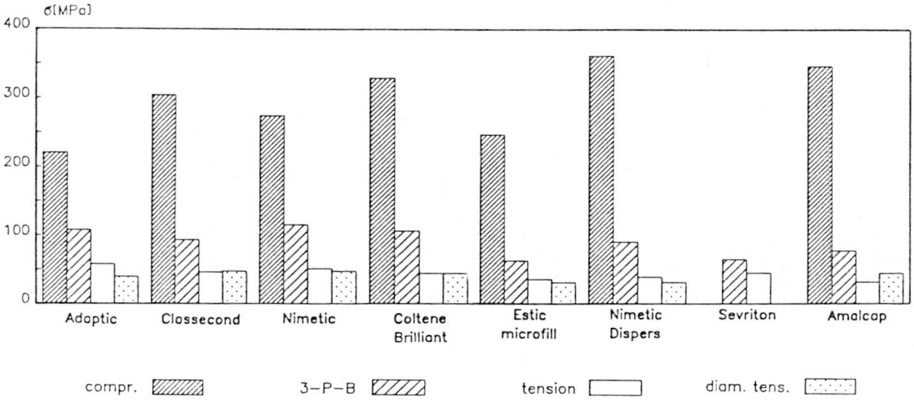

Fig. 1 Comparison of the strength values obtained under different standard testing conditions and under pure tension.

ments for axial compression, 3-point-bending and diametrial tension and additionally pure tension are considered as examples. The columns show the compressive strengths to be the highest ones. The bending values are two to five times smaller, and the tensile strengths - uniaxial as well as diametral - are additionally reduced by a factor of 2 compared to the flexural values.

If comparing, futhermore, the various materials their sequence is changed if one considers different methods. Nimetic Dispers e.g. exhibits the best compressive strength, whereas it becomes the worst material under pure tension.

Looking at the further results for the various specimen sizes and shapes or for the different surface treatments additional details are observed.

Compression testing

Under compressive loads an obvious influence of the specimen size is observed (Fig. 2). Whereas this effect seems to be less for specimens similar in shape (4 x 4 and 8 x 8) in spite of the greatest volume difference in this case, it may be very pronounced for different shapes (comp. e.g. Estic Microfill). Usually the strength values decrease with increasing height-to-diameter ratio. This means that this variation is not,or not only,produced by real volume effects.

Calculations of the failure probabilities following the Weibull-procedure show, too, that the differences generated by pure volume changes would be much smaller [1]. Therefore, further influences which are caused by the special shape of the different specimens and the loading and boundary conditions, and which may depend on various material properties such as stiffness, friction and yielding behaviour must play an important role. The pure polymer Sevriton e.g. could not be tested in this arrangement.

Thus, not only material but also structural properties seem to be determined in these tests. Since furthermore, comparable structures, loading and boundary

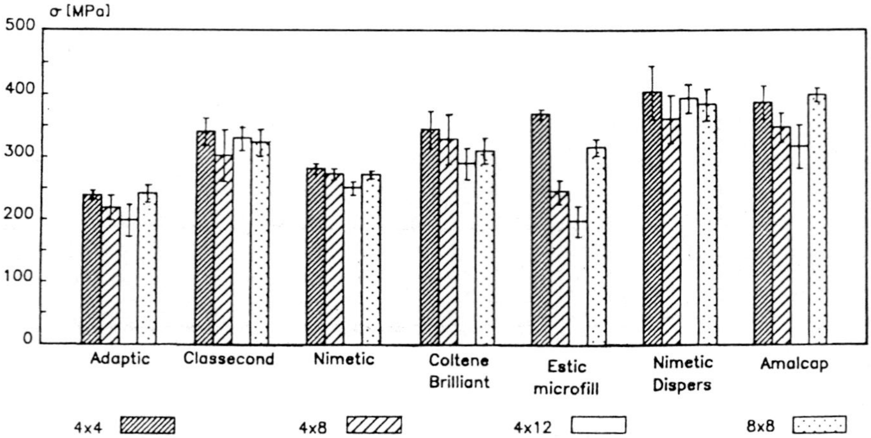

Fig. 2 Compressive strength obtained for different specimen sizes (diameter x height)

conditions are quite unusual in restorative dentistry it must be concluded from these findings that uniaxial compression testing is not useful for filling materials.

Uniaxial tensile testing

From the theoretical point of view pure tension is the most correct procedure to describe the failure of materials due to rupture. It delivers the lowest and most critical values (Fig. 1). Comparison of the materials with higher resolution (Fig. 3) exhibits the macrofilled composites to be stronger than the microfilled ones and amalgam.

There are, however, some disadvantages due to the necessary experimental procedure: Relatively large specimens, more complicated in shape, have to be prepared, the load has to be applied by some clamping device which leads to 20 to 30 % of non-valid tests with fractures initated by the clamping device.

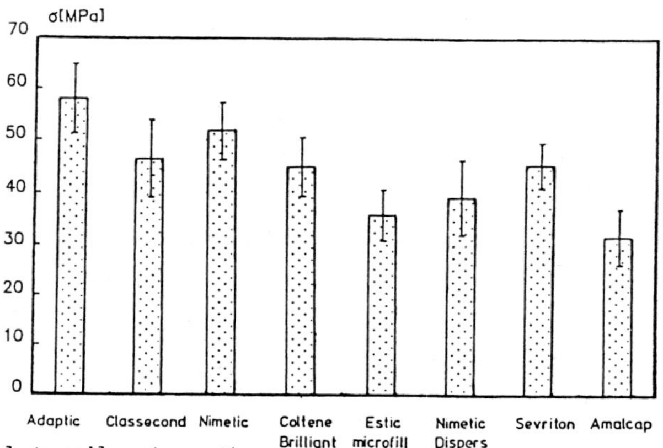

Fig. 3 Uniaxial tensile strengths

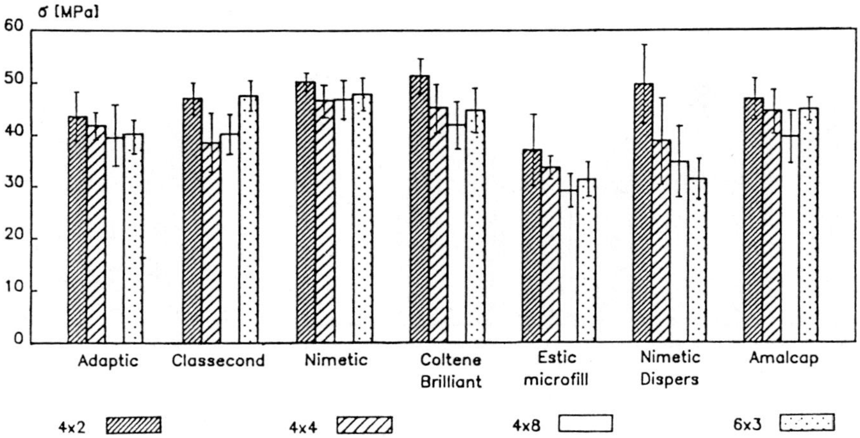

Fig. 4 Diametral tensile strengths obtained for different specimen sizes (diameter x depth)

Diametral tensile testing

Diametral tensile tests result in very similar values as under uniaxial tension (Fig. 1). The sequence of the materials is also comparable.

The examination of different sizes and shapes of the specimens leads to systematical differences in the values (Fig. 4). It can, however, be shown that these differences can be explained by the volume changes and that the values of one material can be calculated from another considering the failure probabilities according to the Weibull procedure [1].

As an additional advantage, it should be mentioned that testing procedure and specimen preparation are easier than in uniaxial tension. Furthermore, specimen size and shape are similar to a filling so that the polymerization processes of polymers and composites initiated by mixing or by light as well as condensing amalgams can be performed close to reality.

Bend testing

3-point-bending. The usual way, according to the standards, of utilizing a 3-point arrangement leads to values about twice that found under tension (Fig. 1). This can mainly be explained by volume effects [1]. In this case the highly stressed volume is very small and restricted to a region near the surface.

4-point bending. Under 4-point loading the strengths are normally slightly reduced (Fig. 5) due to the larger stressed volume. Such values appear to be more critical and more representative for the material because the natural distribution of defects is involved more realistically in the failure process.

Influence of surface treatment. Because of the special stress distribution under bending with high stresses only near the surface this test may be used to describe influences of surface treatments. Grinding of the composites normally

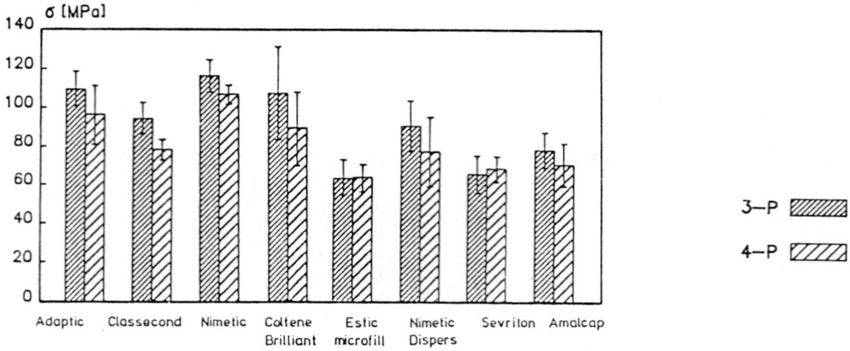

Fig. 5 Comparison of 3- and 4-point flexural strengths

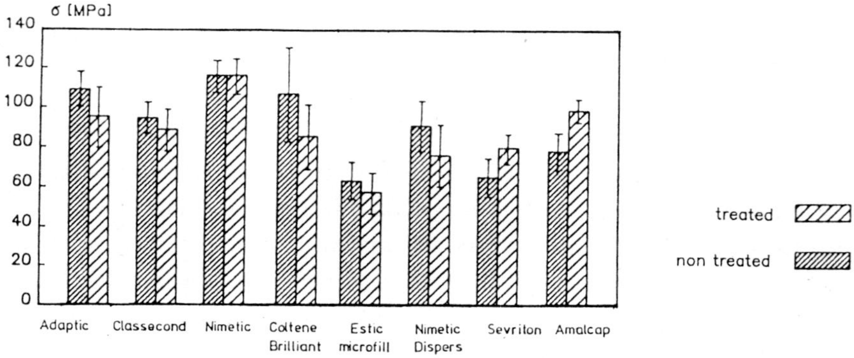

Fig. 6 Influence of surface treatment on 3-point flexural strengths

reduces the strength whereas polishing of the amalgam leads to an increase (Fig. 6). This is true as well for 3- as for 4-point bending. The more pronounced influence under 3-point loading shows again its extreme sensitivity to special features of the defect distribution.

CONCLUSIONS

From these findings it must be concluded that compression tests do not seem very useful for strength characterization of filling materials. To determine real material properties tensile tests should be applied, and with regard to specimen preparation and experimental procedure the diametral loading appears to be easier and more convenient. If, however, the influence of treating and finishing of the surface is of interest, a 4-point-bending arrangement should be used.

REFERENCES

1 J. Sander, U. Soltész and B. Klaiber, Zur Festigkeitsprüfung von Füllungsmaterialien - Ein Vergleich verschiedener Verfahren und Probenformen, Fraunhofer-Inst. f. Werkstoffmechanik, Report No. W 8/86, 1986

Biomaterials and Clinical Applications, 119
edited by A. Pizzoferrato, P.G. Marchetti, A. Ravaglioli and A.J.C. Lee
Elsevier Science Publishers B.V., Amsterdam, 1987 — Printed in The Netherlands

CORROSION AND PROTECTION OF SURGICAL AND DENTAL METALLIC IMPLANTS

C. SELLA, J.C. MARTIN[1], J. LECOEUR, J.P. BELLIER[2] and J.P. DAVIDAS[3]

[1]Lab. de Physique des Matériaux, C.N.R.S., MEUDON 92195 (France)

[2]Lab. Electrochimie Interfaciale, C.N.R.S., MEUDON 92195 (France)

[3]Univ. Paris VII, Soc. Fr. des Biomatériaux et Systèmes Implantables (France)

SUMMARY

Corrosion resistance of metals and alloys can be enhanced by protective coatings or by special alloying additives. In this paper the protection efficiency of Al_2O_3 coatings, deposited by RF sputtering onto NiCr and CoCr alloys, is tested. An intermediary layer of Al_2O_3 cermet is deposited and this enables the stresses at the interface metal-coating to be reduced. Electrochemical studies, in different biological media (synthetical blood plasma and artifical saliva) are performed. The potentiodynamic current potential curves analysis is carried out. Using the faradic currents amplitude, the corrosion resistance of different metals and also the efficiency of the protective coating can be rapidly and simply tested.

INTRODUCTION

Most of metals used for orthopaedic and stomatologic implants and prostheses belong to the families of nickel base and cobalt base superalloys elaborated for the industries of advanced technology (space - aeronautic - nuclear, ...) and have been experimented as biomaterials.

Metal corrosion in biological electrolytes, such as saliva and blood plasma, is mainly due to electrochemical process resulting from several oxidation reactions occuring simultaneously. All anodic surface reactions are not always corrosion reactions, a partial oxidation of some products of the solution can occur, so that the measured current corresponds to the addition of both an oxidation and a corrosion current.

EXPERIMENTAL TECHNIQUE

The corrosion resistance is evaluated from potentiodynamic current-potential curves I(E). A standard three electrode system is used. The working electrode is the specimen, the reference electrode, with a constant potential, is a saturated calomel electrode (sce) and the counter electrode is made of vitreous carbon. Potential is imposed on the working electrode versus the reference electrode and the current flowing between the specimen and the counter electrode is recorded continuously on a linear scale. The potential range used is (-1,2 ; + 1,5)V/SCE and the scan rate 20 $mV.s^{-1}$.

This technique permits the study of a lot of experimental conditions :

- metals : chemical composition, casting, heat treatment, internal stresses, machining, grinding, sandblasting, surface quality, roughness, superficial contamination, coating defects ...

- solutions : chemical composition, temperature, pH, aeration, stirring, organic or biological substances adsorption...

Test specimens consist of disks with a thickness of 1 to 3 mm and a diameter of 12 mm. The surface was polished to a mirror finish using standard metallographic techniques, with fine diamond plastes down to 1 μm. The specimens are studied using a scanning electron microscope, both before and after corrosion tests. A compositional analysis is made for each specimen using an electron probe microanalyser.

The in vitro experimentation required the use of artifical saliva and synthetic blood plasma. The composition of these solutions is in conformity with recommendations of "Association Française de Normalisation (AFNOR).

The artificial saliva was buffered with lactic acid to a pH of 6.7 and maintained at 37°C.

CORROSION BEHAVIOUR OF NiCr AND CoCr ALLOYS USED IN ORTHOPAEDIC SURGERY AND STOMATOLOGY

Polarization curves

The potentiodynamic polarization curves for different alloys are shown in fig. 1 for artificial saliva solutions and in fig. 2 for artificial plasma. For alloys of similar composition (fig. 1c,2) the shape of the curves are very similar, demonstrating that in a given alloy, corrosion is not very different whether it occurs in artificial saliva or plasma. Furthermore, the corrosion in a given solution, depends strongly on the alloy studied. For example, fig.1 shows the curves for different NiCr and CoCr alloys. In the case of Ni based alloys, including a wide variety of compositions having a Nickel content ranging between 64 and 74 weight % and a chromium content of between 16 and 22 %, the shape of the curve depends strongly on the composition.

These alloys may contain up to 10-12 % of molybdenum and minor alloying elements like Fe, Si may be added. The passivation domain is reduced for alloys with less than 16 % Cr and without Mo and an important hysteresis is seen (fig. 1a). This hysteresis could be due to the kinetics of the formation of corrosion products. The addition of Mo increases the passivation domain (fig. 1b) and a larger passivation domain is obtained by the addition of Mo plus W (fig. 1c).

In this last case, the hysteresis is greatly reduced.

For CoCrMo stellites all polarization curves are very similar for all of the alloys studied. No hysteresis is observed and the passivation domain is roughly the same for all of them so only one type of curve is given (fig. 1c, 2). Corrosion resistance of these alloys can be attributed to the cumulative effect of chromium plus molybdenum.

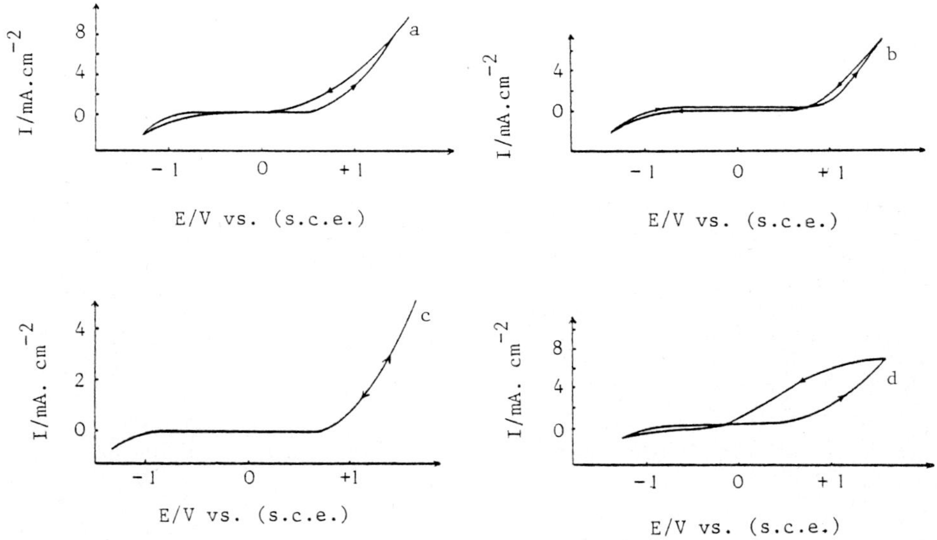

Fig. 1 : Current potential curves in artificial saliva
Sweep rate : 20 mV.s^{-1}, T° = 37°C, pH = 6,7
(a) NiCr (AD-1 : 72 Ni - 20 Cr - 6 Mo - 1.26 Si)
(b) NiCr (BiO 21 : 64 Ni - 18 Cr - 6,2 Fe - 8,5 Mo - 1.3 W - 1.2 Si)
(c) CoCrMo (67 Co - 27 Cr - 3 Mo - 1 Si)
(d) NiCr (Platinel : 74 Ni - 16 Cr - 8 Fe - 1 Ti - 1 Si)

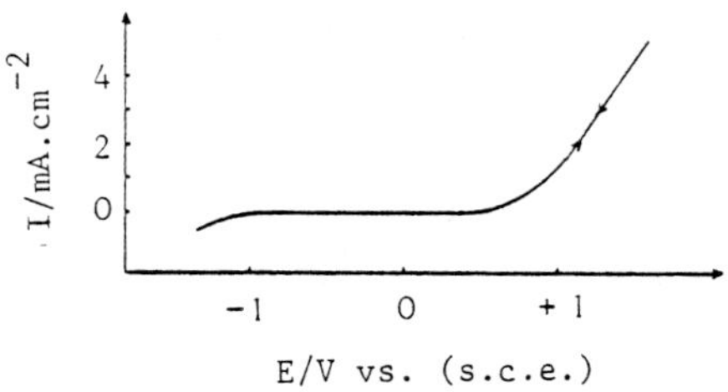

Fig. 2 : Current potential curves in artifical plasma
Sweep rate : 20 mV.s^{-1}, T° = 37°C
CoCrMo alloy (C 60 - 66 Co - 28 Cr - 5.5 Mo)

Scanning electron microscope studies of the alloys surface in corrosion

After electrochemical corrosion the surface of NiCr alloy is covered by the corrosion products. After removing this layer, corrosion pits are observed in the case of Platinel (fig. 3) which has a low chromium content and no molybdenum.

For CoCrMo alloy after electrochemical corrosion in a thin layer of corrosion produits appears. After removing this layer the precipitated $M_{23}C_6$ carbides are more visible (fig. 4).

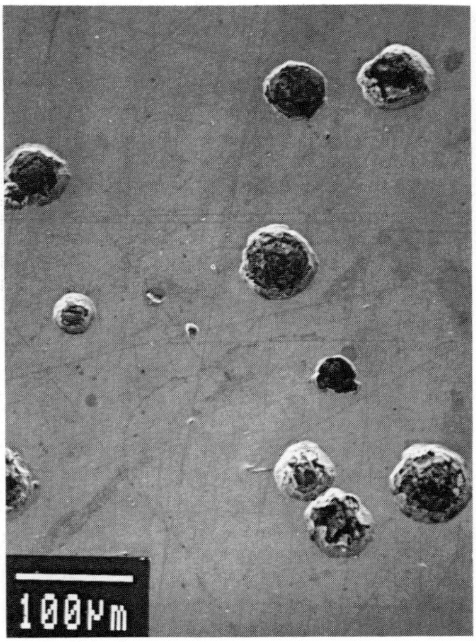

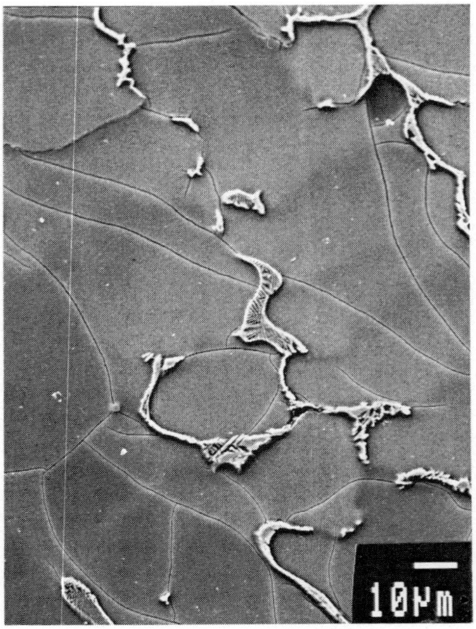

Fig. 3 : Corrosion pits observed after removing the corrosion products on NiCr alloys (Platinel, Fig. 1d).

Fig. 4 : Surface aspect of CoCrMo specimen after removing the corrosion products layer. The corrosion rate within Mo rich carbides (in relief) is lower than it is on the metal grains.

The addition of Mo or Mo + W and an increase in the Cr content greatly enhance the resistance to pitting and crevice corrosion : no pits are observed after electrochemical corrosion of such alloys (fig. 5,6). However intergranular Mo rich carbide precipitates are observed in relief since the corrosion rate is lower within these carbides than it is on the metal grains (fig. 5).

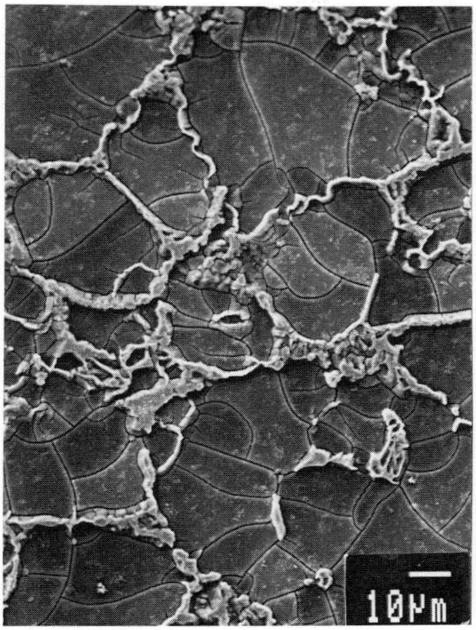

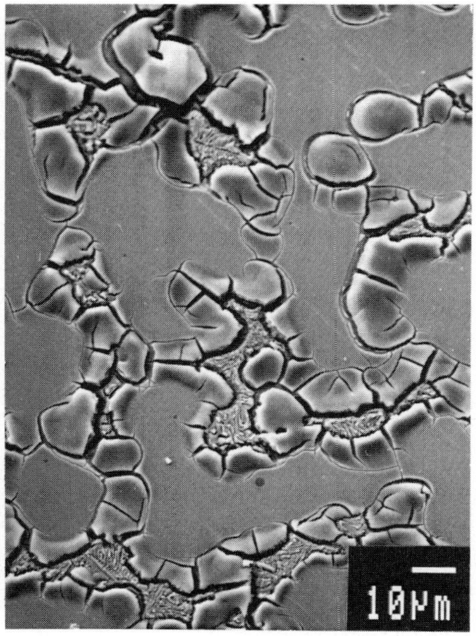

Fig. 5-6 : The addition of Mo or Mo + W enhances the resistance to pitting and crevice corrosion :
Fig. 5 : 67 Ni - 27 Cr - 6 Mo - (AD-1 alloy in saliva. Fig. 1a)
Fig. 6 : 64 Ni - 18 Cr - 8.5 Mo - 1.3 W (BiO 21 in saliva. Fig. 1b)

PROTECTIVE COATINGS

Corrosion resistance of metals and alloys can be enhanced by protective coatings or by special alloying additives (i.e : Al added in hot corrosion resistant superalloys provides the constant presence of an Al_2O_3 protective surface layer).

In this paper the protection efficiency of Al_2O_3 coatings deposited by RF sputtering onto NiCr and CoCr alloys is tested. The protective efficiency of the coatings is evaluated rapidly and simply from the potentiodynamic current-potential curves.

Using a sputtered intermediary layer of Al-Al_2O_3 cermet, the stresses at the interface are reduced, the cermet plus Al_2O_3 coating becomes strongly adherent and the corrosion current is strongly reduced (fig. 7). Moreover the free Al in the Al + Al_2O_3 cermet reinforces the Al_2O_3 layer in parts susceptible to weakness.

The two main problems in the protective efficiency are due to the adherence of the coating and the surface quality and porosity of the metal. For example if a surface cavity has not been perfectly protected by the coating, a corrosion pit could be induced.

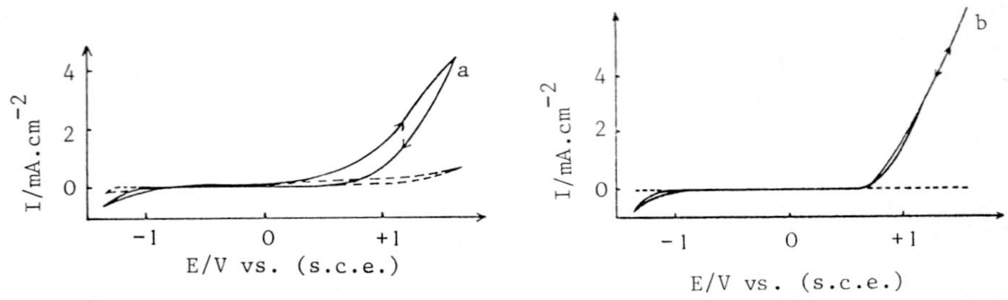

Fig. 7 : Current-potential curves in artificial saliva
Sweep rate : 20 $mV.s^{-1}$, T° = 37°C, pH = 6,7
(a) NiCr (SP 20 : 66 Ni - 22 Cr - 9 Fe - 3 Si)
(b) CoCr (SP 2000 : 60 Co - 30 Cr - 4 Ni - 4 Si - 1.5 Fe - 0.5 Mo)

CONCLUSION

New deposition techniques are now experimented, such as ion plating and ion vapour deposition, in which the adhesion of the film is improved by high energy ion bombardment of the growing film.

New multilayer coatings such as TiN plus Al_2O_3 or TiC plus Al_2O_3 turn to be a better solution because their adhesion to the NiCr or CoCr substrate seems to be better than that of a cermet plus Al_2O_3 coating.

These in vitro corrosion test results are confirmed by cell culture as well as by clinical experience. Signs of corrosion have not been observed on any of the Al_2O_3 coated dental implants removed several years after implantation.

The electrochemical corrosion tests allow us to identify and quantify (by atomic absorption) all released materials which are susceptible to be diffused from metals implanted in vivo, both in situ and in the general circulation. Such release products might induce cytotoxic effects, allergic effects.

Biomaterials and Clinical Applications, 125
edited by A. Pizzoferrato, P.G. Marchetti, A. Ravaglioli and A.J.C. Lee
Elsevier Science Publishers B.V., Amsterdam, 1987 — Printed in The Netherlands

THE INFLUENCE OF CAVITY DIAMETER ON THE IN VITRO TOXICITY TESTING OF DENTAL MATERIALS

S.D. MERYON

Department of Oral Pathology, Dental School, University of Birmingham, UK.

SUMMARY

The influence of the surface area of dental materials on their resulting toxicity was investigated in vitro by assessing the cytotoxicity of equal volumes of nine materials in artificial cavities of three different diameters, chosen to cover the range found in vivo. With most of the materials there was a significant increase in toxicity with increasing surface area with a uniform pattern of response within specific groups of materials. Most materials, particularly in large diameter cavities, exhibited significant toxicity relative to control cultures. An additional study of the effect of volume on the cytotoxicity of dental materials with a constant surface area demonstrated almost no effect. From this study it is apparent that the range of cavity diameters in which a dental material may be used clinically must be considered when evaluating their toxicity.

INTRODUCTION

In the general testing of dental materials little attention has been paid to the influence of cavity diameter on the response obtained. This applies in vivo where burs of similar size are generally used forming cavities of uniform diameter, although the depth may vary with consequent variations in the thickness of residual dentine. The possible influence of both, the surface area of test material in contact with the residual dentine and the total volume used, cannot be dissociated from the biological response observed. Thus it is feasible that a material will elicit only a slight response in a small cavity but a much larger response in a larger cavity. However, due to the many variables which exist in in vivo testing, such a study would be difficult to undertake. Similarly, in vitro testing has paid little attention to the specimen size of test materials used (ref.1). Preliminary studies by Meryon demonstrated an increase in the cytotoxicity of equal volumes of two cements with increasing surface area (ref.2) while increasing the volume had an effect with only one of two materials tested (ref.3).

The model cavity system has been developed in Birmingham for the in vitro toxicity testing of dental restorative materials (ref.4). In this method, designed to simulate the clinical situation, both the cavity diameter and volume of test material used can be varied. Using this method the aim of the present study was to investigate the effect of the surface area of equal volumes of a wide range of dental materials on their toxicity. An additional study of the influence of volume was also carried out.

METHODS

Test Methods

The materials investigated included two amalgams, Dispersalloy and Solila Nova; two glass ionomer cements, AquaCem and ChemFil II; a polycarboxylate cement, Poly-F Plus; two composites, Concise and Occlusin; two calcium hydroxide liners, Dycal and Life; Kalzinol, a resin bonded ZOE cement and two cements containing phosphoric acid, Zinc phosphate and Silicap. All were mixed according to manufacturer's instructions. The first nine were used in surface area experiments, all twelve in volume experiments.

Test Apparatus

This was a modification of that first described by Tyas (refs.4-5). It comprised a 35mm diameter petri dish containing a cell monolayer covered with 4 ml of culture medium. The lid contained a centrally drilled hole beneath which was attached a pyrex cylinder 4 mm in length with a permeable membrane filter at the base (Whatman, UK). The cylinders had i.d. of 3mm, 5mm and 8 mm, providing surface areas of 7.07, 19.63 and 50.24mm^2, forming small, medium and large cavities respectively. In the surface area experiments equal volumes of test material were placed in each cylinder, irrespective of its diameter. In the supplementary volume study 5mm cavities were used filled with three different volumes of material termed half-, standard- and double- volumes of approximately 19.63, 39.25 and 78.50mm^3. Immediately after filling the filters at the base of the cavities were lightly swabbed with alcohol and the lid assembly immediately placed over the base of the dish and agitated so that the culture fluid contacted the filter.

Cell Culture

Suspensions of BHK-21 (C-13) fibroblasts in the Glasgow modification of Eagles MEM (Flow Labs) were diluted to contain 1 x 10^5 cells/ml. 4 ml aliquots of this suspension were pipetted into covered petri dishes and incubated for 24 h followed by placement of the lid assemblies. The cultures were then exposed to the test material for 24h at 37^oC in a humidified atmosphere of 5% CO_2 in air. Following exposure the fibroblasts were washed, detached using trypsin - EDTA (Flow Labs) and counted using an electronic coulter counter.

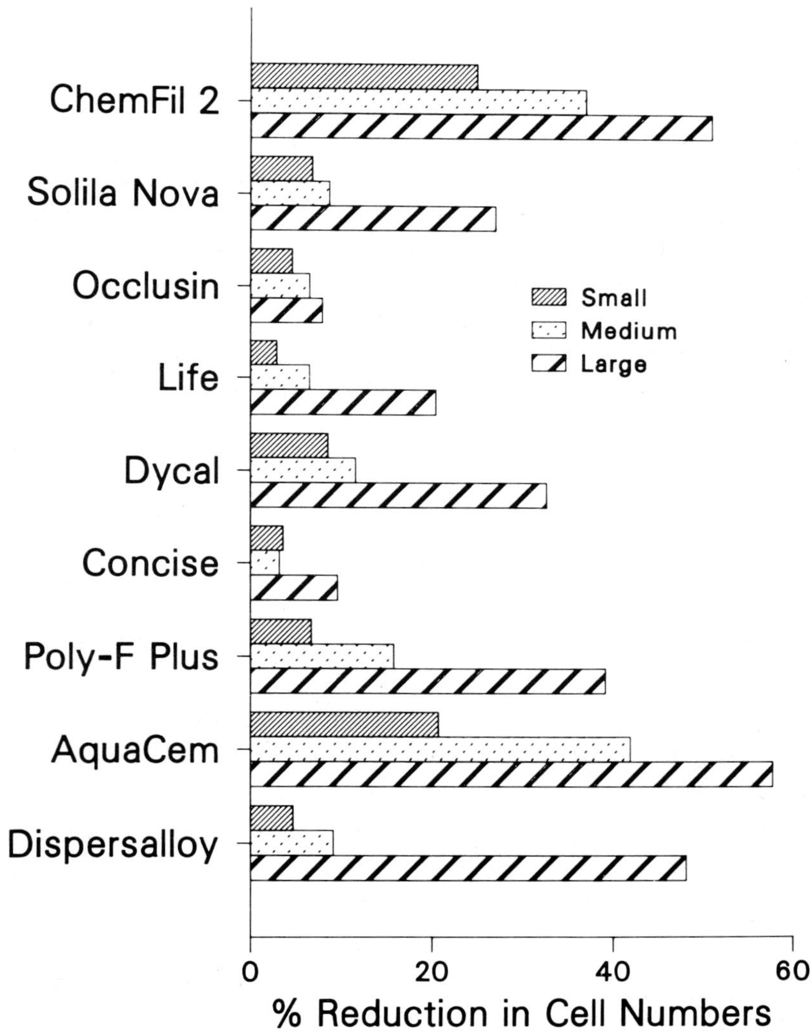

Fig.1: The influence of cavity diameter on the cytotoxicity of nine test materials expressed as a % reduction in cell numbers relative to controls.

Test Method

The materials were tested in a series of experiments, 3 per series and a control. In every series each material was tested in quadruplicate in each cavity size or at each volume and the experiment repeated three times. The effect of cavity diameter and material volume on the cytotoxicity of each material was analysed using a One-way Analysis of Variance test. Cytotoxicity relative to controls was assessed using an unpaired Student t-test.

RESULTS

The effect of the nine test materials in cavities of different diameters is presented in Fig 1. With all the materials tested except for Concise and Occlusin there was a significant increase in toxicity with increasing surface area ($p < 0.01$). Results of a Students t-test of differences between the nine materials in 3 cavity sizes and controls is presented in Table 1. Only AquaCem and ChemFil had a significant effect in small cavities while in addition Poly-F Plus, Dycal and Solila Nova had a significant effect in medium cavities and all materials except Concise and Occlusin were significantly toxic in large cavities.

Cell count determinations following exposure to 12 test materials at 3 different volumes but in cavities of uniform diameter demonstrated a significant effect of volume only with AquaCem ($F = 5.43$, $p < 0.01$). With Kalzinol there was a strong trend towards decreasing cell numbers with increasing volume but this difference was not significant. Most of the materials caused a significant reduction in cell numbers relative to controls.

DISCUSSION

In general increasing the surface area of each of the materials tested without altering its volume led to a significant increase in toxicity to underlying cells as demonstrated previously with zinc phosphate and silicate cements (ref.2). This probably results from the increased release of toxic components with increasing surface area which, when a threshold is reached, leads to cell damage or inhibition of cell growth (ref.6). Zinc, which is released from Dispersalloy and Poly-F Plus (ref.7) and fluoride released from Silicap and the glass ionomers (ref.8) have been shown to be cytotoxic.

The pattern of toxicity varied between different groups of materials (Fig.1). The two composites were non-toxic even in the large cavities. Several materials including the amalgams and calcium hydroxide liners were slightly toxic in medium cavities with a dramatic increase in toxicity in the large cavities. The poly-

TABLE 1

Reduction in cell numbers beneath nine test materials in cavities of increasing diameter relative to controls expressed at "t" and "p" values obtained using a Students t-test.

Material		Cavity Size Small	Medium	Large
Dispersalloy	t	0.957	1.912	4.665
	p	ns	ns	<0.001
AquaCem	t	3.264	6.819	11.572
	p	<0.005	<0.001	<0.001
Poly-F Plus	t	0.934	2.472	5.612
	p	ns	<0.025	<0.001
Concise	t	0.785	0.709	1.975
	p	ns	ns	ns
Dycal	t	1.774	2.827	7.624
	p	ns	<0.01	<0.001
Life	t	0.619	1.510	4.317
	p	ns	ns	<0.001
Occlusin	t	1.658	1.391	1.592
	p	ns	ns	ns
Solila Nova	t	1.835	2.639	8.064
	p	ns	<0.02	<0.001
ChemFil II	t	5.813	10.062	19.292
	p	<0.001	<0.001	<0.001

carboxylate was non-toxic in small cavities but caused a linear reduction in cell numbers with increasing surface area. In contrast the glass ionomers were strongly toxic in all cavity sizes. From these results it is apparent that the pattern of the influence of surface area on the toxicity of materials within groups i.e. amalgams, composites etc. is fairly uniform.

In contrast increasing the volume of several materials while retaining a constant surface area had almost no effect. The positive effect with AquaCem may reflect the ability of the toxic agent to diffuse through the material rather than release only occurring from the area of material in contact with the culture medium. A significant effect of volume on cytotoxicity has previously been demonstrated with zinc oxide eugenol attributed to the release of eugenol (ref.3). A similar but non significant trend was demonstrated by Kalzinol in this study possibly due to the presence of resin in this material limiting the diffusion of free eugenol.

From the data presented in this study, it is apparent that the maximum cavity diameter which is appropriate for the material under test must be taken into account in its biological evaluation. Thus materials such as amalgams, which are frequently used in large diameter cavities, should be evaluated either in vivo or in vitro in cavities which represent the upper size limit. The overall volume of dental materials appears to have little effect on their toxicity.

AKNOWLEDGEMENTS

This study was supported by a grant from the Lord Dowding Fund. The author is grateful to Mr A.J.C Potts and the Photographic Unit for assistance in preparing the figure, to Mrs H. Richmond for preparing the manuscript and to Professor R.M. Browne for his help and advice.

REFERENCES

1 A. Hensten-Pettersen and K. Helgeland, Evaluation of biologic effects of dental materials using four different cell culture techniques, Scand. J. Dent.Res., 85 (1977) 291-296.
2 S.D.Meryon, The importance of surface area in the cytotoxicity of zinc phosphate and silicate cements in vitro, Biomaterials, 4 (1983) 39-43.
3 S.D. Meryon, The influence of dentine on the in vitro cytotoxicity testing of dental restorative materials, J. Biomed.Mater.Res., 18 (1984) 771-779.
4 S.D.Meryon and R.M. Browne, Test methods for assessing the cytotoxicity of dental materials using an in vitro model cavity system, In: P. Vincenzini (Ed.) Ceramics in Surgery, Elsevier, Amsterdam, 1983, pp 127-135.
5 M.J. Tyas, A method for the in vitro toxicity testing of dental restorative materials, J.Dent.Res., 56 (1977) 1285-1290.
6 S.D.Meryon, A.J. Smith, R.S.Tobias and R.M. Browne, Fluoride as the possible cytotoxic component of Silicap. 1. Fluoride release, Int.End.J. 16 (1983) 20-25.
7 S.D.Meryon and K.J.Jakeman, The effects in vitro of zinc released from dental restorative materials, Int.End.J. 18 (1985) 191-198.
8 S.D.Meryon and A.J.Smith, A comparison of fluoride release from three glass ionomer cements and a polycarboxylate cement, Int.End.J.17 (1984) 16-24.

Biomaterials and Clinical Applications,
edited by A. Pizzoferrato, P.G. Marchetti, A. Ravaglioli and A.J.C. Lee
Elsevier Science Publishers B.V., Amsterdam, 1987 — Printed in The Netherlands

CEMENTLESS PROSTHESIS: CLINICAL EXPERIENCE

Jorge O. Galante, M.D.

Department of Orthopedic Surgery, Rush-Presbyterian-St. Luke's Medical Center, 1753 West Congress Parkway, Chicago, Illinois 60612 (U.S.A.)

INTRODUCTION

Our approach to cementless total hip prosthesis has been based on the use of a porous material to serve as a means of attachment to bone via bone ingrowth into its open pores. The material we have used is a fiber titanium composite made from unalloyed titanium fibers. These fibers are made into porous pads that are attached to the surface of the prosthetic device by means of a sintering process (refs. 1,2).

A review of some of the basic processes that take place following the implantation of a porous prosthetic device is critical to understand the principles of clinical application (refs. 1,3,4,5,6,7,8). Immobilization of the prosthetic device and intimate contact with the surrounding bone are two essential prerequisites to obtain bone ingrowth. These two prerequisites translate themselves into the need for an excellent press fit. They imply that accurate instrumentation is required to prepare an ideal site in the intramedullary cavity of the bone or to ream an ideal hemispherical site in the acetabulum. It is not the patient that is immobilized but the prosthesis by virtue of an interference fit and the use of whatever additional elements of internal fixation such as screws might be required. Immobilization is critical (refs. 9,10). Under the influence of motion, fibrous tissue rather than bone will form, a development that is not ideal for the fixation of a major weight bearing device. Intimate contact is also important and perhaps more critical in some areas than others (refs. 11,12,13). Bone has the ability to bridge some gaps in the intramedullar cavity of the bone, where spaces may be present between the prosthesis and the endosteum in some areas and intimate contact present in others. On the other hand, in the acetabulum it appears that intimate contact is an important prerequisite throughout if bone ingrowth is to occur (ref. 14). These details mandate that in addition to excellent instrumentation, precise surgical technique be used to obtain the kind of fit and fixation that is desired.

Experimental studies have indicated that within the first two or three weeks, primary bone formation occurs in the interstices of the porous material. Appositional bone formation leads to thickening and strengthening of these immature bone trabeculae, and within six weeks the process of bone remodelling takes place, leading eventually to the appearance of mature bony trabeculae with haversian type structures. The bony surfaces come into close contact with the interweaving titanium fibers and in many histological fields it is possible to see very intimate apposition between bone and metal without an intervening soft tissue layer (refs. 15,16,17).

The process of stress induced bone remodelling is critical to the success of the arthroplasty and also to the health and function of the surrounding bone (refs. 13,18,19,20,21). Diffuse cortical osteoporosis has been a phenomenon that is seen routinely in our canine total hip replacements. It appears to be self limited, nonspecific and, at least in the experimental animal at six months, the cortex appears to be completely healed. This form of diffuse cortical osteoporosis is probably related to the trauma of surgery and may be based on vascular phenomena or related to the initial disuse atrophy that follows the surgical trauma.

Bone remodelling processes, probably related to the patterns of stress transfer, induce the development of an entirely different type of cortical resorption. This phenomenon is characterized primarily by periosteal bone resorption, and it has been called, clinically, stress shielding. The process seems to be related in part to the extent of porous coating, to the manner of stress transfer from the prosthetic device to the surrounding bone and finally in some degree to the stiffness of the prosthetic device. In the experimental animal, devices fully coated with porous material exhibited a much higher degree of bone resorption than those that were partially coated (ref. 21). In addition, the bone resorption was much more severe in the proximal than in the distal portion of the shaft indicating an effect from the mechanism of stress transfer and loading on the prosthetic device. The process of stress shielding is therefore partly interpreted as distal stress transfer leading to proximal bone resorption. The conclusion from these studies is that the porous material should be limited to the proximal portion of the prosthetic device in the femoral canal. An additional advantage of using this configuration is that it assures and facilitates removal of the prosthetic device with minimal damage to the surrounding cortex should it ever become necessary.

MATERIAL AND METHODS

We have used a prosthetic device made from Ti6Al4V alloy in its solid portions and from unalloyed titanium fiber composite in its porous layers. The femoral component is available in 9 sizes and additional custom made devices are available with special dimensions for unusual revision surgery cases or congenital hip problems with dysplastic femurs. The component is straight, incorporates a distal cylindrical portion and a proximal triangular like segment that fills the metaphyseal cavity of the bone. The prosthesis is symmetrical, one device serves right or left femurs. The anteversion is provided by orienting the device according to the natural geometry of the upper femur. The porous composite is limited to the anterior, posterior and medial aspects of the prosthesis where it is sintered onto preformed slots. The process of diffusion bonding is used for sintering the porous composite to the solid shaft. This precludes the use of high temperatures that result in changes on the internal structure of the metal with a consequent decrease in the fatigue strength of the prosthesis.

The acetabulum is a hemispherical shell, fully coated with the porous unalloyed titanium composite. It has a modular polyethylene insert and it is fixed to the pelvis with cancellous type screws. The acetabulum is available in 2 mm increments from 40 mm to 80 mm.

Patient selection included the following criteria. In general young active patients, which we define as being below the age of 70, were considered candidates for cementless fixation. Below the age of 60 we usually indicated cementless arthroplasties. Between the ages of 60 and 70 the decision was made primarily on the basis of the patient wishes, the degree of activity, the quality of the bone stock and other local factors. Consideration of the presence of bilateral disease, the presence and severity of osteoporosis and not necessarily the presence of systemic disease, were important factors in the selection of a cemented or a cementless technique. We feel that above the age of 70 there is little indication for the use of a new and experimental technique when a time tested reliable technique for patients in that age group is available with the use of acrylic cement. In addition to these indications in primary hip surgery, we use cementless prosthesis almost exclusively in revision surgery for failed cemented total hip arthroplasties. In these instances the use of cementless techniques in conjunction with the use of bone grafts can lead to the solution of very severe problems.

We recently reviewed 104 patients who were operated on at our institution and who had a follow-up from 12 to 24 months. Procedures were done under general epidural anesthesia. Autologous blood transfusions were used routinely. An anterolateral approach with the patient in the lateral decubitus was used for the vast majority of our patients. Prophylaxis for thromboembolic disease was begun the night before surgery using dicumarol with the intention of maintaining the prothrombin at a 50% level. Postoperative recovery included ambulation with crutches with the aim of maintaining the weight bearing to 50% of the patients weight for the first six weeks. Additional use of crutches for another six weeks but with allowance of full weight bearing on the affected extremity was allowed until full weight bearing without supports if feasible was permitted three months after surgery.

All the procedures were performed in laminar air flow equipped operating rooms. We used routinely antibiotic prophylaxis with intravenous cephalosporins.

RESULTS

There were 104 hips in 98 patients equally divided between male and female. The average age for this population was 49 years (20-72), somewhat younger than the usual candidate population for total hip surgery. This reflects to a great extent the criteria used for the selection of patients. The diagnosis included 57 patients with osteoarthritis, 27 patients with avascular necrosis, 5 patients with failed surface replacements, 5 patients with rheumatoid arthritis, 3 with ankylosis spondylitis and 1 patient with traumatic arthritis. Only 8% of the patients had some form of polyarthritis. The distribution of diagnosis reflectsthe careful consideration given in the patient selection to the quality of bone stock The vast majority of patients represent patients with osteoarthritis and other diagnostic categories where adequate cortical and trabecular structure was present. This was deemed essential to obtain satisfactory fixation and initial support for the femoral component.

The preoperative Harris hip score for this group of patients was 55 (12-79). The postoperative hip score was 94 (57-100). Evaluation of pain indicated that 76 patients (73%) had no pain, 21 (20%) had slight pain, 6 (6%) had mild pain and 1 had severe pain. 54 patients (52%) had no limp, 39 patients (37%) had a slight limp, 10 patients (10%) had a moderate limp and 1 patient had severe limp. Ninety patients, (86%) used no support, 9 patients (9%) used a cane for long distances, 4 patients (4%) used a cane full time and one patient used a crutch.

The following complications were observed. One dislocation (1%), 3 wound hematomas (2.8%), 3 undisplaced longitudinal fractures of the femoral neck (2%), 2 pulmonary embolism (1.9%), 2 deep vein thrombosis (1.9%), 1 death presumed pulmonary embolism.

As of the time of this write-up there have been two reoperations. One was a revision for a loose femoral component and the second was performed for removal of massive heterotopic bone formation.

A complete radiographical evaluation was possible in 83 patients who had between 12 to 24 months follow-up. The femoral stem was positioned in neutral in 35 patients (42%) in varus in 27 patients (33%), in valgus in 21 patients (25%). There were two patients who exhibited subsidence. One 2 mm and the other one 3 mm. Both were asymptomatic, one had a Harris hip rating of 95 and the other one 97. Six patients exhibited resorption of the calcar of two or more millimeters. Decreased density of the medial femoral cortex was observed in a large number of patients. It was considered minimal in 28 patients (34%) and moderate leading to cancellisation of the medial femoral cortex in 33 patients (40%).

There were no complete radiolucencies or cortical erosions seen at the femoral interface. Radiolucencies were commonly seen around the convex portion of the prosthesis proximally in the trochanteric region and at the tip of the device. In these two areas there are no porous composites and a finding of a radiolucent area in contact with a solid metalic surface is not an uncommon event. On the other hand, in the lateral view radiolucencies in contact with the porous pads were seen in 4 patients. This may well indicate lack of bone ingrowth. They were present in the 2 patients that exhibited subsidence.

Distal bone formation at the tip of the stem was seen complete in 7 patients (8.4%) and partial bone formation in that region was seen in 12 (14%). There was no correlation between the presence of sclerosis at the tip of the stem and the clinical rating observed. Femoral cortical thickening was seen around the distal portion of the stem in 22 patients.

There were no cases of acetabular migration. There was 1 patient in which complete acetabular radiolucency was observed.

Heterotopic ossification observed in 42 patients (50%), was of grade 1 in 29 patients, grade 2 in 9 patients, grade 3 in 4 patients and grade 4 in 2 patients. These two patients with grade 4 heterotopic ossification exhibited significant clinical symptoms with the presence of pain and limitation of motion. One patient had the bony mass surgically excised and on the other patient surgery is pending.

There is one patient in this population who had severe pain and a Harris hip score rating of 57. This patient exhibited an abnormal bone scan with markedly increased uptake at the tip of the prosthesis. Previous surgery was performed for a nonunited femoral neck fracture and femur exhibited considerable thinning of the lateral cortex due to the presence of a plate that had been used for internal fixation. It is currently felt that she has a loose femoral component although there are no radiographic findings that are diagnostic at this time. Revision is contemplated.

DISCUSSION AND CONCLUSIONS

One of the basic questions that one must consider in the evaluation of a new cementless prosthetic system is whether it is as good or better than the currently used cement techniques. In the short term results are probably not comparable to those that can be obtained today with contemporary cement techniques. Recovery is faster using cement and a potential failure rate within the first two years of 2% may not be seen with the use of contemporary designs and cement pressurization techniques. If we separate considerations regarding fixation of the femur to those of the acetabulum it appears that fixation of the acetabulum is reproducible and reliable. We have had the opportunity to review in our laboratory 16 prosthesis that were removed for instability. In every single one of those cases fixation by bone ingrowth was present although the extent of bone ingrowth varied extensively from patient to patient. It is our current feeling that fixation of the acetabulum is as reliable as that which can be obtained using cemented techniques. The femur is a more critical area and is closely related to the quality of the bone stock present preoperatively, to details of the surgical technique and to biological variables that may be outside the control of the surgeon.

The long term results of cementless total hip replacements are not known. The potential advantages may include the ease of revision due to the absence of cement and a potential lower incidence of failure over a long term.

Specific areas where cementless surgery may have advantages are in the revision of failed cemented hip arthroplasties and in the younger patient population. This is a new technology that requires careful clinical scrutiny and planned long term studies to ascertain its advantages over contemporary cement techniques.

Areas that require continued research include those of bone remodelling, studies of long term biocompatibility, issues of design and material selection. All of these are problems that can affect the long term function of these prosthetic devices.

REFERENCES

1 J. Galante, W. Rostoker, R. Lueck and R.D. Ray: Sintered fiber metal composites as a basis for attachment of implants to bone. J. Bone Joint Surg. 53A (1971) 101-114.

2 W. Rostoker, J.O. Galante and G. Shen: Some mechanical sintered fiber metal composites. J Test Eval. 2 (1974) 107-112.
3 P.Q. Chen, T.M. Turner, H. Ronningen, J. Galante, R. Urban and W. Rostoker: A canine cementless total hip prosthesis model. Clin. Orthop. 176 (1983) 24-33.
4 E. Lembert, J. Galante and W. Rostoker: Fixation of skeletal replacement by fiber metal composites. Clin. Orthop. 87 (1972) 303-310.
5 D.P. Rivero, J. Fox, A.K. Skipor, J.O. Galante and W. Rostoker: Enhancement of early bone ingrowth into titanium fiber metal implants. Surg. Forum 235 (1984) 517-519.
6 D.P. Rivero, J. Fox, A.K. Skipor, R.M. Urban, J.O. Galante and W. Rostoker: Effects of calcium phosphates and bone grafting materials on bone ingrowth in titanium fiber metal. Trans. Orthop. Res. Soc. 1985.
7 D.P. Rivero, A.K. Skipor, M. Singh and J.O. Galante: Effect of EHDP on bone ingrowth in a porous material. Trans. Orthop. Res. Soc., 1985.
8 H. Ronningen, P. Lereim, J. Galante, W. Rostoker, T. Turner and R. Urban: Total surface hip arthroplasty in dogs using a fiber metal composite as a fixation method. J. Biomed. Mater. Res. 17 (1983) 643-653.
9 P. Ducheyne, P. Delport and M. Martens: The initial stability of wire mesh porous coated tibial components of knee prostheses. Trans. Orthop. Res. Soc. 9 (1984) 175.
10 P. Ducheyne, P. DeMeester and E. Aernoudt: Influence of a functional dynamic loading on bone ingrowth into surface pores of orthopedic implants. J. Biomed. Mater. Res. 11 (1977) 811-838.
11 G.B.J. Andersson, A. Gaechter, J.O. Galante and W. Rostoker: Segmental replacement of long bones in baboons using a fiber titanium implant. J. Bone Joint Surg. 60A (1978) 31-40.
12 H.U. Cameron, R.M. Pilliar and I. Macnab: The effect of movement on the bonding of porous metal to bone. J. Biomed. Mater. Res. 7 (1973) 301-311.
13 A.K. Hedley, M. Kabo, W. Kim, I. Coster and H.C. Amstutz: Bony ingrowth fixation of newly designed acetabular components in a canine model. Clin. Orthop. 176 (1983) 12-23.
14 W.H. Harris, R.E. White, J.C. McCarthy, P.S. Walker and E H. Weinberg. Bony ingrowth fixation of the acetabular component in canine hip joint arthroplasty. Clin. Orthop. 176 (1983) 7-11.
15 L.D. Anderson: Compression plate fixation and the effect of different types of internal fixation on fracture healing. J. Bone Joint Surg. 47A (1965) 191-208.
16 R.L. Cruess, Healing of Bone, Tendon and Ligament, in: C A. Rockwood, Jr. and D.P. Green (eds), Fractures in Adults, Vol. 1, J.B. Lippincott Co., Philadelphia, 1984, pp. 147-160.
17 B. McKibbin: The biology of fracture healing in long bones. J. Bone Joint Surg. 60B (1978) 150-152.
18 J.D. Bobyn, H.U. Cameron, D. Abdulla, R.M. Pilliar and G.C. Weatherby: Biologic fixation and bone remodeling with an unconstrained canine total knee prosthesis. Clin. Orthop. 166 (1982) 301-311.
19 J. Miller, D.L. Burke, J. Stachiewicz and L. Kelebray: The fixation of major load-bearing metal prostheses to bone - An experimental study comparing smooth to porous surfaces in a weight-bearing model. Trans. Orthop. Res. Soc. 1 (1976) 52.

20 R.M. Pilliar, H.U. Cameron, A.G. Binnington and J.A. Szivek: Bone ingrowth and stress shielding with a porous surface coated fracture fixation plate. J. Biomed. Mater. Res 13 (1979) 799-810.
21 T.M. Turner, D.R. Sumner, R.M. Urban, D.P. Rivero and J.O. Galante: A comparative study of porous coatings in a weight bearing total hip arthroplasty model. J. Bone Joint Surg. 68-A (1986) 1396.

Biomaterials and Clinical Applications,
edited by A. Pizzoferrato, P.G. Marchetti, A. Ravaglioli and A.J.C. Lee
Elsevier Science Publishers B.V., Amsterdam, 1987 — Printed in The Netherlands

DESIGN RATIONALE OF INTERFERENCE-FIT TOTAL HIP PROSTHESES

INDONG OH, M.D.

Joint Implant and Orthopaedic Surgery
800 Fairmount Ave. Suite 313
Pasadena, CA. 91105

SUMMARY

It is apparent through the animal experimental as well as human clinical studies that the prerequisites of bone ingrowth fixation are initial interference fit, intimate apposition of bone and maintenance of these two conditions until the bone grows in. So far about 10 percent of the porous area of the total hip implant has shown bone ingrowth under ideal circumstances. Load transfer through such a small area of ingrowth fixation may lead to a high stress concentration to a local area. On the other hand, stress shielding of the majority of non-ingrown area may result in severe bone resorption on long term use. Removal of porous surfaced implants caused severe damage to the remaining bone stock. It is also well known through the past clinical experience that when the implant was fixed tightly to the bone, such fixation has been maintained for a long time without adverse effects. Thus, a well designed femoral stem with wedge shape in two planes for proximal loading and a tight fitting stem in the canal for stability will induce a stable fibrous tissue interface. Also, a partially threaded metal shell acetabular component will achieve immediate stable fixation. A series of macro and microscopic examinations of the surrounding fibrous tissue and bone revealed inactive, bland looking connective tissue which is quite different from the histiocytes laden tissue of the loose cemented stem. This fibrous tissue will transfer load more physiologically over the entire implant - bone interface obviating the chance of stress shielding or concentration and will facilitate removal of the implant without damage to bone. Clinical experience with interference fit implants have been gratifying in primary and in secondary revision cases.

INTRODUCTION

Cemented total hip arthroplasty is one of the most consistently successfull orthopaedic procedures with a clinical success rate of more than 90 percent. However, among those arthroplasties that have failed, late loosening of the fixation has been identified as the major cause of failure (ref. 1-6). Despite the promise of better results with improved cementing techniques and superiorly designed components, it is conceivable that aseptic loosening will eventually occur in young or active patients.

Loosening of the cemented prosthesis with loss of bone stock, difficulties with revision of such failed hip arthroplasty, relatively low success rate of revision surgery and the need for longer-lasting fixation in young or active patients directed attention to total hip arthroplasty in which no bone cement is used. Current cementless implants include those with porous surfaces for bone ingrowth fixation and implants designed to achieve an interference-fit with ensuing fibrous tissue stabilization.

HISTORICAL BACKGROUND

Cementless hip prostheses are not new. Austin-Moore and Thompson prostheses have been used since the 1950's for many arthritic conditions of the hip joint and for displaced femoral neck fracture in the elderly. The erosion of acetabular cartilage by the metallic head over long-term use often produced protrusion and disabling groin pain. Frequently, there also was thigh pain caused by a loose fitting stem and/or torsional motion of a small stem in a large medullary canal. Stem undersizing was frequently unavoidable because essentially there was only one stem size despite variations in stem length.

Despite these limitations, many patients have done well when fitted tightly with the stem remaining stable in the medullary canal over a long period of time. However, many patients required conversion to total hip implants because of acetabular erosion and groin pain. During removal of the well-fitted and stabilized Austin-Moore stem, one usually finds a layer of fibrous tissue between the stem and canal wall. Examined microscopically, this fibrous tissue is very bland inactive, with a scant number of inflammatory cells (ref. 7). A very stable, thin layer of fibrous tissue apparently transmitted the dynamic joint load from the implant to the surrounding bone for a long time. This is a striking contrast to the fibrous tissue, laden with histiocytes and giant cells from a loose cemented femoral component (ref. 8). Apparently, the tightly fitted cementless metal stem reaches a cerain degree of equilibrium with surrounding bone through the fibrous tissue. Another remarkable finding in one postmortem strain gauge study was that a femur implanted with an Austin-Moore prosthesis had a similar stress pattern, as did the nonoperated hip of the same patient (ref. 9).

MECHANICAL AND BIOLOGIC CONSEQUENCES OF INTERFACE FIT IMPLANTS

It is highly likely that fibrous tissue will always form between the bone and nonbiologic implant material as a natural biologic defense barrier. As long as the implant is stably fixed under dynamic load without macromotion, the patient would not experience thigh pain and the fibrous membrane will remain thin, inactive and stabilized. Thus, this fibrous tissue acts as an interposing medium to absorb the impact of loading through the implant to the surrounding bone, transferring load in a more physiologic manner over a larger area of bone-implant interface. This load transfer characteristic would probably obviate stress concentration and help prevent stress-shielded bone resorption. Furthermore, removal of such an implant, should it become necessary, will be less difficult than removal of a cemented or bone ingrowth prosthesis with less chance of damaging surrounding bone. In fact, a long-term follow-up study of well fixed cementless implants shows adaptive bone remodeling around the lengths of the stems (ref. 10).

The author has had extensive experience in revision surgeries for failed cemented or non-cemented hip arthroplasty. In many revision cases with severe osteolysis and deficiency of bone stock, it has not been possible to use cement because of inadequacy of fixation and the risk of further loss of bone in the future. Prompted by the conviction that a well fitted cementless femoral stem will function satisfactorily, the author used custom made long-stemmed prostheses in conjunction with auto or allograft in a series of revision cases (ref.11) The long-stemmed implants provided adequate stability by achieving multiple area contact with the bone along the length of the stem. This group of patients had done very well with little or no thigh pain and radiographs of femurs have shown adaptive bone remodeling around the stem.

Since the 1960's, British surgeon, P.A. Ring, has done extensive series of cementless total hip arthroplasty using a modified Austin-Moore type prosthesis with a high rate of success in over 3,000 cases (ref. 12). Furthermore, Mittelmeier (ref. 13) and Lord (ref.14) who used respectively, ceramic and metal-backed screw-in acetabular cups, reported excellent clinical results after follow-up periods of 7-10 years. These implants were all tight fitting acetabular cups used without cement.

BONE INGROWTH FIXATION BY POROUS IMPLANTS

Another approach to cementless fixation is by bone ingrowth into the porous surface implant. Numerous animal studies have shown that the bone will grow into the optimal pore size provided that implant fixation is rigid, without motion and that the porous surface is in intimate apposition to the bone for 6-12 weeks (refs. 15-18). Experimental studies also have shown that fibrous tissue will grow in when there is motion, a prosthesis gap of even 1 mm or so not permitting bone ingrowth (ref. 19). It is speculated that the best circumstance for bony ingrowth is when the implant is subjected to a compressive mode of loading with negligible shear of tension loading. The complex loading mode of a stem type implant in the femoral medullary canal - mainly shear, tension and little compression loading - makes complete bone ingrowth difficult. In fact, in studies of currently used implants, retrieved from animals and humans, the area of bone ingrowth is minimal and spotty (refs.19-21). The remainder of the large area is filled with fibrous tissue. Histologic analysis of tissue grown into 56 retrieved humans total joint porous prostheses showed minimal (10 percent or less) bone ingrowth into femoral and acetabular component (ref. 22). One third of the cases showed no ingrowth and non-ingrown area showed marked bone resorption with numerous area of osteoclastic activity (ref. 22). Since cementless prostheses are primarily for young or active patients, long term consequences of such a rigid yet spotty fixation is a crucial issue. The potential problems associated with such bone ingrowth fixation with a porous-surface implant are numerous:

Bone Remodeling by Wolff's Law

When bone ingrowth is achieved by the porous implant, load will be concentrated through a small area of rigid fixation and will by-pass a large area without growth. Thus, will there be stress shielded bone resorption around the large area without bone ingrowth or will there be a local area of bone hypertrophy around the small area of bone ingrowth according to Wolff's law (ref.23)? Ring reported severe proximal bone resorption in seven out of 10 cases, nine years after implantation of porous stems (ref. 24) due to rigid distal fixation. The greater and lesser trochanters had gradually avulsed and fractured because of severe bone resorption.

Difficulty of Implant Removal

Can one remove a spottly fixed stem with resorptive area without damaging the surrounding bone stock? Removal of such a stem without destruction of bone will be difficult. Lord abandoned his own porous femoral stem design after 7-8 years of use because of the disastrous difficulties and destruction of bone during stem removal (ref. 25). Ring claims similar difficulty of stem removal with his fully porous-coated stem (ref. 24).

Fatigue Strength of Porous Implant

The sintering process for porous surface fibrication requires varying degrees of heat treatment. This heating process substantially reduces the fatigue strength of the implant due to various microstructural as well as other transformations (refs. 26-28). In addition, the resulting porous area creates notch sensitivity at the sintered surface, a possible stress-raising characteristic that could cause crack initiation and propagation (ref. 18). The porous layer itself also reduces the section modulus of the stem of the porous coated area. The combined effect of these factors raise substantial concerns about femoral stem fatigue fracture, especially in implants intended for long-term use in young, active, heavy patients.

Corrosion and Metal Ion Release

Porous layers substantially increase the surface area of the metal. Consequently, the enlarge metal surface accelerates the corrosion process that it may lead to prosthesis loosening and increases metal ion release (ref. 29). Accumulated metal ion may cause adverse systemic effect as well as toxic effect on the adjacent tissue. Instances of tumor formation from smooth surfaced implants have also been reported (ref. 30).

EARLY CLINICAL EXPERIENCE OF POROUS COATED IMPLANTS

These potential problems associated with porous-surfaced implants became apparent during early clinical trials in Europe. The macroporous Judet prosthesis (ref. 31) is no longer used because of acetabular bone resorption, stem breakage, stem removal difficulty and severe stress shielded bone loss. Likewise, Lord himself has taken off a porous layer from the Madreporique femoral stem after eight years of clinical trials (ref. 25). After 10 years of experience with a full-length porous surface stem, Ring recommended not using such a stem because of similar problems (ref. 24).

In North America, Cameron first reported his experience with a fully porous-coated modified Matchett-Brown prosthesis (ref. 32). Because of many interrelated factors of stem design and patient group, this three-year follow-up study showed no evidence of bone ingrowth. In fact, most of the stems were stabilized with fibrous tissue and had no evidence of stress relief osteoporosis at six-year follow-up (ref. 33). Engh and others reported their experience with fully porous-coated Austin-Moore type stems (ref. 34). Their five-year follow-up study indicated a combination of fibrous and bony tissue ingrowth but without localized stress concentration or bone resorption. It will be interesting to see how this group of patients will do at 10 years compared to those with the similarly designed porous-coated stem of P.A. Ring (ref. 24).

EVOLVING CHANGES OF POROUS IMPLANTS

Long and short-term follow-up studies on porous implants indicate that some of the potential problems are becoming actual concerns. Thus, the current versions of porous-coated implants are going through rapid and serious design changes. Some stems are long and others, short. Some are curved and others, straight. Some have a collar and others do not. Some have a porous coating laterally or medially and some do not. However, the most notable evolution is in the area of porous coating along the stem and the number of porous layers. Initially, there was a full-length coating, but with increasing concern on the effect of bone ingrowth fixation in recent years, it has progressively diminished toward proximally so that certain current prostheses have only minimal coating around the collar of the femoral stem. In addition, fear of firm bone ingrowth fixation into two to three layers of porous area led to a single layer of beads for simple stabilization. The conceptual terminology is also gradually evolving with the increasing knowledge. Only a few years ago, it was a dire wish to achieve bone ingrowth fixation. It is now shifting to bone ingrowth, bone and fibrous tissue ingrowth, and now, tissue ingrowth to tissue stabilization. The author believes that such conceptual expansion is righteous in view of our rapidly increasing knowledge of porous-surface implants. Ironically, if these trends continue, there may be no porous coating on the stem other than a degree of structured surface.

CURRENT CLINICAL TRIAL OF POROUS IMPLANTS

Unlike the early European version of macroporous implant or American version or microporous implants, current porous implants are much more refined in their pore size, layers and area of porous coating. The basic design features of recent cementless prostheses are much more anatomic and comes in many different sizes to achieve initial interference fit. Surgically, recipient bones are prepared much more precisely and the implant is chosen from 7-8 different sizes. It is almost inevitable that most of the implant will achieve interference fit. At the clinical level, short term results with porous implants are reported very favorably. Among many patients who were implanted with porous coated stem which showed definite fibrous tissue interposition on roentgenographs have not changed its appearance in many years nor had any pain according to Engh (ref. 35). The author believes that the reason why most of the patients are doing well is due to this interference fit and stability of fixation.

The cause of pain in a certain number of patients after implantation of cementless prostheses is probably secondary to improper interference fit and of course no bone ingrowth. Even this group of patients generally do well with the passage of time due to secondary stabilization of the prostheses with a certain degree of subsidence. In this case, bone ingrowth to the porous stem is not conceivable and fibrous tissue interposition is a natural consequence. It is well known that once the fibrous tissue forms, no bone will subsequently penetrate through this barrier into the porous area.

Interestingly, the current version of porous total knee prostheses have been used in the belief that the coaptative geometry and the compressive loading nature of knee anatomy will achieve bone ingrowth fixation. After clinically successful trials of such prostheses over the past five years, it has become apparent from many retrieval analyses that no bone ingrowth occurs in the tibial component. Yet this group of patients also did well clinically without appreciable pain. Most of these patients achieved optimal mechanical fit and subsequent fibrous tissue stabilization. If so, is it proof that bone ingrowth fixation is not necessary to achieve a pain free joint?

RATIONALE OF INTERFERENCE FIT IMPLANTS

The ultimate goal of hip arthroplasty is a pain-free joint with lasting fixation. To achieve this goal in a young, active, heavy patient and certain cases of revision total hip, porous implants and interference fit implants are being tried.

Judging from the multiple interrelated factors of fixation and durability as described earlier, it is the author's belief that what is needed presently seems to be a tight-fitting prosthesis that stabilizes itself and achieves equilibrium. Since fibrous tissue interposition is an inevitable biologic consequence under dynamic load against implant material that the crucial issue is how one can make the fibrous tissue remain stable, thin and inactive. Absence of macromotion of the implant will do this, and interference fixation will achieve this goal. Thus, if the design of the implant follows the anatomic shape and size of the recipient bone, an interference fit is possible. Absence of macromotion under dynamic loading will result in a pain-free joint. Likewise, in acetabular reconstruction, a screw-in type of cup achieves immediate firm fixation simply because the threads carve into the sturdy bone structure to make a tighter fit than that possible when a correspondingly shaped cup is fitted to a reamed acetabulum.

Short and long term clinical results of press-fitted, stabilized non-porous prostheses have shown favorable outcomes compared to numerous problems already identified on short and mid-term follow-up porous implants (ref.11). Until proven otherwise, it seems much safer to use interference-fit prostheses to avoid the many potential biologic and mechanical problems associated with the long-term use of porous implants.

DESIGN CONSIDERATIONS OF INTERFERENCE FIT FEMORAL STEM

The design feature of an implant is crucial to achieve interference fit. Even with non-porous prostheses, if the stem is only fixed distally, stress-shielding will occur proximally. Thus, desirable design objectives include; stabilization all along the stem length with loading through the proximal part of the femur.

To achieve this goal, the following design features should be included among others. The wedge-shaped posts at the proximal part of the stem in frontal and sagittal planes will achieve a tight fit and proximal loading (Fig1) The antero-posterior dimension of the stem has to be particularly well matched with the medullary canal geometry by substantially increasing the stem dimension. The midpart of the stem should gradually taper distally according to the medullary canal geometry. The distal part of the stem cross-section may be a crude rectangle, larger in AP than medial-lateral dimension, as in the medullary canal geometry. The dimension of the distal stem should allow maximum contact for stem stability. The length of each stem should reach down to the isthmus area of the medullary canal for neutral positioning and stability.

The four corners of the stem should be rounded to have maximum contact in the medullary canal and to help prevent point contact or point loading.

To further augment stable fixation and torsional stability, locking wings may be placed on the AP surface of the wedge-shaped proximal stem to direct the stem straight down into the medullary canal. In addition, a lateral fin added to the lateral surface of the most proximal stem area will provide torsional stability. Structuring of the anterior and posterior stem surface by small recesses or grooves will accept the cancellous bone debris left along the medullary canal wall during stem insertion. Such structure area increases the surface area without porosity and provides secure fixation and stabilization by fibrous tissue interdigitation.

Anatomically shaped collar on the medial side can be adapted in certain cases. The 20 to 30 degrees collar angle is normal to the resultant joint force and will transfer compression force to the medial neck area. The neck cross-section of the circulotrapezoidal shape provides a large range of motion for stability of the hip joint. The Morse-type taper neck design can accept many different neck lengths and different OD femoral heads for versatility of the system.

The moment arm of abductors and the head-stem offset should be anatomical and proportioned to the stem size and neck length.

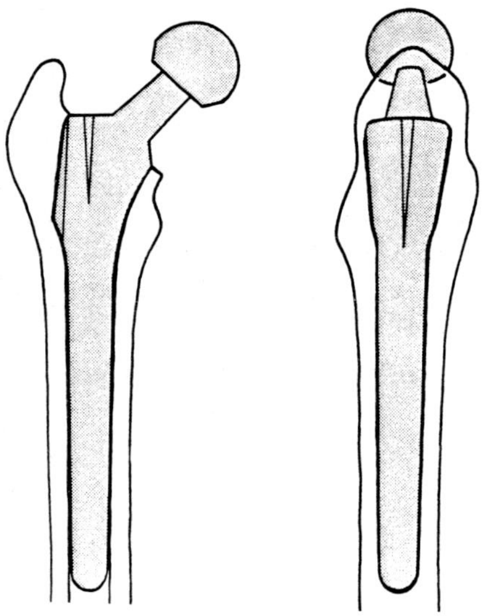

Fig. 1 Double wedge shape design in two planes.

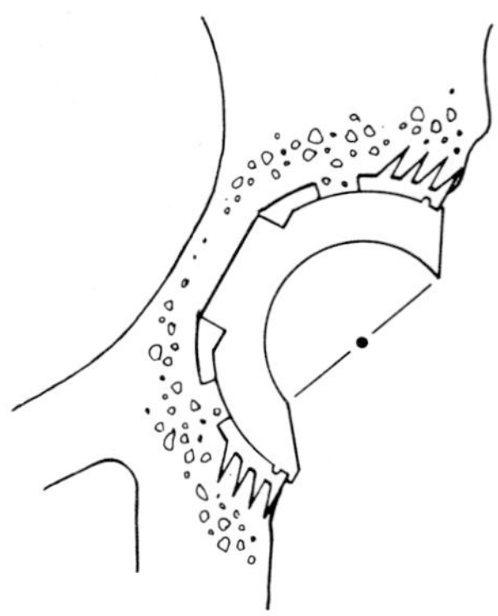

Fig. 2 Partially threaded, open domed, side windowed hemispherical cup.

DESIGN CONSIDERATION OF ACETABULAR METAL SHELL

In order to achieve an immediate rigid fixation and lasting stability of an acetabular component, multiple factors including stable geometry, amount of bone removal, ease of preparation, flexibility in positioning, complete containment of the cup with intimate apposition, capacity to monitor the seating and load transfer pattern were considered. Based on these factors, a partially threaded, open domed, side windowed, low profile, hemispherical metal shell acetabular component seems to satisfy most of these considerations in designing an acetabulum metal shell (Fig. 2). Cylindrical, chamfered-cylindrical, truncated cone and hemispherical metal shells with additional pegs, screws and threads were carefully analyzed. Generally, a hemispherical cup makes its preparation easy and flexible in positioning. In any design, complete containment of the metal shell within the bony acetabulum is desirable to provide lasting fixation under dynamic load. Thus, the metal shell should not be more than hemisphere, otherwise it will protrude beyond the rim of the acetabulum. The metal shell can be slightly less than the hemisphere at the periphery and at the same time the dome area can be cut off to make the shell low profile. When porous coating is adapted, it is essential to expose the bleeding cancellous bone for bone ingrowth fixation. This means more bone has to be removed from the acetabulum and usually the remaining bone surface is a relatively weak cancellous structure. However, for interference fit, removal of only the remaining cartilage and osteophytes are necessary. The remaining bone is a mechanically sturdy structure into which the threads carve for rigid fixation. As the shell is driven further, it makes complete contact with the bone. Generally, only the last one or two rows of thread contributes secure fixation of the implant in engineering principle. Thus, the non-threaded portion of the metal shell can be utilized for some other beneficial design features such as viewing windows that provide the ability to see the direct apposition of cup to bone during implantation. After complete insertion, the bone graft can be packed through them to provide further fixation and stability during future implant life. The open dome of the metal shell will also serve as the driving platform of the metal shell. When implanted correctly into the acetabulum together with the articulating insert, the load transfer should occur radially through the smooth and threaded area of the metal shell as well as through the bone grafted area for lasting durability.

DESIGN FEATURES OF ARTICULATING INSERT

In order to provide an articulating surface for the prosthetic femoral head, a separate insert is desirable. When the metal shell is less than a hemisphere, then the articulating insert can take up the rest of the hemispheric dimension peripherally. The articulating area should at least be hemispherical, to help prevent easier dislocation of the prosthetic femoral head. Further, the articulating insert should be slightly more than a hemisphere to provide bevelling toward the articulating area. This design creates a self-seeking feature facilitating reduction of the prosthetic femoral head.

Anatomically, the abduction and anteversion angles of the natural acetabulum are 50 to 70 degrees and 10 to 20 degrees respectively.

When an acetabular cup is fixed in 60 degrees of abduction, it is likely that the femoral head would dislocate superiorly. Thus, it is desirable to have 20 degrees or so of tilted overhang superiorly in a separate articulating insert itself to achieve a resulting abduction angle of 40 degrees or so. Extending the hemispheric insert laterally makes the overhang protrude substantially out of the metal shell and more importantly displaces the hip rotation center laterally (Fig. 3). This lateralization of the center of hip rotation increases the body weight moment arm and relatively decreases the abductor moment arm. Thus, the resultant joint force will increase and at the same time the resultant joint force direction will lateralize. The lateralized joint force will act on the large overhang portion of the articulating insert which is not covered by the metal shell or under the bony acetabulum. This will tend to rock the insert and may lead to eventual early loosening of the metal shell-polyethylene composite. Furthermore, the laterally protruded large overhand makes the reduction of the femoral head component extremely difficult during surgery and after dislocation.

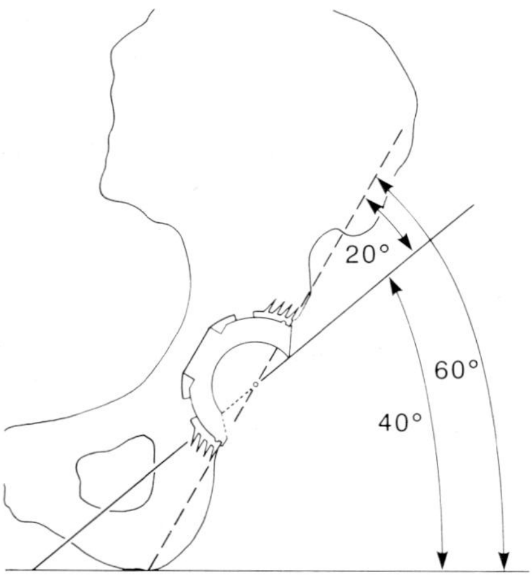

Fig. 3 Maintenance of the same center of hip with minimal overhang.

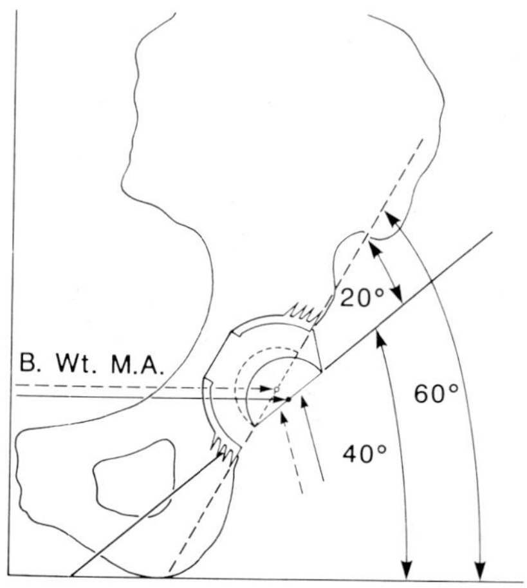

Fig. 4 Biomechanical analysis of lateralization of the center of hip rotation.

In order to achieve a desirable degree of abduction while maintaining the same center of hip rotation, the articulating surface is tilted 20 degrees and the directly opposite portion of the articulating area is recessed (Fig. 4). The resulting overhang becomes quite small without much protrusion. Thus, the cup does not lateralize the center of hip rotation and reduction manuver becomes easy due to the small overhang and self-seeking feature of the insert.

One additional consideration on this separate polyethylene cup is its orientation when inserted into the already implanted metal shell. To provide maximum stability of the joint, the insert can be positioned in any of 12 different positions of 30 degree increments, after trial range of motion testing prior to final locking of the articulating insert. Thus, the gear design at the dome of the polyethylene insert allows optimum orientation of the overhang portion.

CONCLUSION

While cemented total hip arthroplasty in a discreetly selected group of patients will continue to do well, some will loosen with time. The pathophysiological mechanism of loosening is a combination of mechanical as well as biological factors along with wear debris of implant materials.

Despite the numerous potential concerns associated with the bone ingrowth fixation by porous surfaced prostheses in long-term use, the early clinical results in the U.S. have been reported to be favorable. The early clinical results of non-porous interference fit prostheses are also good and equilvalent to that of the porous implant. It is conceivable that both groups of prostheses will do reasonably well because most of the current cementless prostheses are far better designed in regards to anatomic geometry and are available in a wide variety of implant sizes. This makes initial interference fit possible and hence a good result. But it must also be pointed out that as long as cementless prostheses, porous or non-porous, are used there will always be a certain number of patients with incomplete relief of pain until the prostheses achieves an equilibrium status with surrounding bone. Thus, crucial factors in reducing the incidence of painful hip arthroplasty are the design features of the prosthetic component which will provide an interference fit that will last over a long period of time.

The controversial issues at present evolves around porous or non-porous and bone ingrowth fixation or fibrous tissue stabilization. When a porous surface implant is used, bone ingrowth fixation area will be spotty and minimal at best. Will the bone react favorably to this small area of firm fixation through which a majority of the joint load will have to be transferred? Or will the bone resorb severely secondary to stress shielding of a larger area? When a non-porous interference-fit implant is used, such concerns as with the porous implants would not exist. However, will the fibrous tissue remain inactive and carry joint load effectively over a long period of time?

While orthopaedic communities are pursuing two different avenues of implant fixation bone ingrowth vs. interference fit, respective results in these two modes of fixation in the coming years will enrich our knowledge on implant durability. However, given the material characteristics of today, fixation and durability of an artificial implant will depend on the design features of such an implant. All of these features must be throughly thought out and justified.

REFERENCES

1 J. Charnley and Z. Cupic, The nine and ten year results of the low friction arthroplasty of the hip, Clin. Orthop. Rel. Res. Ref.,95(2) (1973) pp.9-25.
2 R.D. Beckenbaugh and D.M. Ilstrup, Total hip arthroplasty: A review of three hundred and thirty-three cases with long follow-up, J. Bone and Joint Surg., Ref., 60-A(1) (1978) pp. 306-313.
3 M.J. Griffith, M.K. Seidenstein, D. Williams and J. Charnley, Eight year results of Charnley arthroplasties of the hip with special reference to the behavior of cement, Clin. Orthop. Rel. Res., Ref., 137(2) (1978) pp. 24-36.
4 P.M. Pellicci, E.A. Salvati and H.J. Robinson, Mechanical failures in total hip replacement requiring reoperation, J. Bone and Joint, Ref.,61-A(1) (1979) pp. 28-36.
5 R.N. Stauffer, Ten year follow-up study of total hip replacement: With particular reference to roentgenographic loosening of the components, J. Bone and Joint Surg., 64-A(1) (1982) pp 983-990.
6 B.F. Kavanagh, D.M. Ilstrup and Fitzgerald, Revision total hip arthroplasty, J. Bone and Joint Surg., 67-A(1) (1985) pp 517-526.
7 S.C. Kozinn, N.A. Johnson and P.G. Bullough, The biological interface of cementless hip endoprostheses. The Journal of Arthroplasty, Vol. 1 #4 1986.
8 J. Charnley, Low friction arthroplasty of the hip, Theory and practice, Springer-Verlag, Berlin, 1979.
9 S.B. Murphy, P.S. Walker and A.L. Schiller, Adaptive changes in the femur after implantation of an Austin-Moore prosthesis, J. Bone and Joint Surg., 66-A(1) (1984) pp 437-443.
10 F. Vandnedriessche, R. Verdonk, J. Ven Dooren and H. Claessens, The Austin Moore prosthesis. A long term follow-up, Acta Orthop. Belg, 49 (1983) pp. 483-494.
11 I. Oh, Total hip replacement arthroplasty update: Cementless and revision with smooth stem, AAos Summer Institute, Monterey, CA. Sept. 22-26, 1986.
12 P.A. Ring, Ring UPM total hip arthroplasty, Clin. Ortho. Rel. Res., ref. 176(2) (1983) pp. 115-123.
13 H. Mittelmeier, J. Heisel and E. Schmitt, The first decade of clinical experience with a cemented ceramic total hip, AAOS Program, Las Vegas, NE., 1985.
14 G. Lord and P. Bencel, The madreporic cementless total hip arthroplasty. Clin. Ortho. Rel. Res., Ref. 176(2) (1983) pp 67-76.
15 U.H. Cameron, R.M. Pilliar and I. Macnab, The rate of bone ingrowth into porous metal, J. Biomat. Res., Ref. 10(1) (1976) pp 295-302.
16 S.D. Cook, K.A. Walsh and R.J. Haddad, Interface mechanics and bone growth into porous Co-Cr-Mo alloy implants, Clin. Ortho. Rel. Res., Ref. 193(2) (1975) pp 271-280.
17 R.P. Welsh, R.M. Pilliar and I. Macnab, Surgical implants. The role of surface porosity in fixation to bone and acrylic. J. Bone and Joint Surg. 53-A(1) (1971) pp 963-977.

18 R.M. Pilliar, Powder metal-made orthopedic implants with porous surface for fixation by tissue ingrowth, Clin Ortho. Rel. Res., Ref. 176(2) (1983) pp 42-51.
19 M. Jasty, S.P. Rogers, E.H. Weinberg and W.H. Harris, The role of uniform surgical fit on bone ingrowth into porous-coated canine acetabular replacement, Trans. 31st Ann. ORS, ref.10(1) (1985) pp. 167.
20 R. Rosenquist, B. Bylander, K. Knutson and et al., Loosening of the porous ing of biocompartmental prostheses in patients with rheumatoid arthritis, J. Bone and Joint Surg., Ref. 68-A(1) (1986) pp. 538-542.
21 P.K. Buchert, B.K. Vaughn, T.H. Mallory, et al., Excessive metal release due to loosening and fretting of sintered particles on porous-coated hip prostheses. Report of two cases, J. Bone and Joint Surg., Ref. 68-A (1) (1986) pp. 606-609.
22 K.A. Thomas, S.D. Cook, R.J. Hadad, et al., Histologic analysis of tissue growth into retrieved human total joint components, Trans of ORS, Ref. 12 (1) (1987) pp. 432.
23 R.W. Treharne, Review of Wolff's law and its proposed means of operation, Ortho. Rev., Ref. 10(1) (1981) pp 35-47.
24 I.W. Brown and P.A. Ring, Osteolytic changes in the upper femoral shaft following porous-coated hip replacement, J. Bone and Joint Surg., Ref. 67-B(1) (1985) pp. 218-221.
25 G. Lord, "G. Lord universal polarized prosthesis cementless biological fixation, yet extractable." Translation of Sanortho Company Publication, 1985.
26 "Fatigue and porous-coated implants." Technology in Orthopaedics Services, Zimmer Publication 85-000-0000-0287, 1984.
27 S.D. Cook, F.S. Georgett, H.B. Skinner and R.J. Haddad, Fatigue properties of carbon and porous-coated TI-6Al-4V alloy, J. Biomater, Res., Ref. 18 (1) (1984) pp. 497-512.
28 F.S. Georgette and J.A. Davidson, The effect of hip'ing on the fatigue and tensile strength of a cast, porous-coated Co-Cr-Mo alloy. Soc. Biomater Trans., Ref. 8(1) (1985) pp. 118.
29 T.J. Jorgensen, F. Munno, T.G. Mitchell and D. Hungerford, Uninary cobalt levels in patients with porous Austin-Moore prostheses, Clin. Ortho. Rel. Res., Ref. 176(1) (1983) pp 124-126.
30 H.G. Penman and P.A. Ring, Osteosarcoma in association with total hip replacement. J. Bone and Joint Surg., Ref. 66-B(1) (1984) pp. 632-634.
31 R. Judet, M. Signier, B. Brumpt and T. Judet, A non-cemented total hip prosthesis, Clin. Ortho. Rel. Res., Ref. 137(2) (1978) pp. 76-86.
32 H.U. Cameron, The results of early clinical trials with a microporous coated metal hip prosthesis, Clin. Orthop. Rel. Res., Ref.165(2) (1982) pp. 188-190.
33 H.U. Cameron, six-year results with microporous-coated metal cup prosthesis, Clin. Orthop. Ref. 208(2) (1986) pp. 81.
34 C.A. Engh, Hip arthroplasty with a Moore porsthesis with porous coating: A five year study. Clin Ortho. Rel. Res., Ref. 176(2) (1983) pp. 52-66.
35 C.A. Engh, Total hip replacement arthroplasty update with cementless and revision - ingrowth - collared, AAOS Summer Institute, Monterey, CA. Sept. 22-26, 1986.

Biomaterials and Clinical Applications,
edited by A. Pizzoferrato, P.G. Marchetti, A. Ravaglioli and A.J.C. Lee
Elsevier Science Publishers B.V., Amsterdam, 1987 — Printed in The Netherlands

STEM-BONE MICROMOTION IN NON-CEMENTED HIP PROSTHESES

H. McKELLOP, E. EBRAMZADEH, A. SARMIENTO, P. NIEDERER

Orthopaedic Biomechanics Laboratory, Department of Orthopaedics, University of Southern California, 2400 S. Flower Street, Los Angeles, California, U.S.A., 90007

SUMMARY

The relative motion between total hip prostheses and the surrounding femoral bone were measured for cemented and non-cemented designs in a laboratory model. Considerable tightening of the non-cemented stems occurred during cyclic loading, with final micromotions on the order of hundreds of microns or less. Firm distal wedging of one stem design significantly reduced micromotion.

INTRODUCTION

The purpose of this study was to measure the bone-prosthesis motion in cemented and non-cemented prostheses to determine the effects of stem designs and implantation techniques on the resultant micromotion. Although Cameron and colleagues (ref. 1) stated in 1973 that bone ingrowth will occur in the presence of "micromovement" but not of "macromovement", these terms have not been defined on a quantitative basis. With porous-coated or press-fit prosthetic joints excessive motion between the implant and surrounding bone may lead to tissue necrosis, bone resorption, pain and implant loosening. It may prevent bone ingrowth and even cause separation of the coating material from the implant through a fatigue process (ref. 2).

PROCEDURE

The prostheses were inserted into potted proximal femurs using appropriate instruments and surgical techniques. Synthetic plastic femurs were used to reduce the experimental variation caused by differences in bone quality and geometry among human cadaver femurs. The plastic femurs were formed by copying the outer geometry of a human femur using silastic moulds (Dow Corning Type E). The femur was then sectioned length-wise and the cancellous bone carefully removed, leaving an intact cortical shell. The inner cancellous geometry was then copied using silastic, with locating pins embedded, and a cancellous mater mould constructed. Multiple cancellous cores were then formed using polyurethane foam (Polyol Isocyanate) and cast with fiber-glass reinforced epoxy resin (Ciba Geigy 6010 resin with 956 hardener and Owens Corning fiberglass powder) to form the cortex (Fig. 1). The elastic modulus of the polyurethane was 75 to 100 MPa, compared to a range of 13 to 300 MPa that has been measured for cancellous bone in the trochanteric region (ref. 3). The modulus of the epoxy was 7 to 10 Giga Pascals, about one-half that of cortical bone. Three to seven tests were run in plastic bone for each stem design, with at least two cadaver femurs included for comparison.

We tested a cemented Muller stem to provide a minimum micro-motion baseline. The non-cemented stems included an Austin Moore press-fit hemiarthroplasty (Howmedica), a design that has been in clinical use for about 35 years, a newly developed CLS press-fit stem (Protek) that achieved fixation by combined wedging of the stem and cancellous interdigitation of fins on the anterior and posterior faces, and the PCA stem (Howmedica) with porous bead coating on the proximal portion. The PCA differed from the other stems in that it had an anterior-posterior bow to match the curvature of the proximal femur.

After stem insertion a rigid aluminum frame was fastened to the bone using pointed screws (Fig. 2). Three displacement transducers mounted on this frame contacted the prosthesis to record axial sinking, medial shifting and A-P motion of the head during torsional loading (i.e., rotational motion). A 2000N load was applied to the femoral head while the axial and medial displacements were recorded. The axial load was then held constant while $\pm$ 10 Nm torque was applied about the shaft and the rotational displacements were recorded. The prosthesis was then subjected to 5000 walking load cycles of zero to 2000N (sinusoidal at 1 Hz) while the sinking and medial shifting were recorded. Axial, medial and rotational motion under 2000N and $\pm$ 10 Nm torque were again measured after the 5000 walking cycles.

RESULTS

Fig. 3 shows the axial motion due to 2000N load on the first load cycle compared to after 5000 cycles. The "x" symbols represent plastic bone experiments, other symbols represent cadaver tests. The bars represent mean values for plastic bones only. The cemented stem showed minimal motion. The negative axial motion recorded in one experiment probably corresponded to slight tilting of that prosthesis under load. The non-cemented CLS and Moore stems displaced up to several millimeters on the initial load but only a few tenths of a millimeter or less after cycling. Clearly, micromotion should be compared only after sufficient cyclic loading to firmly seat the prostheses. This is the motion that will have clinical significance. Comparing the three non-cemented designs after cyclic, none of the differences were statistically significant ($p < 0.05$ by the Student t-test).

The magnitudes of the medial motions were comparable to those in the axial direction and will not be discussed here. The motions measured with cadaver femurs tended to fall into the low end of the range with plastic femurs, possibly due to the higher elastic modulus for the cadaver cortical bone. In general, the trends exhibited in the plastic bones were the same as those with cadaver femurs, although we do not yet have sufficient cadaver data to assess this statistically.

Fig. 4 compares the rotational motion of the stems due to 10 Nm torque. There was little difference before versus after cyclic loading, due to the fact that the torque measurements were taken after a 2000N axial load had seated the prosthesis. The differences in rotational motion for the various stem designs were not statistically significant ($p > 0.05$).

An example of the effect of insertion technique is shown in Fig. 5, comparing the micromotion of the CLS prosthesis for proximal compared to distal wedging. That is, the CLS stems were initially inserted with only minimal wedging of the distal stem in the intramedullary canal. In a second series the prostheses were inserted several millimeters more distally and firmly impacted to jam the stem in the canal. The motion on the left in each box in Fig. 5 represents proximal wedging and the right distal wedging. The motions were significantly less for distal wedging. For this particular stem secure distal wedging improved initial stability.

CONCLUSION

The plastic bone and micromotion apparatus provided a valuable tool for quantifying the initial stability of non-cemented prostheses. The same techniques could be applied to total knee replacements. The model appeared to be more useful in evaluating the effect of alternate design features on a single type of stem, as opposed to rating the micromotion of two very different stem designs.

It is recognized that these measurements cannot include effects due to long term bone remodelling. Rather, the experiment is intended to assess the initial stability that will likely effect ingrowth or bone resorption.

We are continuing to experiment with other epoxy formulations to more closely approximate cortical bone properties. Detailed instructions for fabrication of the model bones can be obtained by contacting the author (H. McKellop).

We would like to acknowledge financial support from Protek of Bern, Switzerland and the Doctor's Education and Research Foundation of Orthopaedic Hospital, Los Angeles, California, U.S.A.

REFERENCES

1 H.U. Cameron, R.M. Pilliar and I. McNab, The effect of movement on the bonding of porous metal to bone, J. Biomed. Mat. Res., 7, (1973) 301-311.
2 R. Rosenqvist, B. Bylander, K. Knutson, U. Rydholm, B. Rooser, N. Egund and L. Lingren, Loosening of the porous coatings of bicompartmental prostheses in patients with rheumatoid arthritis, J. Bone Jt. Surg., 68-A(4) (1986) 538-542.
3 M. Martens, R. Van Andekerche, P. Delport and P. De Meester, The mechanical characteristics of cancellous bone at the upper femoral region, J. Biomechanics, 16, (1983) 971-984.

Fig. 1. Photograph showing plastic femur (top) & potted cadaver femur (bottom).

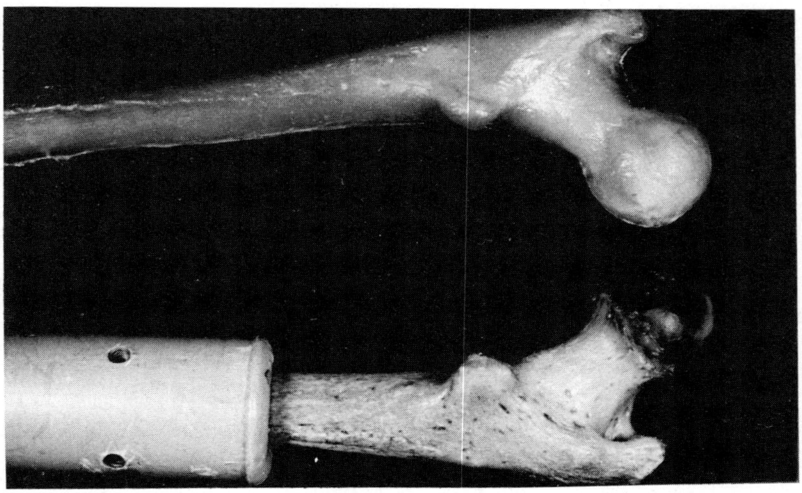

Fig. 2. Photograph showing transducers mounted on femur inside load frame.

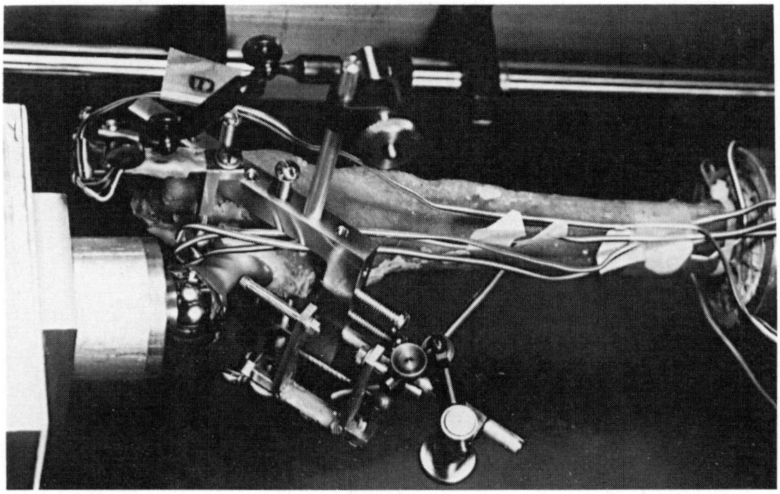

Fig. 3.

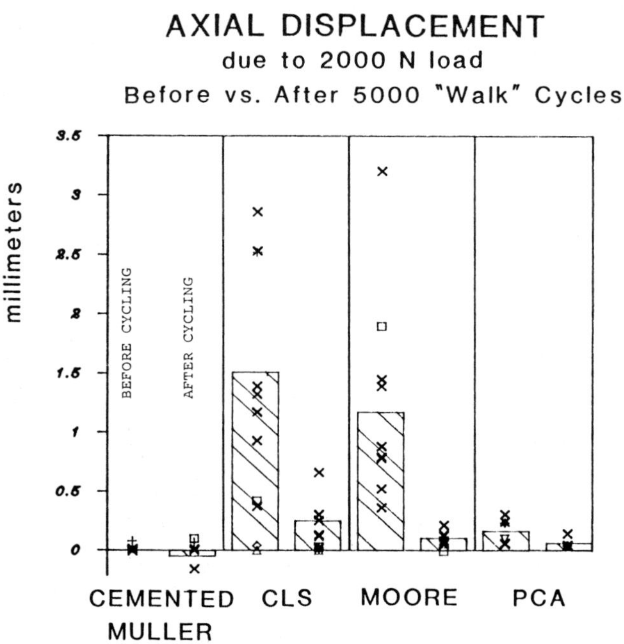

Fig. 4.

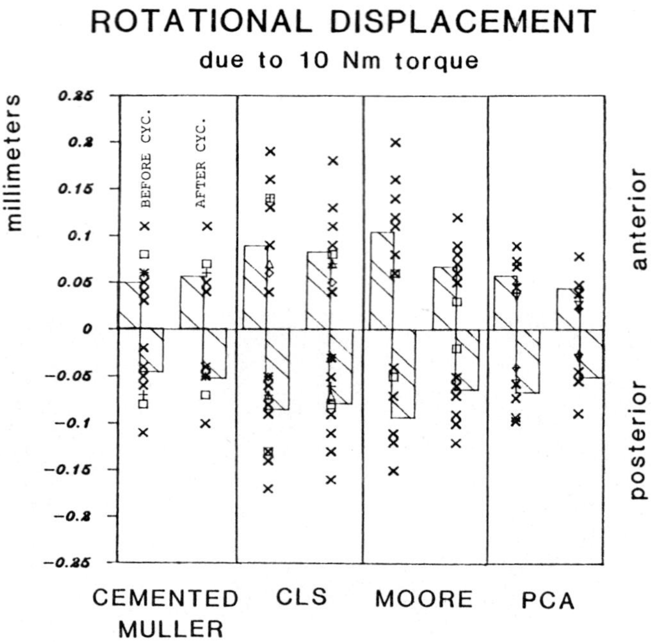
ROTATIONAL DISPLACEMENT
due to 10 Nm torque
millimeters
0.25
0.2
0.15
0.1
0.05
0
-0.05
-0.1
-0.15
-0.2
-0.25
BEFORE CYC.
AFTER CYC.
anterior
posterior
CEMENTED MULLER
CLS
MOORE
PCA

Fig. 5.

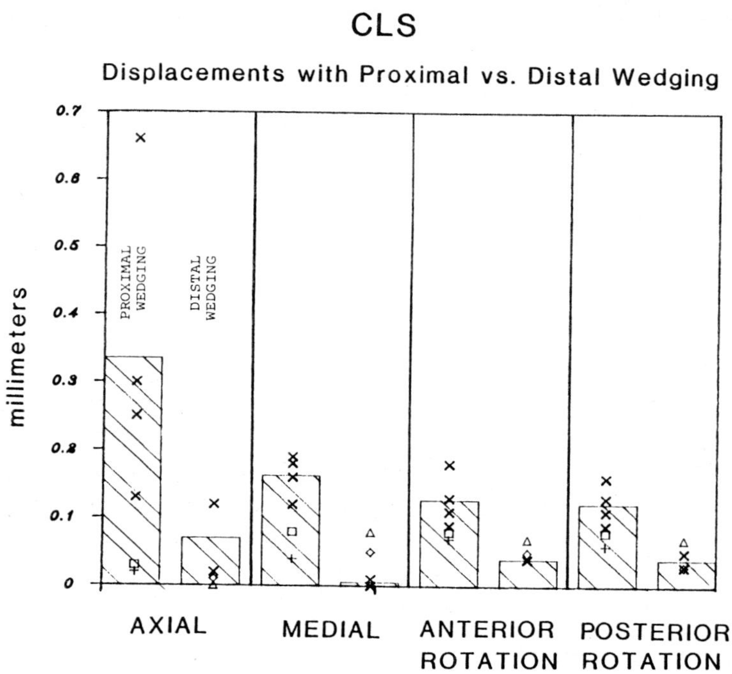
CLS
Displacements with Proximal vs. Distal Wedging
millimeters
0.7
0.6
0.5
0.4
0.3
0.2
0.1
0
PROXIMAL WEDGING
DISTAL WEDGING
AXIAL
MEDIAL
ANTERIOR ROTATION
POSTERIOR ROTATION

Biomaterials and Clinical Applications,
edited by A. Pizzoferrato, P.G. Marchetti, A. Ravaglioli and A.J.C. Lee
Elsevier Science Publishers B.V., Amsterdam, 1987 — Printed in The Netherlands

PRELIMINARY EXPERIENCE WITH CEMENTLESS POROUS COATED ANATOMIC (P.C.A.) TOTAL HIP REPLACEMENT: THE FIRST 180 CONSECUTIVE CASES

P.G.MARCHETTI*, R.BINAZZI*, V.VACCARI* and L.PONZIANI*

* 2nd Orthopaedic Dept. University of Bologna - Istituto Ortopedico Rizzoli - Via Codivilla 9 - Bologna (Italy)

SUMMARY

Cementless fixation is a very satisfactory solution for Total Hip Replacement. In this paper we describe our experience with Porous Coated Anatomic (P.C.A.) Total Hip Arthroplasty, in the first 70 consecutive cases. In all patients, the prosthesis was applied without the use of cement.

The clinico-radiographical results have been very good, even if the technique had to be partially modified with time.

Absolutely indispensable is the initial stability of the implant, in order to allow complete bone ingrowth.

Key words: Hip Arthroplasty, Cementless fixation

INTRODUCTION

Several years ago, when considering the great problems associated with the use of cement, we tried other proposed solutions for the fixation of total hip replacement components.

In this field, there have been a number of studies introducing the concept of "biological fixation", based on the bone ingrowth into porous metallic materials. These studies led to the production of prosthetic models, to be applied without the use of cement, which gave extremely encouraging results. (ref. 1) .

MATERIALS and METHODS

We have employed, in all our cases, the Porous Coated Anatomic (P.C.A.) Total Hip Replacement, which consists of three separate components.

The acetabular component has an outer shell of Vitallium alloy, coated with a double layer of sintered beads, providing three-dimensional porosity. Along the rim of this component there are two fixation pegs providing stability against rotation movements.

The femoral component is also covered with a porous coating, but only in the proximal one third, to eliminate the possibility of proximal stress shielding. The stem has an anatomical design with an anteverted neck.

We think that the P.C.A. Hip has a certain number of advantages: the anatomic stem increases the surface area contact between the prosthesis and bone, with a more uniform stress distribution. The femoral head components are available in two styles, each with an internal taper of different depth, allowing a choice of two effective neck lengths with each size stem.

The two types of cups (Low profile and Deep socket) allow the restoration of the normal center of rotation of the Hip joint.

The instruments are simple and valid, even if we have never used the devices designed for the neck cutting, which, in our opinion, are completely useless.

The porous coating is applied only to the proximal third of the stem, allowing biological stabilisation of the prosthesis. The distal two thirds of the stem, though, are smooth, to avoid stress shielding.

From June 1984 to September 1986, we have implanted 180 P.C.A. Hip Prostheses. All prostheses have been implanted without the use of cement.

We evaluated the first 70 cases.

The average follow-up was of 18 months (RANGE = 12-27 months). One patient has been operated on bilaterally; most of our patients were female and their average age over 55 years.

The etiology of the first 70 cases we have considered was: Osteoarthritis 39 cases (56%), Dysplastic Arthritis 14 (20%), Osteonecrosis 8 (11%), Trauma 5 (7%), Rheumatoid Arthritis 2 (3%), Tubercular Arthritis 1 and Revision 1.

All our patients have been evaluated pre- and post-operatively with the protocol of Hungerford.

Almost 30% of the cases showed an evident Trendelenburg and 51% of them showed a limb shortening over one centimeter (RANGE = 1-4 cm.).

The average pre-operative flexion was 66 degrees.

No patient could walk for more than 500 metres and 82% could not negotiate stairs normally.

SURGICAL TECHNIQUE

The patient is in the supine position, and the skin incision is almost linear.

We isolate and retract the Glutei muscles which are divided anteriorly from the Trochanter. Once the capsule is removed and the femoral head dislocated, we cut the neck fairly long. We then start to prepare the acetabulum.

Along the supero-lateral margin we prepare the seating of the two pegs of the acetabular component, which is then inserted.

We then pass to the femoral side, using the flexible reamers, if necessary.

It is always better to perform a trial reduction before inserting the definitive stem.

We reinsert the Glutei muscles very accurately and then we apply a below-knee cast in internal rotation, to avoid post-op. dislocation, which, however, we have never observed.

We allow ambulation with partial weight-bearing in the fifth post-op day. Full weight-bearing is allowed at one month and a half.

RESULTS

Regarding the results obtained with the first 70 cases, only three patients have complained of mild and intermittent pain; the limp showed by 5 patients was due to diseases involving the controlateral limb.

No case showed Trendelenburg; only 9 patients had residual shortening of the limb, however inferior to 1 and a half centimeters.

The average flexion rose from 66 to 100 degrees.

All patients could walk for more than two kilometers, except the 5 previously mentioned, with controlateral limb pathology and a sixth patient, who, post-op, had a severe myocardial infarction.

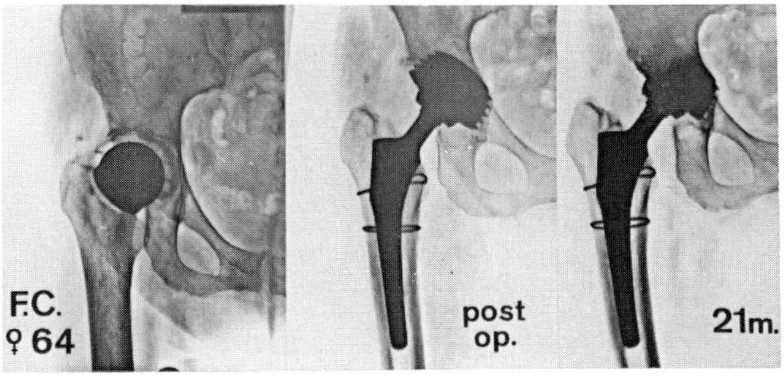

Fig. 1. Female, 64 year-old. The patient had a cemented surface replacement performed 4 years before, successively loosened and painful.
Revision with cementless P.C.A. stem and self-locking screw-ring. During the insertion of the stem, a vertical fracture of Calcar occurred, requiring a double circular wiring. Excellent clinical result.

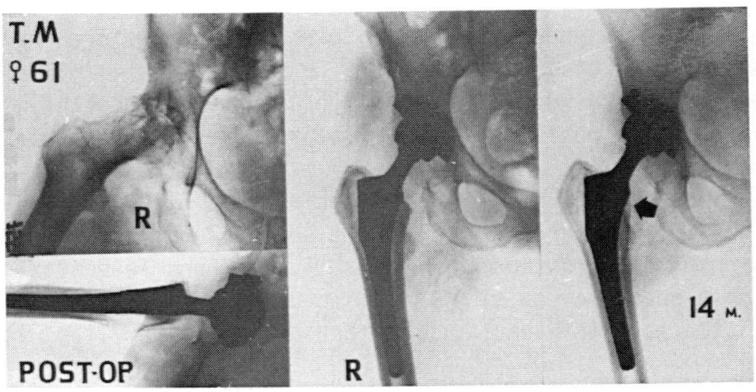

Fig. 2. Female, 61 year-old. Correct size and placement of the prosthetic components. Notice the atrophy of Calcar. Excellent result at 14 months.

All patients, except the same 5 ones, were negotiating stairs correctly and only 6 used a support

COMPLICATIONS

Regarding complications, we observed 3 vertical cracks of the medial Calcar

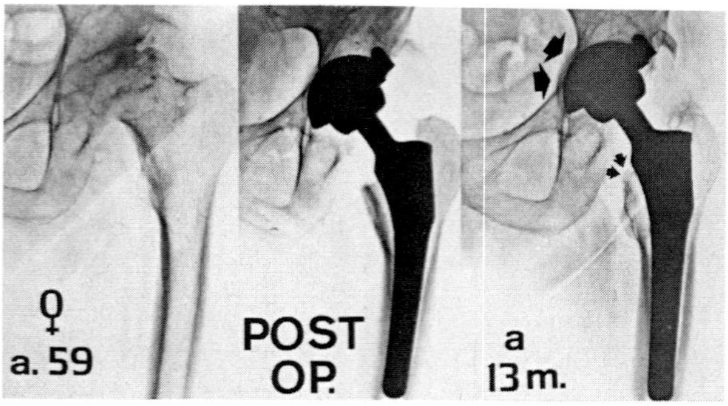

Fig. 3. Female, 59 year-old. Notice, at 13 months, the atrophy of the Calcar and the evident covering of the acetabular component with new bone. In this case the Lamina Quadrilatera had been broken through during the operation. The clinical result was excellent.

region (Fig. 1), fixed with circular wiring, one Phlebitis, 4 urinary tract infection, 4 deep hematomas and periarticular ossification. All cases healed completely and ossifications did never interfere with Hip function.

Regarding the vertical wiring of fracture of the Calcar, today, we do not advise such procedure any more, since our experience has taught us that the wiring is totally useless.

CONCLUSIONS

Considering our fairly short average follow-up, we cannot draw definitive conclusions, but only make some observation;

1) the lateral approach we always have used is very satisfactory, because the patient is in the supine position and does not require any particular positioning;

2) the partial detachment of Glutei muscles did not give us, as we thought, any complication, but the surgeon must take a special care to resuture it;

3) positioning of the prosthesis requires minimal bone resections, leaving good chances for a possible revision (which we never had to do);

4) the operation is fairly short, once the surgeon is familiar with the instruments;

5) it is absolutely mandatory for the initial stability of the implant that, especially in the femoral side, the right size is used. (Fig. 2-3)

Regarding this, we found the flexible reamers absolutely indispensable, allowing a perfect seating of the stem inside the femoral canal;

6) this prosthesis is well tolerated by the patients that, in particular, do not complain of any pain localised at the anterior-upper third of the femur, as they do with other prosthetic models having a different conception.

REFERENCES

1 D. Hungerford, Total Hip Arthroplasty: Clinical Results with the P.C.A. Hip, in: Williams & Wilkils, Baltimore, 1986.

Biomaterials and Clinical Applications,
edited by A. Pizzoferrato, P.G. Marchetti, A. Ravaglioli and A.J.C. Lee
Elsevier Science Publishers B.V., Amsterdam, 1987 — Printed in The Netherlands

SOME ASPECTS OF FAILURE ANALYSIS OF EX VIVO CEMENTLESS IMPLANTED CERAMIC TO CERAMIC TOTAL HIP JOINT PROSTHESES

A. WALTER, TH. MITTLMEIER and G. WASMER

Labor für Biomechanik und experimentelle Orthopädie, Orthopädische Klinik und Poliklinik der Universität München, Staatliche Orthopädische Klinik München, Harlachingerstr. 51, D-8000 München 90, FRG

SUMMARY

At present estimated 3 to 5 per cent of the total number of total hip replacements performed in the FRG make use of the alumina-alumina ceramic material combination.

Despite some encouraging clinical observations in vitro testing and damage analysis of retrieved self-paired alumina ceramic hip joint prostheses have shown that subsurface contact stresses in the tribo-contact zone could initiate a surface deterioration with eventual formation of massive abrasive wear or even inductionof component fracture. The subsequent investigation demonstrates that in 13 total hip joints out from 46 retrieved couples (4 different prosthesis designs) rim contact or subluxation phenomena had occurred in vivo which presumably are not the consequence of obvious component loosening or prosthesis dysfunction. This could primarily be ascribed to the particular prosthesis design characteristics or the unfavourable implant position.

INTRODUCTION

Clinical experience with polycrystalline alumina ceramic to ceramic total hip replacement (THR) exists now for periods up to 15 years (ref.1)

This type of self-paired bearing had once been supposed to solve the life-time limiting problem of tribologically stressed load bearing couples of bio-aterials owing to its outstanding wear-resistance and the good biocompatibility of the bulk material and its wear particles within a wide range of size distribution (ref.2).

Though experimental and, in particular, clinical results on the wear performance of various ceramic THR designs are quite contradictory (survey at ref.3) wear has repeatedly been denied to play an essential role in ceramic to ceramic THR dysfunction or loosening (ref.1,4). The occurrence of wear has been regarded as a consequence of loosening (ref.1) or had been attributed mainly to "clinically exceptional" situations as an obvious malposition of the implant at insertion or a subluxation of the prosthesis components (ref.5).

Now the objective of the present analysis was to correlate specific implant design characteristics and available clinical parameters with material properties and wear phenomena found in retrieved total ceramic THR components.

Since the mechanism of wear generation of self-paired alumina THR, or, at worst, the mechanism of component fracture in vivo and in vitro had already been discussed in detail (ref. 6-9) our main present interest was directed to the analysis of ex vivo total ceramic THR regarding contact areas and wear phenomena beyond the common tribo-contact zone which usually means a type of rim wear or the contact between non-polished ceramic or between ceramic and metal surfaces.

MATERIAL AND METHODS

Our retrospective retrieval collective consists of 46 explanted alumina couples implanted between 1975 and 1982 (implantation period ranging from 0.25 to 9.5 years). 4 different types of prosthetic design corresponding to 4 different manufacturers had been included (table 1). The main indication for reoperation had been aseptic loosening of one or both prosthesis components. Due to the way of supply of the retrieved components the collective can not represent a statistically relevant distribution regarding the number of failures with respect to the prosthesis model.

The verification of wear included the registration of the deviation from sphericity of both components which only represents minimum wear depth data since this method can not establish a concentric loss of material. Wear areas and "extra-articular" contact zones were registered by planimetry and examined by stereomicroscopy and, in part, by SEM and EDX analysis.

All objects regarded met the requirements of ISO 6474 with respect to the chemical composition and the standard average grain size of 7 microns within a confidence limit (ref. 10).

The clinical investigation included a radiographical analysis of the primary implant position and an examination of an eventual component migration during

TABLE 1
Description of the retrieval collective (n=46)

MODEL	NUMBER	CAUSE OF REVISION					
		LOOSENING			FRACTURE		INFECTION
		CUP	STEM	CUP+STEM	CUP	BALL	
A	11	3	2	3	0	2	1
B	26	3	6	11	4	0	2
C	07	0	5	2	0	0	0
D	02	1	0	0	0	1	0
TOTAL	46	7	13	16	4	3	3

the implantation period and a registration of the implant bed reaction as visible on the X-ray.

RESULTS AND DISCUSSION

Sphericity deviation in cup specimens varied between 0.0 and 3,700 microns and in retrieved balls between 0.0 and 840 microns. The ample range of values prevented us from calculating a constant wear rate which would imply a linear correlation of material loss and implantation period. This appears rather unlikely according to our results from wear quantification in wear-screening and hip joint simulator studies (ref.7). In our opinion, the conclusion from single wear data to wear kinetics is not allowed.

Clear evidence of a correlation of the implant period and our wear data was not demonstrable apart from the fact that increasing wear at the cup side corresponds to an increasing wear on the femoral ball side (p 0.0001, Spearman rank correlation test) which may point to boundary lubrication conditions in vivo. This fact is little surprising since the registration of sphericity deviations - in contrast to direct wear data as a gravimetrical wear quantification - may comprise rather complex and even contrary wear processes: in simulator specimens even a cup sphericity improvement had become evident with increasing number of loading cycles (ref. 7). There is no indication of a plain correlation between the mean grain size and the wear data; the same applies to the density which characterizes, as a material constant, the strength-determining porosity.

A correlation of the implant position as defined by the acetabular (AC) angle and the femoral shaft- prosthesis stem (CCD) angle and the wear data did not point to the importance of an "exceptional implant position" for the generation of wear. Moreover, 80 per cent of our retrieved implants correspond to the recommendations for an adequate implant position (AC angle 30 - 55 deg., CCD angle 125-140 deg.). There exists no unequivocal proof of wear caused by loosening in acetabular cups with central wear.

On the other hand, 13 out of 46 THR specimens show clear signs of rim wear. The depth and the constant direction of the wear tracks let it appear quite unlikely that the wear phenomena happened accidentally as one would expect in predominantly loose THR components. Fig.1 visualizes that the implant position, essentially the inclination of the cup in the frontal plane (beside the ante- or retroversion in the horizontal plane) and the design characteristics of the stem neck and the cup rim determine the range of motion possible without rim contact or subluxation phenomena. In our opinion, rim contact phenomena may predominantly occur at the anterior aspect of the joint during everyday activities of the patient, primarily in taking a seat or rising from a chair or

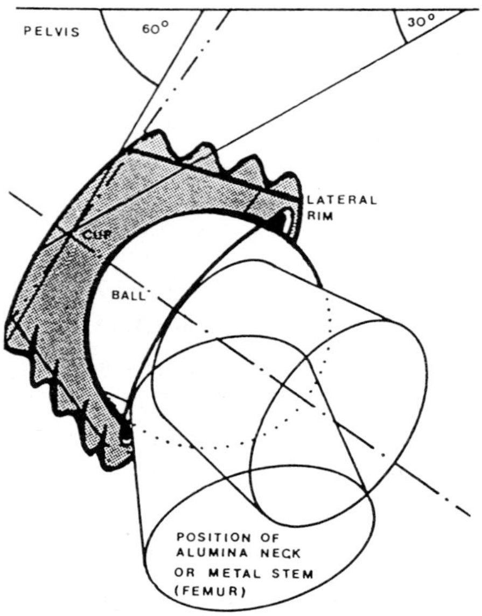

Fig.1: Schematic representation of a ceramic couple demonstrating the limits of motion due to design or alignment

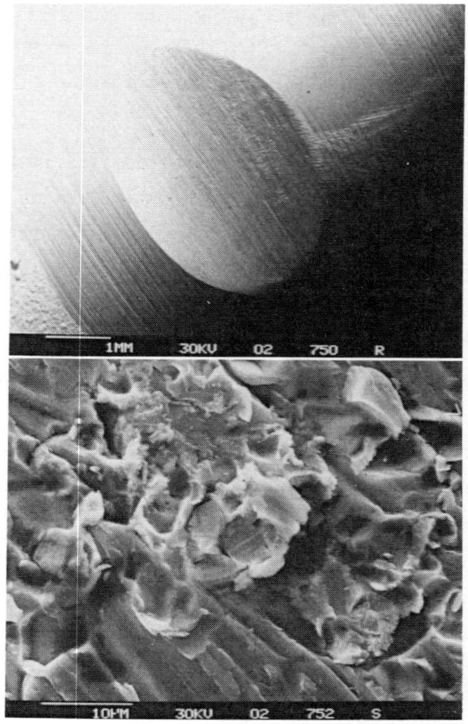

Fig. 2: Extra-articular circumferential contact between a CoCr-alloy neck and the cup rim (no subluxation)

during ascending or descending stairs where a higher degree of flexion and adduction is needed. A flat position of an acetabular cup as recommended for an optimized load distribution in the main load-bearing area at the supero-lateral part of the cup will limit the degree of flexion possible even more in the prosthesis models discussed here.

Up to 40 per cent more motion angle may be provided if the cup rim is not contacted by a large-dimensioned femoral component with a projecting collar which nowadays has become obsolete in a prosthesis model included in our analysis.

Theoretically, in rim contact phenomena we can expect ceramic-to-metal (e.g. contact between the metal neck or collar and the ceramic cup) and ceramic-to-ceramic wear (e.g. contact between the ceramic neck or collar and the cup).

Fig.2. depicts a 200 microns deep notch in the metal neck of a ceramic THR which had been implanted for 9.5 years. The upper part of the micrograph demonstrates the wear tracks running in a predominantly circumferential direction which does not point to any luxation phenomenon. The sharp-edged particles on

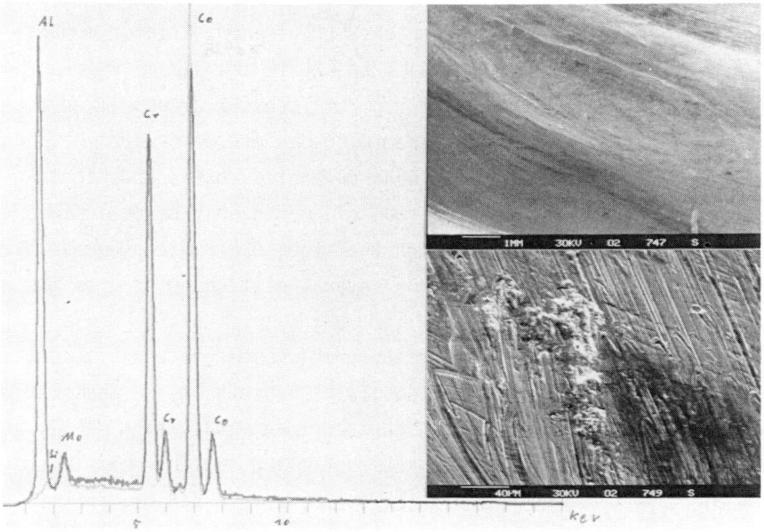

Fig.3: Extra-articular wear mark on a CoCr-alloy stem collar; preferentially circumferential wear direction. Oxydic particles in the wear tracks correspond to alumina particles derived from the cup rim (see EDX diagram).

the lower micrograph had induced a three-body abrasive wear.The impression in the left lower corner shows the configuration of an alumina grain.

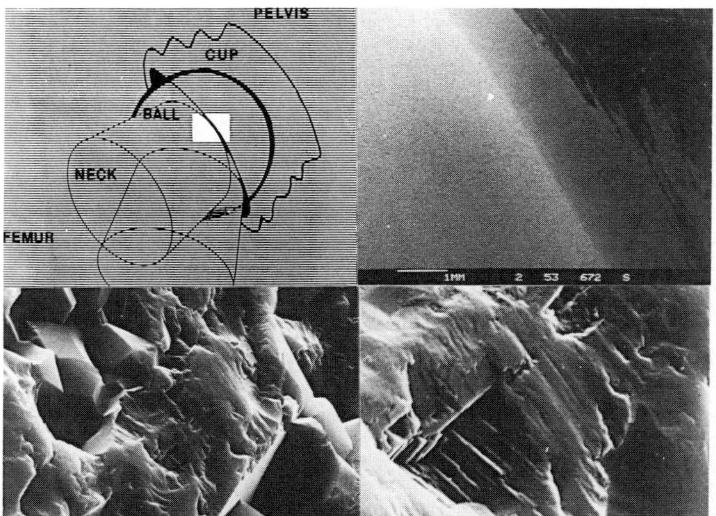

Fig.4: Extra-articular ceramic-to-ceramic wear at the ball-neck junction showing preferentially trans-and intercrystalline fractures.

Fig.3 shows an extra-articular wear zone on the metal collar of a ceramic THR which had been implanted for 3.2 years; the wear direction is preferentially circumferential. The deviating wear tracks occurred at a later moment. Oxydic particles visible within the wear tracks in the SEM micrograph correspond to alumina particles derived from the cup rim (see EDX diagram).

Fig. 4 represents an example of ceramic-to-ceramic wear which happened at the femoral ball-neck junction. The main wear mechanism corresponds to trans- and intercrystalline fractures. The direction of wear cannot be determined exactly, but the low magnification micrograph on the right upper side demonstrates that the region of contact affects a zone of several millimeters due to the geometry of the cup rim and the ball neck.

Since extra-articular rim wear and subluxation phenomena exert additional forces at the bony implant bed, they should be avoided. As we observed rim wear phenomena in more than 25 per cent of our retrieval collection it may be concluded that the recommendations for an optimized implant position do not suffice in the case of alumina implants. Any change in design, in particular, a reduction of the material thickness at the cup rim or abrupt changes in wall thickness, is limited by an increased danger of ceramic component fracture, as can be supposed from results in joint simulator testing (ref.3).

REFERENCES

1 P.M.F. Boutin, A 15 years follow-up with a ceramic endoprosthesis, Proc. 6th CIMTEC, World Congress on High Tech Ceramics, Milan, Italy, June 24-28, 1986, in press.
2 J. Harms and E. Mäusle, Biokompatibilität von Implantaten in der Orthopädie, Hefte zur Unfallheilkunde,83 (1983),1.
3 Th. Mittlmeier and A. Walter, The influence of prosthesis design on wear and loosening phenomena, CRC Crit. Rev. Biocompatibility, 2 (1986), in press.
4 H. Mittelmeier, J. Heisel and E. Schmitt, 10 Jahre Erfahrung mit Keramikhüftprothesen, Z. Orthop., 123 (1985), 657-662.
5 G. Heimke and P. Griss, Five years experience with ceramic-metal-composite hip endoprostheses, Arch. Orthop. Traumat. Surg., 98 (1981), 165-171.
6 A. Walter, Fracture phenomena in orthopedical alumina, Proc. Conference on the Fractography of Glasses and Ceramics, Alfred, New York, U.S.A., August 4-6, 1986, in press.
7 A. Walter, Wear-screening of ceramic-to-ceramic components for total hip replacement by ring-on-disc device and joint simulator test, Proc. 6th CIMTEC, World Congress on High Tech Ceramics, Milan, Italy, June 24-28, 1986, in press.
8 A. Walter and W. Lang, Al_2O_3 fatigue fracture of ceramic-to-ceramic total hip replacements, Fall Meeting 1985, Mat. Res. Soc., Boston, U.S.A., December 2-6, 1985, in press.
9 A. Walter, G. Wasmer and W. Plitz, Untersuchung der Versagensvorgänge von Hüftpfannen aus Aluminiumoxidkeramik, VIII. Münchner Symposium für experimentelle Orthopädie, München, FRG, February 7-8, 1986, Georg Thieme, Stuttgart,1986, in press.
10 A. Walter and W. Plitz, Wear mechanism of alumina-ceramic bearing surfaces of hip-joint prostheses, in P. Ducheyne, G. Van der Perre and A.E. Aubert,(Eds.), Biomaterials and Biomechanics 1983, Elsevier, Amsterdam,1984, 55-60

Biomaterials and Clinical Applications,
edited by A. Pizzoferrato, P.G. Marchetti, A. Ravaglioli and A.J.C. Lee
Elsevier Science Publishers B.V., Amsterdam, 1987 — Printed in The Netherlands

ADAPTIVE BONE REMODELLING IN MADREPORIC HIP PROSTHESES

M.PORTIGLIATTI BARBOS[1], F.BAUDROCCO[2], P.IULITA[2], P.ROSSI[1]

1)Clinica Ortopedica dell'Università - Torino ITALY

2)FIAT AUTO Direzione Tecnica Laboratori Centrali - Torino ITALY

SUMMARY

Human histology of bone remodelling in madreporic surfaced prostheses is rare, due to the difficulty in obtaining and processing human specimens.

Therefore in order to evaluate resorptive and formative changes in bone tissue around a Lord prosthesis, three cases were histologically examined at different time lapses from implant: i.e. at 40 days, 11 months and 2$\frac{1}{2}$ years respectively after surgery.

The first two specimens were right and left femur with hip prostheses excised from a 70 year old male, who died from natural causes . The other was a Lord prosthesis removed from a 62 year old woman because of a rotational defect .

In all three cases the prostheses were well fixed with no clinical signs of loosening .

The specimens were cut into pieces at various distances from the hip joint and prepared for S.E.M. examination . Particular care was taken in order to avoid fractures or other artefacts at the bone-metal interface during the cutting procedure .

The results obtained from the S.E.M. examination of the sections from the three prostheses, allowed us to make the following conclusions :

- Adaptive bone remodelling varies along the prosthesis stem;
- Both resorptive and formative changes occur in the femoral diaphysis with a particular topographic distribution and in relation to the time lapse from implant ;
- New bone formation is made up of woven bone which can be found very close to the madreporic surface .

INTRODUCTION

Over the past few years orthopaedic experience with cementless prostheses and experimental research on biological fixation of bone implants have supported the concept that bone will provide an interlocking surface by direct ingrowth into the spaces of porous or madreporic surfaced metal implants(refs 1 -7). Experiments on animals have established that mechanical interlock does occur as a direct consequence of bone ingrowth at bone-metal interface . Histologic sections and microradiographs revealed extensive mineralized bone growth deep inside the spaces within the metallic surface . Both mature haversian bone and less mature woven bone were found at this level .

Bone remodelling around madreporic surfaced prosthesis was particularly studied by Lord in an experimental model in dogs (ref 8).

However, due to the difficulty in obtaining and processing human specimens , human histology of bone remodelling around madreporic surfaced prosthesis is rare .

Here three madreporic implants were evaluated at different time lapses .

METHOD

Two femurs were explanted from a 70 year old male who had died from natural causes in order to obtain the specimens for histological examination. Due to advanced bilateral arthritis the patient had been operated on the left hip 11 months previously and then on the right 40 days before death . Two Lord prostheses were implanted.

Further observations were carried out on another Lord prosthesis removed with longitudinal osteotomy of diaphysis from a 62 old woman $2\frac{1}{2}$ years after surgery, because a rotational defect .

In all three cases the prostheses were well fixed without clinical

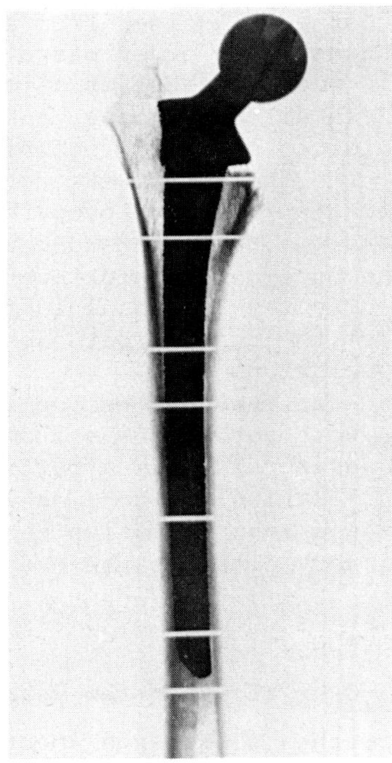

Fig.1 For all specimens S.E.M. studies were performed on transverse sections from levels shown on radiograph .

signs of loosening.

The specimens were radiographed with high definition film and then cut into pieces at various distances from the hip joint,as shown in fig.1 . Particular care was taken in order to avoid fractures or other artefacts at the bone-metal interface during the cutting procedure . All samples were fixed and dehidrated in graded ethyl alcohol solutions and embedded for study without decalcification . They were then placed directly into plastic blocks for simultaneous cross-sectioning of bone and metal to avoid any artificial changes of the bone-metal interface. Cutting procedure was performed with a water cooled diamond cut-off wheel. Transverse bone-metal specimens were prepared under vacuum for study by scanning electron microscopy . The polished surfaces of specimens were etched with N/10 HCL for 1 minute in order to make more detectable the details of distributions of lamellae which could not be seen in untreated surfaces (ref 9) and finally coated by sputtering with silver .

RESULTS

40 DAYS POSTOPERATIVELY

The vast majority of the madreporic surface of the implant was void of bone tissue formation (fig. 2 and 3) .

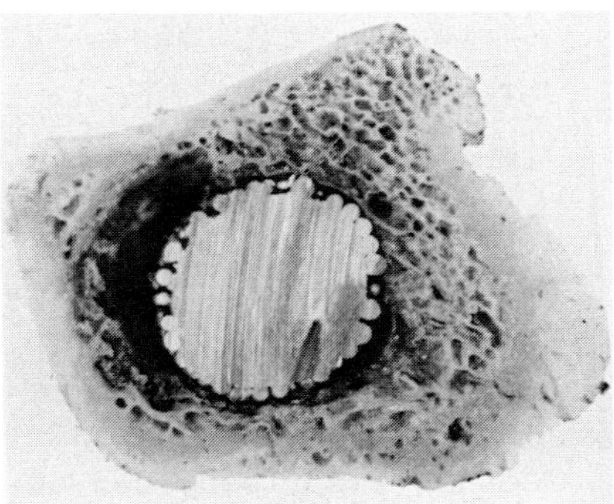

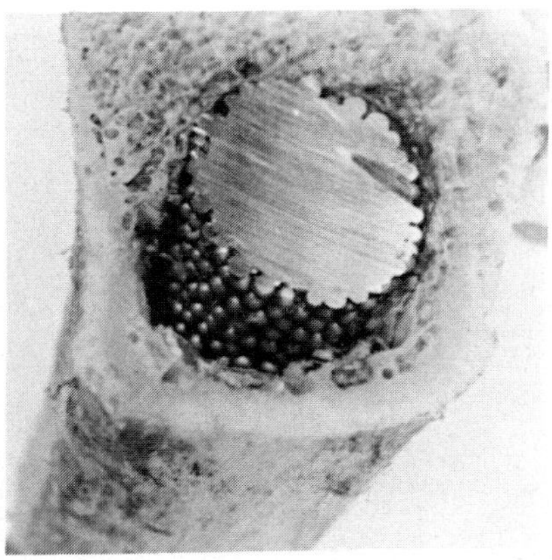

Fig.2,3 and,next page, 4,5: at 40 days postimplantation madreporic surface is void of bone-tissue formation. B = bone P = prosthesis

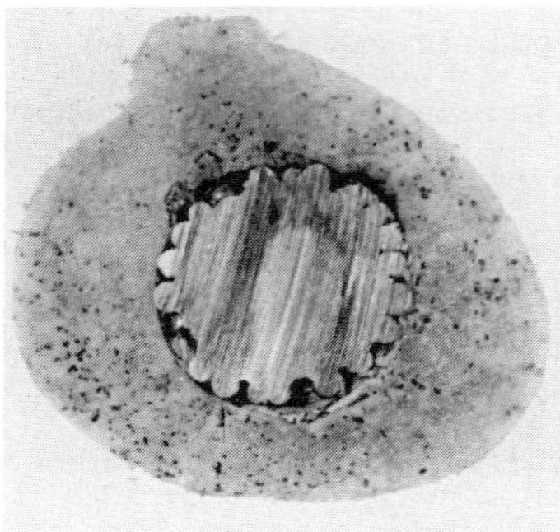

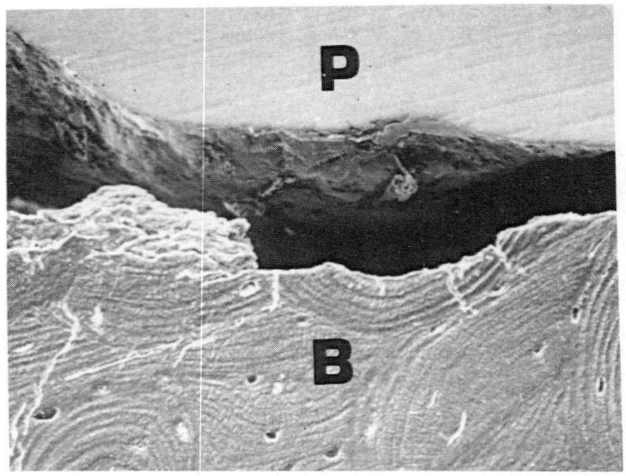

The lower part of the stem is sorrounded by old cortical bone with very extensive macroscopic bone-implant contact, but without sign of new bone apposition (fig. 4) . S.E.M. shows that between old osteonic bone and madreporic surface there is no new bone formation (fig. 5) . Neither is there any evidence of significant bone resorption at any level in the femur .

11 MONTHS POSTOPERATIVELY

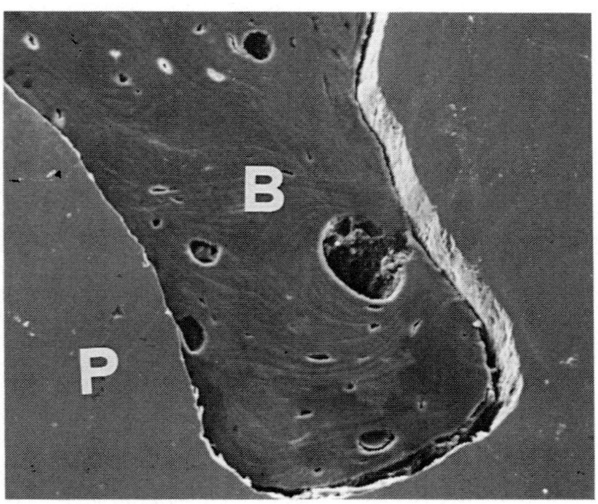

Fig.6: initial bone ingrowth on madreporic surface at 11 months postop.

Bone apposition and growth on the madreporic surface is macroscopically detectable in a narrow zone of the posterior and lateral region of the upper part of the implant (fig. 6) .

In the lower part of the implant initial bone ingrowth around madreporic surface is also evident .

Connective tissue can be seen filling the remainder of the non-bone-ingrown spaces of the madreporic surface. Old cortical bone seems to be some more osteoporotic than in the sample at 40 days postoperatively .

$2\frac{1}{2}$ YEARS POSTOPERATIVELY

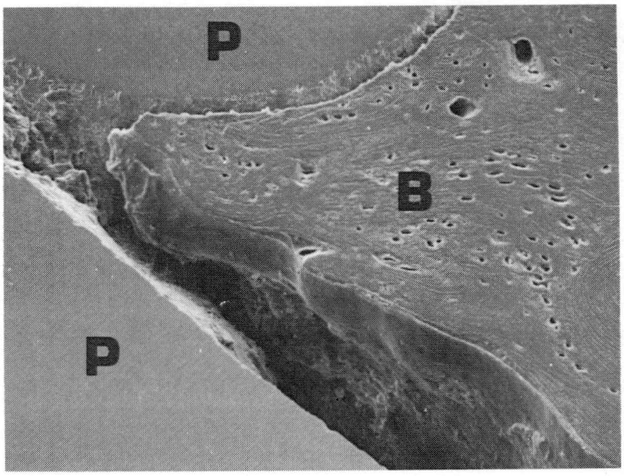

S.E.M. shows extensive bone ingrowth often extending to the core of the madreporic surface (fig.7) . However in some areas bone is not totally filling the madreporic surface and many points of the interface show some distance between metal and bone (fig.8) . Moreover,although bone tissue is observed in apparent direct contact with the implant surface in some areas, it is most often separated by a thin fibrous tissue membrane .

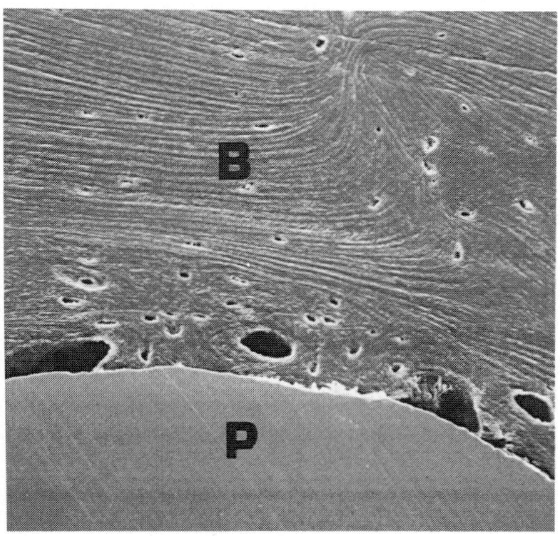

New bone formation is characterized by type of tissue :immature woven bone is tipically found at the interface and within the madreporic space (fig.9) .

Fig.7,8 and,next page, 9: see text
B=bone P=prosthesis

CONCLUSIONS

The results of this study indicate that extensive remodelling is still under way at 11 months postimplantation and that the madre-

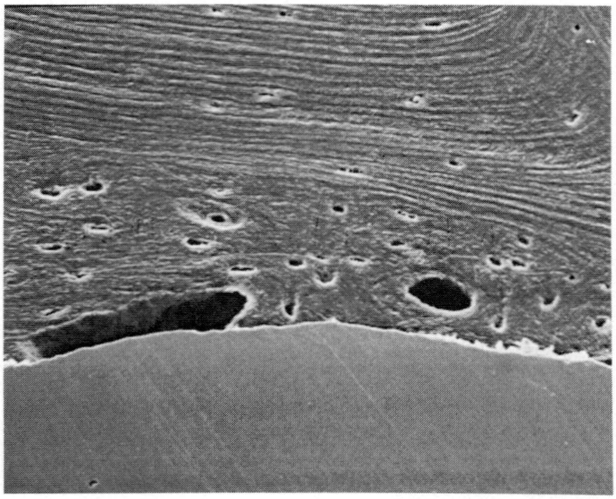

poric surface is diffusely infiltrated by osseus tissue at $2\frac{1}{2}$ years. Furthermore: the closer the contact between diaphysis and implant, the greater is the new bone ingrowth on madreporic surface .

REFERENCES

1 R.P. Welsh, R.M. Pilliar and I. MacNab, The role of surface porosity in fixation to bone and acrilic, J. Bone Joint Surg. 53A (1971) 963-967 .

2 C.A. Hosmy, T.E. Cain, F.B. Kessler, M.S. Anderson and J.W. King, Porous Systems for prosthesis stabilisation, Clin. Orthop 89 (1972) 220-235 .

3 C. Kenesi, P. Touzet and M. Martraire, Un nouveau type de stellite réhabitable; étude mécanique et histologique, Acta Orthop. Belg. 42 , (1976) 16-21 .

4 A. Patel, G. Guillemin, J.L. Patat and le G.U.E.P.A.R., Resultats des tests mécanique aprés implantation de métaux poreux ou à surface irréguliére, Rev.Chir.Orthop. 63Suppl.II (1977) 116-119

5 F.V. Rhinelander, A flexible composite as a coating for metallic implants; Microvascular and histological studies,International Orthop. , SICOT I (1977) 77-86 ·

6 J.D. Bobyn and C.A. Engh , Human histology of the biological fixation of porous coated hip prostheses, Transactions of the fifth European Conference on Biomaterials, Paris 192, (1985) .

7 J.D. Bobyn, R.M. Pilliar, A.G. Bonnington and J.A. Szivek, The effect of porous coated hip stem design on bone formation and resorption in a canin model, Transactions of the fifth European Conference on Biomaterials, Paris 193 (1985) .

8 G. Lord, J.H. Marotte, J.P. Blanchard, J.L. Guillamon and M.Gory Etude expérimentale de l'ancrage des arthroplasties totales madréporiques de hanche, Rev. Chir. Orthop. 64(1978) 459-470 .

9 A. Boyde, Scanning electron microscope studies of bone in: The Biochemistry and Phisiology of bone, Ed. G.H. Bourne Academic Press New York S. Francisco london, Vol I-II (1972) 259-310 .

Biomaterials and Clinical Applications,
edited by A. Pizzoferrato, P.G. Marchetti, A. Ravaglioli and A.J.C. Lee
Elsevier Science Publishers B.V., Amsterdam, 1987 — Printed in The Netherlands

TEN YEAR FOLLOW UP OF UNCEMENTED TOTAL HIP PROSTHESIS WITH ALUMINA ACETABULUM AND TITANIUM FEMORAL STEM BY PLASMA JET TECHNIQUE.

C.TRENTANI[1] and A.MONTAGNANI[2] and G.VICENZI[2]

1 University of Chieti. Section of Traffic Injuries
2 2nd Orthopaedic Clinics, "Rizzoli" Orthopaedic Institute University of Bologna

SUMMARY

A report is given of five cases of uncemented total hip replacements with the acetabulr component made of ceramic and the stem made of titanium coated with alumina oxide. After ten years experience no revision of the prosthetic components has been necessary. Clinical and X-ray results are good.

INTRODUCTION

Following an interdisciplinary study on ceramic materials undertaken in 1971 at the Rizzoli Orthopaedic Institute (ref.4) a total hip prosthesis without cement was developed. Experimentally it was proved that prosthetic fixation is stable if a continuous connection between bone tissue and alumina is formed in such a way that it is impossible to extabilish where alumina ends and bone tissue starts (Fig.1). A titanium stem (ref.11) covered with alumina oxide through plasma jet technique (ref.1-6-15-16) was devised in order to overcome the obstacle of fragility of pure ceramic implants (ref.9) and of tissue reaction between metal, plastic materials and bone. By covering titanium with alumina, this stem takes the positive properties of metal resistance and ceramic endurance (ref. 2-8). The implant material should resist static and dynamic weight-bearing forces (ref.10) and the action of biological fluids and should be modelled into the proper shapes (ref.3-17). The stem shape was planned to enable the widest possible contact surface between the prosthesis and the femoral cavity to be obtained through suitable instruments and to realize the best coupling between bone and implant(ref.5-7).

The proximal part of the stem has an elliptical shape in transverse section, with a shelf support on the resected femoral neck and, with a good approximation, it imitates the shape of the upper femoral extremity. The distal part is cylindrical in section and the unitary stresses conveyed to the bone are studied in such a way as to reduce the possibility of relative sliding between the bone and the implant.

In 1975, during a meeting at the Rizzoli Orthopaedic Institute when the Eu-

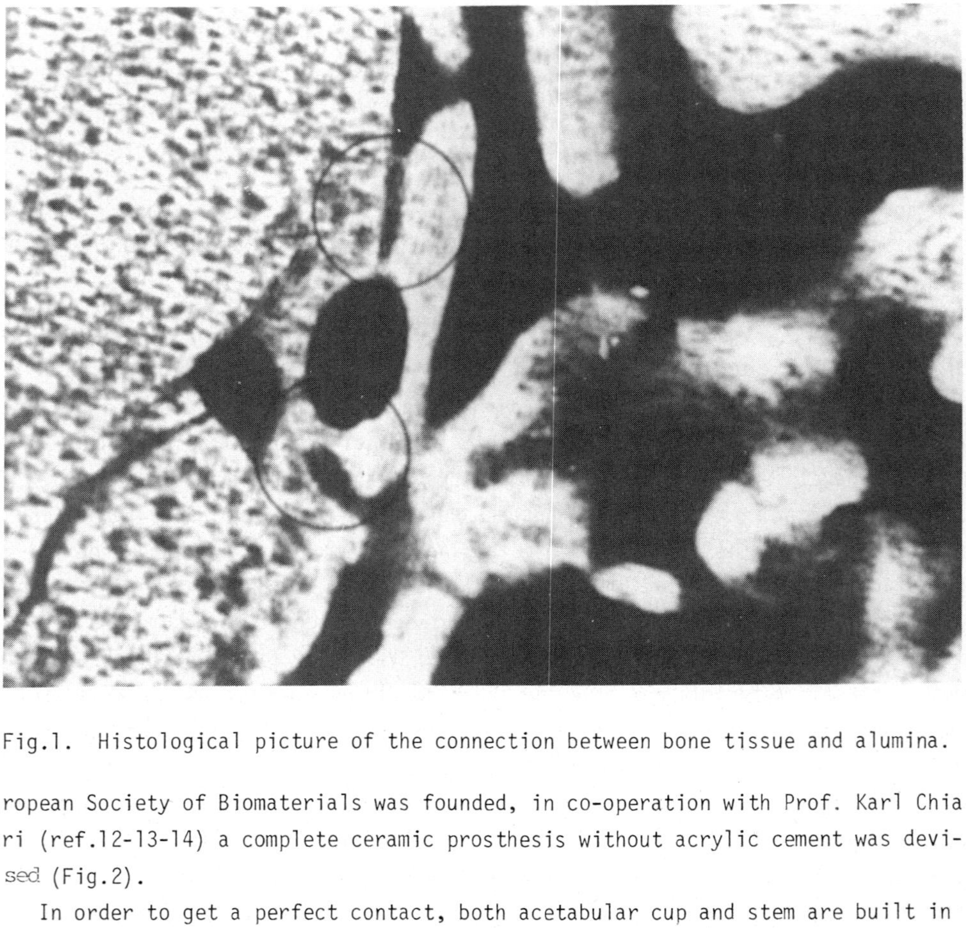

Fig.1. Histological picture of the connection between bone tissue and alumina.

ropean Society of Biomaterials was founded, in co-operation with Prof. Karl Chiari (ref.12-13-14) a complete ceramic prosthesis without acrylic cement was devised (Fig.2).

In order to get a perfect contact, both acetabular cup and stem are built in five different sizes, according to the different anthropometric constitutions.

Five patients are presented who were operated upon in 1976-77 with the ceramic prosthesis: the results achieved were successful, both from a clinical and X-rays point of view (ref.18).

CASE REPORT

Case No 1: H.G.- 53-year-old woman operated on at the age of 43 by Chiari's osteotomy for congenital dislocation of the right hip. A ceramic prosthesis was then applied in 1976: 10 years later there is no pain but a slight limp, which

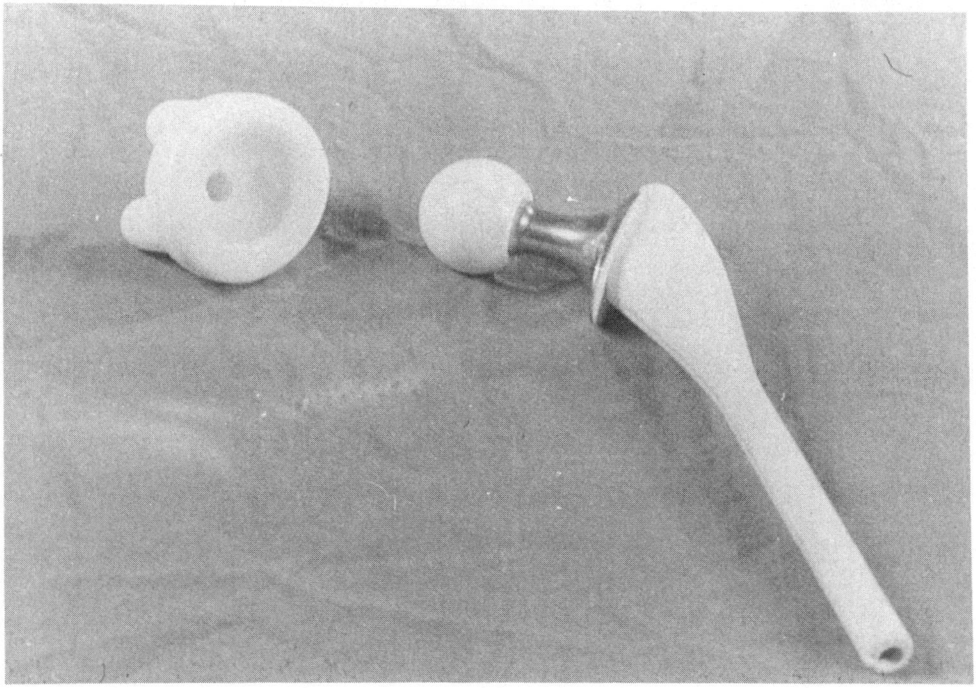

Fig.2. Ceramic total hip prosthesis.

was also present before the operation. X-rays follow-up shows the perfect stability of the implant. There is no bone resorption at the calcar level and, at the apex of the infundibulum a good supporting bone tissue can be observed closing the medullary canal (Fig. 3).

Case No 2: M.H.- 55-year-old man operated in 1976 on the left hip. X-rays post-operative follow up shows the good position of the prosthetic component. After ten years there is no pain, good walking ability and complete hip mobility. The acetabular cup is completely covered with bone tissue. There is no bone resorption at the calcar level and at the apex of the infundibulum there is a good supporting bone tissue formation (Fig.4).

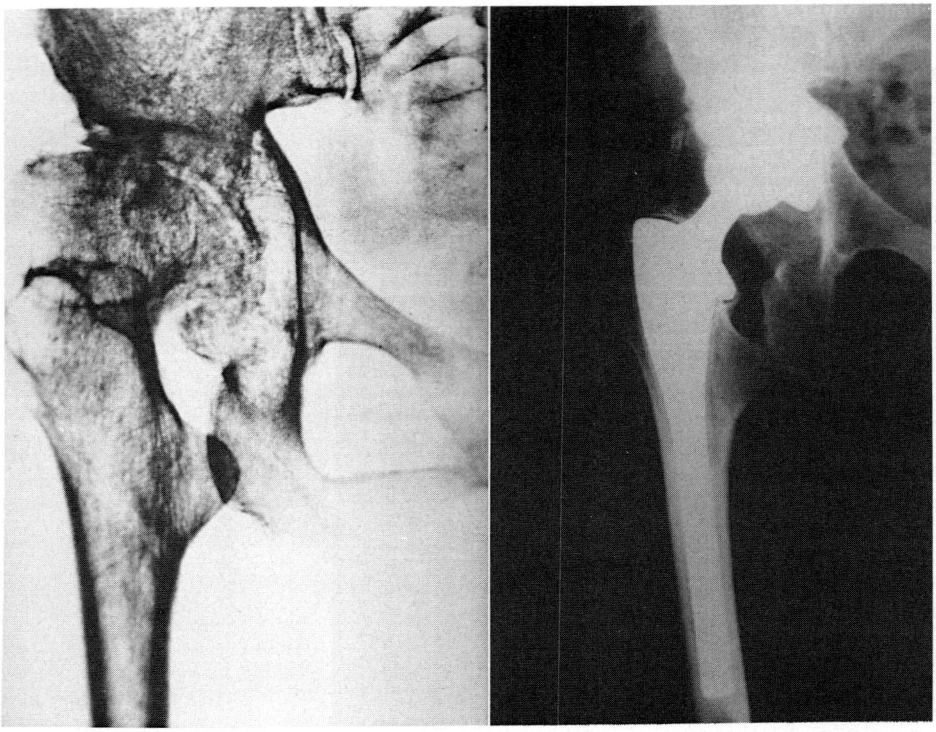

Fig.3. X-rays pre-operative follow up and X-ray follow up after 10 years of case No 1.

Case No 3: H.T. - 57-year-old man operated in 1976 on the left hip. After ten years there is no pain, walking is good and hip mobility is complete. Radiographically there is no change in the position of the prosthesis, no stem sinking, while support at the calcar level is still defective. Contact areas present no signs of impairment and at the apex of the infundibulum there is a good supporting bone tissue formation.

Case No 4: A.F. - 58-year-old woman, operated in 1977 on the right hip. X-ray post-operative follow up shows the good setting of the components. After ten years there is no pain, good walking ability and complete hip mobility. There no bone resorption at the calcar level and at the apex of infundibulum there

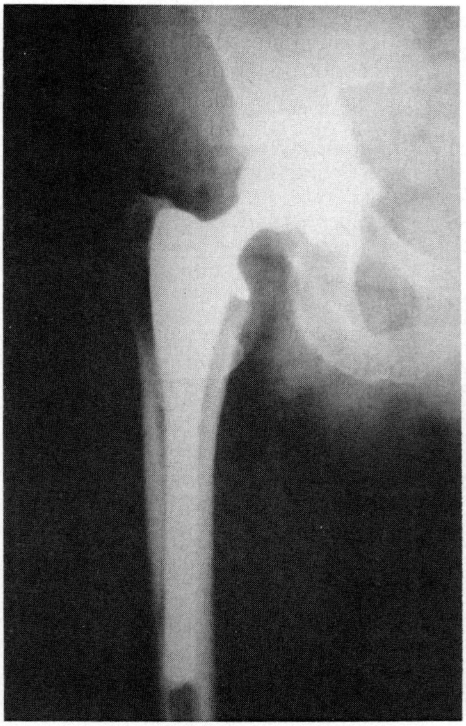

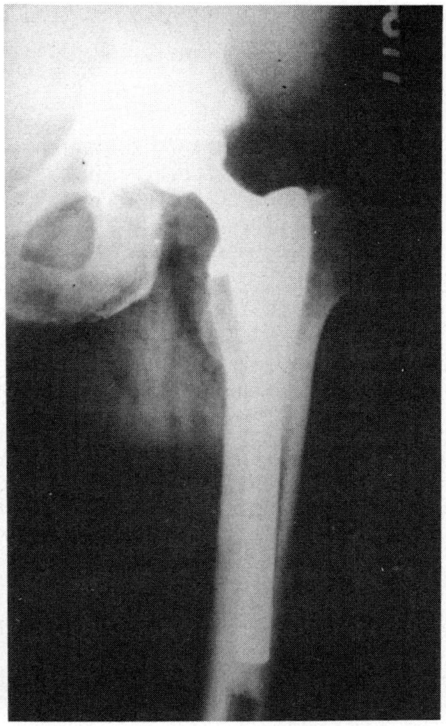

Fig. 4. Ten year follow up of case No 2.
Fig. 5. Ten year follow up of case No 4.

is a good supporting bone tissue formation (Fig.5).

Case No 5: C.C. - 64-year-old woman operated in 1977 on the left hip. In performing hip reduction after the prosthetic fitting, a fracture of the medial lower third of the femur occurred, treated by screw--plate. X-rays post-operative follow up shows the good setting of the prosthetic component. After ten years there is no pain, good walking ability and a complete hip mobility. There is no bone resorption at the calcar level and at the apex of the infundibulum there is a good supporting bone tissue formation.

A 10-year-follow up of our first group of five implanted total hip ceramic prosthesis is reported. Owing to the flattering clinical and radiographic rerults, with the same evolution in all the cases, the age limit could be lowered as to the indication of total hip prosthesis.

The moderate wearing between the two ceramic sliding surfaces did not produce any granulomata from foreign body, because of the high degree of superficial finishing and the lack of toxicity of the material. No seizure between the two ceramic surfaces took place. The careful study in the preparation of the frustum of cone of the upper femoral extremity and the exact design of the ceramic ball and socket did not lead to their breaking off.

This kind of prosthesis is still in use with the same good results.

REFERENCES

1 A.C. Allen, Plasma-jet. A new tool for ceramics, Ceram.Ind., 4 (1964) 112-114.
2 C.A. Beckham, T.K.Greenlee jr., A.R. Crebo, Bone formation at a ceramic implant interface, Calcif.Tissue Res., 8 (1971) 165-171.
3 P. Boutin, Arthroplastie totale de la hanche par prosthèse an alumine frittée. Etude expérimentale et premières applications cliniques, Rev.Chir.Orthop.,58 (1982) 229-246.
4 L. Cini, M.Paltrinieri, A. Pizzoferrato, S.Sandrolini, C. Trentani, Materiali bioceramici in funzione sostitutiva. Nota preventiva, Chir.Org.Mov., 60 (1971) 423-430.
5 L.Cini, M. Paltrinieri, A. Pizzoferrato, S. Sandrolini, C. Trentani, C.Zolezzi, Impianto senza cemento di artroprotesi d'anca con riporto superficiale di allumina. Chir.Org.Mov, 62 (1975) 1-27.
6 L.Cini, M.Paltrinieri, A. Pizzoferrato, S.Sandrolini, C.Trentani, Implant without cement of arthroprosthesis with superficial covering of alumina by means plasma-jet, 7th Annual Biomaterial Symposium, Clemson, 1975.
7 L. Cini, A. Pizzoferrato, C.Trentani, S. Sandrolini, M.Paltrinieri, Thermodifferential analysis of ceramic implants, J. Biomed.Mater.Res., 9 (1975) 441-451.
8 S.F.Hulbert, Prosthesis and tissue, the interface problem, 5th Internat.Biomaterials Symposium, Clemson, 1973.
9 M.Jäger, W. Plitz, Tribologie von Al_2O_3-keramik, Symposium über Biomaterialen Stuttgart, 1981.
10 J.J.Klawitter, S.F.Hulbert, Application of porous ceramics for the attachment of load bearing internal orthopaedic application, J.Biomed.Mater.Res.Symposium 2 (1) (1971) 161.
11 H.Mittelmeier, Selbsthaftende Keramik-Metall Verbund Endoprothesen, Med.Orthop.Technik. 6 (1975) 152.
12 M.Paltrinieri, C.Trentani, K.Chiari, K.Zweimüller, Artroprotesi di anca di materiale ceramico, Chir.Org.Mov., 63 (1976) 409-421.
13 M.Paltrinieri, C.Trentani, Artroprotesi d'anca di materiale ceramico, Bull. Sci.Med., 149 (1977), 162-177.
14 M.Paltrinieri, Artroprotesi d'anca di materiale ceramico. Atti Acc.Scienze Istituto di Bologna, XIII,Tomo V, 1978.
15 G.Perugini, Plasma tecnologie: plasma e getto di plasma, Ingegneria Meccanica,2 (1970), 51-52.
16 M.Salzer, K. Zweimüller, Further experimental and clinical experience with aluminium oxide endoprosthesis, J.Biomed.Mater.Res. 19 (1976), 847-856.
17 S.Sandrolini, L.Cini, M.Paltrinieri, A.Pizzoferrato, C.Trentani, Wear in hip arthroprosthesis evaluation by means of a walk cycle simulating machine, 2nd Annual Meeting Soc. Biomaterial, Philadelphia, 1976.
18 C.Trentani, A.Montagnani, Revisione a distanza delle artroprotesi d'anca di materiale ceramico realizzate dalla collaborazione italo-austriaca, Chir. Org.Mov., 68 (1982-83), 213-223.

Biomaterials and Clinical Applications,
edited by A. Pizzoferrato, P.G. Marchetti, A. Ravaglioli and A.J.C. Lee
Elsevier Science Publishers B.V., Amsterdam, 1987 — Printed in The Netherlands

MODELLING OF THE REAMED PROXIMAL FEMUR BY SIMPLE GEOMETRICAL MODELS

B. HOORNAERT, J. PUTZEYS and E. SLEECKX
K.U.Leuven, Analytische Mechanica, 3030 Heverlee (Belgium)

SUMMARY

By making moulds of the femoral cavity we get an accurate reproduction of the geometry of the canal. The antiloosenings are taken away. Parametrized models are proposed to describe as near as possible the moulds. A small number of parameters is preferred because we wish to standardize the final model. Our final model has a volume ratio model vs. mould of 70 %, where the proximal part of the cavity was filled for 80 %.

INTRODUCTION

The technique of peroperative mouldmaking is until now the only way to get an accurate 3D reconstruction of the reamed proximal femoral canal (see also "A new technique for the design and fabrication of custommade hip prostheses" by E. Sleeckx, et al.).

The present research is an attempt to design a model for the prosthetic stem that is anatomically shaped. A better anatomical fit between cavity and stem is very important. It is generally accepted that a cementlayer with controlled thickness would increase the lifetime of the cement. Concerning the cementless prostheses, it is essential that the support is assured in well known areas, such as the calcar zone, to get enough stability.

The geometry of the cavity differs highly from patient to patient and is also strongly influenced by the reaming technique. To meet the great geometrical differences, the dimensions of the models are parametrised, they are determined for each individual separately. It is our intention to propose, after a statistical study,a finite series of conventional hip prostheses with a standardized anatomical design. To make standardization possible, it is necessary to limit the number of parameters.

THE GEOMETRY

After resecting of the head and greater trochanter, the proximal femur is reamed. A very thin polyethylene bag is inserted, together with a guiding pin. A medical grade elastomer is then injected in the bag and when the cavity is filled, a dummy prosthesis is introduced. After hardening the mould is withdrawn from the canal. In this way one gets a very accurate negative copy of the canal.

For manipulation with a computer it is necessary to describe the moulds by means of a limited series of coordinates. At 10 mm intervals the circumference of the mould is digitized in 40 points, the central pin serves as axis. Starting from these data the plots of fig. 1 can be made.

The cavity is not straight nor constantly narrowing, but shows on the contrary protrusions and bends. Therefore a perfect model could never be placed in the cavity, or a mould in a non-elastic material could never be taken out (antiloosenings : fig. 2).
A simulation program adapts the data taken from the mould to make the antiloosenings disappear. We therefore have developed a very simple simulation technique : only a pure translation is permitted to take the adapted form out of the original. The direction of the translation is determined by the axis of the least square through the centers of gravity of each section. The ratio between the volume of the adapted and the volume of the original mould is very high : 94 % (s = 5 %, n = 50). The axis of the least square was choosen in all the later models as axis of symmetry.

THE MODELS

The geometrical properties of the moulds were calculated. The volumes vary between 9 ml and 35 ml (mean : 24 ml; σ = 7 ml). The measured length varies between 70 mm and 140 mm. The area of the first section varies between 200 mm^2 and 1000 mm^2 (mean : 490 mm^2; σ = 150 mm^2) and no fixed type of shape of these sections can be found.

A first series of models (fig. 3) contains very simple geometrical volumes, such as a cylinder, a cone, a cone with an elliptical section, and composition of these models.
An elliptical cone is the only way to approximate the most proximal sections. A cone can be defined in such way that is gives a good contact in the underlying part. The cylinder type gives a very close fit in the most distal part (starting from 40 mm under the smaller trochanter). The composition of these three leads us to a model that gives a good approximation of the cavity. The only disadvantage is the number of parameters we need to

describe the model (7: the major axis at the top, the ratio major axis vs. minor axis, the slope of the major axis, the radius at the top of the cone, the diminution of these radius, the radius of the cylinder and the length). A second series of models contains solids of revolution with either a circular or an elliptical base. Both types of models give promissing results with only 3 or 4 parameters.As the elliptical base provides an intrinsic stability against rotation, these types of model were chosen for our further investigations.

The radius (or the major and minor axes) diminish by following a linear, an exponential, a power or a logarithmic function. After evaluation of the results, the logaritmic function was preferred (the mean regression is 96 % , number of moulds : 50).

FINAL MODEL

The model (fig. 4) begins on the level of the smaller trochanter and has a length of 70 mm. The axis of symmetry is the axis of least square through the centers of gravity of the individual sections.

The uppermost 40 mm consists of a solid of revolution with an elliptical cross-section. The major and minor axes diminish independently, they follow a logarithmic function. These logarithms are a kind of least square approximation through the "greatest possible" inner ellipses, calculated for each section. These "greatest possible" were the greatest who satisfied the following conditions :

- point of gravity of the ellipse is the intersection point of the section with the axis of symmetry of the model.
- the orientation of the major and minor axes is the orientation of the mean axes of inertia in the upper sections.
- the ratio major-minor axis is equal at the square root of the ratio of the mean moments of inertia.

The undermost 30 mm are cylindrical . The same axis of symmetry is used.

EVALUATION OF THE MODEL

The quality of the model is determined by the volume ratio of model vs. mould.

The mean ratio rises from 35 % for the cylindrical model to 70 % for the final model, whereby the proximal part of the cavity was filled for 80 % (s = 7 %, n = 25).

When comparing our parametrized model with the Charnley Extra Heavy, the ratio volume Charnley vs volume mould (without checking if the Charnley-model fits) gives an estimation of 45 %.
The final model counts 5 parameters (major axis, minor axis, slope of the major axis, slope of the minor axis, radius). To reduce these number, a linear mathematical relationship was searched between the different parameters

major axis	- minor axis	84 %
major axis	- shape minor axis	81 %
minor axis	- shape minor axis	77 %

This is not high enough to eliminate parameters.
(Probably it is possible to eliminate the slope of the minor axis, by requiring that the minor axis at the end of the upper part is equal to the radius).
A model with a broken axis (the axis of symmetry of the uppermost part does not coincide with the axis of the undermost part), gave only a minimal improvement (the volume ratio increased only 2%). Therefore, and because of the two extra parameters we need to describe an angle in the 3D-space,this was excluded.

CONCLUSION

The final model gives a good approximation of the reamed femur cavity starting from the smaller trochanter. The models are not yet implantable. (A close contact is also required in the sections above the lesser trochanter. The transition between the upper and the lower part must be smoothed.)
This kind of prosthetic stem design is probably superior to the existing prostheses since it gives a much beter filling of the cavity, especially in those areas where a close fit is necessary. Since the model can be described by only 5 parameters it is likely that a standardization is possible.
It is possible to support the reaming technique on these calculations. By doing this we will surely get an even more favourable situation.

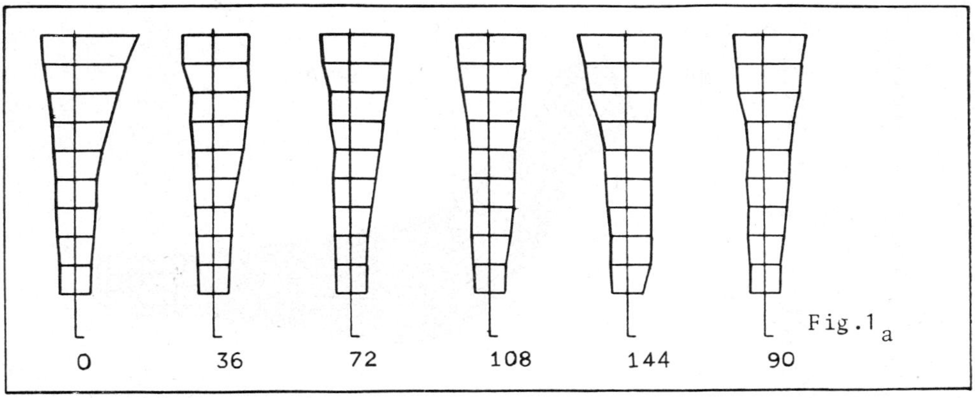

Fig.1 a

Fig.1 At 10 mm intervals the circumference of the mould is digitized (40 points).

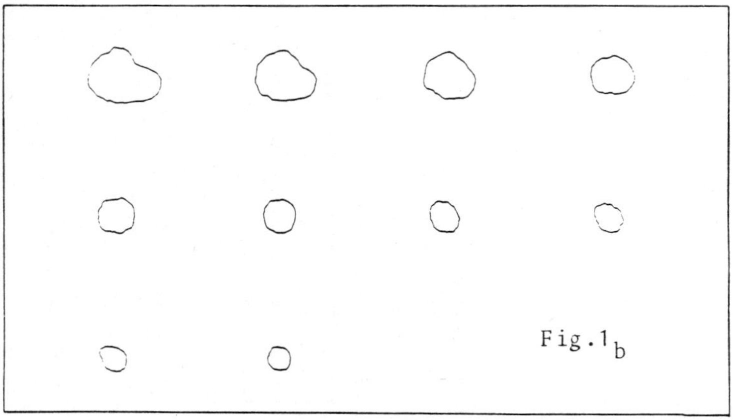
Fig.1 b

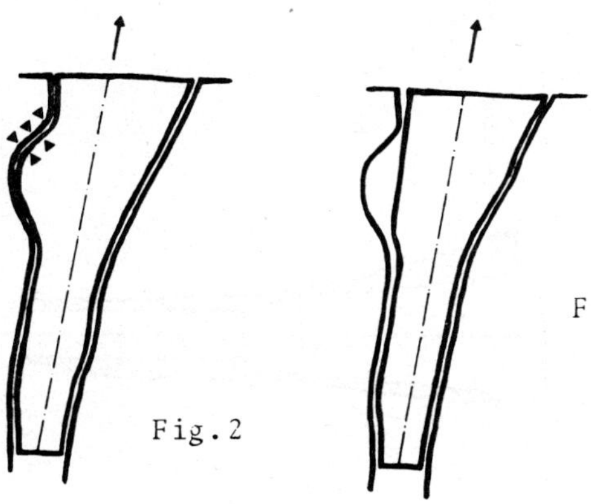
Fig.2

Fig.2 Antiloosenings.
A simulation program adapts the data taken from the mould.

Fig.3 The first moulds

Fig.4 The final model

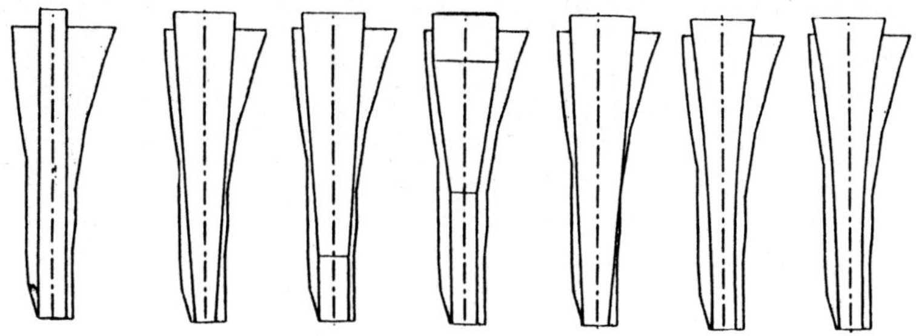

Fig.3 ↑ Fig.4a ↓

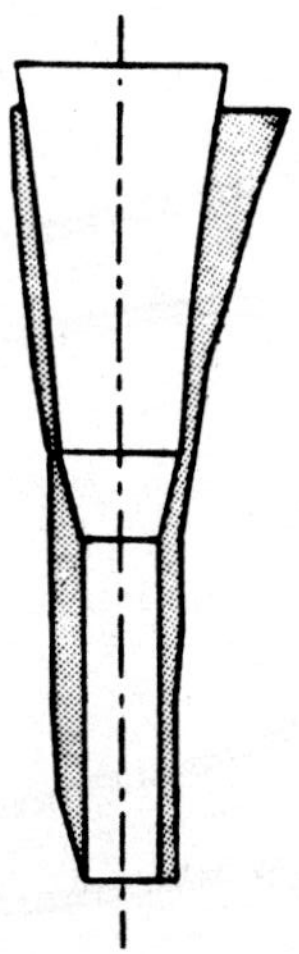

FINAL MODEL

Section : uppermost 40 mm : elliptical
undermost 30 mm : circular

Axis of symmetry : axis of least square

Parameters : 5 -major axis at the top
-slope major axis (logarithmic decrease)
-minor axis at the top
-slope minor axis (logarithmic decrease)
-radius

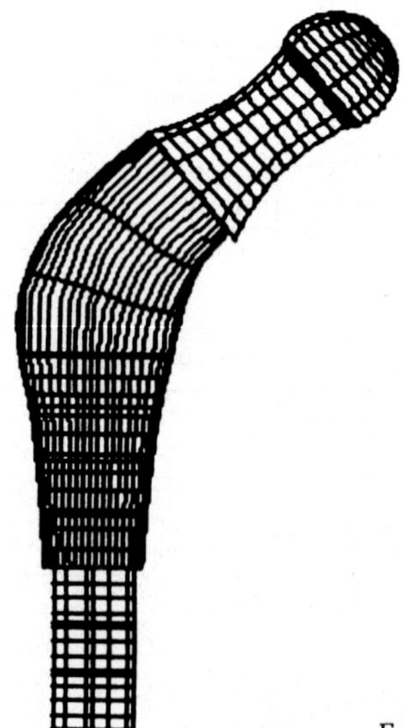

Fig.4b

Biomaterials and Clinical Applications,
edited by A. Pizzoferrato, P.G. Marchetti, A. Ravaglioli and A.J.C. Lee
Elsevier Science Publishers B.V., Amsterdam, 1987 — Printed in The Netherlands

TRICALCIUM PHOSPHATE CERAMICS IN PERIODONTAL THERAPY : HISTOLOGICAL RESULTS

P. PASSI* , A. MIOTTI** , V. TERRIBILE WIEL MARIN***

University of Padua
Institute of Dental Surgery* (Prof. B. Miotti)
Dental School ** (Prof. G.P. Giron)
Institute of Pathological Anatomy and Histology***
(Prof. V. Terribile Wiel Marin)

SUMMARY

An infra bony pocket of a second mandibular molar, with a third degree furcal involvement, was surgically treated with a tricalcium phosphate ceramic graft.Three months later, the mesial root was removed with part of the surrounding tissues, and the block section was prepared for histologic examination. The root resection was carried out for the incomplete healing of the furcation, in spite of a noticeable improvement of the lesion.
Several osteoid spicules were detected, in contact with the graft material, elsewhere included in a collagen fibril texture.
Newly formed ligament fibers were present,but no new cement was seen. The epithelial attachment was not longer than the normal one, even if it showed signs of proliferation and phlogosis.
Tricalcium phosphate ceramics may therefore be helpful in periodontal therapy, because they probably stimulate osteogenesis, as this investigation and other experimental and clinical studies support.

INTRODUCTION

Tricalcium phosphate (TCP) ceramics are commonly utilized today, in the treatment of bone defects in oral, maxillo-facial and periodontal surgery (1).

Synthesised TCP is resorbed in several months, mainly by chemical dissolution, and partly by phagocytosis. It is then replaced by newly formed tissue (2).
Hydroxyapatite is another bone graft material, which is commonly considered nonresorbable, even if it is very slowly partially degraded, over many years (3,4,5).
Some Authors pointed out that calcium phosphates are able to activate the complement 'in vitro'; these findings would indicate an activation of the immune system (6). However, in spite of this, no significant clinical complication was reported after the use of these materials, which are generally considered to be 'bioinert' and very well tolerated by the tissues.

From a biological point of view, TCP ceramics , for their relatively fast resorption, are specially apt for grafting.
Here some histological results are reported, that were obtained in treating an infrabony pocket in a patient.

CLINICAL CASE

A 52 years old man was suffering from a periodontal infrabony defect of a second lower molar, with mesial root and third degree furcation involvement (fig. 1).
The probing depth was 7 mm, on the mesial side of the tooth.
After performing root scaling and planing, and soft tissue 'curettage', a surgical flap was raised, and a tricalcium phosphate ceramic (Synthograft, Johnson & Johnson) was inserted into the bony defect (fig.2).
After surgery, tetracycline therapy was carried out for fifteen days.
Three months later, the probing depth on the mesial side appeared to be reduced to 4 mm; the furcal involvement was evaluable as a second degree (3 mm horizontally in both buccal and lingual directions);
Radiologically, the radiotransparency of the defect looked to be reduced, specially in the furcation; the graft material seemed to be integrated in a radiopaque texture, though less dense than the surrounding bone (fig.3).
This result appeared to be good enough, particularly with regard to the gain in bone level mesially to the distal root, that could be utilized as fixed bridge abutment. However, the mesial root was not to be considered reliable, owing to the residual furcal involvement.
The removal of the mesial root was then carried out, and its resection with part of the surrounding tissues was accomplished.
The patient, who had previously been consulted , agreed with this procedure.
The block section was fixed in salt neutral formalin for 72 hours, then decalcified by means of pure hydrate sodium citrate, and included in paraffin melting at low temperature.
Slices 7 micron thick were cut with a microtome, stained with hematoxylin-eosin and Azan-Mallory, and examined at light microscope.

HISTOLOGICAL RESULTS

Crevicular and junctional epithelium were seen to be almost normal in size, though the junctional epithelium was curled and proliferated buccally :its apical limit appeared to be closed to the tricalcium phosphate ceramic granules. The gingival chorion was affected by a chronic nonspecific phlogosis (figs.4-5).
The ceramic granules were surrounded by a collagen fibril texture in which some osteoid spicules, with active osteogenesis, were evident (figs. 5-6-7-8).

It was possible to observe some newly formed collagen fibrils, entering the cement.
These findings were more marked on the distal side of the root, where many newly formed ligament fibers were detected (fig. 9).
No new cement was seen, but residual cement was detected over the whole surface of the root; therefore, the scaling and planing, even if accurate, didn't cause the complete removal of this tissue, in any zone of the treated root.

DISCUSSION

The numerous osteoid spicules in contact with the TCP ceramic particles are probably the most significant finding of this investigation.
Some other studies pointed out the apparent osteogenetic ability of calcium phosphates (7,8,9,10,11), while on the contrary other investigations showed that they are inglobated by connective tissue (12,13,14).
In some experimental trials on animals, the osteogenetic ability of TCP ceramics was verified, in the weeks after its surgical insertion in bone (15,16,17).
Other histologic human findings ascertained osteoid tissue nearby hydroxyapatite particles (18), even if the main aspect was a fibrous encapsulation, without any sign of phlogosis (19).
These inconsistent histological results may probably be explained considering the different biological features of the bone in which the material is inserted. The more the bone is cancellous and endowed with osteoblasts, the greater is the osteogenetic ability of calcium phosphates grafts.
However, nearby the alveolar ridge, the bone is generally rather compact, and scarcely endowed with medullary tissue, as often occurs in periodontal therapy.
The evidence of an epithelial attachment of almost normal size, is certainly an interesting finding, because most of the infrabony pockets that recover, usually heal by means of a long epithelium.
The observation of newly formed ligament fibers is equally noticeable, even if no cemental regeneration was seen; however, this finding might not be caused by the TCP graft. Indeed, it is well known that healing of a periodontal infrabony pocket with a new attachment may occur even without any graft, but only by careful preparation of the hard and soft tissues, and skilled plaque control (20).
This histological investigation, however, supports the usefulness of calcium phosphate ceramic grafts, which at least are able to supply a matrix for the blood clot that follows the surgical therapy; but it is also probable that these materials take part in stimulating the conversion of the collagen fibrils into osteoid tissue.
According to the results of this study and several other works ,

calcium phosphate ceramics seem to be helpful in periodontal therapy, and certainly devoid of any risk for the patients.

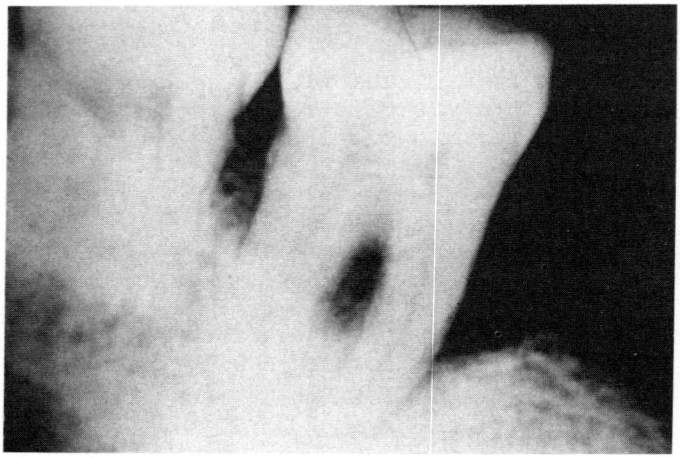

Fig.1. Second mandibular molar with an infrabony defect involving the mesial root and the furcation

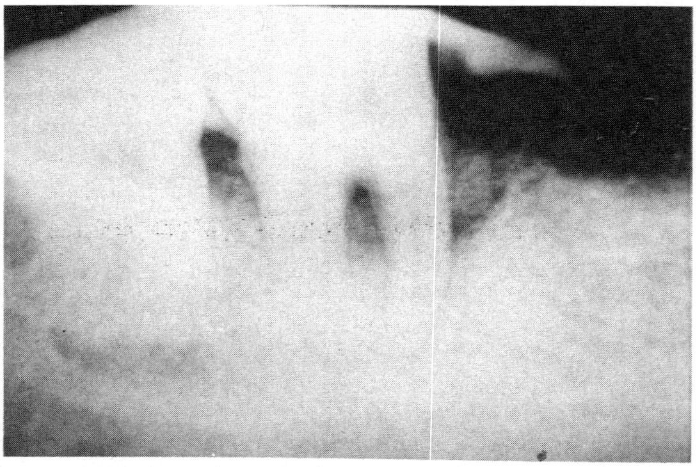

Fig.2. Intra-operating radiograph, showing the granular texture of the TCP ceramic graft

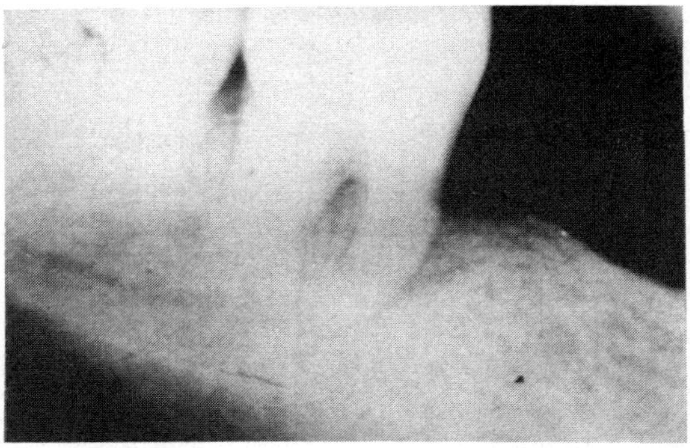

Fig. 3. Radiograph taken after 90 days: the granular structure of the graft is no longer visible. The radiotransparency of the defect looks to be lowered.

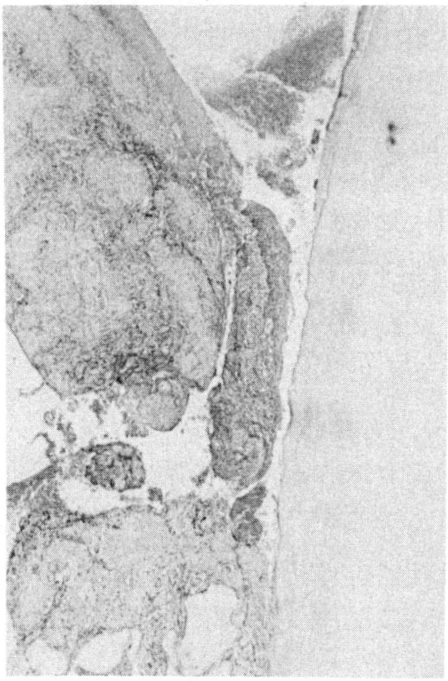

Fig.4. The crevicular epithelium appears to be almost normal in size; the junctional epithelium invaginates until the ceramic granules, and curls in the direction of the gingiva.
An intense phlogosis of the chorion is visible. Mesial side. (Hematoxylin & eosin, 40 X).

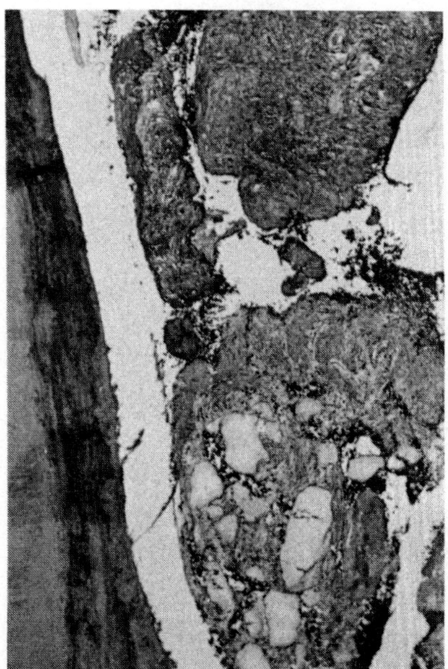

Fig. 5. The TCP ceramic is included in a fibrillar texture with hemorrhagic signs; the graft material appears to delimit the apical border of the junctional epithelium. A newly formed osteoid trabecula is visible. Mesial side.
(Azan-Mallory, 62 X).

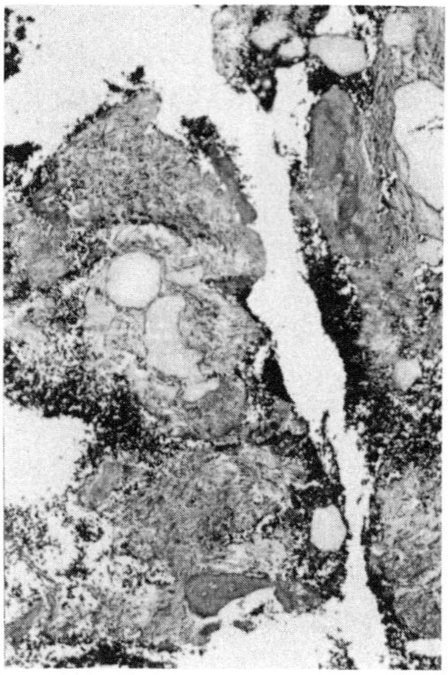

Fig.6. More apically, TCP ceramic particles surround osteoid trabeculae, with osteogenetic activity. Mesial side.
(Azan-Mallory, 62 X)

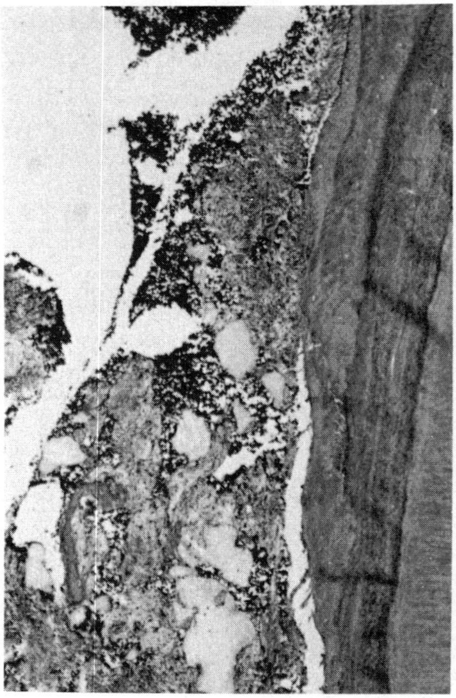

Fig.7. An osteoid trabecula nearby a ceramic granule; some newly formed ligament fibers are visible. Mesial side.
(Azan-Mallory, 50 X)

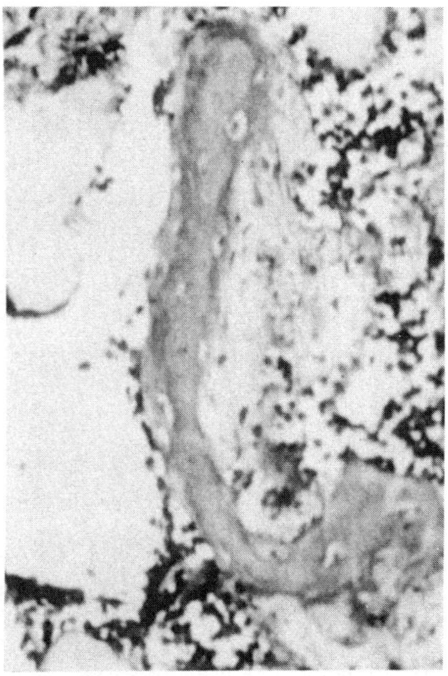

Fig.8. A close-up view of the osteoid tissue shown in Fig. 7. It is surrounded by TCP ceramic and red blood cells.
(Azan-Mallory, 250 X)

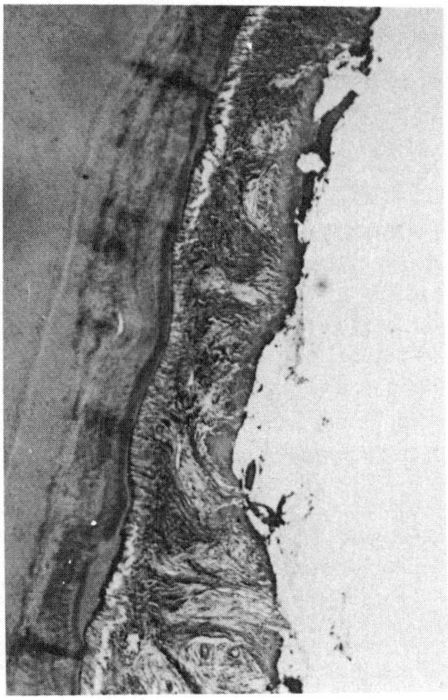

Fig. 9. Many newly formed ligament fibers, entering the root cement. There isn't new cement, but it is residual from the root scaling and planing.
Distal side, closed to the furcation.
(Azan-Mallory, 50 X)

REFERENCES

1) Snyder A.J., Levin M.P.,Cutright D.E.: Alloplastic Implants of Tricalcium Phosphate Ceramic in Periodontal Osseous Defects. J. Periodontol.,55(5):273-277,1984
2) Jarcho M.: Biomaterial Aspects of Calcium Phosphates.Properties and Applications. Dent. Cl.N.Am., 30(1):25-47,1986.
3) Yukna R.A.,Mayer E.T.,Brite D.V. : Longitudinal Evaluation of Durapatite Ceramic as an Alloplastic Implant in Periodontal Osseous Defects after 3 Years. J. Periodontol.,55(11):633-637, 1984.
4)Meffert R.M., Thomas J.R., Hamilton K.M., Brownstein C.N.: Hydroxyapatite as an Alloplastic Graft in the Treatment of Human Periodontal Osseous Defects. J. Periodontol.,56(2):63-73,1985
5) Yukna R.A., Harrison B.G.,Caudill R.F.,Evans G.H.,Mayer E.T., Miller S.: Evaluation of Durapatite Ceramic as an Alloplastic Implant in Periodontal Osseous Defects.II.Twelve Month Reentry Results. J. Periodontol., 56(9):540-547,1985.
6) Klein C.P.A.T.,Van Kamp G.,de Groot K.,Vermeiden J.P.W. : Possible Involvement of the Immune System in the Degradation of Hydroxyapatite Implants. In : G. Heimke, Dental Implants.Materials and Systems. pp.41-46, C. Hanser Verlag, München,1980
7) Kenney E.B.,Lekovic V.,Sa Ferreira J.C.,Han T.,Dimitrijevic B., Carranza F.A.:Bone Formation within Porous Hydroxyapatite Implants in Human Periodontal Defects.J. Periodontol.,57(2) : 76-83,1986.

8)Levin M.P., Getter L.,Cutright D.E.,Bhaskar S.N.:Biodegradable ceramic in periodontal defects.Oral Surg.,38(3):344-351,1974
9) Palattella G.,Ruggeri B.,Corbelli V.,Massi C.,Palattella E., Palattella A.: Fosfato tricalcico sinterizzato:risultati clinici di alcuni casi e studio istologico.Dental Cadmos,n.19:55-64,1985.
10) Sapkos S.W.: The Use of Periograf in Periodontal Defects. Histologic Finding. J. Periodontol.,57(1):7-13,1986.
11) West T.,Brustein D.D.:Freeze-Dried Bone and Coralline Implants Compared in the Dog. J. Periodontol.,56(6):348-351,1985.
12)Baldock W.T., Hutchens L.H.,McFall W.T.,Simpson D.M. : An Evaluation of Tricalcium Phosphate Implants in Human Periodontal Osseous Defects of Two Patients.J. Periodontol.,56(1):1-7,1985.
13) Cordioli G.P., Favero G.A.:Il trattamento di difetti ossei parodontali con materiale non riassorbibile. Il Dentista Moderno, n.5:571-575, 1984.
14) Moskow B.S., Lubarr A.:Histological Assessment of Human Periodontal Defect after Durapatite Ceramic Implant.Report of a Case. J. Periodontol., 54(8):455-462, 1983.
15) Bhaskar S.N.,Brady J.M., Getter L.,Grower M.F.,Driskell T. : Biodegradable ceramic implants in bone.Electron and light microscopic analysis. Oral Surg., 32(2):336-346, 1971.
16) Getter L.,Bhaskar S.N.,Cutright D.E.,et al.:Three biodegradable calcium phosphate slurry implants in bone.Oral Surg., 30(4):263-268, 1972.
17) Passi P., Miotti A.,Terribile Wiel Marin V.:La risposta del tessuto osseo a innesti di fosfato tricalcico ceramizzato. Il Dentista Moderno, n.7:1266-1275,1985.
18)Grigolato P.,Ferrari Parabita G.,Derada Troletti G., Zanetti V.,Berenzi A., Marocolo D.: L'impiego dell'idrossiapatite di calcio in chirurgia oro-maxillo-facciale.Nota I.Generalità e valutazione istochimica ed istofisica. Minerva Stomatol.,34:587-594 , 1985.
19) Miotti A., Terribile Wiel Marin V.,Passi P.:L'impiego dell'idrossiapatite in chirurgia orale. Il Dentista Moderno ,n.5: 877-886, 1986.
20) Ramfjord S.G.: The Role of Surgery in the Treatment of Periodontal Pockets. Quintessence Int.,15(10):1051-1056, 1984.

Authors' address : Dr. Pietro Passi - Clinica Odontoiatrica - Via Giustiniani 2 - 35100 Padova - Italy.

Biomaterials and Clinical Applications,
edited by A. Pizzoferrato, P.G. Marchetti, A. Ravaglioli and A.J.C. Lee
Elsevier Science Publishers B.V., Amsterdam, 1987 — Printed in The Netherlands

PHYCOGEN HYDROXYAPATITE - A NEW INTERCONNECTING POROUS BIOMATERIAL

C. KASPERK*, R. EWERS*
*Department of Oral-Maxillo-Facial Surgery,
Christian-Albrechts-University Kiel (West-Germany)

SUMMARY

The healing potency of three different hydroxyapatite implant materials into osseous tissue was investigated. Coralline hydroxyapatite, synthetic hydroxyapatite and a hydroxyapatite that derives from marine algae (phycogen) were used. The implant materials derived from coralls or from algae posess an interconnecting porosity. After 21 days all materials showed bone apposition on the implant surfaces. The coralline and phycogen hydroxyapatite granules developed a more intensive bone - implant compound and seemed to accelerate the bone formation which could be found after 28 days. These observations are due to the unique natural structure (surface morphology and interconnecting porosity) of both materials of marine origin. The phycogen hydroxyapatite material has an interconnective m i c r o p o r o s i t y whereas the coralline hydroxyapatite implant shows an interconnective m a c r o p o r o s i t y . The cortical bone is important for the biomechanic stability. Morphology and the unique porosity of the phycogen material resemble this natural component of bone. Surface porosity and morphology seem to attract bone - forming cells. Bone formation directly on the implant surface takes place earlier than on the other investigated implant materials.

INTRODUCTION

Different hydroxyapatite materials show clinically entirely different healing potencies. This observation indicates that besides the chemical structure of the material several other important parameters are of importance. Surface structure, microporosity, grain size, degree of cristallinity and solubility of the applied hydroxyapatite may diverge distinctively despite an identical basic material. It is not yet possible to estimate the importance of the different grain size or of the other parameters in regard to a better biocompatibility. The present investigation deals with the examination of three different hydroxyapatite materials which differ significantly in specific surface,structure and origin of the material.

MATERIAL AND METHOD

In our investigation a solid hydroxyapatite granulate, produced synthetically (Calcitite R) and two natural interconnective porous,hydrothermally transformed hydroxyapatite granules were applied into osseous defects. The porous materials are of coralline (Interpore 200 R) or phycogen origin (derived from algae) and differ mainly in the size of their interconnective pore-system.The granulate transferred from coralls has an average pore diameter of 200 micron according to the manufacturers information. An average pore diameter of 10 micron was found with the phycogen material. All materials are of hydroxyapatite. The three implant materials were brought into two drillholes of 3 mm size each in the diaphyses of femurs of 600 gr.rats . After 21 respectively 28 days the animals were sacrificed and the diaphyses were prepared to histological sections according to DONATH and BREUER (1982) resp. EWERS et al. (1983). The biocompatibility , healing tendency, bone - formation on and within the implant as well as the osseous integration of the material was evaluated for all the three different bioceramics.

RESULTS

All implant materials healed into the holes without any complications and showed first ossifications on the implant material after 21 days. After 28 days lamellar organized bone was found on and around the implants.

Solid hydroxyapatite material

Ossification does not take place simultaneously on the surfaces of all granules. Only partially we observed complete bone covering. We found granules showing no signs of ossification along the surface as well as merely punctuate contacts with newly formed bone. A fluorochrome penetration into the surface of the solid hydroxyapatite material at the implant-tissue-border was not observed. 28 days after the implantation no resorptive or biodegradative changes (KLEIN et al. 1983 and 1984) of the implant material were found.

Coralline hydroxyapatite material

The bone deposition on the implant begins at the periphery of this porous material and proceeds centripetally. The bone ingrowth into the implant is furthest advanced to the centre of the granule in that region next to the adjacent cortical bone. At the periphery as well as at the centre of the material an extremely narrow 20 micron wide zone of fluorochrome penetration is visible. After 28 days no resorptive or disintegrative changes in the meaning of biodegradation could be observed with this material.

Phycogen hydroxyapatite material

With this material the bone ingrowth also proceeds around and into the implant. The cavities on the surface are filled out completely with bone (Fig. 1). Within the peripheral cavities of the granule the staining also shows coloured structures down to a depth of the implant of 200 micron. Bone bridges which have developed between the granules provide an early compound osteogenesis in spite of the distance between the granules. The bone defect has been substituted completely by bone. The phycogen material shows a complete fluorochrome penetration of the granules.

DISCUSSION

The three examined hydroxyapatite granulates show the familiar implant characteristics (WINTER et al. 1981, DENISSEN et al. 1980, DONATH et al 1985) of this bioceramic material: non - irritant healing, tendency to compound osteogenesis, so - called osteotropic impact, osseous substitution and uncomplicated application.

The phycogen hydroxyapatite shows a defined highly organized surface pattern and seems to catalyse the cell differentiation from monocytes to macrophages.In our investigation the phycogen bioceramic only showed advanced bone formation in interparticular regions which were originally filled with embedding soft tissue around the implant already after 21 days. Another eminent difference of the phycogen matrial compared to all other known hydroxyapatite ceramics is the interconnecting microporosity which reveals itself with complete fluorochrome penetration in the granule particles under the fluorescence microscope. Surface structure and interconnective microporosity of this material lead to an enormous enhancement of the specific surface. This parameter is important for the ionic exchange which takes place immediately after the implantation between the implant material and the tissue fluid (NEUMANN and NEUMANN 1953 and 1958). This process of equilibration adapts the implant material to the individual, ionic environment and increases its biocompatibility. The adsorption of proteins to the hydrophilic hydroxyapatite surface turns the purely physicochemical interactions between implant and tissue to biochemical interactions and finally to the integration into hard tissue. The protein film on the

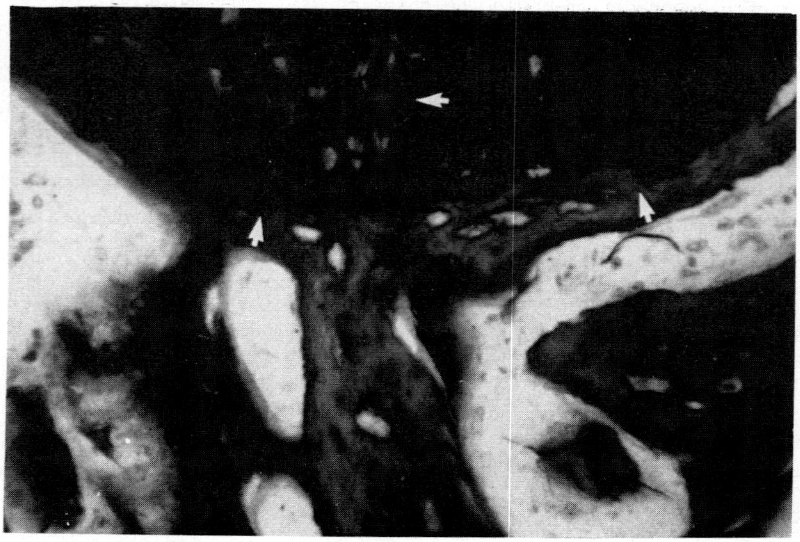

Fig.1:
Apposition of bone (stained blue) on and within the implant (arrows), phycogen material. (Polarisation, 1:350, undecalcified ground section 25 micron).

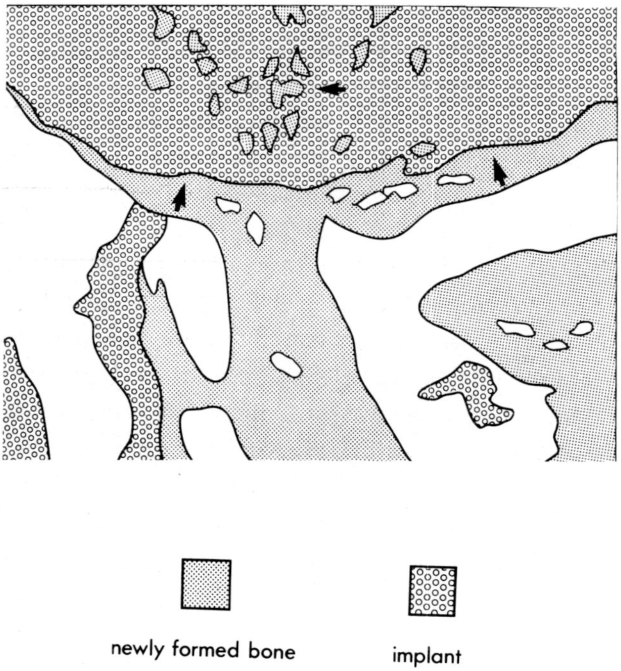

surface functions as a transmitter for osteoid adsorption on to the implant. On the other hand an opsonine function of adsorbed proteins is discussed (von OSS et al. 1974 and 1978). The interconnective microporosity intensifies the implant-tissue interactions and its healing as well.

The coralline hydroxyapatite has interconnective macropores of about 200 micron width which allow an ingrowth of bone into the ceramic material. This results in an implant-bone-compound that is very resistant to stress conditions. The 20 micron wide zone of fluorochrome penetration into the surface of the material shows that there is no microporosity with the coralline and the solid hydroxyapatite ceramic (Fig. 2-4). The coralline hydroxyapatite has a macroporous interconnective canal system within a solid hydroxyapatite material.

A disadvantage especially of larger solid hydroxyapatite implants is the brittleness of this bioceramic. A compound out of solid implant blocks and bone cannot have the same biomechanical qualities as the original bone structure. The covering of the surface (which is relatively small compared to its volume) of solid hydroxyapatite bodies means a superficial implant - bone - adhesion, hinders the implant biodegradation and the ingrowth of bone. The original elasticity of the bone structure can be established only by an intensive implant bone compound and a quick implant integration into osseous tissue.

The biodegradation of the coralline hydroxyapatite is significantly delayed after osseous ingrowth as Holmes showed in 1979 and confirmed in 1985 so that initially no sufficient stability within the bone can be guaranteed. The osseous integration of the phycogen hydroxyapatite which starts shortly after the implantation seems suitable to reestablish the elasticity and continuity of the bone structure.

ACKNOWLEDGEMENTS

For their kind support and constructive cooperation we wish to thank Dr. D. Ackermand (Institute for Mineralogy of the Christian-Albrechts-University, Kiel), P.H. Sahling (Institute for Biology, Helgoland) as well as Prof. Dr. K. Müller (Center for Biological Studies of the Christian-Albrechts-University, Kiel).

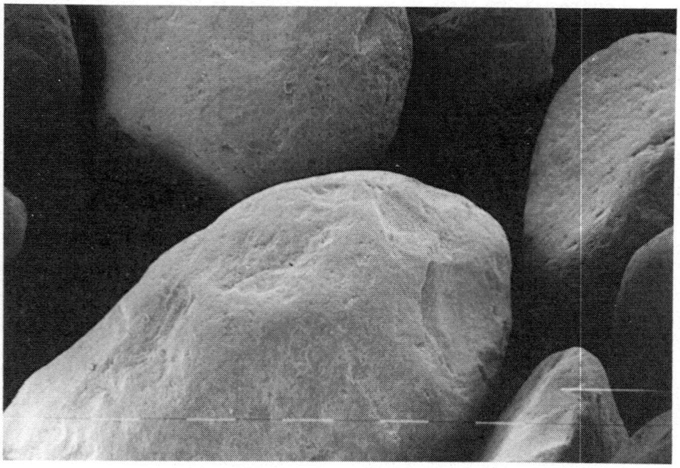

Fig.2:
Solid synthetic material.
(Scanning electron microscope, 1:80)

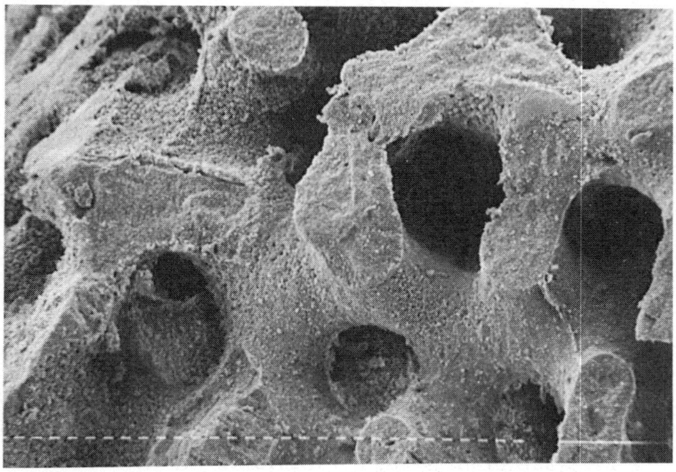

Fig.3:
Coralline material: interconnective macroporosity
(Scanning electron microscope, 1:160).

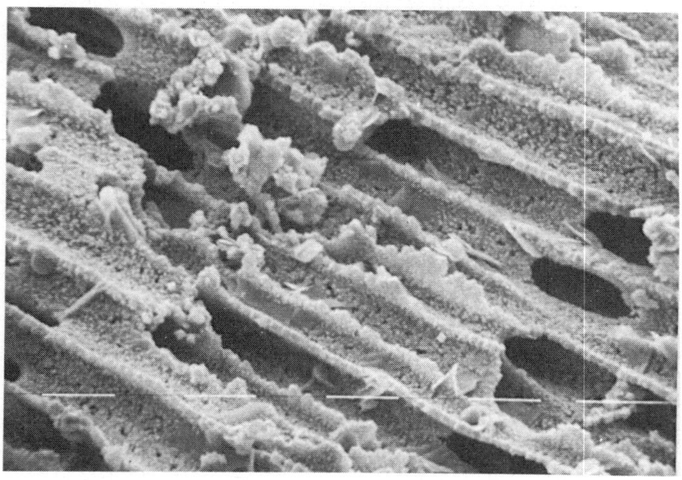

Fig.4:
Phycogen material: interconnective microporosity
(Scanning electron microscope, 1:1250)

REFERENCES

1 H.W. Denissen, K. de Groot, P.C.H. Makbes, Tissue response to dense apatite implats in rats, J Biomed Mat Res 14, (1980) 713-721.
2 K. Donath, G. Breuer, A method for the study of undecalcified bones and teeth with attaches soft tissues, J Oral Pathol 11, (1982) 318-326.
3 K. Donath, K. Hörmann, A. Kirsch, Welchen Einfluß hat die Hydroxylapatitkeramik auf die Knochenbildung? Dtsch Z Mund Kiefer GesichtsChir 9, (1985) 438-440.
4 R. Ewers, S. Meier, U. Ingrisch, Ch. Schönfeldt, W. Alai-Omid, Die histologische Aufarbeitung von Hautgewebsstrukturen, Dtsch Zahnärztl Z 38, (1985), 1085-1087.
5 R.E. Holmes, Bone Regeneration Within a Coralline Hydroxylapatite Implant, Plastic & Reconstructive Surg 63, (1979) 626-633.
6 R.E. Holmes, Mandible Contour Augmentation Autograft vs. Porous HA Implant. Annual Meeting of the American Association of Oral and Maxillofacial Surgeons 1985.
7 C.P. Klein, A.A. Driessen, D. de Groot, Biodegradation behaviour of various calciumphosphate materials in bone tissue, J Biomed Mater Res 17, (1983) 769-784.
8 C.P. Klein, A.A. Driessen, K. de Groot, Relationship between the degradative behaviour of Calciumphosphate ceramics and their physical-chemical characteristics and ultrastructural geometry. Biomaterials 5, (1984) 157-160.
9 W.F. Neumann, M.W. Neumann, The chemical dynamics of bone mineral Chemical Reviews 53, (1953) 1-45.
10 W.F. Neumann, M.W. Neumann, The chemical dynmaics of bone mineral University of Chicago Press 1958.
11 C.J. von Oss, C.F. Gillmann, O.M. Bronson, J.R. Border, Opsoniac properties of human serum alpha -2-HS-glycoprotein, Immun Commun 3, (1974) 329-335.
12 C.J. von Oss, Phagocytosis as a surface phenomeron, Ann Rev Microbiol 32, (1978) 19-39.
13 M. Winter, P. Griss, K. de Groot, H. Tagai, G. Heimke, H. Dijk, K. Sawai, Comparative histocompatibility testing of seven calciumphosphate ceramics, Biomaterials 2, (1981) 159-160.

Biomaterials and Clinical Applications,
edited by A. Pizzoferrato, P.G. Marchetti, A. Ravaglioli and A.J.C. Lee
Elsevier Science Publishers B.V., Amsterdam, 1987 — Printed in The Netherlands

OSSEOUS REGENERATION INDUCED BY POROUS HYDROXYLAPATITE AROUND PERIODONTALLY INVOLVED LOWER MOLARS IN HUMANS

SBORDONE L.*; RAMAGLIA L.*; CIAGLIA R. N. * and KENNEY E.B.**;
*Istituto di Discipline Odontostomatologiche.2a Facolta' di Medicina e Chirurgia,Universita' di Napoli.

**U.C.L.A.,School of Dentistry,Sec. of Periodontics.

SUMMARY

The potential for osseous regeneration induced by granular porous hydroxylapatite (HA) (400-625μ)in the treatment of complete interradicular periodontal osseous defects (Class III) in human lower molars has been investigated.Four patients showing ,at least,two Class III furcation defects in lower molars have been selected .In each patient one furca has been treated with conventional surgical therapy, acting so as control site, while the other has been implanted with the biomaterial and used as experimental site.Pre,intra and six months post-operative clinical and radiographical records have been taken,computed and statistically analyzed for significance. Results suggest that,due to differences in maintaining the marginal bone level post-operatively between experimental and control sites, porous HA might be active in counteracting bone resorption induced by the surgical trauma.In addition osseous regeneration induced by porous HA might be dependent on the anatomical configuration of the defect, that is on the presence of vertical bone walls.Finally complete clinical integration of the material in the surrounding bone together with absence of inflammation in the overlaying gingival tissue suggests that porous HA could be fully biocompatible.

INTRODUCTION

Periodontal destruction is widespread among the adult population with approximately 90% of persons over 50 years old having periodontal disease (Ref.1).Periodontitis is associated with bacterial infections of a chronic nature which lead to ongoing destruction of the periodontium (Ref.2).The advancement of periodontal destruction leads in many cases to intrabony defects of the supporting bone.In multirooted teeth these areas of bone destruction are most frequently found in the area of furcations.Previous reports of therapy of this Class III furcation defect (complete interradicular bone loss) have not yielded any predictable procedure to take care of this particular lesion.Therefore,we are investigating the use of a synthetic bone implant material as a mechanism for resolving these periodontal conditions.The porous hydroxylapatite (HA) implant material derived from the coral of the Genus Porites has been developed (Ref.3).This material has been used in various anatomical sites and has shown itself capable of inducing bone formation throughout the implant material. A good rate of success has been reached in the treatment of periodontal defects with such a material.West and Brustein (Ref.4) created chronic intraosseous periodontal defects in dogs and used porous HA as an implant to fill these defects.At six months the implant was completely infiltrated with connective tissue and bone.A clinical study by Kenney et al.(Ref.5) using also porous HA,in human interproximal vertical defects demonstrated significant pocket reductions,attachment level gains and radiographic evidence of defect obliteration.

The present study has been undertaken to investigate the use of granular porous HA (400-625 μ) as a synthetic bone implant material for the osseous regeneration in the complete interradicular bone loss in human lower molars.

MATERIALS AND METHODS

Four adult patients,35-55 y.o.,have been selected for the present study,each patient having,at least,two class III furcation defect of the intrabony type in lower molars,and showing in such teeth at least 4mm of pocket depth,a mobility of 2 or less and no gingival recession over 1mm.At least four weeks after an initial therapy,patients have been subjected to a standard Widman flap surgical procedure to gain access to the two furcas involved in the study.One furca has been thoroughly root planed and curetted acting so as control site,while the other has been implanted with granular porous HA,400-625 μ,(Interpore 200 R) and used as an experimental site. Prior to the surgery the following clinical measurements have been taken in both experimental and control sites:1)Plaque Index(Pl.I.)by Loe and Silness;2)Gingival Index(G.I.)by Silness and Loe;3)Pocket Depth(P.D.)in the midfurcal area and 4)Probing Attachment Level(P.A.L.)using a self cured acrylic occlusal stent with grooves to reposition the probe for subsequent measurement;5)Mobility according to the criteria of Lindhe (Ref.6);6)Precision standard periapical radiograph. Intraoperative Bone Level(B.L.)assessment from the occlusal stent have also been registered. Patients have then been recalled for a standard clinical maintenance and six months later the measurements repeated and a reentry surgical procedure performed to assess bone level and clinical integration of the material. Pooled data have been statistically analyzed for significance according to the Student's t-test.

RESULTS

Plaque Index (Pl.I.) values recorded show that all the patients have maintained a satisfactory level of personal oral hygiene throughout the study in both experimental and control sites,allowing good wound healing and maintenance of the surgical results obtained.Gingival Index (G.I.) also remained very low during the study reflecting the absence of local inflammatory agents,such as plaque accumulation,or local toxicity of the implant material. Tooth mobility has not shown clinical variation before and after either experimental or control surgery. Data collected for all these parameters and for the furcation involvement for control as well as for the experimental sites are reported in Table 1 and 2.

CASE \ time		Pl. I.		G.I.		furcation involvement		tooth mobility	
		t_0	t_6	t_0	t_6	t_0	t_6	t_0	t_6
1 (37)	B	1	0	2	1	III	III	0	0
	L	2	1	2	1	III	III		
2 (46)	B	1	2	2	2	III	III	1	1
	L	1	2	1	2	III	III		
3 (47)	B	0	0	0	1	III	II	1	1
	L	0	1	0	1	III	II		
4 (46)	B	0	0	2	1	III	III	0	0
	L	1	1	2	2	III	III		

Table 1

CASE \ time		Pl. I.		G.I.		furcation involvement		tooth mobility	
		t_0	t_6	t_0	t_6	t_0	t_6	t_0	t_6
1 (36)	B	1	0	2	1	III	III	1	2
	L	2	1	2	1	III	III		
2 (36)	B	1	1	1	1	III	III	1	1
	L	1	1	1	2	III	III		
3 (48)	B	0	0	0	0	III	III	1	1
	L	0	1	0	1	III	III		
4 (36)	B	1	1	1	1	III	III	0	0
	L	2	2	1	2	III	III		

Table 2

Table 1: Clinical parameters recorded for Experimental sites before (t0) and six months post surgery (t6). In the first column : tooth number (W.H.O. identification); B:buccal,L:lingual.

Table 2: Clinical parameters recorded for control sites before (t0) and six months post-surgery (t6).In the first column: tooth number (W.H.O. identification); B:buccal,L:lingual.

Means of the differences for P.D.;P.A.L. and B.L. measurements registered before and six months post surgery ($\Delta$to-t6)have been calculated and analyzed for significance in a Student's t-test.Control sites show an average decrease of P.D. of 1mm,an average loss of P.A.L. of 1mm and of B.L. of 1.62mm.Experimental sites show as well an average decrease in P.D.of 1.12mm,an average loss of P.A.L.of 0.75mm and a gain in B.L.of 0.37mm.Variations are not statistically significant for either group of sites.Fig.1 reports a comparison of mean changes of P.D.,P.A.L.and B.L.of experimental sites versus control sites.When computing P.D.and P.A.L.differences results are not significant while the differences in the response of the bone level in the experimental versus the control group are statistically significant ($p<0.05$).

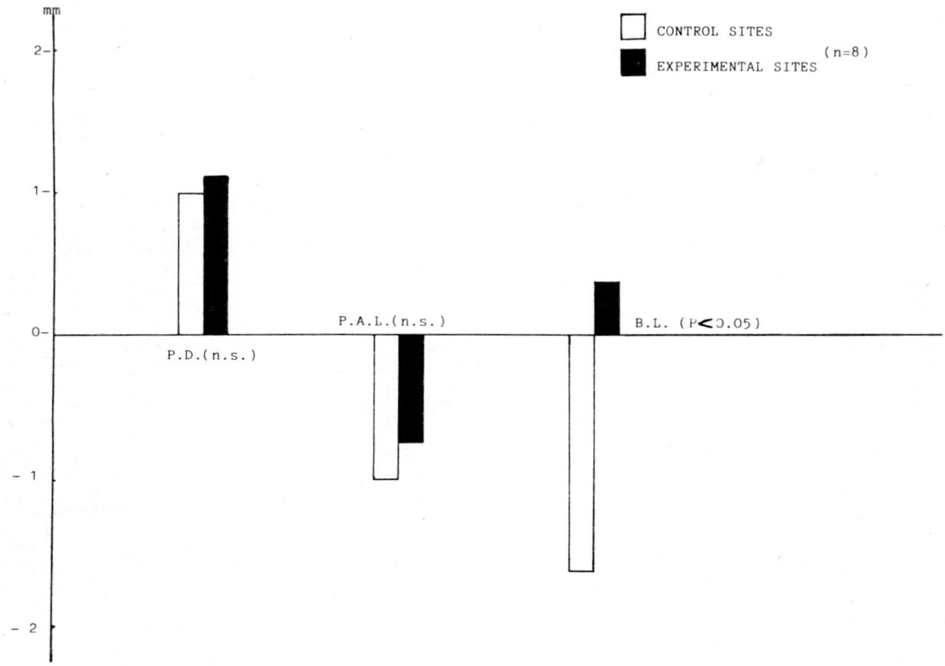

Fig. 1: Mean of changes (Δt0-t6) in mm of P.D.;P.A.L.;B.L.before (t0) and six months after surgery (t6).Control sites versus experimental sites (n=8).

X-rays taken immediately after experimental surgery show a complete filling of the defects with HA.After six months only one,out of four cases,in the experimental group,maintained such a closure of the furcation,while control sites,of course,did not show any bone formation in the furcation area at all During the reentry surgery in the experimental sites all the remaining porous HA appeared to be clinically fully integrated in the remodeling crestal bone.

DISCUSSION

To evaluate from the clinical standpoint the potential for osseous regeneration of porous HA the most conclusive parameter to look at seems to be the comparison of the means of the changes in B.L.,following the reconstructive technique,in the experimental versus the control sites.Values obtained are statistically significant ($p<0.05$) and point out particularly a loss of B.L. in the control group with a contemporary slight increase of the same parameter in the experimental.The results might suggest that porous HA could be active in counteracting bone resorption that usually follows the elevation of a surgical flap (Ref.7). A positive result might also be considered the clinical and radiographical healing of one,out of four,Class III furcation defect,in a Class II,showing,in such a way an horizontal regeneration.Unfortunately experimental measuring method was not designed to quantitate the horizontal bone regeneration.The radiographical data,six months post-surgery,support anyway the finding of a complete furcation healing and rule out the possibility of only a partial healing just sufficient to stop the progression of the clinical probing in the furcation area.Comparing the results obtained in this study with that ones of Kenney et al.(Ref.5) and of Meffert et al.(Ref.8),who successfully used various forms of HA in treating interproximal periodontal defects,it must be considered primarily the anatomical differencs between an interproximal defect and a complete interradicular furcation involvement,showing the latter,in contrast to the former,two avascular walls,i.e. the two root surfaces within the furcation that will not take part in the formation of the osseous coagulum (Ref.9),and the remaining two bony walls,buccal and lingual,very often unfavorably oriented for an effective retention of the implant material and for the organization of the osseous coagulum. Speculations about this point might conclude that the amount of osseous regeneration induced by porous HA is dependent on the anatomical configuration of the periodontal defect and that vertical vascular bone walls should be present to support a successful guided osseous regrowth. Regarding the biocompatibility of the material used,the reported complete clinical integration of the implant material in the surrounding bone at the surgical reentry experimental time,together with the absence of inflammation in the overlaying gingival tissue might suggest that porous HA could be fully biocompatible. Further studies are anyway needed on a larger clinical sample and on human block sections for hystologic evaluation to fully understand the dynamics involved in the healing of periodontal defects implanted with granular HA before any definitive statement concerning the exact nature of the periodontal response can be made.

REFERENCES

1 Kelly J.E. and van Kirk L.E..Periodontal Disease in Adults,U.S.1960-62, U.S.P.H.S.,National Ctr. for Health Statistics Pubbl.n.1000,Series11, n.12;1966

2 Dzink J.L.;Tanner A.C.R.;Haffajee A.D.;Socransky S.S..Gram negative species associated with active destructive periodontal lesions.J. Clin. Periodontol. 12:648;1985.

3 White E.W.;Weber J.N.;Roy D.M. et al..Replamineform porous biomaterials for hard tissue implant affections.J. Biomed. Mater. Res. Symp.6:23;1975.

4 West T.L. and Brustein D.D..Comparison of replamineform coral and bone alloplants in dog periodontal pockets.J. Dent. Res. 57:101;1978.

5 Kenney E.B.;Lekovic V.;Han T.;Carranza F.A.Jr.and Dimitrijevic B..The use of a porous hydroxylapatite implant in periodontal defects.I.Clinical results after six months.J. Periodontol. 56:82;1985.

6 Lindhe J. Textbook of Clinical Periodontology 1st Ed.,Munksgaard, Copenhagen,1983.

7 Donnenfeld O.W. and Glickman I..The apically repositioned flap-a clinical study.J. Periodontol.35:381;1964.

8 Meffert R.M.;Thomas J.R.;Kent M.H.and Brownstein C.N..Hydroxylapatite as an alloplastic graft in the treatment of human periodontal osseous defects.J. Periodontol. 56:63;1985.

9 Hiatt W.H. and Schallhorn R.G..Intraoral transplants of cancellous bone and marrow in periodontal lesions.J. Periodontol. 44:194;1973.

Biomaterials and Clinical Applications,
edited by A. Pizzoferrato, P.G. Marchetti, A. Ravaglioli and A.J.C. Lee
Elsevier Science Publishers B.V., Amsterdam, 1987 — Printed in The Netherlands

CO-ADSORPTION OF SALIVARY MUCINS AND PHOSPHOCOMPOUNDS TO HYDROXYAPATITE

A.V.NIEUW AMERONGEN, C.H.ODERKERK, E.C.I.VEERMAN and K.DE GROOT

Department of Biomaterials and Biochemistry, ACTA, Vrije Universiteit, van der Boechorststraat 7, 1081 BT Amsterdam (The Netherlands)

SUMMARY

The adsorption to hydroxyapatite (HAP) of human whole salivary mucins (HWSM), was studied in comparison with that of ovine submandibular mucin (OSM). The maximum binding capacity of HAP for HWSM was about 20-fold higher than that for OSM. Because in saliva several phosphoproteins binding strongly to the tooth enamel surface are present, the adsorption of both mucins was also studied in competition with model phosphocompounds, such as phytate and phosvitin.

Phytate (200 µg/ml) is able to desorb OSM completely from the HAP surface, in contrast to HWSM, which remained bound for the greater part. Phosvitin can desorb OSM completely at low concentrations (400 µg/ml), while for complete desorption of HWSM high concentrations of phosvitin (1000 µg/ml) are necessary.

Apparently, human salivary mucins bind stronger than OSM to HAP and are able to compete with phosphoproteins for the HAP surface. It is suggested that the combination of sulphate and sialic acid residues in HWSM is responsible for the higher affinity for HAP, compared to that of OSM.

INTRODUCTION

In saliva several proteins and glycoproteins are present, which adsorb rapidly and strongly to mucosa and apatite surfaces of the teeth. To these salivary glycoproteins belong the high molecular weight mucins, which are secreted from the acinar cells of the mucous salivary glands, particularly the submandibular and sublingual glands. The mucins consist of a long polypeptide backbone, densely packed with covalently bound oligosaccharide side chains. Because of the high content of hydrophilic sugars, the mucins have a high contribution to the viscoelasticity of saliva. In addition, the mucins are involved in aggregation of oral bacteria (ref. 1) and in protection of teeth against demineralization (ref. 2) and of the mucosa against microbial and viral infiltration. All these functions require the attachment of mucins to oral surfaces, which under physiological conditions takes place in competition with other salivary components, such as phosphoproteins (ref. 3).

We are interested in the physiological functions of the human salivary mucins in the oral cavity, e.g. for the preparation of appropriate artificial salivas.

METHODS

Isolation of human salivary mucins

From unstimulated human whole saliva the mucin fraction was isolated by sedimentation, due to their high molecular weight, in an ultracentrifugation technique (ref. 4). The final mucin preparation, designated HWSM, consisted for 18% of protein, 74% of carbohydrate and of 1.4% sulphate, and has been used to study its adsorption to HAP (ref. 5).

Adsorption experiments

Portions of 10 mg of synthetic hydroxyapatite (Biogel-HTP) were washed three times with distilled water and incubated up to 20 h with a suitable amount of adsorbate in a glass stoppered tube. Incubation was performed by rotating the tubes at 6 r.p.m. at room temp. After incubation the HAP was sedimented by centrifugation and the adsorbed amount was calculated by measuring the concentration of sialic acid, protein and/or phosphate in the supernatant. For calculation of the maximum binding capacity, N (μg/m^2 HAP), and the affinity constant, K (ml/μg), the Langmuir adsorption equation was used: $C_e/A = 1/K.N + C_e.N$.

Coadsorption experiments

To investigate the influence of the phosphocompounds, phytate and phosvitin, on the adsorption of the mucins to HAP, three different incubation schemes were followed:

1. mucins (400 μg/ml) were preincubated with HAP for 20 h, followed by coadsorption with a phosphocompound (0 to 1000 μg/ml) for 4 h,
2. phosphocompound (0 to 1000 μg/ml) was preincubated with HAP for 20 h, followed by coadsorption with mucins (400 μg/ml) for 4 h,
3. phosphocompound (0 to 1000 μg/ml) and mucins (400 μg/ml) were incubated together with HAP for 4 h. The pH in all three experiments was 6.3.

RESULTS

Adsorption of HWSM

Because the adsorption of mucins decreased sharply between pH 6 and 7, the adsorption experiments were performed at both pH 6.3 and pH 7.0. When 10 mg HAP was incubated with 400 μg HWSM/ml the adsorption at pH 5.5 was about 65%, at pH 6.3 45% and at pH 7.0 only 20% (ref. 5). In Fig. 1. adsorption isotherms at pH 6.3 and pH 7.0 of HWSM are shown. As can be seen the affinity of HWSM to HAP is higher at pH 6.3 than at pH 7.0. It seems that at pH 7.0 a plateau of adsorption is reached with a lower

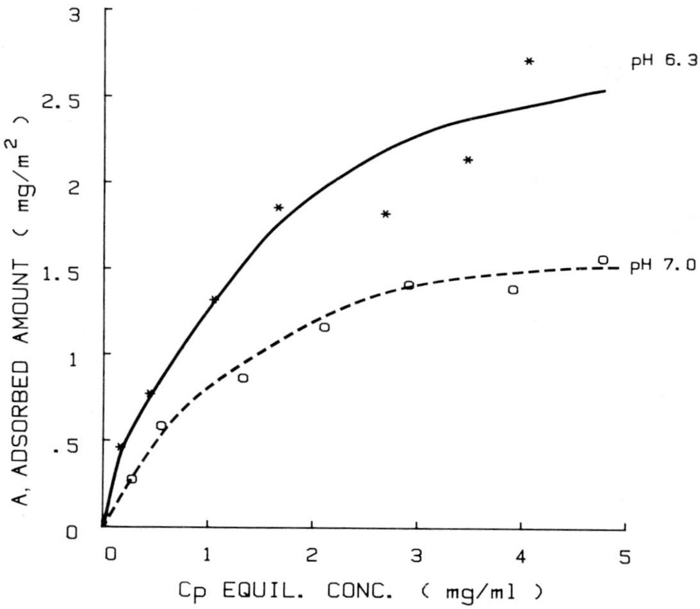

Fig 1. Adsorption isotherms of HWSM as a function of the equilibrium concentration of HWSM. Various amounts of HWSM, in the range of 0.5 to 6 mg/ml, were incubated with 10 mg of hydroxyapatite for 4 h at pH 6.3 (*----*) and 7.0 (o----o).

concentration of HWSM than at pH 6.3. Plotting the data of Fig. 1 according to the Langmuir adsorption equation yielded in both cases straight lines with high correlation coefficients. From such a plot it could be calculated that the apparent maximum binding capacity of HAP for HWSM (N) at pH 6.3 and 7.0 was 2,640 μg/m^2 and 2,050 μg/m^2, respectively, and that the affinity constant (K) at these pH's was 1.11 and 0.65 ml/mg, respectively.

When similar experiments were performed with ovine submandibular mucin (OSM), the calculated maximum binding capacity was about 20 - fold lower, namely 113 μg/m^2 HAP (Boerman et al., submitted for publication).

To study whether mucins are able to adsorb to HAP in competition with phosphocompounds, phytate and phosvitin were taken as a model. Phytate is hexakis phosphate of myoinositol and phosvitin is a major phosphoprotein from egg yolk. The adsorption of OSM decreased dramatically, even by the addition of small amounts of phytate or phosvitin. In the presence of 400 μg/ml of a phosphocompound hardly any OSM was still adsorbed. On the other hand, HWSM could be desorbed by phytate only for about 25%, even at phytate concentration of 1 mg/ml (Fig. 2). In the presence of 400 μg phosvitin/ml about 50% of the HWSM remained adsorbed, whereas OSM was desorbed for 100%. However 1 mg/ml phosvitin desorbed HWSM almost completely.

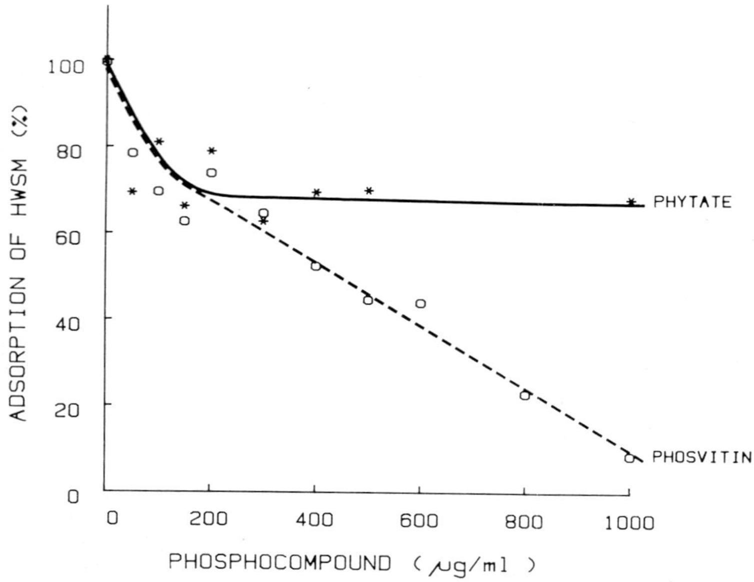

Fig. 2. Desorption of HWSM by phytate and phosvitin. HAP (10 mg) was preadsorbed at pH 6.3 with HWSM (400 µg/ml) for 20 h, followed by coadsorption with phytate (*——*) or phosvitin (o——o) for 4 h.

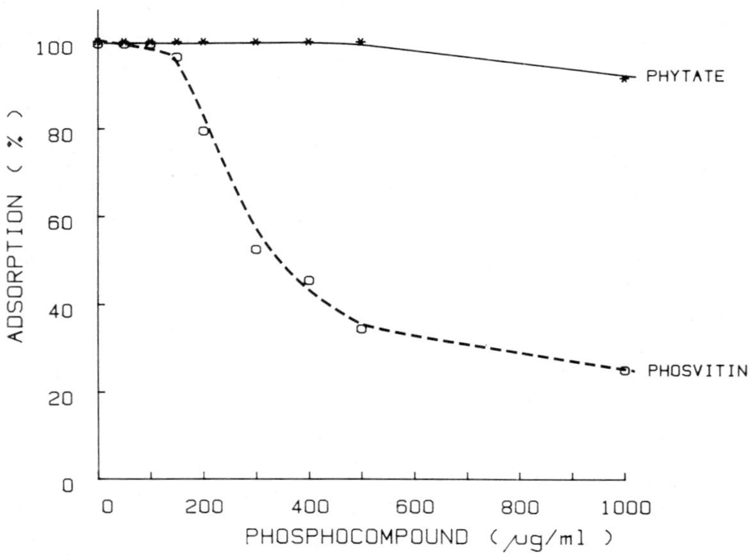

Fig. 3. Influence of preadosrbed HWSM on the coadsorption of phytate (*——*) and phosvitin (o——o). See legends of Fig. 2.

It appeared that in the same experiment HWSM affected hardly the adsorption of phytate (Fig. 3). Up to its maximum amount of binding (500 µg/10 mg HAP) the adsorption of phytate was nearly 100%. On the other hand, the adsorption of phosvitin decreased in the presence of HWSM, as is illustrated in Fig. 3. Apparently, HWSM and phosvitin can prevent mutually their adsorption, possibly by interacting with each other in solution.

DISCUSSION

From this study it is clear that human salivary mucins bind stronger to HAP than the animal mucin OSM. This was also the case for porcine submandibular mucin, PSM, and porcine gastric mucin, PGM (Boerman, personal communication). In comparison to the animal mucins, the human salivary mucins can compete with phosphocompounds better for the HAP surface (Fig. 2). The reason for the differences of the mucins in binding to HAP might be due to the difference in chemical composition, particularly of the carbohydrate side chains (Table 1). From these data the relative numbers of negatively charged groups can be calculated (Table 2). It is shown that OSM and PSM have as negatively charged groups mainly the carboxylic group of sialic acid, whereas PGM has only a low content of sialic acid but has sulphate residues in addition. In the HWSM preparation sulphate and phosphate were detected in addition to sialic acid.

TABLE 1. CHEMICAL COMPOSITION OF THE MUCINS (per cent of dry weight)

	Protein	Sialic acid	Fucose	Sulphate	Phosphate
Porcine Submandibular mucin (PSM)	19.4	14.0	6.0	---	---
Ovine Submandibular mucin (OSM)	20.6	22.4	---	---	---
Porcine Gastric mucin (PGM)	21.1	1.0	5.5	1.0	---
Human whole salivary mucin (HWSM)	18.2	5.1	17.4	1.4	0.14

Furthermore, it is known that OSM (ref. 7) and PSM (ref. 8) have only disaccharide chains and pentasaccharide chains, respectively, whereas human salivary mucins may contain more complex carbohydrate structures (ref. 9).

TABLE 2. INDICATION OF THE NUMBERS OF NEGATIVELY CHARGED GROUPS OF THE MUCINS (assuming for mol. wt. 500,000)

	Numbers of residues / molecule			
	PSM	OSM	PGM	HWSM
Phosphate ($-PO_3H_2$)	---	---	---	7
Sulphate ($-SO_3H$)	---	---	62	88
Sialic acid (-COOH)	227	362	16	82

In conclusion, the sulphate-containing sialomucins bind more strongly to hydroxyapatite than the sialomucins lacking sulphate residues. Therefore, in artificial saliva the sulphosialomucin PGM should be preferred to the sialomucins OSM, PSM or BSM. However, because of the much better adsorption properties of HWSM, this compound can not be substituted adequately in artificial saliva by the animal mucins studied.

REFERENCES

1. H.M.Koop, M.Valentijn-Benz, A.V.Nieuw Amerongen, P.A.Roukema and J.de Graaff, Aggregation of oral bacteria by human saliva, human salivary mucins and animal mucin preparations, submitted for publication.
2. A.V.Nieuw Amerongen, C.H.Oderkerk and A.A.Driessen. The role of mucins from human whole saliva in the protection of tooth enamel against demineralization in vitro, submitted for publication.
3. A.Bennick, G.Chau, R.Goodlin, S.Abrams, D.Tustian and G.Madapallimattam, The role of human salivary acidic proline-rich proteins and their fate after adsorption to the human enamel surface, Archs Oral Biol., 28 (1983) 19-27.
4. P.A.Roukema, C.H.Oderkerk and M.S.Salkinoja-Salonen, The murine sublingual and submandibular mucins. Their isolation and characterization, Biochim. Biophys. Acta, 428 (1976) 432-440.
5. A.V.Nieuw Amerongen and C.H.Oderkerk, Adsorption of human salivary mucins onto hydroxyapatite and the effect of the phosphocompound phytate, submitted for publication.
6. J.W.Boerman, M.Valentijn-Benz, P.A.Roukema and A.V.Nieuw Amerongen, On the adsorption of sialomucins to hydroxyapatite and the role of sialic acid in their binding, submitted for publication.
7. W.Pigman, Submandibular and sublingual glycoproteins, in: M.I.Horowitz and W.Pigman (Eds.), The Glycoconjugates, Vol. I, Academic Press, New York, 1977, pp. 137-152.
8. H.v.Halbeek, L.Dorland, J.Haverkamp, G.A.Veldink, J.F.G.Vliegenthart, B. Fournet, G.Ricart, J.Montreuil, W.D.Gathmann and D.Aminoff, Structure determination of oligosaccharides isolated from A^+H^+ and A^-H^- hog-submaxillary gland mucin glycoproteins, by 360-MHz ^1H-NMR spectroscopy, permethylation analysis and mass spectrometry, Eur.J.Biochem. 118 (1981) 487-495.
9. M.S.Reddy, M.J.Levine and A.Prakobphol, Oligosaccharide structures of the low molecular weight salivary mucin from a normal individual and one with cystic fibrosis, J. Dent. Res. 64 (1985) 33-36.

Biomaterials and Clinical Applications,
edited by A. Pizzoferrato, P.G. Marchetti, A. Ravaglioli and A.J.C. Lee
Elsevier Science Publishers B.V., Amsterdam, 1987 — Printed in The Netherlands

THE BONE-HYDROXYLAPATITE INTERFACE

G.L. DE LANGE, C. DE PUTTER, E.H. BURGER and K. DE GROOT

Dept. of Oral Cell Biology, Academic Center of Dentistry, P.O. Box 7161, 1007 MC Amsterdam, The Netherlands

ABSTRACT

The interface between bone and dense sintered hydroxylapatite (HA) was investigated by light microscopy, electron microscopy and microradiography. The study was performed on biopsies derived from a) subperiosteally placed granules for jaw augmentation with or without hip bone, b) loaded endosteally placed permucosal dental implants for tooth substitution, c) subperiosteally placed implant blocks for alveolar bone correction and d) endosteally placed artificial toothrooths for reducing residual ridge resorption. The light microscopical results showed extensive bone apposition on the infrabony parts of the HA surface. A direct bone contact was also observed by microradiography on thin undecalcified ground sections. At the ultrastructural level a thin electron dense layer of organic bone material was observed at the bone-implant interface, which may be related to the lamina limitans of bone tissue. Substantial degradations or phagocytosis were not observed at the bone-implant interface.

INTRODUCTION

Many recent reports deal with clinical results obtained by the use of hydroxylapatite (HA) as an implant material for hard tissue replacement. (Ref. 1,2,3). In general it can be stated that besides physical or biomechanical factors, the success of implantation is strongly dependent on a favourable tissue reaction at the implant-tissue interface. Although clinical observations provide much information, an accurate judgement of the tissues at the tissue-implant interface is only possible by microscopical examination. This study deals with implants of dense sintered hydroxylapatite which had functioned for a certain period of time in dogs and in humans.

MATERIALS AND METHODS

Biopsies were investigated from patients who had been treated for mandibular ridge augmentation six months before. (Ref. 4). For augmentation a 1:1 mixture was used of fresh autologous hip bone with dense HA granules or granules only. The implants were placed subperiosteally. Permucosal implants, made of dense sintered HA (Ref. 5) were placed in edentulous parts of the lower jaw of beagle dogs (Ref. 6). The implants were loaded and left in situ for six months to five years and inspected monthly. Subperiosteally placed blocks of dense HA used for alveolar bone correction (Ref. 7) and endosteally placed dental root implants (Ref. 8) were also investigated in dogs. These implants were applied unloaded and were left in situ for six months and five years respectively. The dogs were sacrificed and their jaws fixed by vascular perfusion. Tissue blocks were prepaired for light microscopy and electron microscopy. Contact microradiographs were made of thin non-decalcified ground sections. The mineral density at the bone-implant interface was measured in steps of 1 um. (Ref. 9). During all procedures care was taken not to damage the original tissue-implant interface.

RESULTS

The healing of the HA implants in the dogs passed without complications. Fixation of the smooth cylindrical permucosal implants was obtained as a rule within one week, despite the lack of protective measurements. The wear on top of these implants indicated that they had been loaded by occlusal forces. In light microscopical sections the bone surrounding the permucosal implants was of the normal lamellar type, with horizontally orientated trabecules. At the interface with marrow spaces in between, these trabecules were connected by a bone layer, deposed at the implant surface (Fig. 1). As a rule the whole implant surface was covered with bone, which was continuously connected with alveolar bone. The endosteally placed root implants showed a similar bone-implant interface. Bone was deposed on the whole surface, including the top of the implant. The subperiosteally placed implants in dogs showed a thin layer of bone, sometimes entirely covering the implant, sometimes partly. Occasionally small bony bridges were observed, connecting the deposed bone with the outher layer of alveolar bone. At other sides a dense capsule of connective tissue fibers surrounded the subperiosteal implant. Collagen fibers had grown into the finest surface irregularities of the implant. Macrophages were observed and occasionally multinuclear giant cells.

Apposition of bone occurred also on HA granules used for jaw augmentation in patients (Fig. 2). The latter occurred mainly when the granules had been mixed with hip bone. Below the mandibular bone level, the granules were surrounded by bone and interconnected by bony bridges. However, above this level the granules showed only occasionally bone apposition. Most of the granules were then surrounded by a dense connective tissue. At the bone-HA interface no space could be observed light microscopically. Calcified bone matrix filled the finest irregularities of the implant surface. Differences between loaded and non-loaded implants were not observed. Contact microradiographs made of thin non-decalcified ground sections showed also a very intimate implant-bone interface. Although the high mineral density of the implant gave rise to a higher absorption of the x-rays, no interruption or discontinuity could be observed at the HA-bone interface. Measurements in steps of 1 um also showed no discontinuity.

At the ultrastructural level the very intimate bone-implant interface could be confirmed. Intrinsic collagen fibres of the bone tissue could be followed into the finest surface irregularities of the implant. An electron dense layer of organic bone material was observed at the bone-implant interface (Fig. 3). It had a thickness varying between 20-80 nm. This layer had many similarities with the lamina limitans of bone as described elsewhere (Ref. 10). In contrast to the bone interface, we always observed macrophages or multinuclear giant cells at the connective tissue-HA interface.

DISCUSSION

One of the most obvious results was the fact that the smooth permucosal cylinders became so well fixed in the dog and so soon. Immobilization could be obtained without special mechanical protection during bone healing provided there was a good initial fit. Fixation must be based on a quick and extensive apposition of bone on the implants. This results in a relative large amount of bone contact (Ref. 11). This means that loading forces can be distributed over a large volume of supporting bone. Fixation is also based on a very intimate bone contact giving rise to an interlocking by microretention. The results obtained from the measurements of microradiographs showed that the distance between the calcium phosphate crystals of bone and implant did not exceed 1 um. Thin sectioning (< 0,1 um) of HA was not possible without severe mechanical damage and artefacts. We demineralized little section blocks, prior to ultrasectioning. The free coming space was then refilled with epoxy resin. By doing these procedures very carefully, it is possible to remove the ceramic component and to preserve the organic components at the interface. This was clearly demonstrated by the presence of a thin electron dense layer between bone and implant which we also observed at spots where the HA was not completely removed and remnants of implant material were still present due to the incomplete demineralization. A similar layer has been described in foetal and adult bone tissue (Ref. 10) between the mineralized and non-mineralized parts of the bone matrix.

From the morphological observations several conclusions can be drawn:

1. Presence of HA seems not to disturb the normal process of bone tissue maintenance.

2. There is no direct contact between bone crystals and implant crystals.

3. The mineral phases of bone and implant are connected by organic material.

The presence of this layer is an indication that a normal physiologic bone reaction has occurred at the bone-implant interface. Although the ultrastructural results were derived from dogs, it may be assumed that human bone reacted similarly.

If there was bone apposition, even if this layer was very thin, macrophages were absent. In contrast, when a non-calcified connective tissue bordered the implant, a wide variety of macrophages, fibroblasts and/or multinuclear giant cells were observed. From these results we may conclude that due to bone apposition a high degree of biological stability can be obtained at the bone-implant interface. This may be seen as the best condition for the successful use of HA as a bone or tooth substituting material.

REFERENCES

1 J.N. Kent, M.F. Zide, M.J. Jarcho, J.M. Ouinn, I.M. Finger and S.S. Rothstein, Correction of alveolar ridge deficiences with non resorbable hydroxylapatite, JADA, 105 (1982) 993-1001.

2 C. de Putter, K. de Groot and P.A.E. Sillevis Smitt, Transmucosal implants of dense hydroxylapatite, J.Prosth. Dent. 49 (1983) 87-95.

3 C.A. van Blitterswijk, J.J. Grote and W. Kuijpers, Hydroxylapatite in the infected middle ear in: J.J. Grote (Ed) Biomaterials in Otology, Martinus Nijhoff Publishers, 1984.

4 P.J.W. Stoelinga, P.A. Blijdorp, R.R. Ross, H.A. de Koomen and T.J.M. Huijbers, Augmentation of the atrophic mandible with interposed bone grafts and particulate hydroxylapatite, J.Maxillofac. Surg., 44 (1986) 353-360.

5 K. de Groot, Bioceramics consisting of calcium - phosphate salts, Biomaterials, 1 (1980) 47-50.

6 C. de Putter, Permucosal dental implants of dense hydroxylapatite, an animal experimental study, Free University Press, Amsterdam, 1984.

7 F.L.J.A. de Wijs, G.L. de Lange, C. de Putter and K. de Groot, Korrektur von Resorptionsdefekte im Oberkiefer Frontgebied. Die Quintessenz, 4 (1985) 647-656.

8 H.W. Denissen and K. de Groot, Immediate dental root implants from synthetic dense calcium hydroxylapatite, J. Prosth. Dent., 42 (1979) 551.

9 J.M. Ten Cate and P.P.E. Duysters, Influence of fluoride in solution on tooth demineralization II. Microradiographic data, Caries Res., 17 (1983) 513-519.

10 J.P. Scherft, The lamina limitans of the organic matrix of calcified cartilage and bone, J. Ultrastruct. Res., 38 (1972), 318-331.

11 G.L. de Lange, C. de Putter, R. de Vos, R. de Laat and K. de Groot, Permucosal dental implants. The relationship between bone anchorage and the quality of surrounding gingival tissues in: P. Christel, A.Meunier and A.J.C. Lee (Eds), Biological and Biomechanical Performance of Biomaterials, Elsevier, Amsterdam, 1986, p 519-524.

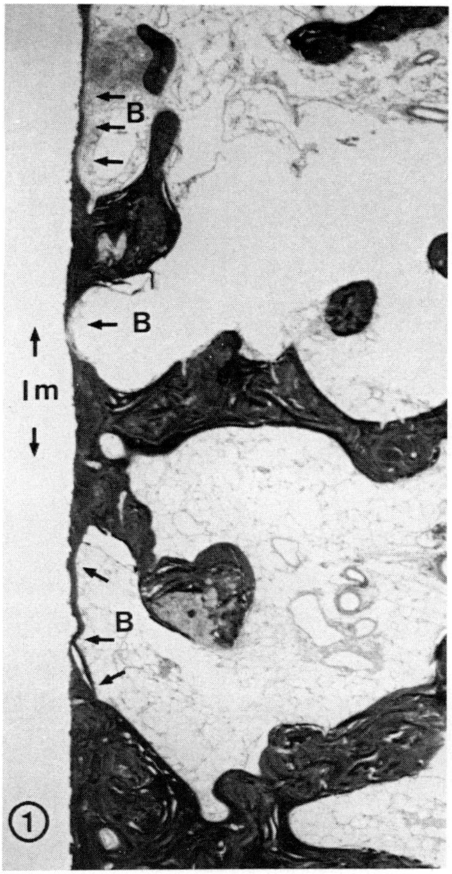

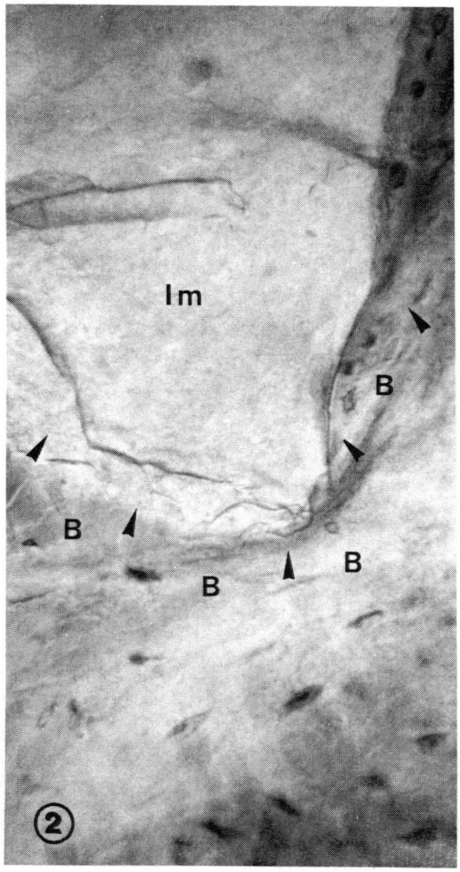

Fig. 1 Light micrograph of a two year loaded permucosal dental implant (Im). The bone surrounding the implant is of the normal lamellar type. Horizontal lying trabecules are connected by a bone layer (B) deposed at the implant surface. Decalcified dog specimen. Van Gieson, x 40.

Fig. 2 Light micrograph of a subperiosteally placed HA granule for jaw augmentation. There has been extensive bone apposition (arrows) on the surface around the implant (Im). Notice normal appearing osteocytes in the bone (B). Undecalcified human specimen, x 500.

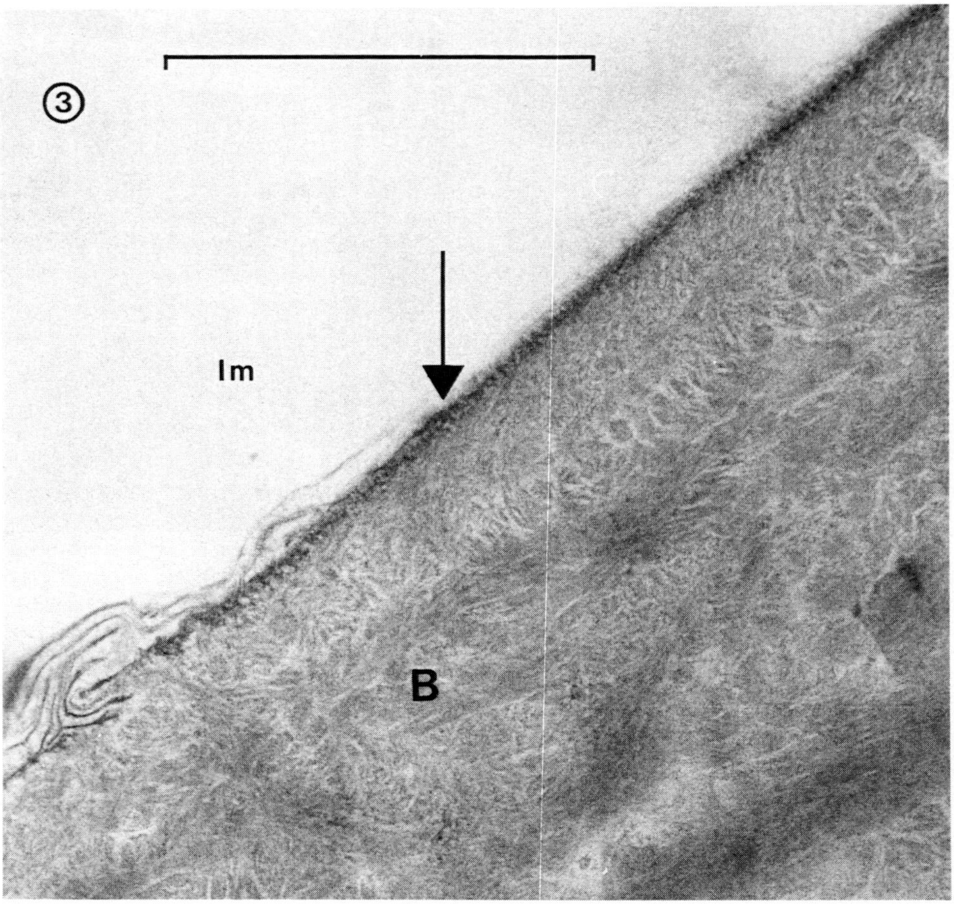

Fig. 3 Electron micrograph of the bone-HA interface. The implant (Im) is removed by decalcification. There is an electron dense layer of organic material (arrow) between the mineralized bone matrix (B) and the implant crystals. Bar is 1 µm.

Biomaterials and Clinical Applications,
edited by A. Pizzoferrato, P.G. Marchetti, A. Ravaglioli and A.J.C. Lee
Elsevier Science Publishers B.V., Amsterdam, 1987 — Printed in The Netherlands

BIOACTIVE MATERIALS FOR PERIODONTAL TREATMENT: A COMPARATIVE STUDY.

JUNE WILSON[1], S. LOW[2], A. FETNER[2] and L.L. HENCH[3]

[1]Program Manager, Bioglass® Research Center, University of Florida, Gainesville, FL 32610
[2]College of Dentistry, Department of Periodontics, University of Florida, Gainesville, FL 32610
[3]Director, Bioglass® Research Center, Professor, College of Engineering, University of Florida, Gainesville, FL 32610

INTRODUCTION

Calcium phosphate ceramics have been proposed and used in many dental applications including osseous augmentation. Particulate materials are presently in use as treatment for periodontal defects (ref. 1). These ceramics may be of hydroxylapatite or tricalcium phosphate providing a non-degradable and degradable source of calcium phosphate respectively, all contribute to the restoration of normal alveolar bone and reattachment of the periodontal membrane. Bioglass® , a bioactive glass material has been shown to bond to bone and to soft tissues in many different situations,(refs. 2,3) and has been applied to surgically created periodontal defects in this study. The Bioglass® was prepared in two formulations and in three particle size ranges and its efficiency in restoration of the defect assessed and compared with presently available calcium phosphate materials used for this purpose.

MATERIALS

Bioglass® - 45S5 formula (ref. 4).

Bioglass F® - 45S5 with substitution of 12.25% CaF_2 for some of the CaO.

Hydroxylapatite - commercially available particulates for treatment of periodontal defects

Tricalcium phosphate - commercially available particulates for treatment of periodontal defects

All materials were within a range of comparable particle sizes.

EXPERIMENTAL

Materials were mixed with saline and packed into infrabony defects created surgically in Patus monkeys. Root surfaces were planed to simulate true periodontal lesions. Both Bioglass® materials had markedly superior handling and manipulative properties and were noticably haemostatic (ref. 5).

Tissues were taken and examined microscopically after 1, 4, 6 and nine months.

RESULTS

Bioglass®

After one month the particles are present in soft tissues and above the alveolar bone, only occasional particles have bone at the interface. A foamy macrophage response is associated with particles at the lower end of the particle size range. Repair of the defect has begun with cementoid lining the defect and a cellular osteocementum extending from the normal cementum at the base. For remaining time periods of up to nine months the tissue response has more bone at the interface and particles are seen within repairing alveolar bone (Fig. 1). Particles are also within the new osteocementum which, by 9 months, lines the whole defect and which permits epithelial growth only to its upper limit, which is generally close to the original, normal level.

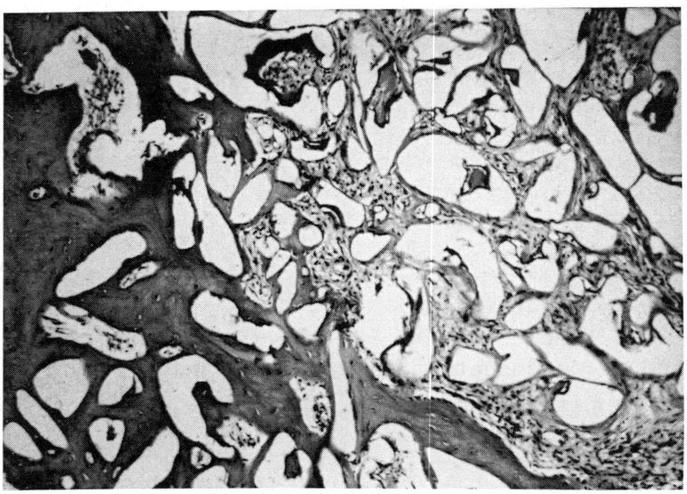

Figure 1. Bioglass® particles in bone and soft tissues after 4 months.

Insertion of transgingeval fibers into the repaired cementum is clear above the defect level. Association of foamy macrophages with the smallest particulate is still seen after 9 months.

Bioglass F®

At one month the tissue response is similar to that for Bioglass® except that those macrophages which are present are fewer in number and are not foamy in appearance. The number of particles with bone at the interface is greater than for Bioglass® alone.

By nine months the defects are filled by osteocementum as for those with Bioglass® alone. Particulates are present within bone and osteocementum and bone has formed by osteoconduction from the cemental repair but also by osteoproduction in the center of the defects

Hydroxylapatite

At one month there was early repair in the defects with cementoid. Particles at the base of the defect had bone at the interface by osteoconduction. By nine months the repair had not completely relined the defect and epithelial downgrowth was seen. (Fig. 2) Repairing alveolar bone had particles incorporated in it and particles adjacent to osteocementum had bone by conduction.

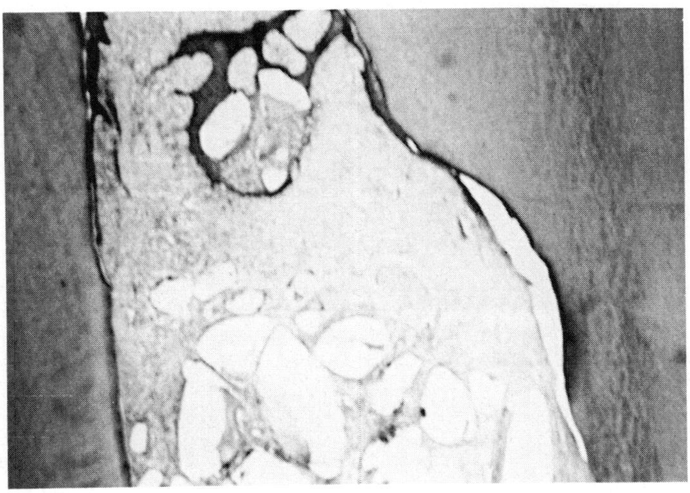

Figure 2. Hydroxylapatite after 4 months.

Particles in the connective tissue above the bone had giant cell and macrophage responses.

Tricalcium phosphate (TCP)

At one month there was early repair extending halfway up the defect. Some particles had bone at the interface and were incorporated within the repairing alveolar bone. The particles were most often surrounded by macrophages and giant cells with particles of TCP within them, as is normal for this material However, a band of tranverse fibers of the periodontal membrane separated most particles from the repairing bone (Fig. 3). By 9 months the defect was repaired but with some slight epithelial downgrowth. There was bone by osteoconduction from osteocementum and particulate incorporated into the regrowing bone, which had only repaired to approximately half of the original level. Particles in soft tissue were associated wth giant cells, macrophages and with bone.

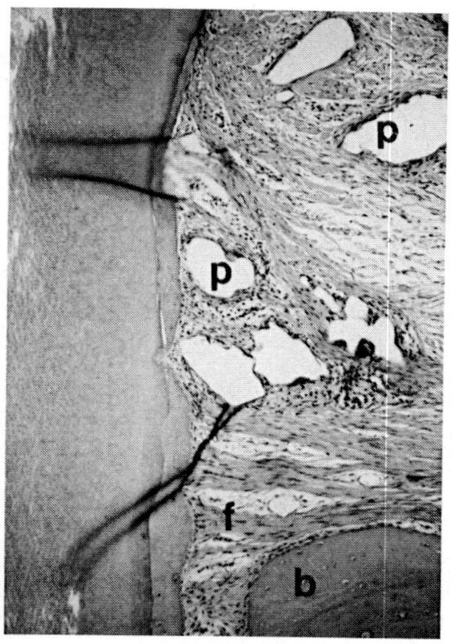

Figure 3. TCP after 4 months. B = bone; F = transverse fibers; p = particles.

DISCUSSION

All materials in this study allowed repair of the defect and restoration of the alveolar bone. Repaired cementum and bone contained particulates and osteoconduction was a feature of the repair mode. Bioglass® materials achieved the repair more quickly and completely with reattachment of the periodontal ligament and little or no epithelial downgrowth. In the case of Bioglass® materials the presence of bone at the interface of particles occurred with and without demonstrable osteoconduction. This has been previously described (ref. 3) and is considered to be due to colonisation of the bioactive surface by osteogenic cells free in the environment as a result of surgical intervention. This is referred to as osteoproduction. An advantage of Bioglass F® over Bioglass® may be that the early cellular tissue response is more limited allowing repair to progress more quickly.

The foamy macrophages associated with Bioglass® in the smallest particle size suggest that these are biodegradable and that the equivalent size in Bioglass F® is not, thus allowing transition from the cellular to the fibrous stage of the interfacial response at an earlier time. This is in accordance with the increase in chemical stability associated with fluoride addition (ref. 4).

CONCLUSIONS

Bioglass® and Bioglass F® can provide effective materials for restoration of periodontal defects, which allow repair to proceed more rapidly than with hydroxylapatite or tricalcium phosphate materials already available. A mechanism of osteoproduction is proposed. The smallest size particles tested appear to affect the early stage of tissue response, but this may be outweighed by the advantage which they give to the cohesive properties of the particulates and their handling ability in the operating room. This effect on tissue response is reduced when the Bioglass® F is used.

Acknowledgment

This work is supported by American Biomaterials Corporation, Princeton, N.J. The authors thank Mrs. Mary Stone for her patience in dealing with a difficult histological study.

REFERENCES

1. R.M. Meffert, J.R. Thomas, K.M. Hamilton, C.N. Brownstein, Hydroxylapatite as an Alloplastic Graft in the Treatment of Human Periodontal Osseous Defects. J. Periodontology 56 (1985) pp. 63-74
2. L.L. Hench and J. Wilson, Surface-Active Biomaterials, Science Vol. 226 (1984) pp. 630-636.
3. J. Wilson, G. Merwin, L. Rogers, R. Martin and D. Spilman Facial Bone Augmentation Using Bioglass® in Dogs, Biological and Biomechanical Performance of Biomaterials (Eds.) P. Christel, A. Meunier and A.J.C. Lee, Elsevier Science Publs. (1986) pp. 93-98.
4. L.L. Hench, D.B. Spilman, D.R. Nolletti, Fluoride Bioglasses® Biological and Biomechanical Performance of Biomaterials, (Eds.) P. Christel, A. Meunier and A.J.C. Lee, Elsevier Science Publs. (1986) pp. 99-104.
5. A.E. Fetner, S.B. Low, J. Wilson, L.L. Hench, Comparison of Various Synthetic Implant Materials for Periodontal Osseous Repair, Abstract, J.Dental Res., 65 (1986) p. 347.

Biomaterials and Clinical Applications,
edited by A. Pizzoferrato, P.G. Marchetti, A. Ravaglioli and A.J.C. Lee
Elsevier Science Publishers B.V., Amsterdam, 1987 — Printed in The Netherlands

RIB-CONNECTING PINS PREPARED FROM POLY-L-LACTIDE

S.-H. HYON[1], Y. IKADA[1], H. KATO[2], T. NAKAMURA[1], S. WATANABE[1], AND Y. SHIMIZU[1]

[1]Research Center for Medical Polymers and Biomaterials, Kyoto University, 53 Kawahara-cho, Shogoin, Sakyo-ku, Kyoto 606 (Japan)

[2]Shiga University of Medical Science, Seta, Otsu, Shiga 520-21 (Japan)

SUMMARY

For intramedullary fixation of rib fractures, bioabsorbable pins were prepared from poly-L-lactide(P-L-LA) with different molecular weights ($\overline{M}n$). The bending strength of the pins from P-L-LA with $\overline{M}n$ of 7 x 10^4 decreased virtually to zero upon hydrolysis in vitro for three months, whereas the pin from P-L-LA with $\overline{M}n$ of 2 x 10^5 showed no significant reduction in bending strength after three months hydrolysis in vitro. A similar effect of the molecular weight of the P-L-LA was also observed on the animal experiment using dogs. The pins prepared from P-L-LA with $\overline{M}n$ of 2 x 10^5 were able to maintain the strength required for connecting the fractured ribs until complete reunion.

INTRODUCTION

Metallic wires and plates as well as ceramic pins have been commonly used for fixation of disconnected ribs (refs. 1,2). However, these materials have some disadvantages. For instance, the extremely high rigidity of these materials in comparison with that of a rib prevents the flexing motion of the rib, often accompanying respiratory distress. In addition, these implants that permanently continue to remain inside the rib even after healing, may weaken the bone tissue and, especially for children, hinder the normal growth of ribs.

Such disadvantages may be surmounted if the rib-connecting pin is made from biodegradable materials that have mechanical properties similar to those of the rib tissue (refs. 3,4). Based on this consideration we have prepared rib-connecting pins from poly-L-lactide(P-L-LA), a biodegradable aliphatic polyester.

EXPERIMENTAL

P-L-LA

The L-LA monomer synthesized from L-lactic acid of 96 % optical purity was subjected to ring-opening polymerization in bulk at 140 °C to yield P-L-LA with a viscosity-average molecular weight ($\overline{M}n$) of 3.6 x 10^5. The polymer was shaped to a plate by compression molding with a hot-press machine.

By changing the thermal hysteresis during compression molding we could obtain P-L-LA plates possessing different molecular weights. Additional heat treatment at 120 °C for 4 hr resulted in crystallization of P-L-LA molecules in the plate.

In vitro and in vivo test

Hydrolytic degradation in vitro was conducted in PBS of pH 7.4 at 37°C for the plate with a volume of $40 \times 6 \times 2$ mm^3 and the resulting plate was subjected to physical measurements after drying. An in vitro test to follow the plate biodegradation was carried out using Japanese rabbits weighing from 2.5 to 3.0 kg. After sterilization with the ethylene oxide gas, the plate was intramuscularly or subcutaneously implanted in the back of rabbit under the aseptic condition.

Implantation in rib

Plates with a length of 2.8 cm, width of 3.0 mm, and thickness of 2.0 mm were used as rib-connecting pins. They were inserted in the bone marrow of fourth, sixth, and eighth rib of the left thorax of mongrel dogs after being cut.

RESULTS AND DISCUSSION

Degradation in vitro

Effects of the initial molecular weight of P-L-LA on the degradation rate were studied in vitro. Changes in molecular weight, bending strength, and weight loss with the hydrolysis time are given in Figs.1 and 2 for the plate from P-L-LA having $\overline{M}n$ of 7×10^4 and 2×10^5, respectively. In both cases the molecular weight drastically decreases in the beginning, but the degradation rate of the P-L-LA with the higher molecular weight slows down with time, compared with that of the lower molecular weight. A similar effect of molecular weight is also seen for the change in strength and weight loss. It should be noted that hydrolysis through the third month virtually accompanies no reduction in bending strength for the plate prepared from P-L-LA with $\overline{M}n$ of 2×10^5.

Degradation in vivo

The in vivo tests were performed to study the influence of the polymer crystallization and the implantation site on the biodegradation rate of plates. The non-crystallized and the crystallized polymer have $\overline{M}n$ of 2.0×10^5 and 1.5×10^5, respectively. The plates were implanted in two different sites; intramuscular and subcutaneous implantation. The results are shown in Fig.3 for the molecular weight change and in Fig.4 for the bending strength

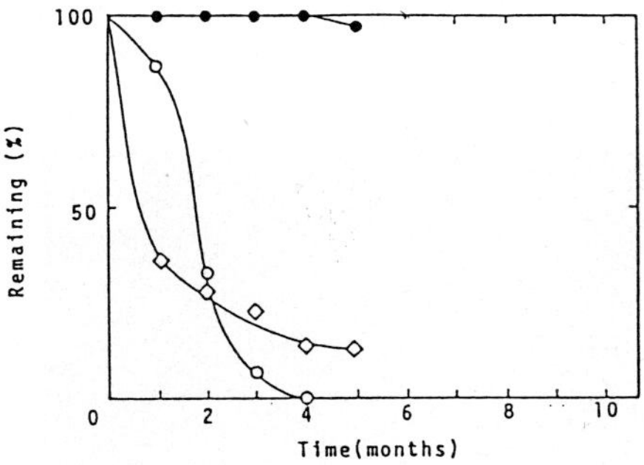

Fig. 1. Molecular weight, bending strength, and weight loss of P-L-LA plate ($\overline{M}n=7x10^4$) as a function of hydrolysis time. (●):weight, (◇):molecular weight, (○):bending strength

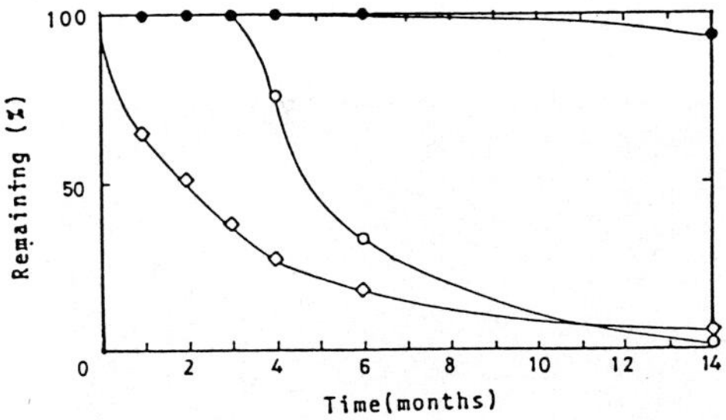

Fig. 2. Molecular weight, bending strength, and weight loss of P-L-LA plate ($\overline{M}n=2x10^5$) as a function of hydrolysis time. (●): weight, (◇):molecular weight, (○):bending strength

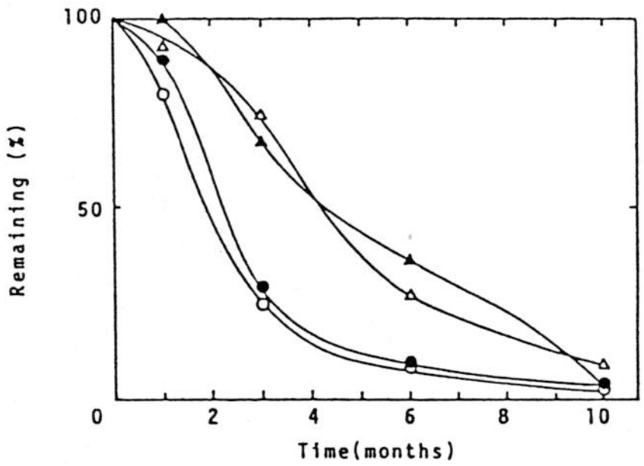

Fig. 3. Molecular weight loss of P-L-LA plate as a function of implantation time.
(△):Non-crystallized polymer,
(○):Crystallized polymer
Open marks;IC Closed marks;IM

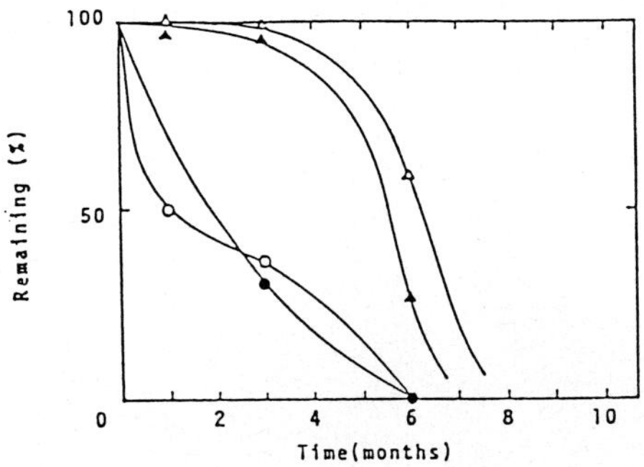

Fig. 4. Bending strength loss of P-L-LA plate as a function of implantation time.
(△):Non-crystallized polymer,
(○):Crystallized polymer
Open marks;IC Closed marks;IM

change. The effect of the difference in implantation site is insignificant at least in this study. On the contrary, the effect of polymer crystallization is remarkable, both for the molecular weight and the strength change. From Figs.3 and 4, crystallization of P-L-LA through heat treatment accelerates the degradation of the plate. The bending strength remains almost unchanged when the plate is not heat-treated, similar to the in vitro test, whereas the bending strength decreases to about 40 % of the starting value after the third month of implantation upon crystallization. The more marked biodegra-

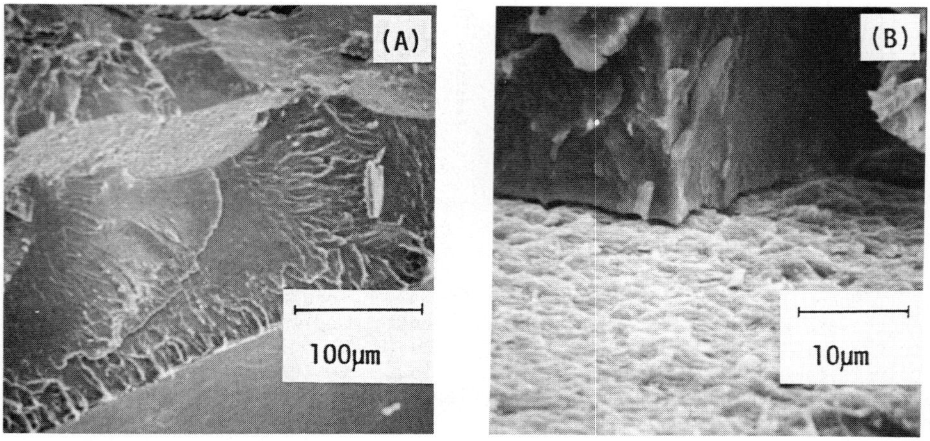

Fig. 5. SEM of P-L-LA plate 10 months after implantation.
(A) Crystallized polymer, (B) Non-crystallized polymer

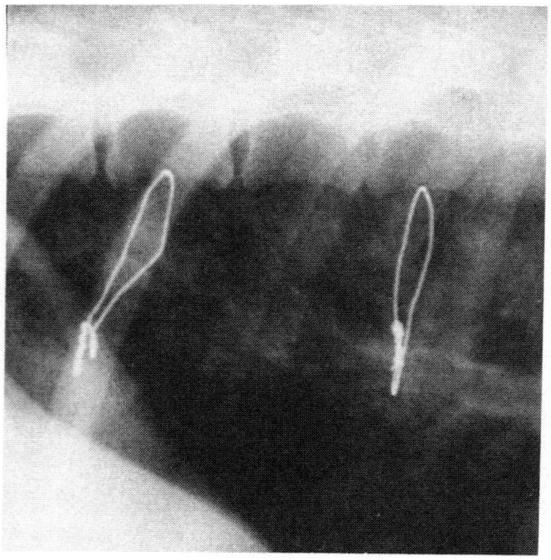

Fig. 6. X-ray photo of the ribs implanted with plates prepared from P-L-LA of $\bar{M}n$ of 2×10^5.

dation of the crystallized plate may be due to a reduction in the molecular weight and the formation of defects by crystallization. The increased crystallinity seems not to contribute to the strength retention.

Fig.5 shows scanning electron microscopic photographs of the plates intramuscularly implanted for ten months. Both the non-crystallized and the crystallized plates are smooth at surface, but the fractured plane of the crystallized plate has sharp crevices while that of the non-crystallized plate has round appearance.

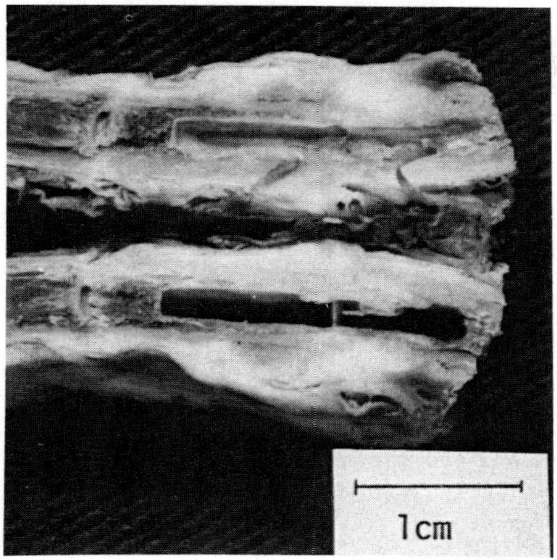

Fig. 7. Longitudinal cross-section of the rib with a P-L-LA plate implanted for one month.

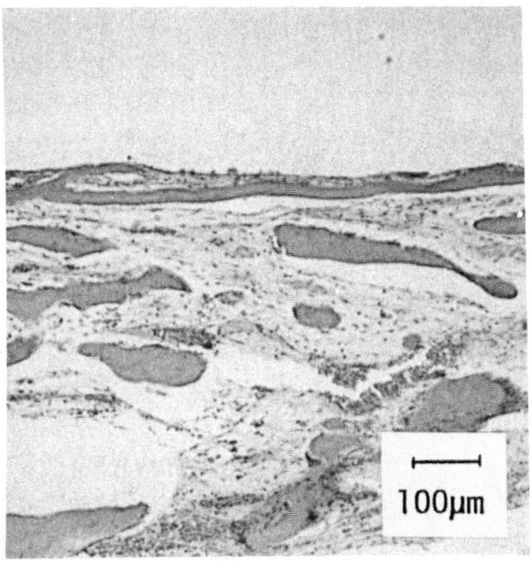

Fig. 8. Light microscopic photo of the rib tissue in contact with the P-L-LA plate implanted for one month.

Application as a rib-connecting pin

Fig.6 shows the X-ray photograph of the dog ribs, in the marrow of which the pins from P-L-LA with $\overline{M}_n$ of 2×10^5 have been inserted for two weeks.

As can be seen, the reunion of the disconnected ribs is satisfactory. However, both of the cut ends of the ribs had been separated from the connected site in two weeks because of breaks in the P-L-LA pins when they were prepared from P-L-LA with $\overline{M}n$ of 7×10^4.

Fig.7 shows the cross-sectional view along the longitudinal direction of the rib with the implanted P-L-LA pin for one month. Ingrowth of the glassy cartilage tissue can be seen at the connected site of the outermost part of the cross-section and the cortical bone at both sides in the cross-section is normal and stays at the same position in the connected region. At the second month of implantation, a continuously connected cortical bone layer has not yet been formed, but a cancellous bone corresponding to the bone marrow has been generated to firmly encapsulate the implanted P-L-LA pin.

To obtain histological information, the surroundings of the implanted pin was fixed one month postoperation and photographed with a light microscope. The result is given in Fig.8. It is seen that a glassy cartilage tissue has grown from the periosteum and is bound to the cortical bone at the connected site. Such a glassy cartilage tissue occupies the gap in the connected region where active bone healing is seen to proceed. After the first month implantation, the tissue surrounding the P-L-LA pin mostly comprises the cancellous bone of normal marrow and there is few inflammatory cells such as foreign-body giant cells. After two months implantation, the cancellous bone around the pin grew further, although the connected site was occupied by a cartilage-like tissue.

REFERENCES

1 H. Kato, M. Mizuno, K. Tamura, S. Watanabe, Y. Shimizu, T. Teramatsu, Y. Kitamura, M. Hirabayashi, Experimental study on artificial ceramic bone for ribs and sternum, Artf. Organs 5, Suppl., 1981, pp. 493-496.

2 S. Watanabe, Y. Shimizu, A. Mitsuoka, K. Tamura, H. Wada, M. Ito, S. Hitomi, Y. Takashima, S. Matsunobe, H. Kato, Clinical experiences with alumina ceramic pin for fracture of ribs, J. Japanese Association for Thoracic Surgery, 34, 1986, pp. 220-225.

3 S.-H. Hyon, K. Jamshidi, Y. Ikada, Spinning of poly-lactide and hydrolysis of the fiber in vitro, ACS Symp. Series, Polymers in Medicine, 51, 1985.

4 K. Jamshidi, S.-H. Hyon, Y. Ikada, T. Nakamura, Y. Shimizu, T. Teramatsu, In vitro and in vivo degradation of poly-L-lactide fibers, 5th European Conference on Biomaterials, Paris, France, 1985.

Biomaterials and Clinical Applications,
edited by A. Pizzoferrato, P.G. Marchetti, A. Ravaglioli and A.J.C. Lee
Elsevier Science Publishers B.V., Amsterdam, 1987 — Printed in The Netherlands

OSTEOSYNTHESIS BY COMMERCIALLY PURE TITANIUM FOR TEMPORARY AND PERMANENT RECONSTRUCTIVE IMPLANTATION IN LIMB SURGERY

H. SCHMID, J. BREME and K. JUNGER

Department of Traumatology, Medical School Erlangen, Maximiliansplatz 1, D-8520 Erlangen (Germany F.R.)

INTRODUCTION

Bundle nailing, as described by Hackethal in 1961, is a method of intramedullary osteosynthesis for shaft-fractures of the humerus and forearm of adults as well as the femur of children. The incidence of complications is low. Good restoration of the shape and function of the injured extremity is usually obtained without any difficulties.

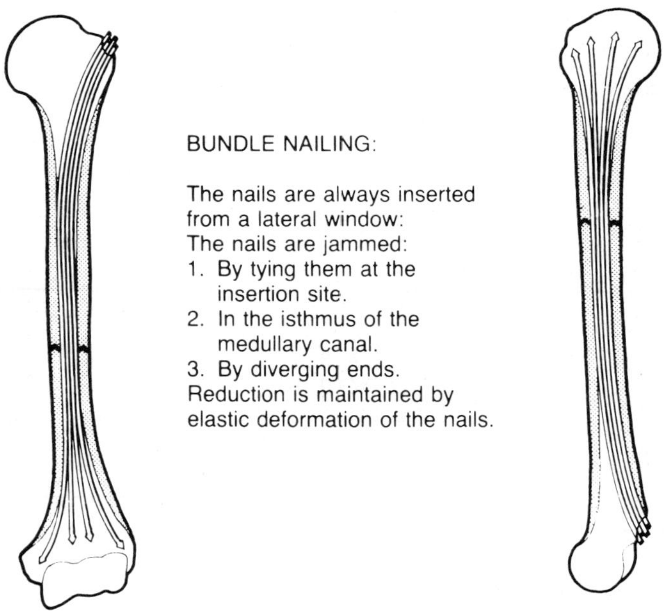

Fig. 1. Bundle Nailing

Bundle nailing provides less stability in the lower extremities than rigid nailing, but has significant advantages for the treatment of fractures of the humerus and forearm of adults. Intraoperative deformities can occur with a rigid nail that can straighten the physiological, often S-shaped curvature of the medullary canal. These deformities do not appear in bundle nailing.

20 years of clinical experience revealed that the stainless steel, which is used for bundle nailing, has some disadvantages. In search of better biocompatible metallic materials, Titanium was introduced and shows the following advantages:

1) High flexibility (Youngs Modulus of 110 000 N/mm^2, which is about half of the elasticity modulus of common materials)
2) Introvital corrosion resistance
3) Lack of allergic reactions
4) No teratogenic, mutagenic or carcinogenic tissue reaction
5) Sufficient mechanical properties (no failures observed)

Material used for the fabrication of the Titanium nails

The nails are produced of Titanium grade 2. Table 1 shows the mechanical properties of a wire in the delivered condition. In order to increase the yield strength of the material, the wire was cold deformed (degree of deformation 75%). The mechanical properties of the cold deformed wire are shown in Table 1.

	R_m (N/mm^2)	$R_{po,2}$ (N/mm^2)	A_5 (%)	Z (%)
as delivered	44o	31o	23	31
cold deform.	825	76o	7	18

TABLE 1 Mechanical properties of Ti grade 2, as delivered and 75% cold deformed

The low Young's modulus increases the stress protection of the bone. While inserting the nails, the high flexibility of the Titanium nails preserve the anatomical shape of the medullary canal. In case of dislocation of the fracture, the flexibility of Titanium nails may even allow a reponation of the fragments.

A severe corrosion reaction is caused by fretting of stainless steel. During and after implantation of bundle nails, the protecting surface layer of the nails is damaged, due to the scratching and close contact of the nails. This corrosion of the steel induces a pathological reaction of the surrounding tissue that is called metallosis. Breaking of the nails and instability may result. Therefore stainless steel nails have to be removed after 4 - 6 month. In contrast to steel, the dissolution of Titanium can be regarded to be extremly low. As shown in an experiment using 0,9% Sodium Chloride, the activated surface will repassivate in a split second (10^{-3}) by the formation of a protecting Oxygen surface layer. Degraded material, too, is rapidly coated, due to its large surface, by an oxide layer and is therefore insoluble. As a result, Titanium bundle nails can be left in the bone, until a complete restoration of the fracture is achieved. In elderly patients a permanent implantation of Titanium nails is justifiable.

An obvious increase in allergic reactions could be observed in the use of stainless steel. Nickel and Chromium are often parts of the alloy. These metals cause a localized allergic reaction in the bone and in the surrounding connective tissue. As a result the nails loosen and stability cannot be maintained anymore. Titanium, on the contrary, is an inert metal without inducing allergic reactions.

RESULTS

3 clinical cases will demonstrate the operative treatment with Titanium bundle nails:

Case 1

A 28 year old man suffered from a transverse fracture of the midshaft left humerus. High stability was achieved with descending bundle nailing. The two right X-rays in Fig. 2 were taken 8 weeks after nailing. A good callus formation across the fracture is visible.

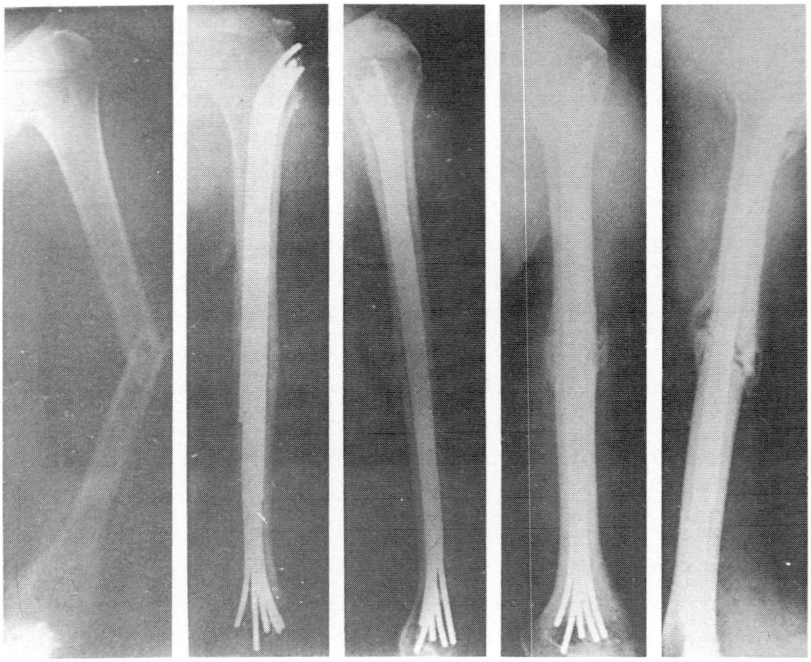

Fig 2. Case 1

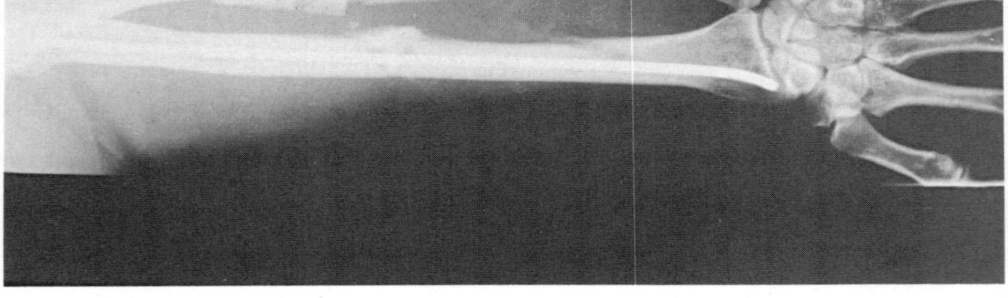

Fig. 3. Case 2

Case 2

A 59 year old woman suffered from a complete forearm fracture, after an accident. The patient was treated with descending bundle nails on the day of the accident. The small diameter of the medullary canal allowed the insertion of only one bundle nail. In addition a plastic cast was applied and removed after 2 weeks. Due to cardiovascular complications, the risk of a removal operation of the nails was too high. Good restoration of the forearm bones was observed and longterm complications did not arise.

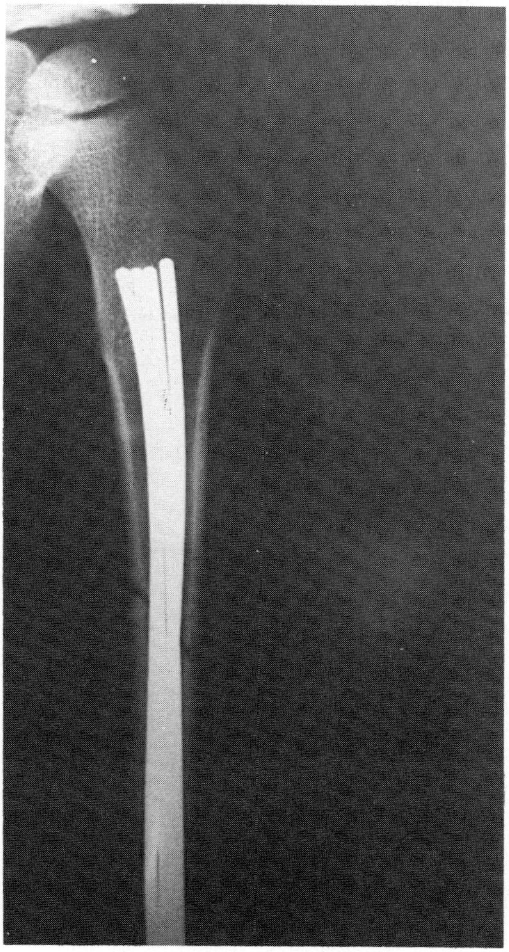

Fig. 4. Case 3

Case 3

A 3 year old girl ran into a car. The femur shaft was broken and a craniocerebral trauma grade 2 was diagnosed. The psychomotoric agitation of the child did not allow the usual conservative treatment of the fracture. Therefore the treatment with ascending bundle nails was indicated. The picture shows the postoperative X-ray.

CONCLUSION

In search of a better biocompatible material for bundle nailing, cold deformed Titanium was introduced. In comparison to stainless steel, the main advantages of Titanium are the high flexibility, corrosion resistance and the lack of allergic reactions. Due to these advantages, a reduction in the rate of postoperative complications could be observed.

REFERENCES

1 R. Maatz, W. Lentz, W. Arens, H. Beck, Intramedullary nailing and other intramedullary osteosyntheses, W.B. Saunders Company, 1986

2 Steinemann, S., S.M. Perren, Gordon Research Conference "Biomaterials", Tilton, 1972

Biomaterials and Clinical Applications,
edited by A. Pizzoferrato, P.G. Marchetti, A. Ravaglioli and A.J.C. Lee
Elsevier Science Publishers B.V., Amsterdam, 1987 — Printed in The Netherlands

COMPOSITE LIGAMENT MADE OF CARBON FIBRE BRAID

David G. Mendes MD, Moshe Roffman MD, Michael Soudry MD, David Angel MD, Mauricio Iusim MD, Dan Mordohovitch VDM, Assa Rotem PhD, Jochanan Boss MD.

Research Center for Implant Surgery, Haifa Medical Center (Rothschild), the Rappaport Family Institute for Research in the Medical Sciences, Technion - Israel Institute of Technology, Haifa, Israel.

ABSTRACT

The evidence gathered in our investigation did not support the concept of gradual take over of the load by the newly formed collagen fibres concurrent with gradual failure or fragmentation of the carbon fibrils. On the contrary it was obvious that the carbon fibrils did not fragment (except for cases of failure) and rather continued to take the tensile load and provided all the tensile strength of the composite ligament. If breakage of the stiff carbon fibrils took place, failure of the collagenous component due to mechanical deficiency of the composite ligament was likely to occur.

INTRODUCTION

In 1977 Jenkins in the United Kingdom reported the use of carbon fibre braid for substitute of tendons and ligaments calling it a temporary scaffold for connective tissue. He assumed that it might be inducing tissue proliferation as well as conducting the direction of growth. Other investigators further developed his concept and in general concurred with his opinion on the mode of action of the carbon braid.

Our group in the Research Center for Implant Surgery in Haifa started in 1980 experimental and clinical studies and have concluded that the carbon fibre composite ligament rather functions as a permanent prosthesis, although it conducts a remarkable proliferation of collagenous tissue.

The natural ligament is a composite made of two kinds of fibres; mostly collagen and minute percentage of elastin embedded within matrix of glycoprotein with a minute number of cells.

The biomechanical properties expressed as the stress-strain ratio can be shown to be non-linear, which, for a predetermined velocity demonstrates a visco-elastic property, that is the relation between deformation and speed of application of force. It also accounts for the crimp which is the dynamic wavy configuration of the fibres under no or low load conditions. The strength of ligaments is age related and the anterior cruciate ligament can carry loads of approximately 50 kg up to 150 kg.

Biocompatibility of the artificial ligament is an essential prerequisite and in general is defined by tissue tolerance, lack of toxicity and lack of carcinogenic effect. Tissue reaction to many synthetic materials when in bulk, is often hardly noticed, manifested by encapsulation with a delicate fibrous membrane. It is the particles and fibres , their chemical structure, shape and size which may provoke various types and intensity of inflammatory reaction.

EXPERIMENTAL MODEL

The clinical challenge was to repair or reconstruct tear of the quadriceps tendon with carbon fibre braid when tissue was deficient and to enhance the speed of recovery and to resume early function of the muscle after repair.

In laboratory animals (dogs) the quadriceps and triceps tendons were cut through. The carbon braid bridged the gap on either side. Evaluation of results was done between 3 and 12 months.

Results

The tensile strength of the 40,000 carbon fibre braid prior to their use in dogs was only 15% of the theoretical strength due to the stiffness of the fibres which failed to reach ultimate length simultaneously (prior to rupture). The ultimate tensile load therefore was on average 660 Newton.

The load extension curve of the composite structure after 1 year in dogs was not dissimilar to the natural tendon and the ultimate load was adequate for in vivo function.

The integrity of the carbon fibres within the functioning composite structure was preserved in its entirety. This was proven by placing the structure after one year in dogs in potassium hydroxide until complete dissolution of the connective tissue component took place. This exposed the entire carbon braid with its original tensile strength.

Conclusions

The carbon fibre braid within the composite structure does not fragment (unless is torn by shear force).

The ultimate tensile load is given by the stiffer and stronger carbon fibres (and not by the collagen).

The tensile strength of the braid of carbon fibres is compromised due to their stiffness.

CLINICAL EXPERIENCE

Material

In 45 Patients replacement of ligament or tendons was undertaken. These were divided into 2 major groups:

1) Ligaments reconstruction in 29 patients: mostly around the knee joint; 2 for ankle instability and 2 for acromio-clavicular joint disruption.

2) Tendon repair and reconstruction in 16 patients: 6 Quadriceps, 3 patella tendon, and 7 Achilles tendon.

Results

Ligaments. The results of ACL reconstruction in 8 patients with over 3 year follow-up is expressed in four parameters - function, motion, stability and power. In general, it was found that improvement occurred in stability and function, that motion was restricted and that power improved or remained unchanged. Results of reconstruction of the medial stabilizers in general was successful, while that of the lateral stabilizers often failed. That was true for natural joints and for artificial joints (total knee arthroplasty).

Tendons. With augumented repair of rupture of quadriceps or patella tendon in 6 patients, the results were uniformly excellent allowing relatively early motion within 3 weeks and early return to full activity.

Repair of Achilles tendon in 7 patients resulted, in two, in infection which compromised the functional results of the excellent healing which took place.

Conclusions.

Reconstruction of ACL gave satisfactory results, but not uniformly so.

Reconstruction of MCL was generally successful.

Reconstruction of LCL was generally unsuccessful.

Reconstruction or repair of tendons gave excellent results but when superficial there was a high incidence of infection.

TECHNIQUE

The carbon braid was anchored to bone through the system of toggle and bollards developed by Strover. In 3 patients radiographic evidence of bone resorption around the expanding rivet was noted compromising the stability of the ligament unless bony ingrowth within the bony tunnel would reinforce the fixation.

It was found that extensive proliferation of connective tissue into the carbon braid had formed a composite structure within the bony tunnel, but the composite ligament was clearly defined by a circumferential fibrous sheath from the wall of the bony tunnel. Therefore, a direct anchorage was not established and the fixation of the composite ligament depended entirely on the fixation devices.

At the start of our clinical experience post operative effusion was noted in ACL reconstruction. In the sediment of the aspirated fluid carbon fibrils were noted.

We have promptly modified the technique by reconstruction of a tissue envelope around the carbon braid which sealed it off the joint space and prevented pollution of the joint due to occasional fragmented fibril. Coating of the braid with protein gel such as gelatin or collagen facilitated easy handling at surgery and prevented pollution during the surgical procedure.

Conclusions

The anchorage of the composite ligament is achieved only by the fixation device. Bone ingrowth does not take place. Intra-articular ligament should be sealed off the joint space.

MORPHOLOGY

Histology, histochemistry and electron microscopy studies of four entire composite ligaments, which were removed from patients 1½ to 3½ years after surgery during a second reconstruction aimed at improving the clinical results, gave us clues for understanding the structure and the mode of action of the composite ligament.

None of the sections showed the histological appearance of normal ligament. The organization of the cellular reaction around the carbon fibres was uniform except for the central area which was not yet organised.

Under high magnification the carbon fibres were surrounded by two to four concentric layers of cells (Figure 1). Most of these cells were fibroblasts and macrophages.

In sections stained by Masson or Silver impregnation the fibroblastic nature of these concentrically arranged cells was readily demonstrated by the formation of reticulin and mature collagen as well (Figure 2).

In contrast to the abundance of collagen fibres, no elastic fibres were found except in walls of blood vessels.

That structure was noted to be consistently oriented in the direction of the carbon fibres with which they were associated and the formations were called units of the composite ligament. These units were separated from each other by small amountsof loosely textured connective tissue.

These features of the units were also well illustrated in the scanning electron micrographs (Figure 3). The combination of collagenous tissue and carbon fibres formed a composite structures that we called composite ligament.

DO CARBON FIBRES FRAGMENT?

Our experimental work has proven that carbon fibres do not fragment unless failure or progressive failure of the composite ligament takes place. Yet in microscopic slides, fragments of carbon fibres were present when these were cut parallel to the direction of the fibres. It seemed that they were distributed in a haphazard fashion in the tissue section. In our opinion they were artefacts caused by fracture of carbon fibres during the sectioning of the paraffin blocks. Carbon fibre has inherent elastic energy and therefore may displace when cut.

There is however no doubt that genuine breakage of carbon fibres also occurred in vivo, though rarely. Carbon debris resulting from this was observed in mononuclear and polynuclear macrophages.

The difference between rupture and fragmentation should be clarified. Rupture is the catastrophic failure of carbon fibres either by excessive tensile load or by shear force. This may occur gradually by rupture of bundles or groups of fibres which simultaneously come into their full length or by a sudden rupture of the entire braid. Fragmentation is the failure of individual fibre during function of the composite ligament and it rarely occurs in the successful case.

Conclusion

Fragmentation during physiological function does not occur. However rupture due to shear forces may lead to failure.

DOES THE COLLAGEN OF THE COMPOSITE UNITS MATURE?

The initial stage of formation of the composite ligament was dominated by an intense inflammatory response producing the cylindrical composite units. Despite the continuous maturation process with time, the cellular response to the presence of the carbon fibres did not subside even 18 months after surgery.

However, portions of that structure lost the pattern of composite units and the wavy parallel collagen was more reminiscent of a ligament.

Polarization microscopy revealed two patterns of birefringence of the collagen fibres: delicate collagen fibres which elicited a uniform and continuous birefringence along the longitudinal axis and striped bands with alternating birefringent segments and short nonbirefringent intervals called crimp.

The crimp is believed to represent the dynamic wavy appearance of the collagen fibres during relaxation and has been noted to have different character in composite and natural ligament.

Conclusion

Inspite of a tendency toward maturation of the tissue the appearance is never of mature ligament.

DOES THE COLLAGENOUS COMPONENT OF THE COMPOSITE LIGAMENT TAKE OVER?

The collagen elongates under tensile load 4-5% prior to reaching the elastic part of its stress-strain curve, probably by straitening its crimp. The stiff carbon fibres which may lengthen about 1% therefore stress shield the collagen continuously and it is only their rupture which may transfer the load to the collagen. However, such transfer in case of rupture is relatively quick and the stress shielded collagen cannot be expected to take over.

In fact, in clinical cases it is expressed as a gradual but clear failure of a previously stable joint, such as the one seen here 3½ years after a good result of reconstruction of the anterior cruciate and the medial collateral ligaments.

Conclusion

The stress shielded collagen remains biomechanically deficient for ever.

SUMMARY

In consideration of the procedure of choice for reconstruction of ligaments, it is general knowledge that instability of a joint leads do degenerative changes. Likewise, compromised reconstruction of the ligaments or failed reconstruction leads to degenerative changes. Therefore the mental approach of the surgeon toward reconstructive procedure should be aggressive provided that he has a reliable method to apply.

In considering reconstruction by carbon fibre composite we emphasize that its function depends on the structural integrity of the carbon fibres.

LEGEND (Reproduced by permission from Clinical Orthopaedics and Related Research 196:51-60), 1985.

Figure 1. The composite unit made of concentric layer of fibroblasts around each carbon fibre.
Figure 2. The cylinders of collagen around the carbon fibrils forming the composite units.
Figure 3. Scan electron micrograph of the composite units.

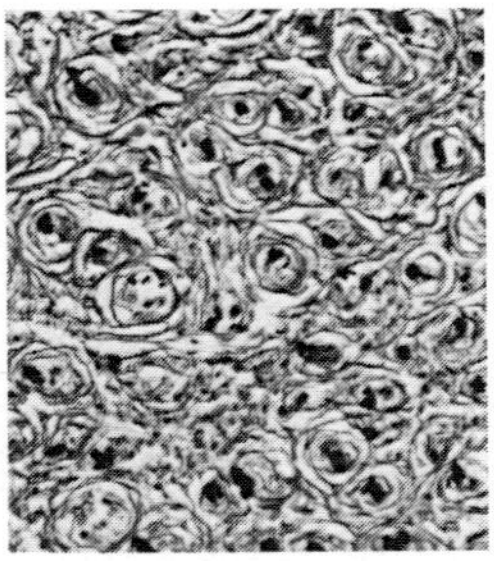

Figure 1

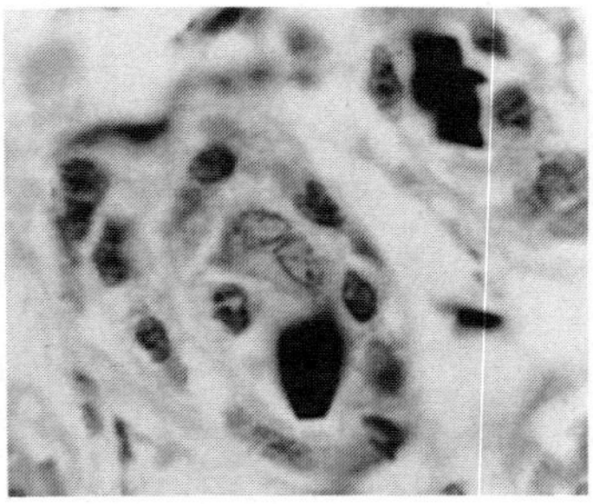

Figure 2

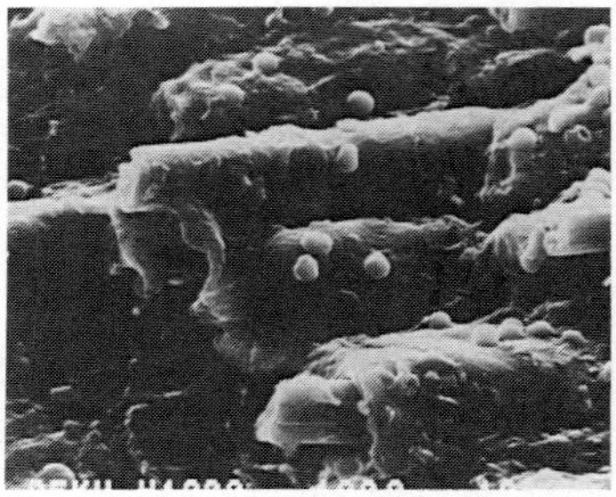

Figure 3

Biomaterials and Clinical Applications,
edited by A. Pizzoferrato, P.G. Marchetti, A. Ravaglioli and A.J.C. Lee
Elsevier Science Publishers B.V., Amsterdam, 1987 — Printed in The Netherlands

ANTERIOR CRUCIATE LIGAMENT SUTURE WITH THE "SELF-ANCHORING CORD" IN ARTHROSCOPICAL TECHNIQUE

A. SCHMID and F. SCHMID

Department of Surgery, Director: Prof.Dr. H.-J. Peiper,
University Clinic, Robert-Koch-Str. 40, 3400 Göttingen (FRG)

SUMMARY

The technique of arthroscopical suture of acute ruptures of the ACL with the "self-anchoring cord" is discussed. After testing the technique on 46 cadaver knees, the results show promise of success. The tensile strengths which were attained in the experiments are sufficient to promote healing. Along with the advantage of avoiding an arthrotomy, the principle of augmentation can also be realized, blood supply to the ACL remains unimpaired.

INTRODUCTION

The advantages of arthroscopic operations as opposed to arthrotomy are already well known in the field of meniscus surgery. For this reason we have developed a new material to be used for arthroscopic sutures of acute ACL ruptures. This material has been tested on 46 cadaver knees.

METHODS

The material conists of a spiked cord, 60 cm long and 1,2 mm in diameter. 20 cm from the top end of this cord, distributed along a length of 4 cm are synthetic spikes 4 mm long pointing in 4 directions. This cord, which we have called "self-anchoring cord", is mounted in an insertion cannula, 24 cm long. The cannula has an external diameter of 3 mm, an internal one of 2,3 mm and the top end is filed diagonally. A so-called extraction cannula filed straight is also employed.

The suture technique will be explained for a proximal ACL rupture.

The operation is performed on the flexed knee with the lower leg hanging freely. The arthroscope is inserted directly medial to the patellar tendon 1 cm below the patellar rim. The marker hook of the Variable Radius VR Drill Guide System is inserted through a ventrolateral portal (Fig. 1). It's point is positioned at the attachment of the ligament to the tibial plateau. An incision is made ventromedially at the head of the tibia. Under arthroscopical

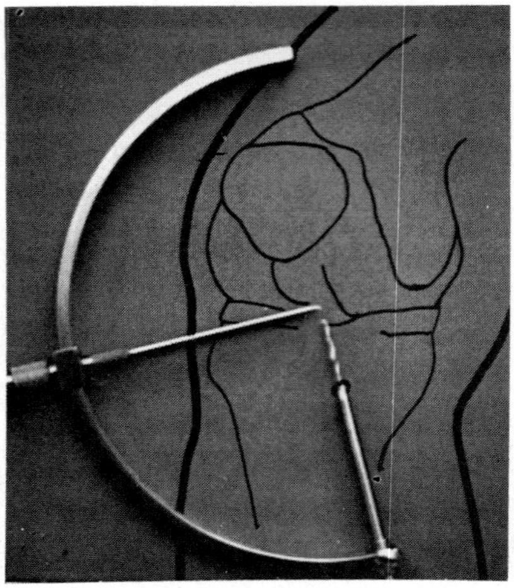

Fig. 1. Exact drilling to the attachment points of tne ACL with the Variable Radius VR Drill Guide System.

control 3 holes are drilled through the head of the tibia towards the point of the marker hook with a 3,2 mm drill. We use a hammer-drill technique to prevent the ligament fibres from winding themselves around the drill.

The point of the marker hook is then positioned at the proximal ligament attachment. From a lateral incision at the distal femur 3 holes are drilled to the points of attachment of the ACL at the lateral femoral condyle under arthroscopic control.

The self-anchoring cords mounted in the insertion cannulas are then introduced into the holes at the head of the tibia and pushed to the ends of the disconnected ACL bundles. The extraction cannulas are inserted into the holes at the lateral femoral condyle. With a forceps inserted ventrolaterally, the cords are pulled out of the insertion cannulas and into the appropriate extraction cannulas (Fig. 2).

When the cords have been pulled right through the holes in the femoral condyle, the extraction cannulas can be removed and the ends of the cords can be gripped by the fingers. The insertion cannulas are then pushed one after the other upto the free end of the ACL stump. The cords are pulled by hand from the transcondylar end into the joint. A colour marker on the cord entering the insertion cannula at the head of the tibia indicates that the first segement of synthetic spikes has passed out of the intra-articular opening

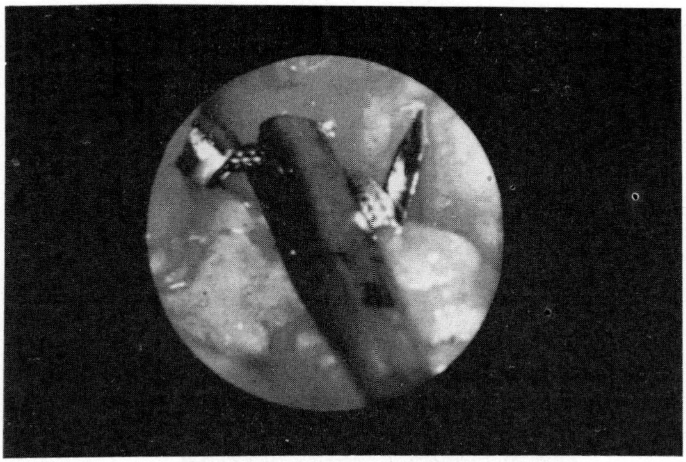

Fig. 2. Pulling through of the cordsunder arthroscopical control.

of the insertion cannula. The insertion cannula can now be extracted. The synthetic spikes, which lie flat in the cannula spread out automatically and anchor themselves in the collagen bundles. Finally the ends of the cords emerging at the femoral condyle are tied tightly together so that the ACL is brought into the correct anatomical position (Fig. 3). Then the cord ends at the head of the tibia are tied together.

We tested our technique on 46 cadaver knees, on 16 cases of proximal disconnections, 16 of distal disconnections and 14 cases of interligamentary disconnection. The technical operational difficulties were assessed and the tensile strength of the sutures was measured.

RESULTS

Cutting the ligament bundles at the proximal or distal end we arrived at a mean load at failure of 45-50 N per cord. In interligamentary cuts the value sank to 35-40 N per cord due to the lesser extent of anchorage.

DISCUSSION

Our results show promise of success for arthroscopical suture of the ACL rupture using the "self-anchoring cord". After some practise the technique is easy to carry out.

By means of the axial central insertion of the cord and the

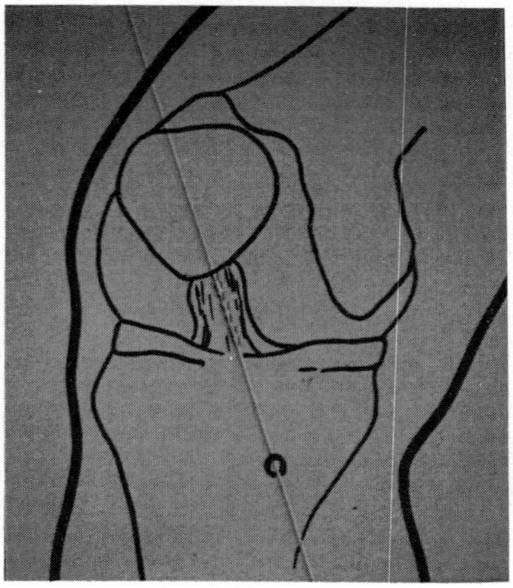

Fig. 3. Anatomical replacement of the ACL with the "self-anchoring cord".

automatic anchorage through the spreading of the synthetic spikes in the ligament, problems such as ligating of vessels through the suture are avoided.

Since the cord is inserted into the ligament the principle of augmentation is taken advantage of. This protective augmentation and a precise drilling of the attachment point of the ACL afford the biomechanical prerequesite for an early postoperative mobilisation treatment (3). The tensile force on the ACL through mobilisation lies below 30 N (1) and according to our results will neither loosen the position of the anchor spikes nor tear the ligatures.

After the cords are knotted a definitive distance of cord is established between the drilled holes. With this the actual ligament suture held by the synthetic spikes is relieved of tension.

According to experimental investigations of other authors, drilling of the ligament attachment points at the tibia and at the femoral condyle may even have a positive effect (2). Fibroblasts can grow through the drilled holes into the sutured ligament. The inserted PDS-cord can act as a guide rail for the ingrowing tissue.

REFERENCES

1 L. Claes, Die Beanspruchung des Kniebandapparates, Hefte Unfallheilkd., 172 (1985) 1-7.
2 K.E. Rehm, K.H. Schultheis, P. Bopp and H. Ecke, Biomechanische Untersuchungen von resorbierbarem Bandersatz und deren klinische Bedeutung, Chirurgisches Forum 84 für experimentelle und klinische Forschung, Springer, Berlin-Heidelberg-New York, 1984, pp 207-211.
3 H. Taruttis, Verletzungen des vorderen Kreuzbandes, in: H. Hempfling (Ed.), Das Knie-Trauma, Medical Concept, München, 1985, pp 47-55.

Biomaterials and Clinical Applications,
edited by A. Pizzoferrato, P.G. Marchetti, A. Ravaglioli and A.J.C. Lee
Elsevier Science Publishers B.V., Amsterdam, 1987 — Printed in The Netherlands

CARBON FIBRE LIGAMENTS IN HUMAN KNEE JOINTS: EVALUATION OF THE REACHED STABILITY IN VITRO

H. Kiefer, L. Dürselen, L. Claes

Laboratory of Experimental Traumatology, University of Ulm, Oberer Eselsberg, D-7900 Ulm (West Germany)

ABSTRACT

In human cadaveric knee joints anterior drawer signs (ADS) were measured in various rotation positions. The specimens were mounted in a special device in 90° flexion position. Section of the anterior cruciate ligament (ACL) increased the ADS to 180%. Additional section of the medial collateral ligament (MCL) raised the ADS to 470%. The replacement of the statically stabilizing ligaments by braided carbon fibre ligament prostheses reduced the anterior drawer signs to initial values. Each of the 3 dynamically stabilizing muscle groups diminished the ADS during the simulated knee bend: the quadriceps femoris by around 20%, the gastrocnemius and the pes anserinus group by about 50% each. In combination the 3 muscle groups minimized the ADS to 20% of the values in the intact knee joint, even when ACL and MCL were cut. Consequently, unstable knee joints can be improved passively by carbon fibre ligament replacement very well. For active stabilisation by postoperative physiotherapy special attention should be paid to the training of the hamstring and calf muscles.

INTRODUCTION

In recent years carbon fibre ligaments (fig. 1) have been used clinically with good success (7). The biomechanical and biological properties of this alloplastic material gained from in vitro and in vivo investigations (1). However, no quantitative data is

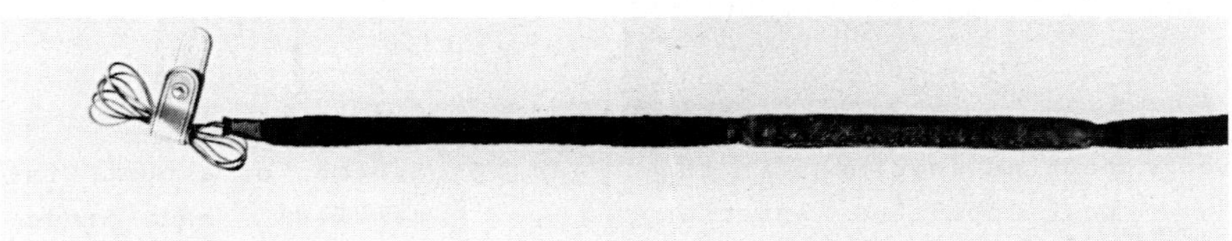

fig. 1: Dura coated carbon fibre ligament prosthesis

available concerning the obtainable stabilizing effect of carbon fibre ligament replacement in human cadaveric knee joints. On the other hand the recovered passive stability can be improved by activity of the knee spanning muscles. Although various experimental studies have been carried out to determine the instability of human cadaveric knee joints (4, 5), presently quantitative effects of the individual muscles on the unstable joint are not known.

MATERIALS AND METHODS

Eight fresh human cadaveric knee joints with a mean age of 44 years, range 18-72 years, were prepared sparing the capsule and the ligaments and stored deep frozen until the date of investigation.

The specimens were clamped in a special mounting support in 90° flexion (fig. 2) allowing free rotation and varus/valgus position (2, 3). The tibia could be set in neutral position as well as in both 15° internal and external rotation. The tibial head was pulled anteriorly by a 40 N force causing an anterior drawer sign (ADS) (fig. 3).

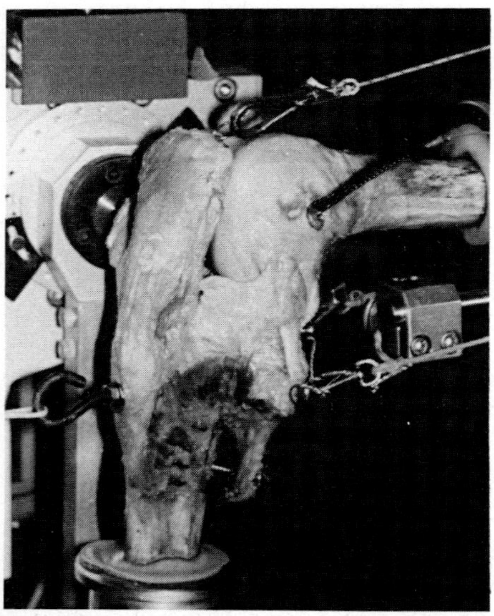

fig. 2: Mounted specimen in the test apparatus. Anterior dislocation of the tibial head is measured.

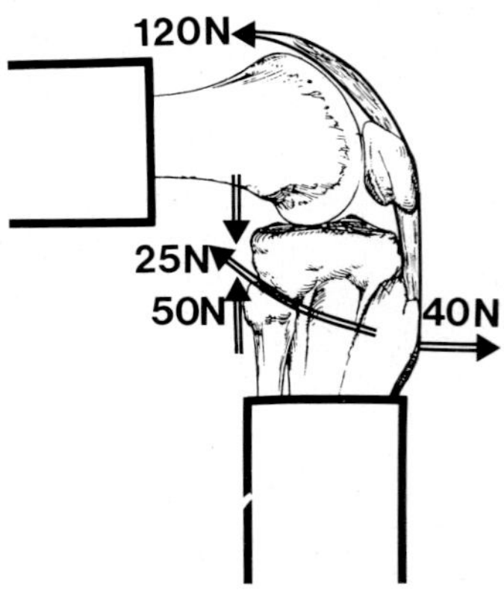

fig. 3: Scheme of amount, insertions, and directions of the muscles and tensile forces.

The active stabilizing muscle forces had been calculated for the knee bend by Röhrle (9). For the load case simulated here single muscle forces could be distributed to 3 major muscle groups as there are quadriceps, gastrocnemius, and semitendinosus-semimembranosus - biceps femoris muscles, the latter here called pes anserinus group. 10% of these physiological tensile forces of quadriceps (120 N), gastrocnemius (50 N) and pes anserinus muscles (25 N) were applied to the normal insertions via cords and cortical screws (fig. 3). These forces were generated by computer controlled pneumatic cylinders (2, 3). Measurements of the anterior drawer signs (ADS) were carried out in neutral, external and internal rotation from the intact knee joint without muscle forces and after application of single muscle groups as well as their combination. After cutting the anterior cruciate ligament (ACL) the ADS determinations were repeated. Commercially available braided carbon fibre ligament prostheses (fig. 4) were used for ACL replacement (fig. 5). The resulting passive stability was compared with the data obtained from transsection and the following replacement of both, ACL and MCL.

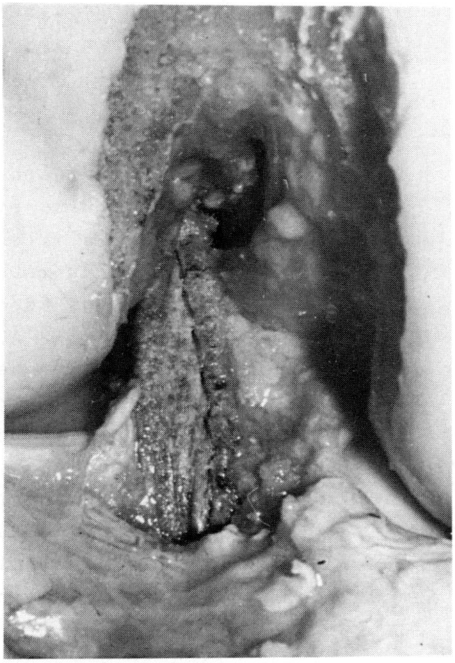

fig. 4: ACL, replaced by a dura-coated carbon fibre lig.

RESULTS

The mean ADS and the SEM was found in NR 2.9 ± 0.6 mm in the intact knee joint. Cutting the ACL increased the ADS to 180% and with an additionally transsected MCL up to 470% in NR. Carbon fibre ligament replacements of the ACL decreased the ADS to 1.2 ± 0.1 mm, i.e. 41%, while after the replacement of ACL and MCL an ADS of 3.0 ± 0.6 mm (equivalently 103%) was found (fig. 5).

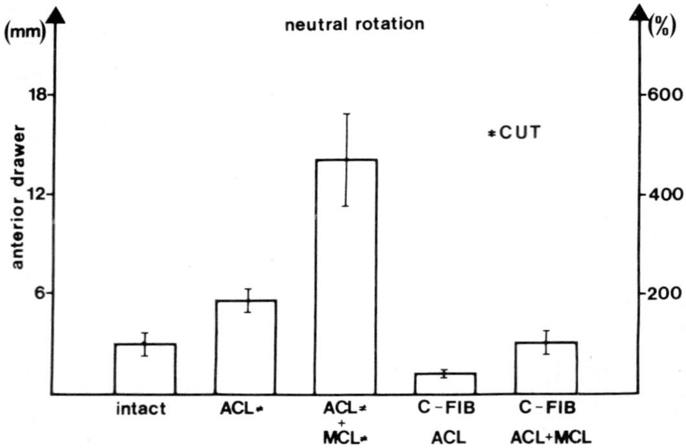

fig. 5

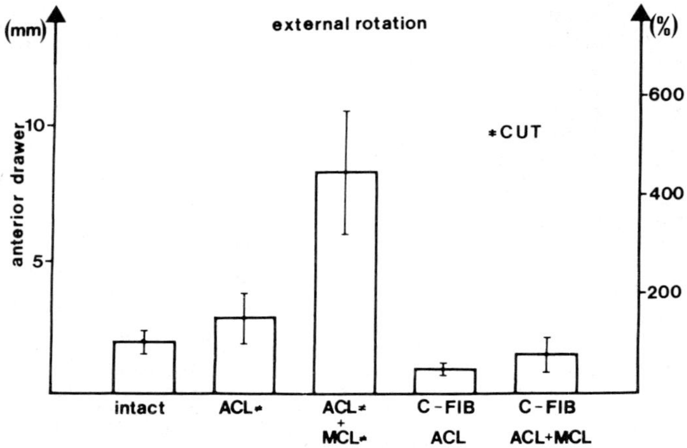

fig. 6

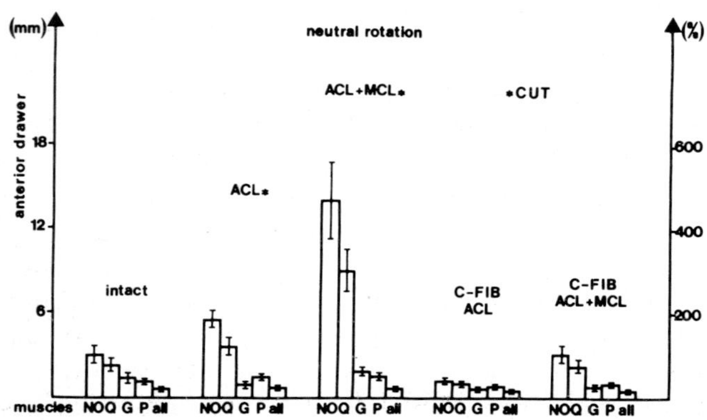

fig. 7

Anterior tibial displacement in ER showed an anteromedial rotatory instability of 2±0.5mm. Carbon fibres led to an ADS of 1.1 ± 0.1 mm and 1.4 ± 0.6 mm, resp. (fig. 6). The corresponding results for IR were similar. In NR isolated quadriceps force reduced the ADS to 76% when ligaments were intact. Gastrocs and pes anserinus muscles decreased the ADS to 45% and 38%. The combination led to a minor ADS of 21% (fig. 7). After resection of the ACL or both ACL and MCL the simulation of the quadriceps reduced the ADS to values, which still remained on the levels of 120% and 300%. However, gastrocs, pes anserinus, and the combined muscle forces diminished the ADS to values of the intact joints (fig. 7). The influence of the muscle forces in ER and IR was only slightly less and qualitatively similar. Thus detailed results are not presented here.

DISCUSSION

Uniform test conditions allowed quantitatively reproducable measurements of the extent of anterior instability in human knee joints after standardized lesions of the passive stabilisers . 90° flexion angle was chosen because the anterior tibial dislocation was most evidently in this test position.

The experimental set up allowed a quantitative evaluation of the influence of muscle forces on the unstable knee joint as well. The magnitude of the muscle forces have been derived from finite element analysis for the knee bend (9). These forces up to 1200 N cannot be introduced into the ligamentous origins since the screws would be pulled out of the bone. However, preliminary tests have shown similar results of the ADS when 5%, 10% or 20% of the calculated muscle forces were applied. Therefore the anterior tensile force pulling at the tibial head could be reduced to 40 N. Thus using 10% of the calculated forces general validity of the obtained results may be assumed.

According to the literature (4, 5), section of the ACL leads to positive anterior drawer signs in all of the tested rotational positions. The ADS was enhanced when the MCL was cut additionally. In this experiment anterior stability of the knee joint could be improved significantly ($p<0,01$) by carbon fibre ligament prostheses for both replacements of the ACL and ACL plus MCL. Under the described test conditions, the gained stability partly was higher than in the intact joints. The reason for this were 3 specimens which were explanted from older individuals. Although they looked macroscopically intact, they were originally somewhat laxer and showed an ADS of 5-6 mm, compared to 1-3 mm of the remaining 5 joints. The high stiffness and tensile strength of the braided carbon fibre ligaments (1) provided high initial stability when the prostheses were tightened correctly. Fatigue of the material, however, is not taken into consideration in this study. This might explain poor clinical results. However, the 86% of good results (7) correlate well to the high mechanical stability of the carbon fibre ligament treated joints in this investigation.

Clinically, training of the thigh muscles commonly means training of the quadriceps (10). Simulating isolated quadriceps muscle force reduces the ADS by about 15-25%, depending on the actual angle of rotation and the extent of injury. This is valid for both the intact and the instable knee joint. The anterior drawer was significantly diminished ($p<0,01$) by isolated tension of the gastrocnemius or the pes anserinus group. The same effect could be observed by a combination of these muscles with the quadriceps group. Here the reduction effect was up to 75-80% for the ADS, even in extended anteromedial instability.

CONCLUSION

From a biomechanical point of view, the anterior instability in human cadaveric knee joints can be treated by carbon fibre ligament replacement with good success. Large anterior drawer signs will disappear in straight and rotation positions in 90° of flexion. This is true for the replacement of both ACL and ACL plus MCL.

In rehabilitation after ligamentous injuries or ligament replacement the dynamic stability should be improved (6, 8). Attention should be paid not only to the strengthening of the quadriceps muscles but to the gastrocnemius and pes anserinus-biceps femoris-semimembranosus muscle groups in particular. In the simulated knee bend, simultaneous contraction of all knee spanning muscles provides maximal dynamic stability, even in severe anteromedial rotatory instability. With carbon fibre ligaments the passive stabilizors can be replaced with good success.

REFERENCES

1 L. Claes, R. Neugebauer, Mechanical properties of ligament replacement with carbon fibres. In C. Burri, L. Claes (eds) Alloplastic ligament replacement. Akt. Probl. in Chir. und Orthop. 26, (1983) pp 58-62
2 L. Claes, L. Dürselen, H. Kiefer, Influence of load, flexion and muscle forces on the stress and strain of knee ligaments. Transactions of the 32nd Annual Meeting of the ORS, (1986), New Orleans : 238
3 L. Dürselen, L. Claes, Simulation und Messung der Beanspruchung des Kniebandapparates, rechnerkontrollierte Steuerung eines Simulators und On-line Meßwertverarbeitung. Biomed Technik 30, (1985), pp 46-47
4 T. Fukubayashi, P. Torzilli et al., An in vitro Biomechanical Evaluation of Anterior-Posterior Motion of the Knee. J Bone Joint Surg 64 A, (1982), pp 258-264
5 W. Furman, J. Marshall, F. Girgis, The anterior cruciate ligament. J Bone Joint Surg 58 A, (1976), pp 179-185
6 W. Müller, Das Knie. Springer, Berlin Heidelberg New York, (1982)
7 R. Neugebauer, H. Kiefer, M. Seling. In C. Burri, L. Claes, G. Helbing (eds) Bandersatz mit Kohlenstoffasern. Hefte z. Unfallheilk. 172, (1985), pp 121-124
8 L. Paulos, FR. Noyes, E. Grood, Die komplexe vordere Knieinstabilität. Thieme, Stuttgart New York, (1981)
9 H. Röhrle, R. Scholten, W. Sollbach, Kraftflußberechnungen in Knochenstrukturen und Prothesen, Phase II, BMFT Bericht 01 VG 106-ZK14MT267, (1977)
10 JS. Smillie, Kniegelenksverletzungen. Enke, Stuttgart, (1985)

Biomaterials and Clinical Applications,
edited by A. Pizzoferrato, P.G. Marchetti, A. Ravaglioli and A.J.C. Lee
Elsevier Science Publishers B.V., Amsterdam, 1987 — Printed in The Netherlands

EVALUATION OF CONTACT STRESSES IN METAL-PLASTIC TOTAL KNEE REPLACEMENTS

M.J. PAPPAS, Ph.D[1], G. MAKRIS, M.S.[1], and F.F. BUECHEL, M.D.[2]

[1]Mechanical Engineering Department, New Jersey Institute of Technology, Newark, New Jersey (USA)

[2]New Jersey Medical School, University of Medicine and Dentistry of New Jersey, Newark, New Jersey (USA)

SUMMARY

On the basis of present knowledge, and use of simple analytical tools a method for evaluation of existing and proposed design replacement knee articulations is presented. Using this method, it appears if peak contact stress in normal walking is below 5 MPa, one can reasonably expect abrasive type low wear rates minimizing potential problems associated with wear debris. If contact stress as predicted by this procedure is in excessive of 10 MPa, one can reasonably expect pitting type high wear rates with attendent high potential for wear-related loosening, infection and other yet unknown complications. A theoretical investigation using the proposed analytical procedure coupled with an experimental study shows that common incongruent knee prostheses are incompetent to perform their intended function in active patients.

INTRODUCTION

The adverse clinical consequences of high wear rates are well documented [1-3]. Very strong clinical evidence relates polyethylene wear debris to aseptic loosening and late infection. Current generation knee protheses which typically employ incongruent surface contact in order to provide needed mobility are a particular hazard. Simulator [4-6] and clinical retrieval analyses [8] clearly demonstrates wear rates in such knees. References [6,] demonstrates the correlation between high contact stress and high wear rates. Thus, the high wear rates observed and expected in most incongruent contact knees is a natural consequence of the excessive stress resulting from highly localized contact.

Since testing is a complex and costly process a need exists for the evaluation of the potential wear resistance of replacement joints. A simple, useful criteria for the qualitative evaluation of wear associated with incongruent contact is feasible. This paper describes this criteria and demonstrates its utility in the evaluation of typical knee protheses currently in use.

II WEAR

The primary wear mode in high contact stress replacement joints is pitting. Pitting is a fatigue related phenomenon primarily existing in incongruent contact bearings [10] When two incongruent bodies are in contact under the action of a compressive load, the maximum fatigue producing stress occurs under the surface as shown in Figs. 1. If this stress is above the fatigue strength of the material, cracks will develop under the contact surfaces and coalesce into pits as shown in Figs. 2-4. Weightman et al. [11] report on what appears to be a classical [10] "transverse" type tibial platform fracture resulting from pitting wear. Such wear is typically present in retrieved polyethylene tibial plateaus of incongruent contact in the prosthesis [7].

Clinical [12] and experimental [5,6,13,] evidence demonstrates that with properly sized prosthetic femoral heads and essentially congruent knee configurations wear can be extremely low and primarily abrasive in nature. For incongruent knees [5,8] and often small (22 mm) femoral heads wear is very high and primarily due to pitting. Thus, from a design view point the avoidance of high wear rates in a metal polyethylene articulation prosthesis is primarily a matter of avoiding fatigue which means avoiding contact stress in excess of the fatigue strength of the polyethylene.

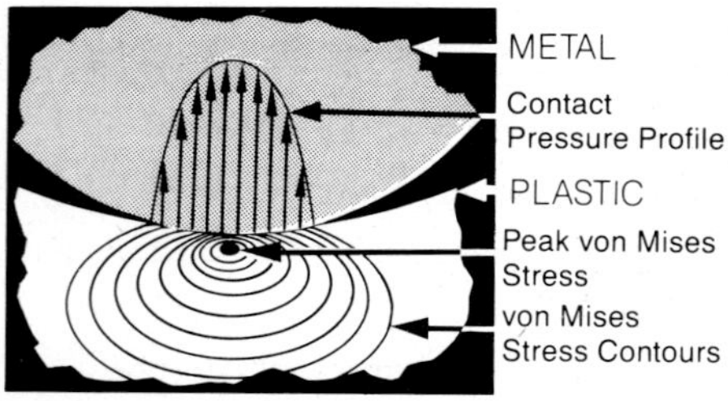

FIG. 1 *Contact Stress*

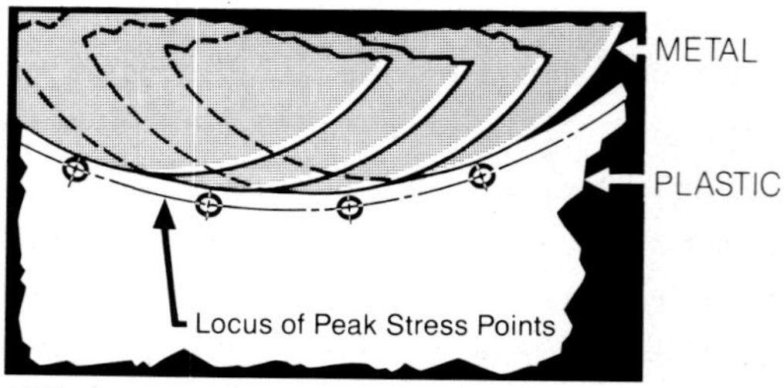

FIG. 2
Movement of Peak Stress Location with Relative Motion of the Bodies in Contact

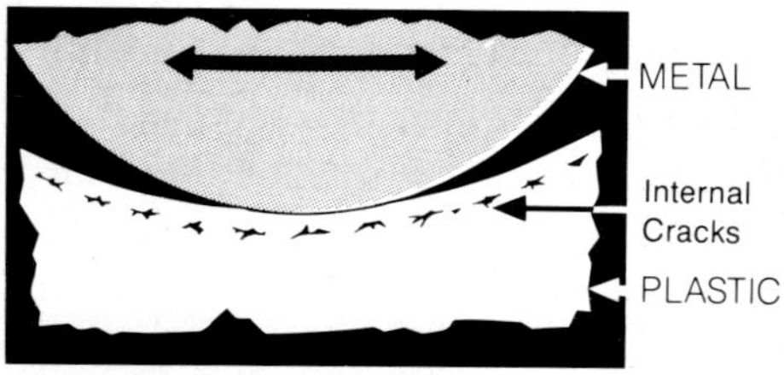

FIG. 3 *Crack Initiation*

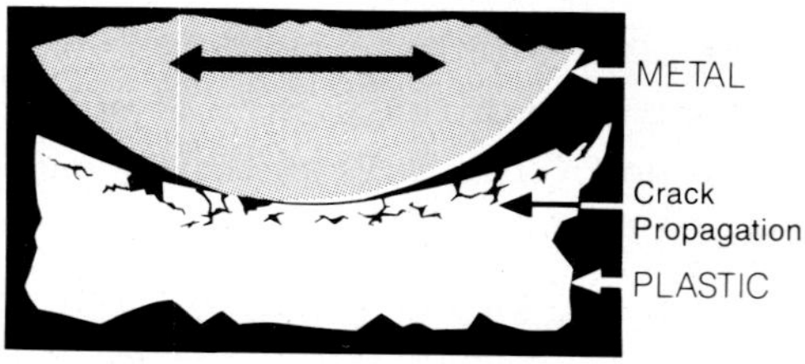

FIG. 4 *Pit Formation*

III COMPUTATION OF CONTACT STRESSES

The equation for the computation of contact stresses under point and line contact are given in [10]. These equations are repeated and the solution process is given in [14].

The principal assumptions used for this analysis are that;

a) the materials are linear and isotropic, a reasonable assumption at safe stress levels, and,

b) the dimensions of the contact patch are small relative to to the principal radii of curvature of the contact surfaces, Thus, these equations should give a reasonable estimate of contact stress given a known geometry loading and material properties, assuming the stress is in the linear region of the stress strain curve as is the case in UHMWPe at safe stress levels.

A BASIC program was developed to implement the method of section III for computing the stresses. The computations were performed on DEC Rainbow 100 personal computer. Contact stresses can also be computed by hand using graphs provided in [10].

IV. THEORETICAL ANALYSIS

One example of each of the typical contact types shown in figs 5-8 are evaluated using the theoretical analysis described above. The properties of UHMWPe are given in [15]. The elastic modulus is taken as 1050 MPa at 23C. The value of the elastic modulus at body temperature can be estimated from information given from [15] as 600 MPa at 37C. A peak load of 2225N at a 15° flexion angle was assumed for these computations. This load is approximately equal to 3 times body weight in a typical patient. The geometry of the articulating surfaces was determined from a 10 to 1 magnification comparator tracings of productions samples obtained from the manufacturer of each device.

The peak Von Mises stresses for each device are computed using values of material properties at 37 C in order to determine the nature of these stresses in the subject devices under in-vivo conditions. The peak compressive surfaces stresses using values of the material properties at 23 C are also computed to allow a comparison with experimentally measured values in order to estimate the accuracy of the analytical methods in this application.

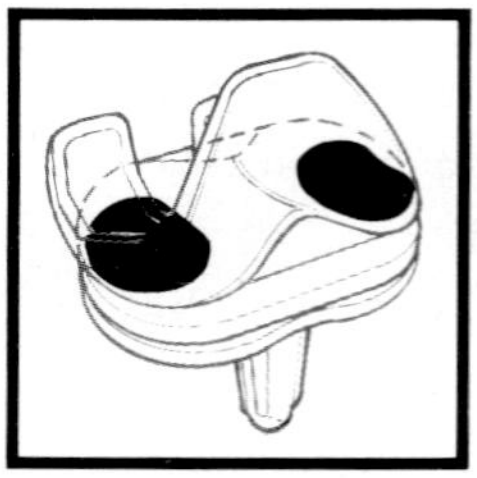

FIG. 5 *Area Contact*

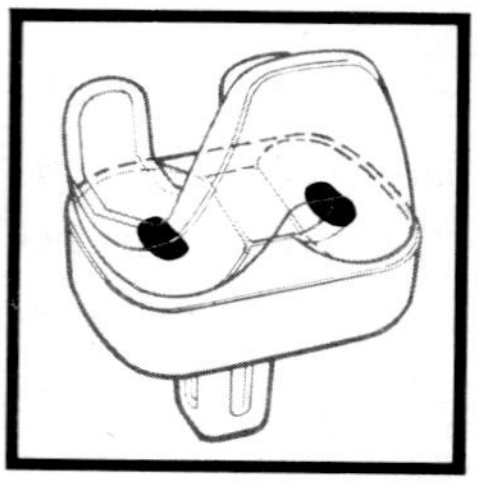

FIG. 6 *Point Contact*

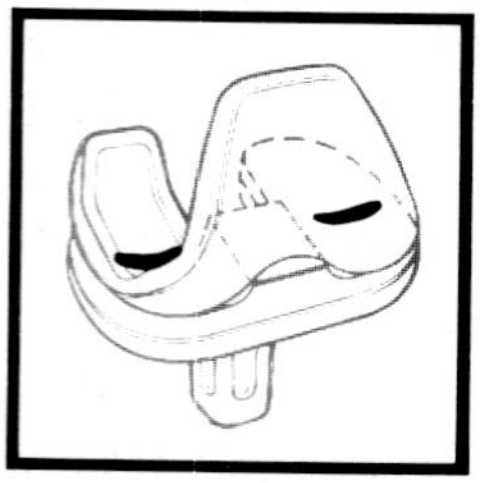

FIG. 7 *Line Contact*

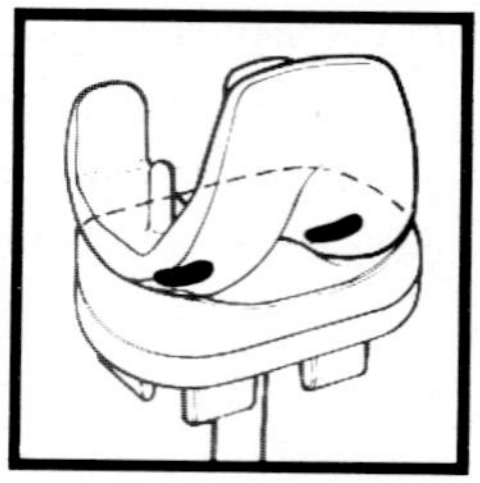

FIG. 8 *Quasi-Line Contact*

V EXPERIMENTAL STUDY

A sample of each of the above knees was loaded to 2225 N at 15° flexion using specially designed fixtures on a Tineus Olson Model 50-62960-6 tension-compression test machine. Loading was applied at the rate of about 100 N/sec and released one second after full load was achieved. The maximum contact stress was determined using Fuji PRESCALE pressure-sensitive film which was read immediately after unloading. The estimated precision of the value read is about 10%. The fixtures employed rollers on both loading surfaces in order to self-centering of the components under loading and to provide symmetrical condyler loading as is assumed in the calculations.

VI RESULTS

The results of the experimental measurement and theoretical computation of contact stress is presented in Figure 9. Comparing the room temperature compressive surface stress values for the area, line and point contact type knees, the theoretical equations can be considered in reasonable agreement with the experimentally determined stress except for the quasi-line contact type.

For the quasi-line contact type knee the computed stress is much higher than measured. This is to be expected for highly incongruent articulations since as the yield point of material is approached, the effective elastic modulus declines dramatically, thus providing a larger contact patch then would be predicted using the elastic modulus at lower stress values [17]. It is interesting to note that the measured contact stress values in all inconquent types are all near the compressive stress that would produce yielding using the Von Mises criteria. Thus, it appears that the similarity in the measured compressive surface stress of the incongruent contact types is the result of the leveling due to yielding indicating that for these three samples local yielding occured.

Notwithstanding the fact that the computational method's not valid for high stresses exceeding the yield point. The method is useful, in evaluating incongruent contact knees since this method under all stress conditions provides either a reasonable or conservative estimate of contact stress behavior. Furthermore, the method provides a means for determing whether a given articulation produces acceptable contact stress levels.

Comparing the computed and measured stress values with the maximum allowable compressive stress of 10 M Pa [15], conventional engineering criteria indicate that only the area contact type knee is competent to support the expected loads. The other knee designs are clearly inadequate, since the computed and measured stress are at least twice the maximum allowable compressive stress for fluctuating load given by the manufacturer of UHMWPe. A contact stress of about half the maximum value given in [15], or 5 M Pa, is probably a more reasonable value for acceptable design stress. Such a lower value is appropriate in light of; the long service life required, expected material and manufacturing variations, body temperature and other environmental effects of implantation, larger loads experienced in stair-climbing, decent, and normal activities, and other unknowns and variables. Thus, from theoretical and experimental data, if one employs conventional engineering criteria, it seems clear that typical incongruent designs can not be expected to perform their

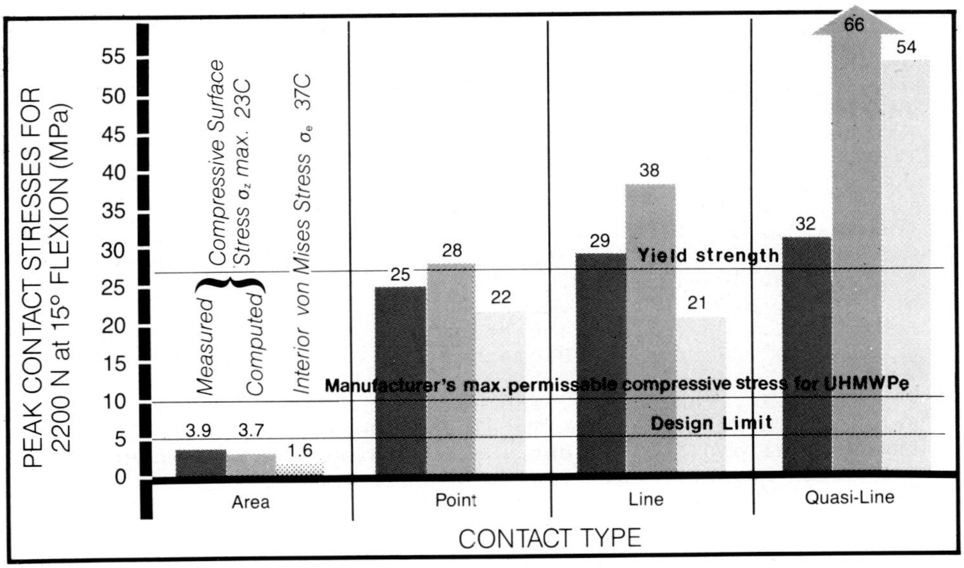

FIG. 9 *Computed and Measured Stresses*

intended function in active adults.

REFERENCES

1 Mirra, J.M. Amstutz, H., Matos, M., and Gold R. "The pathology of joint tissues and its clinical relevance in prosthesis failure" Clinical Orthopaedics and Related Research, NO. 117, pp. 221-240, 1976.

2 Ravell, P.A., Weightman, B., Freeman, M.A.R., and Roberts, B.V., "The production and biology of polyethylene wear debris." Archives of Orthopaedic and Traumatic Surgery, Vol. 91, pp 167-91, 1978.

3 Willert, H.G., and Semlitsch, M., "Relation of the articular joint prostheses" Journal of Biomedical Materials Research, Vol. 11, pp. 134-164, 1977.

4 Rose, R.M. Ries, M.D., Paul I.L. Crugnoia, A.N. and Ellis, E "Wear of the Tibial Component of the knee Prosthesis" Transactions of the 26th Annual Orthopaedic Research Society held at New Orleans, Louisiana on Jan. 19-21, 1982, Vol. 7, p.252.

5 Pappas, M.J. and Buechel, F.F. "New Jersey Knee Simulator" Proceedings of the Eleventh International Biomaterials Symposium held at Clemson, S.C. on april 28-May 1, 1979, p. 101.

6 Treharne, R.W.., Young, R.W. and Young, S.R., "Wear of Artifical Joint Materials III: Simulation of the knee joint using a computer-controlled system" Engineering in Medicine, Vol. 10, pp. 137-142, 1981.

7 Rose, R.M., Crugnoia, A., Ries, N., Cimino, W.R. Paul, I., and Radin, E.L. "On the origins of high in-vivo wear rates in polyethylene components of total joint prosthesis," Clinical Orthopaedics and Related Research, No. 145, pp. 277-287, 1979.

8 Rose, R.M., Goldfarb, E.V. Ellis, E. Crugnola, A.M., "On the pressure dependence of the wear of ultra-high molecular weight polyethylene," Wear vol. 92, pp. 99-111, 1983.

9 Rostoker, W., Galante J.O. "Contact pressure dependence of wear rates of ultra high molecular weight polyethylene," Journal of Biomedical Materials Research, Vol. 13, pp 957-964, 1979.

10 Sealy, F.B., and Smith, J.O. Advanced Mechanics of Materials, Wiley and Sons, Inc., New York, New York, Chapter 14, 1958.

11 Weightman, B., Isherwood, D.P., and Swampson, S.A.V., Fracture of Ultra high Molecular Weight Polyethylene in the Human Body" Journal of Biomedical Materials Research, vol. 13, pp 669-672, 1979.

12 Rose, R.M., and Radin, E.L., "Wear of polyethylene in total hip prosthesis" Clinical Orthopaedic and Related Research, No. 170, p. 107-115, 1982.

13 Weightman, B.O., Paul, I.L. Rose, R.M., Simon, S.R., and Rodin, E.L., "A comparative study of total hop replacement prosthesis", Journal of Biomechanics, Vol. 6, pp. 299-317, 2987.

14 Pappas, M.J., Makris, G., and Buechel, F.F.," Contact Stresses in Metal Plastic Total Knee Replacements: A theoretical and Experimiental Study; Biomedical Engineering Technical Report, Jan. 23, 1986.

15 "Hostalen GUR" Technical publication of Hoechet Plastics, Hoechst Aklenglsellshaft, Verkauf Kirnslstoffe, 6260 Frankfurt am Main 80, Germany, pp 11 and 22, 1982.

Biomaterials and Clinical Applications,
edited by A. Pizzoferrato, P.G. Marchetti, A. Ravaglioli and A.J.C. Lee
Elsevier Science Publishers B.V., Amsterdam, 1987 — Printed in The Netherlands

LONG-TERM-RESULTS OF TOTAL KNEE ARTHROPLASTY WITH THE WALLDIUS- AND THE GSB-PROSTHESES

G. O. HOFMANN [1] and F. - W. HAGENA [2]

[2] Staatliche Orthopädische Klinik Harlaching, Orthopädische Klinik und Polikliniken,

[1] Chirurgische Klinik und Poliklinik, Klinikum Grosshadern, Ludwig-Maximilians-Universität München, Deutschland.

INTRODUCTION

The successful development of the total hip replacement has encouraged and given impetus to bioengineers and surgeons to develop an equally successful total knee replacement. It is apparent that none of the prostheses replacing the knee joint offers results approaching the excellence of total hip replacement in terms of either relief of pain or improvement of function. The majority of the results represent a significant improvement from the preoperative state, but they are far from ideal. It is the aim of this long-term-study to demonstrate the typical problems of total knee arthroplasty due to the special biomechanics of the knee joint.

MATERIAL AND METHODS

During the period from 1967 to 1975, 58 WALLDIUS and from 1975 to 1984 157 GSB-total knee prostheses were implanted at the Staatliche Orthopädische Klinik in Munich (Fig. 1). As shown in table 1 Rheumatoid Arthritis and Osteoarthritis

Fig. 1

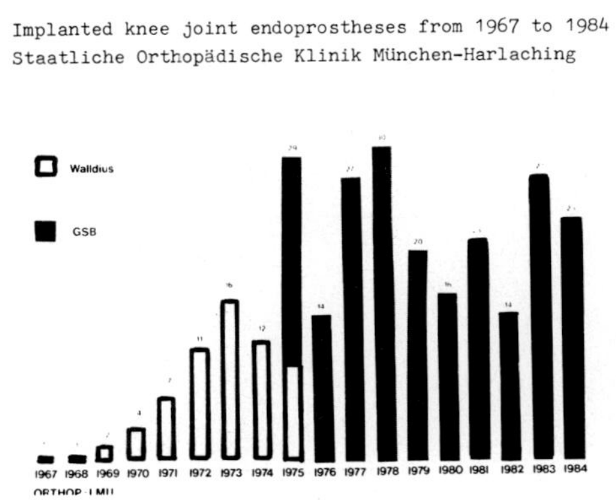

were the most frequent indications for total knee replacement. The distribution of the patients according to their age at the time of the implantation of the WALLDIUS- and GSB- knee endoprosthesis is shown in figures 2 and 3. In the years 1975, 1982 and 1984 review examinations of all living patients with total knee

TABLE 1

Diagnoses for the implantation of 58 WALLDIUS- and 157 GSB-knee endoprostheses

	WALLDIUS Patients		Prostheses		GSB Patients		Prostheses	
Rheumatoid Arthritis	33	63.5%	39	67.2%	53	39.8%	73	46.5%
Osteoarthritis	18	34.6%	18	31.0%	63	47.4%	67	42.7%
Other	1	1.9%	1	1.8%	17	12.8%	17	10.8%
	52	100.0%	58	100.0%	133	100.0%	157	100.0%

Fig. 2

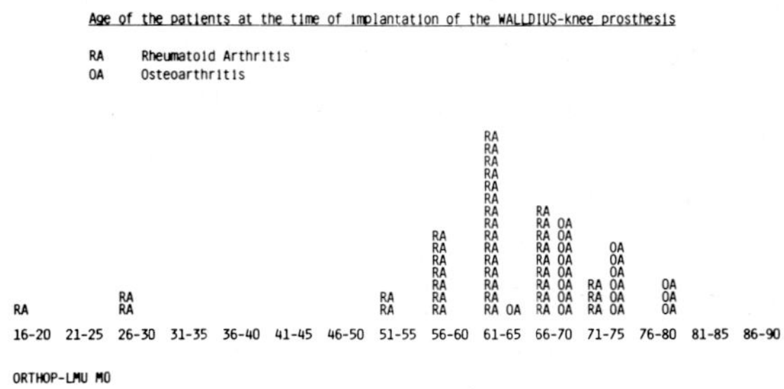

Fig. 3

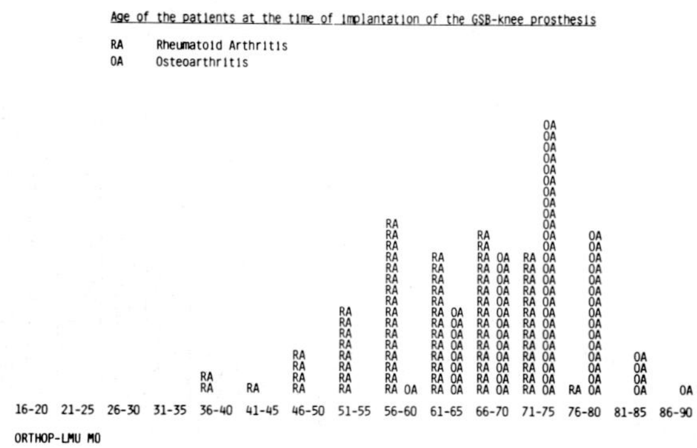

arthroplasties were performed. At the time of the implantation of the endoprosthesis 15.2% of the patients with Rheumatoid Arthritis and 24.7% of those with Osteoarthritis had been operated on the same knee before.

RESULTS

With regard to clinical parameters as range of movement (see tables 2 and 3) postoperative pain (table 4), stability and mobility 61% of the implanted knees were judged as 'very good' and 13.6% as 'well'. Therefore 88.1% of all patients would again undergo the procedure of the operation or would recommend this operation to others in a comparable situation with severely destructed knee-joints. Late complications - 5 years or longer after the operation - counted 20% of all complications. 15% of all implanted knee endoprostheses had to be reoperated. The major late complications were loosening of the tibial or the femoral component, deep infection and persistence of retropatellar pain.

In addition to the patellar problems after total knee arthroplasty such as pain and subluxation described elsewhere we found additional pathologic changes such as an increased incidence of retropatellar erosions and a diminished patellar thickness. By defined measurements of the lateral radiographs we were able to verify and quantify vertical patellar dislocations as an additional pathomechanical factor for patellar problems (Fig. 4). The characteristic changes of the patella following total knee arthroplasty consisted of erosions and reduced patellar thickness. Various bone-resections at the time of the implantation of the prosthesis resulted in different vertical dislocations of the patella lea-

TABLE 2
Results: range of movement - flexion ability

	Rheumatoid Arthritis	Osteoarthritis
90° and more	54	42
70° - 89°	38	36
50° - 69°	18	7
30° - 49°	2	0
	112	85

TABLE 3
Results: Range of movement - extension deficit

	Rheumatoid Arthritis	Osteoarthritis
0°	44	31
1° - 5°	15	10
6° - 10°	30	29
11° and more	23	15
	112	85

TABLE 4

Results: Postoperative Pain

	Rheumatoid Arthitis	Osteoarthritis
No pain, full activity	49	41
Little pain	38	22
Pain after short distances (max.400m)	19	20
Analgesics necessary	5	2
Pain at rest, no activity	1	0
	112	85

ding to the definition of 3 different scenarios (Fig. 5). X-ray radiographs of 82 completely documented cases of total knee replacement with the GSB-prosthesis were studied, consisting of radiographs of both knees in an anterior-posterior direction, in a lateral view with 30° flexion and both patellae in tangential direction. No pre- to postoperative change in 'a' and 'b' led to a physiological position of the patella (case 1 in Fig. 5). This was found in 22 cases (27%). Too large a tibial resection combined with too small a resection of the femur resulted in an increase in 'b' and a decrease in 'a'. This was found in 43 replacements (53%) leading to iatrogenic patella alta. Too large a resection of the femur and too small a resection of the tibia led to an increase in 'a' and a decrease in 'b'. This patella baja was found in 17 cases (20%) (case 3 in Fig. 5).

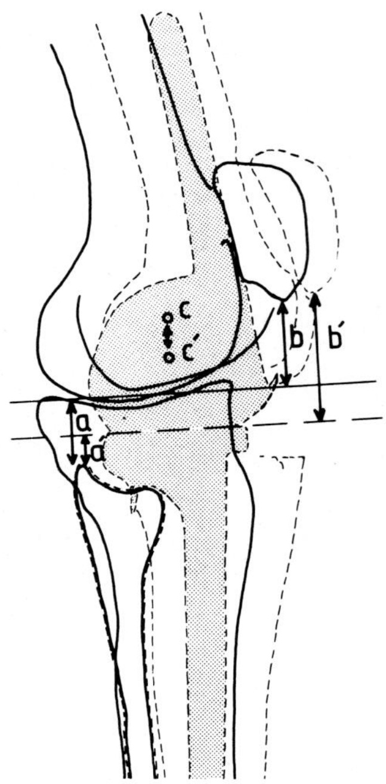

Fig. 4
Patella-dislocation following total knee replacement.

a = distance: head of fibula - joint space

b = distance: apex patella - joint space

c = momentaneous center of rotation

a,b,c: before knee replacement

a',b',c': after knee replacement

Fig. 5

Patella dislocation following total knee arthroplasty. Possible cases depending on position of the components of the prosthesis

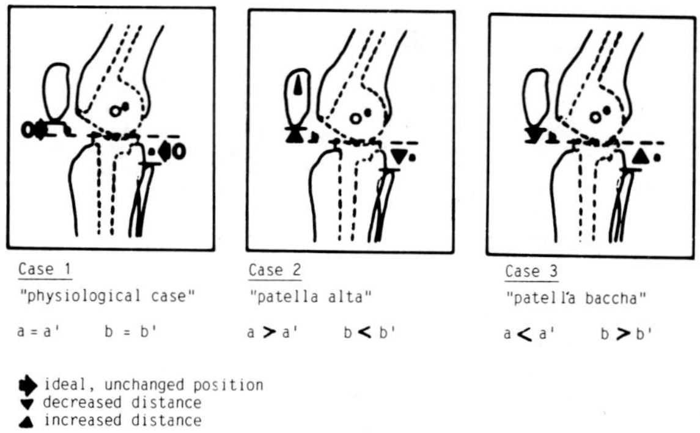

The three patellar parameters and postoperative cranial dislocation of the patella in all 82 of the completely documented cases reveals significant correlation between postendoprosthetic cranial dislocation of the patella and reduction in patellar thickness (Fig. 6). The thickness of the patella at time of evaluation compared to the preoperative state was reduced to more than 1/4 in about 75% of the case 2 knees, while there was only little change of patellar thickness in the case 1 knees. Articular surface erosions of the patellae were detected by tangential radiographs as well as well as quantified by 99m-Tc-scans. The correlation between cranial patella dislocation and retropatellar erosions was even more striking (Fig. 7). 88% of the case 2 knees showed massive defects of the retropatellar joint surface with single or multiple erosions. Case 3 knees were also found to have many retropatellar erosions. There also is a substantial correlation between cranial dislocation of the patella and postoperative persistan-

Fig. 6

Diminution of patellar thickness in correlation to cases of vertical patella-dislocation after total knee arthroplasty

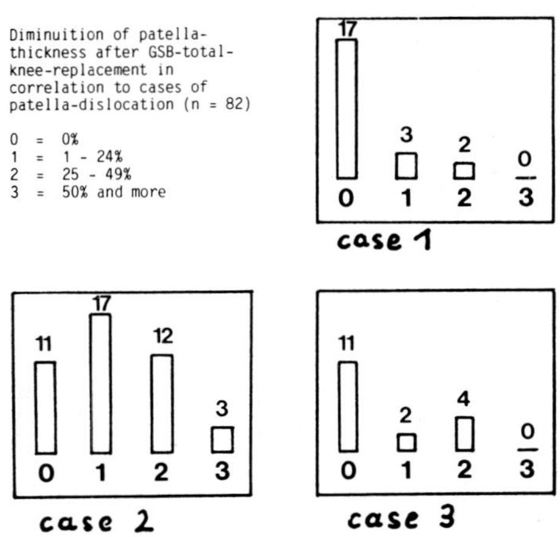

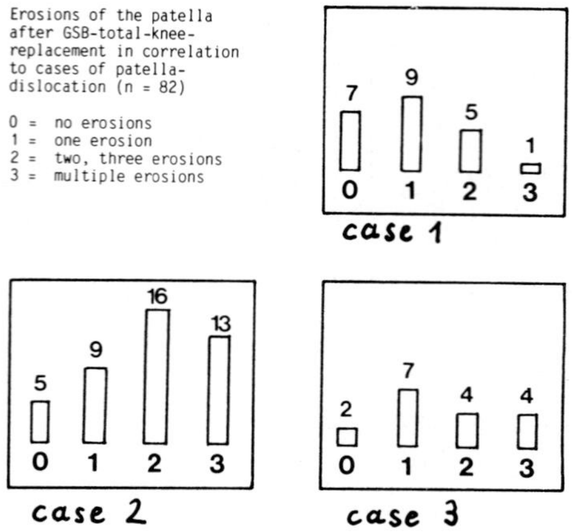

Fig. 7

Erosions of the patella

ce of retropatellar pain (fig. 8). In the total knee arthroplasties of case 2 and 3 the vertical patella dislocation caused discomfort in movement and stress bearing in nearly 50% of the cases. Five out of 22 patients of case 1 showed pain on weight bearing too.

DISCUSSION

Total knee arthroplasty is a successful and preferable alternative to knee arthrodesis. If gross disability is to be avoided, there must be at least one functioning knee. Nevertheless total knee replacement should only be performed in patients with severely destructed knee joints with no other possibility left of improvement by conservative or other operative means.

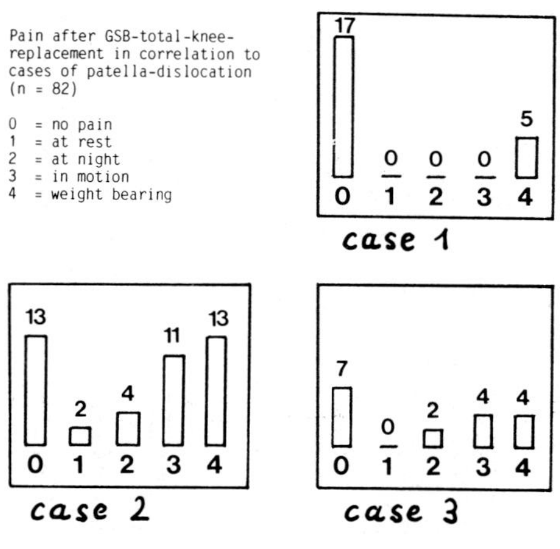

Fig. 8

Pain after total knee replacement

Biomaterials and Clinical Applications,
edited by A. Pizzoferrato, P.G. Marchetti, A. Ravaglioli and A.J.C. Lee
Elsevier Science Publishers B.V., Amsterdam, 1987 — Printed in The Netherlands

BIOMECHANICS OF THE P.C.A. TOTAL KNEE ARTHROPLASTY

P.G. MARCHETTI[1], M. SPINELLI[2] and M. MARCACCI[1]
[1]Clinica Ortopedica, Istituti Rizzoli, Bologna
[2]Clinica Ortopedica IIa, Pisa

Although new cement techniques and designs of prostheses as well as more precise alignment of both the leg and the individual components appear to have improved the longevity of total knee arthroplasty, fixation failure continues to be a serious problem.

Fixation failure is a phenomen which results from a number of factors affecting the fixation interface, including:

a) High shear-stress
b) Micromovement
c) Stress-schielding of bone.

The P.C.A. Total Knee System has been designed to address each of these factors in order to improve the long-term results of total knee arthroplasty. Recognizing that optimal results of total knee arthroplasty are dependent on both the design of the prosthesis and its instrumentation, the P.C.A. Universal Total Knee Instruments have been developed to ensure accurate alignment of the leg and optimal seating of each component to reduce shear stress at fixation interfaces. Anatomically designed components with porous coated fixation surfaces further reduce shear-stresses at fixation interfaces and improve stress distribution to bone.

In the research laboratories of J.H. University in Baltimore (U.S.A.), fresh cadaveric knees with completely intact capsular and ligamentous structures, either in the normal state or after careful implantation of the prosthesis to be studied, were mounted in a knee simulator. This simulator allowed application of a vertical load in an anatomic fashion and permitted rotation of a tibial base plate which produced knee rotation. Rotation was plotted against torque on an x-y recorder. All knees were tested in 0°, 20°, 40°, 60°, and 90° of flexion.

Moreover using this test-apparatus a study on joint stability in fresh cadaveric knees has been performed and particularly postero-lateral instabilities have been tested in various combinations.

Sections have been performed on:

1) Anterior Cruciate Ligament
2) Posterior Cruciate Ligament (with Humphrey and Wisberg and menisco-tibial

ligaments)

3) The Arcuate Complex (with lateral gastrocnemius and popliteus muscles)

4) Lateral Collateral Ligament

Sections had these combinations:

- Sectioning the posterior cruciate affects internal rotation and varus.
- Sectioning the lateral collateral does not affect rotation and only increases varus laxity.
- Sectioning the arcuate complex alone affects neither rotatory or varus/valgus laxities. It would appear that the lateral collateral and arcuate complex are interrelated for rotatory laxity as the sectioning of both would appear to increase external rotation.
- Sectioning the posterior cruciate after sectioning the arcuate and lateral collateral ligament does not affect rotation but markedly increases varus which increases as flexion occurs. The anterior cruciate sectioning always increases internal rotation and valgus and when sectioned after all the other ligaments renders a very lax knee in both rotation and varus/valgus.

A goal of the method is achieving proper alignment.

Joint line is horizontal in monopodalic stance during gait and mechanical axis is normally on the center of the three joints. The difference between the leg and femoral axis is usually 6° and between vertical and mechanical line 3°. This orientation is well achieved with Universal Instruments.

From our experience of more than 100 cases, the average post-oper. score with good alignment is 97,5; on the contrary, malallignment has reduced to 82,5 the average score when there is femoral and tibial malalignment .

Alignment has to be completed with balancement of capsular and ligamentous structures.

There are a number of dependent factors that affect flexion range of motion; patellar thickness, size of the femoral component, and posterior joint space. Patellar thickness and femoral component size are factors that can lengthen the moment arm of the femoro-patellar joint, thus limiting flexion due to tightening of the quadriceps mechanism.

In a few cases reduced patellar resection has increased patellar tracking and produce proximal migration of patellar component; in a more than four years follow-up case, some free beads from porous coating can be seen on the radiograph.

In our opinion the causes of patellar loosening are:

1) a too strong physical activity;
2) an insufficient patellar bone resection;
3) a malalignment of extensor mechanism;
4) a too anatomical patellar and femoral groove design.

This last problem, that's common to other experiences, has induced Hungerford to change the patellar design: the new one has a dome design, symmetrical, with reduced thickness of 5mm and three pegs to reduce shear-stresses.

REFERENCES

1 D.S. Hungerford, K.A. Krackow, R.V. Kenna
Total knee arthroplasty. A comprehensive approach.
Williams E. Wilkins. Baltimore-London 1984.

2 The P.C.A. primary total knee system.
Rutherford, N.J. Howmedica Inc. 1984.

3 P.G. Marchetti, M. Marcalli, M. Spinelli,
La nostra esperienza con la protesi del ginocchio P.C.A.
Il ginocchio, Vol IV, 435, 1985.

Biomaterials and Clinical Applications,
edited by A. Pizzoferrato, P.G. Marchetti, A. Ravaglioli and A.J.C. Lee
Elsevier Science Publishers B.V., Amsterdam, 1987 — Printed in The Netherlands

MECHANICAL PROPERTIES AND BIOCOMPATIBILITIES OF THE NEW GLASS-FIBER COMPOSITE MATERIALS AS ARTIFICIAL BONE

M. MORISHITA[1], M. KOBAYASHI[2], M. SEYAMA[1], S. KONDO[1], K. KAWAUCHI[1], H. ARAI[1]
H. TAGAI[2] and Y. KUROKI[1]

[1]Department of Orthopaedic Surgery, Showa Univ. Fujigaoka Hospital, 1-30 FUJIGAOKA, MIDORI-KU, YOKOHAMA 227 (JAPAN)

[2]Department of Industrial Chemistry, Chiba Institute of Technology, 2-17-1, TUDANUMA, NARASHINO, CHIBA 275 (JAPAN)

ABSTRACT

A glass-fiber composite (CPSA-Composite)(ref.1) molded from CaO-P2O5-SiO2-Al2O3 glass-fiber (CPSA Glass-fiber)(ref.2) and polymethyl methacrylate (PMMA) which the authors developed has excellent mechanical properties and biocompatibilities. The mechanical properties of CPSA-Composite are characterized by its fracture toughness. The maximal bending strength is about 8 times greater than that of human cortical bone, and the elastic modulus and apparent density are equal to or somewhat greater than those of human cortical bone. Additionally, variable bending strength can be achieved by adjusting the volume fraction of the glass-fiber and facilitating secondary processing of the material.
The biocompatibilities of CPSA-Glass and CPSA-Composite were histologically investigated and the cytotoxicity of CPSA-Glass was examined. The results were excellent.

INTRODUCTION

Remarkable progress has been made in the orthopaedic field in biomaterials for joint replacement and artificial bone. Especially, alumina ceramics has been used in the clinical field since it is more stable in the body than conventional materials used thus far, and it has excellent biocompatibilities. However, an alumina ceramic has some problems, such as low fracture toughness and its bending strength, as well as difficulty in processing, although its hardness and compression strength are excellent. On the other hand, the authors have succeeded in fiberizing CaO-P2O5-SiO2-Al2O3 glass (CPSA-Glass) (ref.1) in order to mold it, and polymethyl methacrylate (PMMA) into glass-fiber composite (CPSA-Composite). In this paper the authors report results on mechanical properties and biocompatibilities of the CPSA-Composite.

MATERIALS AND METHODS

Production methods of the CPSA-Composite

Continuously spun CPSA glass-fibers were soaked in an acetone solution of PMMA and dried. After that, cylindrical unidirectional reinforcement with a

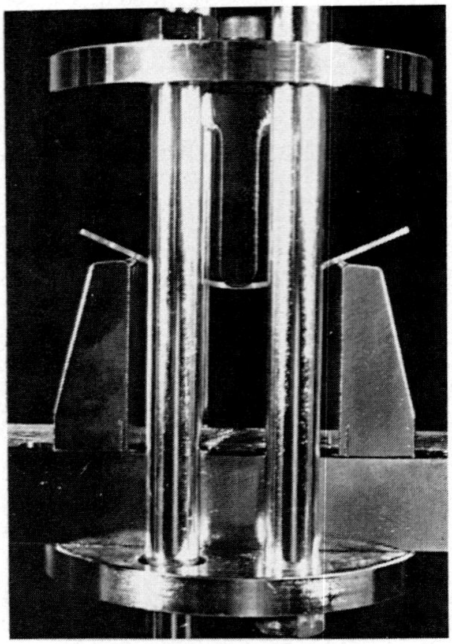

Fig.1 Shimazu Autograph SD-500 and the CPSA-Composite.

diameter of 1.5mm was molded by means of a drawing method employing a molder, the temperature of which was adjusted to 220°C - 250°C. To improve the biocompatibilities of the material, the surface was treated with (NH4)3PO4-H3PO4 solution (25°C) with pH 4 for 30 minutes.

Measurement of mechanical properties of the CPSA-Composite

The measurement of mechanical properties was made by means of a Shimazu Autograph SD-500 (Fig.1) according to Japanese Industrial Standard K 6911 method.

Examination of biocompatibilities of the CPSA-Composite

Each material with a diameter of 1.5mm of CPSA-Composite, CPSA-Glass was implanted into the femur of a mature white rabbit. The bone tissue around the materials was regularly taken out after implantation. The plastic embedded thin section of each material was prepared to examine under an optical microscope after using H-E and Villanueva's bone stain. As for the specimen after implantation at 6 weeks, it was examined for the interface between the bone and materials under an electron microscope.

Examination of cytotoxicities of the CPSA-Glass

As for the cytotoxicities of CPSA-Glass, the growth of the cells on the surface of an 18 x 19 x 2 mm plate was observed. Additionally, CPSA-Glass was compared with SUS-316L stainless steel and poly-crystal almina ceramic. Cells used included Hela S3 cells of the human cervix uteri, Wl-38 cells of the human fetal fibroblast and the neonatal calvarial cells of the mouse.

Each 2 ml of culture fluid containing 1.0×10^4 cells for Hella S3, 2.0×10^4 cells for Wl-38, 2.0×10^4 cells for neonatal calvarium of the mouse was inoculated on the CPSA-Glass plate to be cultured for one week. After that, the number of cells on it was calculated, and a scanning electron microscopic examination was also made on the coadunating condition.

EXPERIMENTAL RESULTS

Mechanical properties of the CPSA-Composite

When a stress-strain curve of the CPSA-Composite (Fig.2-a) was obtained by means of a 3-point bending test, it was found that as the stress increased, the strain also increased, and even when the curve passed the yield point, the material was not suddenly destroyed but only gradually. This fact demonstrated that the CPSA-Composite has fracture toughness.

The relationship between the bending strength and volume fraction (Vf) of the glass-fiber in CPSA-Composite (Fig.2-b) showed that the bending strength was stronger in proportion to the VF of the glass-fiber. The maximal bending strength was 1500 MPa at the moldable upper limit of Vf 0.7 and the material showed bending strength about 8 times greater than that of human cortical bone. Therefore a material with the bending strength of 1500 MPa max. can be obtained by adjusting the Vf of the glass-fiber contained in CPSA-Composite.

When the elastic modulus (Fig.2-c) was obtained from the gradient of the linear part of the stress-strain curve of CPSA-Composite, it was found that

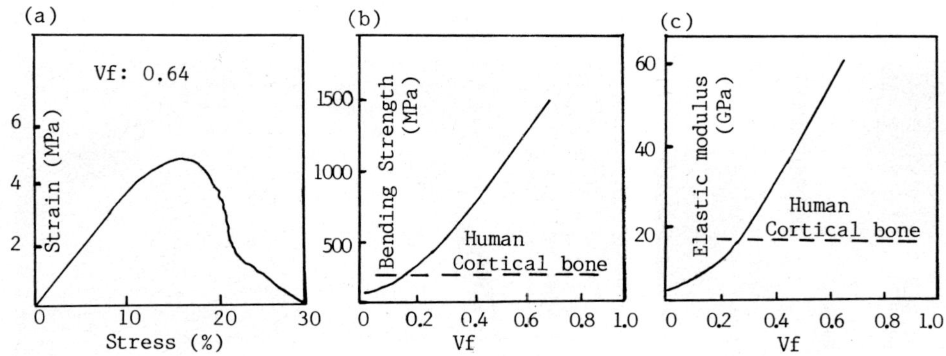

Fig.2
a) Stress-strain diagram of the CPSA-Composite.
b) Relationship between the bending strength and the volume fraction (Vf) of glass-fiber in CPSA-Composite.
c) Relationship between the elastic modulus and the volume fraction (Vf) of glass-fiber in CPSA-Composite.

the elastic modulus increased in proportion to the Vf. The elastic modulus was about 8 - 60 GPa, which is equal to or somewhat greater than that of human cortical bone.

The apparent density of CPSA-Composite was about 1.3-2.3, which is equal to that of human cortical bone, indicating that the material can easily be secondarily processed.

From the above results, it was concluded that the CPSA-Composite has excellent physical properties.

Biocompatibilities of the CPSA-Glass and CPSA-Composite

When the CPSA-Composite was implanted into the femur of a mature white rabbit, from the 2nd week after implantation osteoid formation was observed surrounding the CPSA-composite, (Fig.3-a) and the osteoid formation became clear the 3rd week. New bone formation was observed surrounding part in the 8th week. Osteoid and new bone formation continued to be clearly observed and inflammatory change was not observed surrounding the CPSA-Composite in one year. (Fig.3-b) As for the examination of interface between bone and CPSA-Glass under an electoron microscope at 6 weeks after implantation, there was osteoblast and almost no necrotic tissues at the interface. (Fig.3-c)

(a) (b) (c)

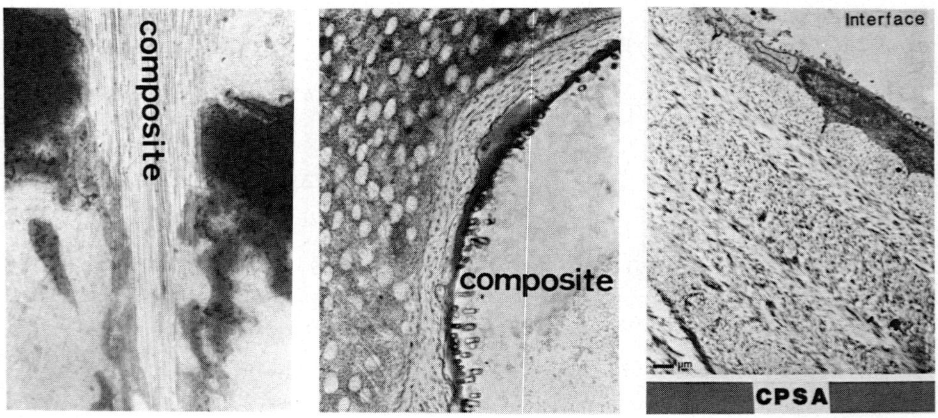

Fig.3
a) The histological findings at 2 weeks after implantation.
b) The histological findings at 1 year after implantation.
c) The examination of interface between bone and CPSA-Glass at 6 weeks after implantation. The black line in the lower part shows the length of 1 micron.

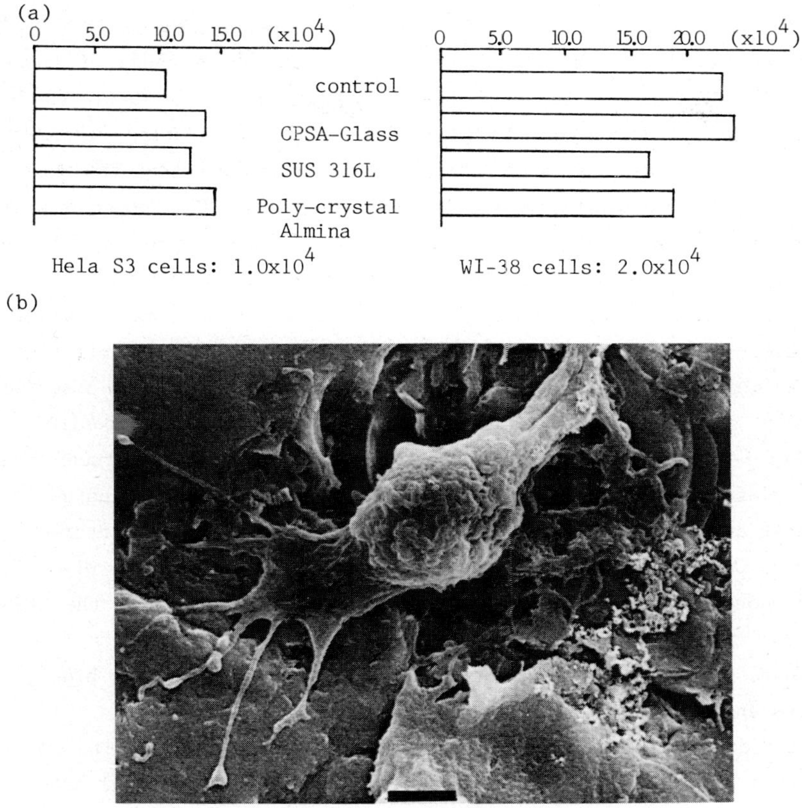

Fig.4
a) The growth of each cell on the CPSA-Glass.
b) The Hela S3 cell coaduation on the CPSA-Glass. The black line in the lower part shows the length of 1 micron.

Plenty of cellular activities were noted since the osteocyte has a large nucleus and rich chromatin. From the above, it was concluded that the CPSA-Composite have better biocompatibilities.

Cytotoxicity of the CPSA-Glass

Excellent growth of Hela S3 cells, Wl-38 cells and neonatal calvarial cells of the mouse were observed on the CPSA-Glass. In comparative study a favorable cell growth on the CPSA-Glass was noted as well as on the poli-crystal almina ceramic. (Fig.4-a) A scanning electron microscopic observation revealed a favorable coadunation of the cells on CPSA-Glass. (Fig.4-b) It was considered that no cytotoxicity would occur on the CPSA-Glass.

DISCUSSION AND CONCLUSION

The mechanical properties of CPSA-Composite are characterized by its fracture toughness. (Fig.2-a) The maximal bending strength is about 8 times greater than that of human cortical bone (Fig.2-b) and the elastic modulus (Fig.2-c) and apparent density are equal to or somewhat greater than those of human cortical bone. Additionally, variable bending strength can be achieved by adjusting the volume fraction of the glass-fiber and facilitating secondary processing of the material. From the above, we have concluded that the mechanical properties of CPSA-Composite are so excellent that CPSA-Composite will be able to be used as artificial bone. It is better to use a Vf of 0.5-0.6 of material since the moldable upper limit of the materials is Vf 0.7.

When the CPSA-Composite was implanted into the femur of a mature white rabbit, we observed the osteoid around the CPSA-Composite at the early time. (Fig.3-a) Osteoid and new bone formation continued to be clearly observed and imflamatory change was not observed surrounding the CPSA-Composite in one year. (Fig.3-b) Furthermore, the examination of interface between the bone and CPSA-glass under an electron microscope at 6 weeks after implantation, osteoblast and almost no necrotic tissues were observed at the interface. (Fig.3-c) On the other hand, excellent growth of Hela S3 cells, Wl-38 cells and neonatal calvarial cells of the mouse were observed on the CPSA -Glass. (Fig.4)

From the above, it was considered that the CPSA-Composite has better biocompatibilities and the CPSA-Glass has no cytotoxicity.

We have reached the following conclusion ; that the CPSA-Composite would be expected to be a good biomaterial since it showed excellent physical properties and biocompatibilities. But we have to wait for further research before use in the clinical field.

(The part of these research funds was provided by THE OHKURA FOUNDATION, TOKYO, and some of the materials were supplied by THE MITSUBISHI MINING & CEMENT COMPANY, TOKYO)

REFERENCE

1) M.Morishita, Y. Kuroki, M.Kobayashi and M. Seyama, The experimental study of properties and histological findings of CPSA-Composite materials, Orthopaedic Research Science, Vol.13, Japan, 1986, pp118-121.

2) H. Tagai, S. Niwa, M. Somiya, M. Ono, T. Takeuchi and M. Kobayashi, Preparation of apatite glass fiber for application as biomaterials, Ceramics in Surgery Elsevier Scientific Pub. Co, Amsterdam, 1983, pp387-393.

Biomaterials and Clinical Applications,
edited by A. Pizzoferrato, P.G. Marchetti, A. Ravaglioli and A.J.C. Lee
Elsevier Science Publishers B.V., Amsterdam, 1987 — Printed in The Netherlands

MECHANICAL STRESSES IN THE CASE OF FIBRE REINFORCED HIP JOINT ENDOPROSTHESES

H. Röhrle and W. Sollbach
Dornier GmbH, D-7990 Friedrichshafen, Germany

INTRODUCTION

The use of implant materials tolerated by the body, as for example carbon and carbon fibre reinforced plastics (CFRP), allows the bone to adhere to or grow into the endoprosthesis (ref. 1). For this reason, the question arises whether or not the mechanical stresses at the boundary surface between the hip joint endoprosthesis and the femur are below the strength of the implant/bone connection known from animal experiments or below values which have still to be determined.

MATHEMATICAL MODEL

The mathematical model for the bone/endoprosthesis combination consists of volume elements with curved surfaces (isoparametric elements) (ref. 2). With a view to an economic processing the structure is subdivided into 4 coupled components which are shown in Fig. 1 and comprise together about 8.800 degrees of freedom.

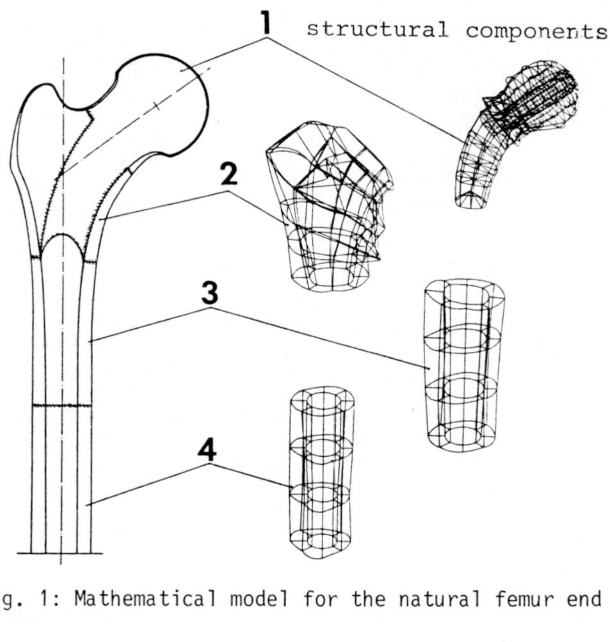

Fig. 1: Mathematical model for the natural femur end

The CFRP-endoprosthesis fills the hollow space of the bone. The upper and central parts of the shaft are in contact on all sides with the corticalis or the spongiosa (see Fig. 2). The splitting effect in the only slightly conical part of the shaft is dependent on the strength of the connection between implant and living bone.

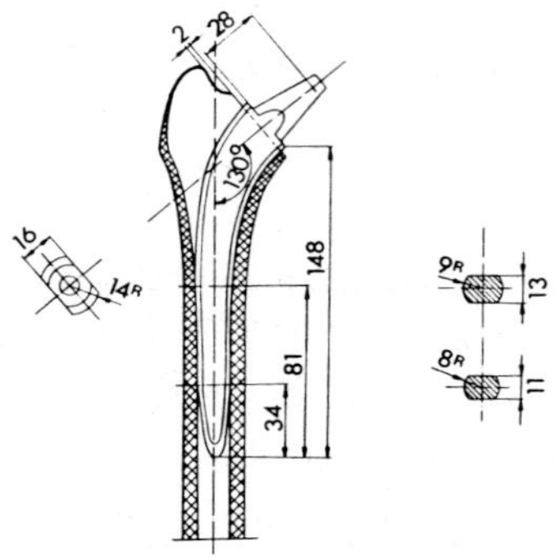

Fig. 2: Endoprosthesis produced by CFRP in the femur

For the description of the material laws for bone and endoprosthesis we assume an orthotrope behaviour. The bone section is subdivided into 7 regions. The values shown in Fig. 3 were partly taken from literature (refs. 3,4) and completed by own investigations (ref. 5).

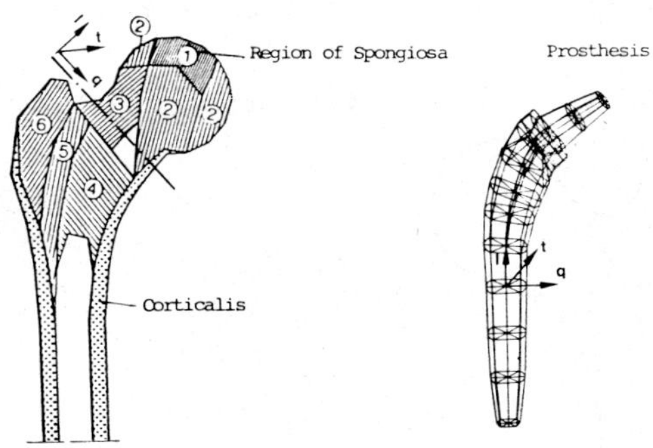

Material properties [N/mm²]	Corticalis	Region of Spongiosa 1	2	3	4	5	6	Prosthesis
E_l	15000	1450	1210	970	390	485	728	100000
E_t	7500	725	605	485	195	242	364	67000
E_q	7500	725	605	485	195	242	364	67000
G_{lq}	5000	484	404	324	130	162	242	2500
G_{lt}	5000	484	404	324	130	162	242	5000
G_{tq}	2500	242	202	162	65	81	121	5000
ν_{lt}	0,3	0,3	0,3	0,3	0,3	0,3	0,3	0,025
ν_{lq}	0,3	0,3	0,3	0,3	0,3	0,3	0,3	0,025
ν_{tq}	0,3	0,3	0,3	0,3	0,3	0,3	0,3	0,35

Fig. 3: Material properties for bone/endoprosthesis compound

The material properties for the prosthesis are hypothetical values which are in the lower range of CFRP. They can be reached for both a core-and-shell structure and a multilayer structure.

We consider a load case which occurs frequently in everyday life, i.e. the terminal stance during horizontal walking. In this case, the hip joint forces are higher than for the pre-stance (ref. 6). From the partly statistically assured data for a gait speed of 1.2 m/sec we take a hip joint force divided by the body weight of H/W = 5.5. The chosen body weight of W = 750 N results in the hip joint force of H = 4125 N. The muscle iliopsoas has a force of M_i = 1.35W = 1021 N due to the balance of moments. The force components are given in Fig. 4.

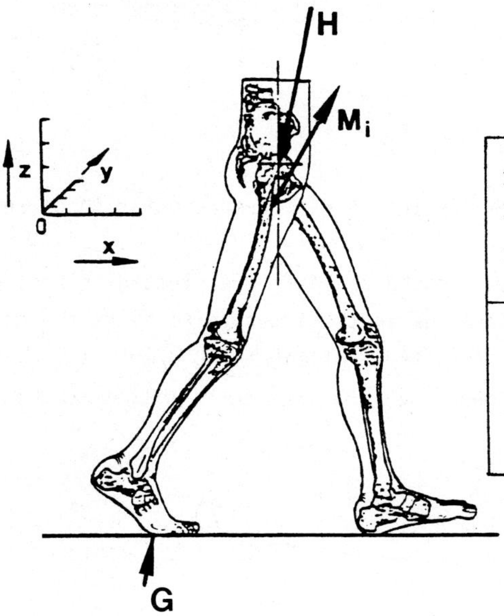

H_x	[N]	- 600
H_y	[N]	- 300
H_z	[N]	- 4050
$M_{i,x}$	[N]	465
$M_{i,y}$	[N]	495
$M_{i,z}$	[N]	750

Fig. 4: Forces in the hip joint and in the muscle iliopsoas for the terminal stance

RESULTS

We consider the longitudinal stresses in the shaft of the endoprosthesis and the shear stresses at the surface of the shaft. The representation in the form of a diagram uses the abscissa scale given in Fig. 5. Due to the three-dimensional bending of the endoprosthesis shaft we consider always 2 points or lines on the medial and the lateral side. The identification is given by the points (1) to (4) in Fig. 5.

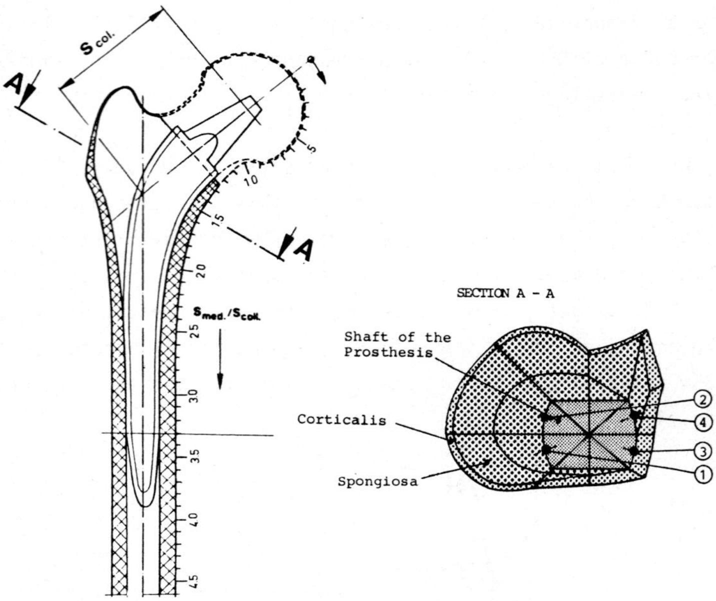

Fig. 5: Definition of coordinates and points for the representation of results

The longitudinal stresses in the prosthesis shaft are plotted in Fig. 6. It can be seen that the maximum values occur in the lower third as in the case of conventional metal endoprostheses. The stress of about 150 N/mm² is very high since it is a cyclic repeating stress level that has to be withstood many times.

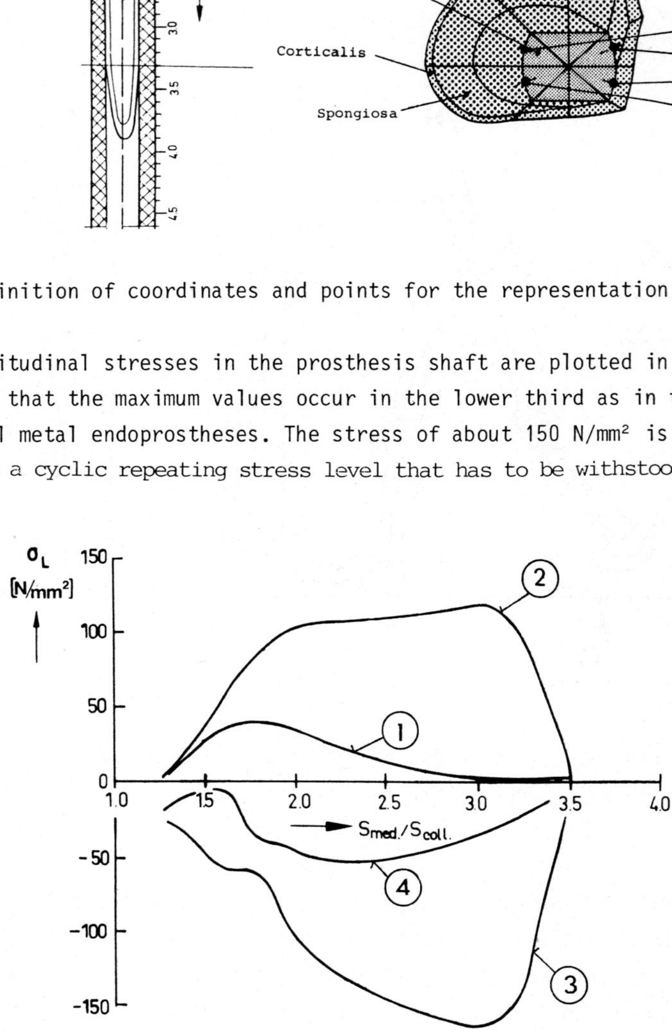

Fig. 6: Longitudinal stresses in the prosthesis shaft during terminal stance

The shear stresses along the medial and lateral contact surface between bone and prosthesis are shown in Fig. 7. It can be seen that the largest stresses are active near of the end of the shaft. The occuring shear stresses with a max. value of 24 N/mm² are extremely high.

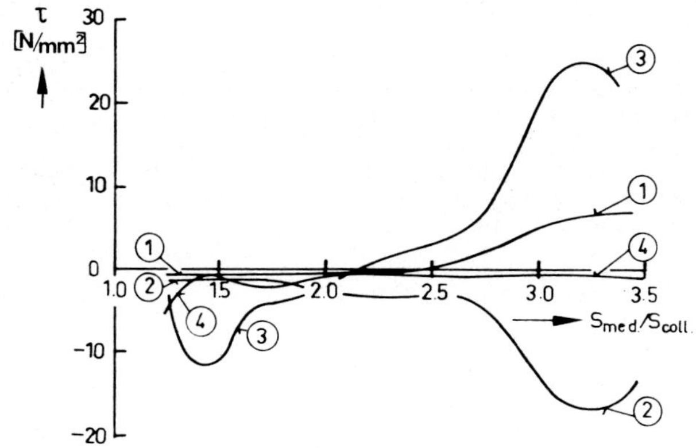

Fig. 7: Shear stresses along the medial and lateral prosthesis contact area during terminal stance

In order to reduce the above mentioned shear stresses to a measure that leads to a bone contact, free, as far as possible, of connective tissue, the stiffness has to be diminished towards the shaft end (ref. 2). This aim can be realized much easier for fibre reinforced plastics than for metal.

ACKNOWLEDGEMENT

This paper was prepared as part of the research project "Die mechanische Beanspruchung im Knochen um die Schaftoberfläche von Faserverbund-Hüftendoprothesen" (BMFT 01 VG 033) sponsored by the West-German Bundesminister für Forschung und Technologie.

REFERENCES

1 W. Scheer, Kohlenstoffaserverstärktes Epoxidharz - ein Werkstoff für Humanimplantate, published in VDI-Taschenbuch "Verarbeitung und Anwenden kohlefaserverstärkter Kunststoffe", VDI-Verlag GmbH Düsseldorf, 1981.

2 H. Stark, Verbesserte FEM-Berechnung zum künstlichen Hüftgelenk, Diplomarbeit TU Stuttgart, Dornier Friedrichshafen, Dezember 1984.

3 D.O. Welch, The Composite Structure of Bone and its Response to Mechanical Stress, Princeton University, Princeton, New Jersey.

4 M.H. Pope and J.O. Outwater, Mechanical Properties of Bone as a Function of Position and Orientation, J. Biomechanics, 1974, Vol. 7, pp. 61-66, Pergamon Press.

5 H. Röhrle, R. Scholten, C. Sigolotto and W. Sollbach, Kraftflußberechnung in Knochenstrukturen und Prothesen, Phase III, BMFT-Forschungsbericht T80-174, Fachinformationszentrum Energie, Physik, Mathematik GmbH, 7514 Eggenstein-Leopoldshafen 2, 1980, ISSN 0340-7608.

6 H. Röhrle, R. Scholten, C. Sigolotto, W. Sollbach and H. Keller, Joint Forces in the Human Pelvis-Leg Skeleton during Walking, J. Biomechanics, Vol. 17, no. 6, pp. 409-424, 1984.

Biomaterials and Clinical Applications,
edited by A. Pizzoferrato, P.G. Marchetti, A. Ravaglioli and A.J.C. Lee
Elsevier Science Publishers B.V., Amsterdam, 1987 — Printed in The Netherlands

PERFORMANCE OF POROUS POLYSULFONE COATED TITANIUM ALLOY FEMORAL STEMS IN DOGS AND HUMAN PATIENTS

M. SPECTOR[1], M. DEMANE[2], J.R. ROBERSON[1], J.R. DE ANDRADE[1], AND R.S. RIGGINS[1]

[1]Department of Orthopaedics, Emory University School of Medicine, Atlanta, GA, USA

[2]Orthopaedic Division, Richards Medical Company, Memphis, TN, USA

SUMMARY

The performance of fully porous polysulfone (PPSF) coated titanium alloy femoral stems was evaluated in dogs and humans for periods up to two years. The performance of canine stems correlated with the canal fill ratio. Femurs exhibiting an acceptable canal fill ratio displayed no evidence of non-anatomic femoral remodeling through two years. Histological evaluation of canine stems revealed considerable osseous ingrowth with bone filling 10-40% of the available porosity. Radiographic analysis of human patients with large fully coated Ti-6Al-4V stems displayed no gross non-anatomic femoral remodeling through two years. Radionuclide imaging revealed near normal bone turnover along the medial femoral and trochanteric regions at two years, with only slightly increased uptake over the prosthesis compared to the unoperated control. The near normal bone remodeling and turnover around these fully porous coated canal filling stems may be due to the low structural stiffness afforded from the use of a porous polysulfone coating.

INTRODUCTION

Recent investigations of porous metal coated devices have confirmed that adequate bone ingrowth stabilization can be achieved (refs. 1,2). The clinical results of these investigations are encouraging. However, the increased toxic metal ion release and reduction in stem strength associated with the application of porous metal coatings to titanium and cobalt alloy stems is cause for some attention. Furthermore, large (canal filling) rigid femoral stems can lead to non-anatomic femoral remodeling due to "stress shielding" effects (ref. 3). The growing demand for exceptionally large diameter devices to provide canal filling in enlarged revision sites may exacerbate this phenomenon.

Porous polymers have been investigated as a low modulus coating on femoral stems (refs. 4,5). Our efforts have concentrated on porous polysulfone, a high strength engineering thermoplastic which can be chemically bonded to a Ti-6Al-4V core. Previous investigations indicate that a porous polysulfone coating on Ti-6Al-4V inhibits the in vitro release of metal ions yet has no adverse affect upon the fatigue properties of the base alloy (ref. 6).

METHODS AND MATERIALS

The performance of porous polysufone coated Ti-6Al-4V femoral stems was evaluated in dogs and human patients. Ti-6Al-4V core stems were fully coated with sintered porous polysulfone to yield a 1.5 mm circumferential coating (250 micron avg. pore dia., 30% porosity). The resin utilized was medical grade polysulfone (Union Carbide Corporation P-1700 MG) with a molecular weight of 25,000. Silyl reactive polysulfone was employed to bond the porous polysulfone layer to the underlying Ti-6Al-4V core.

Animal Study

Twenty-five porous polysulfone coated stems were implanted into 25 dogs (35-40kg; 6-8 yrs. age) with the contralateral limb serving as anatomic control. A polyethylene acetabular component was cemented in the conventional manner. Radiographic and histomorphometric analysis was performed to assess tissue ingrowth at intervals of 1,3,6,12 or 24 months. Radionuclide image analysis was performed on selected animals to assess bone turnover.

Human Pilot Study

In a preliminary investigation, four patients received four large diameter, fully porous polysulfone coated Ti-6Al-4V femoral stems. Ongoing clinical evaluation includes radiographic and radionuclide image analysis for intervals through two years.

RESULTS

Radiographic Findings

The performance of the canine femoral stems correlated with the "canal fill" ratio. Animals with poor canal filling (4 of 13 animals at greater than 5 months post-op) showed radiographic evidence of loosening. Animals with canal filling stems typically displayed a radiodense line at the coating/bone interface, some rounding of the calcar cortex, and an increased radiodensity at the stem tip. Minimal non-anatomic remodeling was observed for periods through two years.

All human patients displayed good canal filling with no evidence of loosening. Radiographic evaluation revealed no gross non-anatomic remodeling through two years. Sequential radiographic evaluation revealed increased radiodensities within the radiolucent coating suggesting bone ingrowth (Fig. 1).

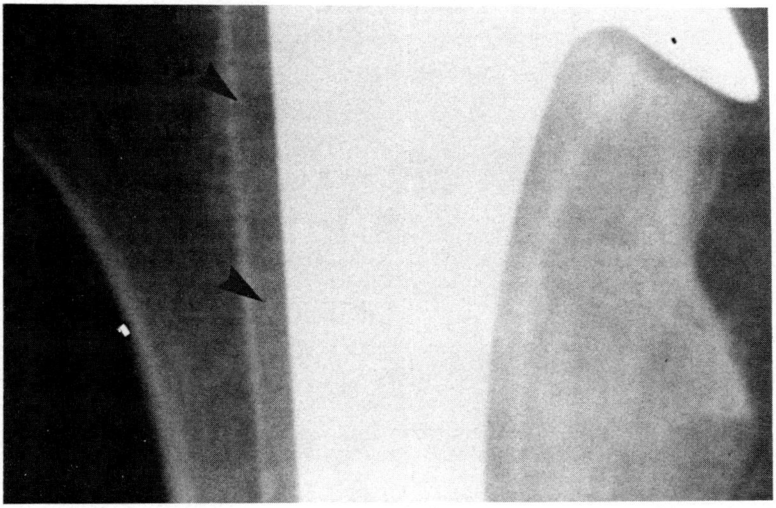

Fig. 1. Radiograph of a portion of a PPSF coated Ti-6Al-4V stem in a human patient (12 mos.) showing radiodensities suggesting bone ingrowth (arrow).

Radionuclide Imaging

Radionuclide imaging of animal and human operated femurs revealed an increased radionuclide uptake during the 4-6 month post-op period which gradually decreased thereafter. Subsequent radionuclide imaging (up to 2 years) revealed near normal bone turnover along the medial femoral and trochanteric regions, with only slightly increased uptake over the prosthesis compared to the non-operated control side.

Histology Results (Animal Study)

Histological evaluation of 13 implants after 14 months of implantation revealed bone ingrowth into 10-40% of the available porosity on stems with an acceptable canal fill ratio (Fig. 2,3). Areas of the porosity not filled with bone were filled with marrow elements and fibrous tissue. A continuous trabecular structure (corresponding to radiodense lines) was occasionally observed at the coating/bone interface. Bony ingrowth could not be correlated as a function of location along the stem. There was a suggestion of more uniform ingrowth along the medial aspect of the femur compared to the lateral region. Histology further suggested increased ingrowth in those regions of the coating that were in close proximity to the endosteal cortex.

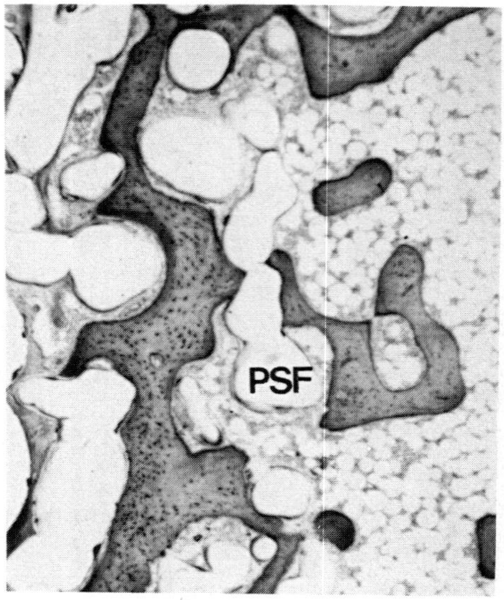

Fig. 2. Histology micrograph displaying bone ingrowth into a PPSF coated canine stem after 1 year.

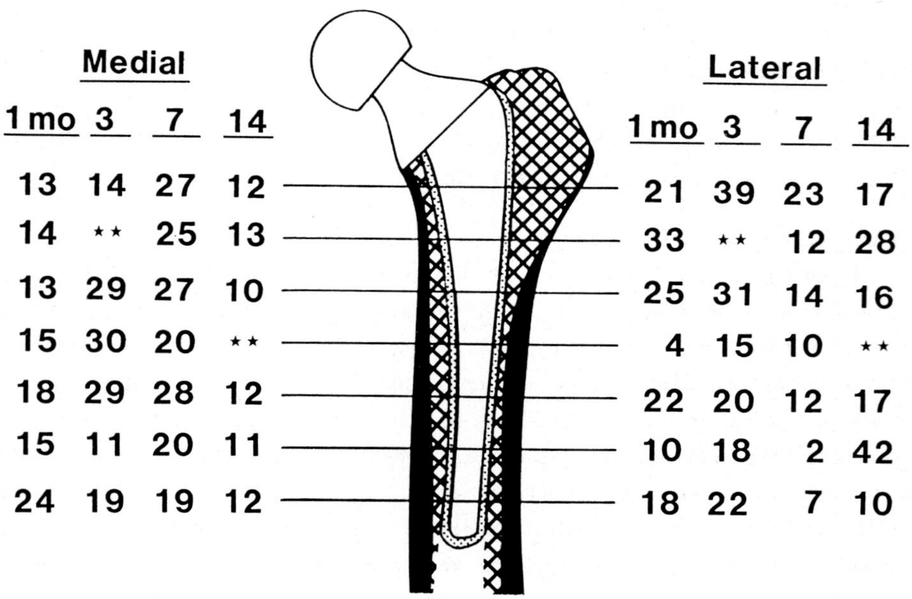

Fig. 3. Percentage of the available porosity (to a depth of 500 micrometers) occupied by bone for 4 typical stems.

DISCUSSION

In the present study, large diameter (canal filling) porous polysulfone coated stems elicited no demonstrable adverse femoral remodeling in dogs and humans through two years. These findings contrast with previous investigations which found gross femoral remodeling associated with fully porous metal coated stems (Refs. 7,8). The lower stiffness associated with porous polysufone coated Ti-6Al-4V stems may result in more favorable adaptive remodeling. For example, approximate calculations (Ref. 7) for the bending stiffness of femoral stems and femora (assuming a typical large stem of circular geometry) revealed a significant difference between a porous polysulfone coated Ti alloy stem and a porous coated Co-Cr-Mo stem of comparable geometry (Table 1). In the dog, implantation of a Co-Cr-Mo alloy stem reduced the stress in the surrounding bone (at the isthmus) to 17% of normal, compared to 60% of normal for the porous polysulfone/Ti alloy stem. In human patients, the Co-Cr-Mo stem caused a 75% reduction in surrounding bone stress, compared to a 38% reduction associated with porous polysulfone coated Ti alloy stems.

TABLE 1

Bending Stiffness* (N m^2)

	Femur	Co-Cr-Mo	PPSF/Ti Alloy
Canine (Proximal)	58	179	24
Canine (Distal)	40	123	14
Human (Isthmus)	279	830	168

*Typical prosthesis for large patient.

Non-anatomic remodeling associated with very large stiff femoral stems may prove to be an important consideration in primary and revision arthroplasty. The canine and human investigations described herein suggest that large diameter low stiffness porous polysulfone coated titanium alloy stems can be utilized to achieve bone fixation without non-anatomic femoral remodeling. However, additional study is warranted to fully ascertain the variables influencing long-term remodeling of the implanted femur.

REFERENCES

1 C.A. Engh and J.D. Bobyn, Biological Fixation of a Modified Moore Prosthesis, Orthopaedics, 7 (1984) 285.

2 A.K. Hedley, D.S. Hungerford, L.S. Borden, E.T. Haberman, R.V, Kenna, Clinical Results with a New Cementless Hip System: Minimum 2 Year Follow-Up, in Proc. 53rd Ann. Mtg. of the Amer. Acad. of Orthop. Surgeons, New Orleans, February, 1986.

3 I.W. Brown and P.A. Ring, Osteolytic Changes in the Upper Femoral Shaft Following Porous Coated Hip Replacement, J. Bone and Joint Surg., 67B, (1985), 218.

4 M. Spector, R. Davis, E.M. Lunceford and S.L. Harmon, Porous Polysulfone Coatings for Fixation of Femoral Stems by Bony Ingrowth, Clin. Orthop. and Rel. Res., 176 (1983), 34.

5 M. Spector, W.R. Flemming, A. Kreutner and B.W. Sauer, Bone Growth into Porous High Density Polyethylene, J. Biomed. Mater. Res., 7 (1976), 595.

6 M. DeMane, N. Beals, D.L. McDowell, K. Greenwood and M. Spector, Porous Polysulfone-Coated Femoral Stems, in: J. Lemons (Ed.), Quantitative Characterization and Performance of Porous Implants for Hard Tissue Applications, in press.

7 C.A. Engh, and J.D. Bobyn, Biological Fixation in Total Hip Arthroplasty, Slack, Thorofare N.J., 1985.

8 T.M. Turner, R.M. Urban, D.P. Rivers, D.R. Summer, and J.O. Galante, A comparative study of porous coatings in a weight-bearing total hip arthroplasty model, Trans. of the 31st Ann. Mtg. of the Orthopaedic Res. Soc., 10 (1985), 169.

Biomaterials and Clinical Applications,
edited by A. Pizzoferrato, P.G. Marchetti, A. Ravaglioli and A.J.C. Lee
Elsevier Science Publishers B.V., Amsterdam, 1987 — Printed in The Netherlands

PERFORMANCE OF ORGANIC AND INORGANIC BONE REPLACEMENT MATERIALS AND THEIR COMBINATIONS IN REPAIR OF BONY DEFECTS IN THE RAT.

J.M. RUEGER, K. WAGNER, R. INGLIS, H.R. SIEBERT, A. PANNIKE.
Unfallchirurgische Klinik, Zentrum der Chirurgie, Universitaetsklinik Frankfurt, Theodor Stern Kai 7, 6000 Frankfurt am Main. Leiter: Prof. Dr. med. A. Pannike.

SUMMARY

Different organic (bone matrix extracts: demineralised bone powder, DMBP, bone gelatine, BG, bovine collagen) and inorganic (calciumphosphate-ceramics: beta-tricalciumphosphate, TCP, hydroxyapatite, HA) bone replacement materials, BRM, and various combinations (n=5) of these substances were implanted in bilateral diaphyseal femoral drill holes in Spraque-Dawley rats. For evaluation of the materials` and the material-combinations` performance, i.e. their ability to stimulate bone formation and repair of the drill holes, histomorphometry of the defects was carried out after implantation periods between seven and 220 days. Maximum values for volume density bone (structural parameter) and volume density osteoid (formation parameter) were to be observed only after the joint implantation of the bone matrix extract BG together with a calciumphosphate compound, either TCP or HA. Minimum values for total surface resorption density (resorption parameter) for the latter combinations were indicative of the maturity of the stimulated new bone. The sole implantation of collagen or particulate, porous hydroxyapatite lead to the worst results after 220 days.

INTRODUCTION

For orthopedic and traumatologic use various substances, labelled as bone replacement materials, are recommended to replace autogeneic and allogeneic cancellous bone in surgery. To use these materials seems to be sensible only if their biologic activity at the implantation site is equivalent to or even better than that of cancellous bone. The aim that is to be achieved by the application of cancellous bone or a BRM in surgery is a positive influence on the healing / repair process via:

1. an osteostimulation, i.e. an increased bone formation rate compared to an untreated defect / fracture,
2. an acceleration of the physiologic repair processes,
3. the induction and formation of bone tissue in preexisting partial or segmental bony defects even though scar tissue may prevail there (viability, biologic responsiveness of the recipient site).

It remains unclear, and this holds true for cancellous bone as well as the different bone replacement materials, by which primary mechanism/s (biochemical, biophysical, biological) the reactivity of and the subsequent biologic activity at the implantation site is triggered.

For classification of the bone replacement materials one can distinguish between biologic, organic substances, which can be extracted out of bone`s organic phase, and inorganic, synthetic BRMs, which are part of bone`s mineral. Part of the first group are the collagens (ref. 1), mineralised and demineralised matrix extracts, especially demineralised allogeneic bone powder (ref. 2), and bone gelatine (ref. 3, 4). Furthermore highly extracted matrix fractions like the bone morphogenetic protein (BMP, ref. 5), the matrix factor (ref. 6) and the sceletal growth factor (SGF, ref. 7).

Collagen supposedly serves as a scaffold for regenerating autochtonic bone and as a nucleus for mineralisation processes in bone formation.

Demineralised matrix extracts contain one or more factors , which after implantation in muscle, i.e. heterotopic, elicite osteoinduction = osteoneogenesis, and after implantation in bone, i.e. orthotopic, stimulate repair of the autochtonic bone tissue. The matrix extracts excert their effects either via the induction, subsequent proliferation and differentiation of on site pluripotent mesenchymal cells (pericytes?), progenitor cells (IOPCs, DOPCs) or - in orthotopic implanation- possibly even through osteoblast-stimulation.

Inorganic bone replacement materials

In the inorganic, synthetic BRM group calciumphosphate-ceramics, the so called`soluble`beta-tricalciumphosphate and hydroxyapatite (ref. 8, 9, 10), are under investigation and especially in maxillo- facial- surgery in clinical use. The biologic value of a calciumphosphate-ceramic depends on (ref.11): 1. the stochiometric Ca/P-ratio, 2. the purity and water-content of the primary powder, 3. the applied sinter-temperatures, 4. micro- as well as macroporosity, 5. its potential for biodegradation, 6. its induction and stimulation of an continuous inflammatory response. The applied sinter-temperature determines microporosity as well as the cristalloid structure; the former, together with the macroporosity, influences significantly the materials biodegradability and incorporability into newly forming bone. Like the collagens, the calciumphosphate-ceramics supposedly serve as scaffolds for regenerating autochtonic bone and sprouting vessels. Via direct incorporation - TCP - mineralisation of newly forming bone tissue is facilitated. HA implantation leads to the early formation of a bone-implant-composite without any connective tissue interface (mechanical properties of these composites unknown!).

Combinations

The joint implantation of an organic BRM together with a synthetic one - collagen / HA - supposedly results in an accelerated multicentric bone formation (ref. 12). The combination of BG together with either HA or TCP results in an acceleration and amplification of BG´s effects via an influence on the velocity of the liberation and prolonged activity of the active fraction/ -s of BG by the calciumphosphate-ceramics.

Aim of our investigation was to check into the biologic activity of different

BRM and their combinations in repair of drill holes in the femoral diaphyses in rats.

METHODS

We implanted:

1. Powderised beta-tricailciumphosphate, particle size 200-350µm.
2. Hydroxyapatite, particulate Ceros 80^R, No. 00, 01, 03, 06, 07 (ref. 14).
3. Bovine collagen, lyophilised, two different forms, particulate, blocks.
4. Bovine collagen, lyophilised, particulate, together with beta-TCP (see 1), ratio 1/1.
5. Bovine collagen, lyophilised, particulate, together with Ceros 80^R, No. 00, ratio 1/1.
6. Demineralised allogeneic bone powder, particle size 35-1000µm.
7. Demineralised allogeneic bone powder together with beta-TCP (see 1), ratio 1/1.
8. Allogeneic bone gelatine, particle size 400-800µm.
9. Allogeneic bone gelatine (see 8) together with beta-TCP (see 1), ratio 1/1
10. Allogeneic bone gelatine (see 8) together with Ceros 80^R, No.00, ratio 1/1.

In 98 Spraque-Dawley rats the above mentioned materials were implanted in bilateral diaphyseal femoral drill holes (2X4mm). Unfilled drill holes served as controls . An intravital tetracyclin double labelling was carried out 14,13 (if applicable) and 2 and 1 days prior to sacrifice. Materials were implanted for 7, 21, 42, 150/180 and 220 days. Evaluation by xeroradiography of the native explants, light- and fluorescent microscopy of undecalcified PMMA embedded micro- and ground-sections after Masson-Goldner, v. Kossa and methylgreen-pyronin staining. (Ground-sections haematoxylin satining). Contact microradiography of the ground-sections. For quantitation, histomorphometry of the micro-sections was carried out, according to the method of Delling 1975 (ref. 15), after 21, 42 and 150/180 days.

RESULTS

Obviously due to biomechanical reasons a cup-like support made of trabecular bone developed between the edges of the drill holes and the opposite untouched cortical bone. These supports were fully developed after 21 days and were demonstrable until the end of the observation period. Depending on the quality, i.e. biologic activity, of the implanted BRM or BRMs-combination this support was either detached from the opposite cortical bone with subsequent re-canalisation of the femur and healing of the defect or remained unchanged with encasement of the implant in scar tissue and absence of a healing of the defect.

<u>Calciumphosphate-ceramics</u>

TCP was partly incorporated into the cuplike support, demonstrable by the coralline like structure of the TCP particles. In most of the sole implants of TCP after 220 days remnants of unchanged TCP particles, surrounded by connective tissue, were demonstrable without neither recanalisation of the medullary cavity nor healing of the defects. Complete resorption of the TCP did not occur.

The implantation of Ceros 80[R], regardless of the batch applied (different particles sizes, different porous volumes), resulted in the development of a partial bone-implant composite already after 21 days. Even after 220 days the HA particles seemed to be unchanged, without any resorption. There was never the formation of a bone-HA composite throughout the defect, whereas the majority of the HA particles were encased in scar-tissue. There were some giant multi-nucleated foreign body cells but no continuous lymphoplasmacellular reaction.

Collagen and collagen/calciumphosphate-ceramic combinations

The implantation of none of these materials or material-combinations led to a recanalisation of the medullary cavity. The application of collagen together with TCP resulted in an excessive scar-formation. Unchanged remanants of the implanted collagen were demonstrable in such scar-tissue inside the drill holes. There were no morphological differences in the incorporation pattern between particulate collagen and the collagen blocks.

Demineralised allogeneic bone powder and DMBP/TCP combination

After the sole implantation of DMBP a recanalisation of the medullary cavity or a healing of the cortical defect did not occur up to 220 days after implantation. At this point in time remnants of the DMBP were not demonstrable. In the DMBP/TCP combination the TCP performed similar to the sole implants of TCP. It was partly incorporated in newly formed trabecular bone that was part of the biomechanically induced cuplike support. Again, remnants of the TCP were demonstrable until the end of the observation period, encased by scar-tissue inside of the defects.

Bone gelatine and its combinations with TCP and HA

In the combination of BG/H^ ¬lready after 21 days a bone-HA composite formation was visible that was superior to that of the sole implantation of HA. An interfaceless direct contact between HA and bone, the amount of it increasing with time, was demonstrable at any point in time. TCP was incorporated at a higher rate into the newly forming bone. Only in the implants of BG together with a calciumphosphate-ceramic a recanalisation of the femurs did occur with healing of the cortical defects completed after 150/180 days. TCP was extensively resorbed and demonstrable only in minute amounts after 220 days, whereas the unresorbable, unsoluble HA remained unchanged until the end of the observation period, thus impeding the recanalisation but not the healing of the cortical bony defects.

Histomorphometry

The histomorphometric analysis after 21 days showed that nine out of 13 BRMs had performed equal or worse than the controls on determination of volume density bone (V_V %) and volume density osteoid (V_{VOS}%), whereas highest values were found for the combination of bone gelatine together with TCP, followed by BG together with HA. After 150 days highest values for the above mentioned parameters were again found in the combination of BG, either together with HA or TCP.

DISCUSSION

The synthetic BRM are partly encased by vital bone, if particulate materials are implanted, in the formation of a bone-implant composite. With histologic techniques a real incorporation of a synthetic BRM is only demonstrable for powderised beta-TCP. According to our own results as well as material published by Lemons, 1985 (ref.16) , HA as well as TCP is demonstrable after orthotopic implantation up to five years after surgery.

Demineralised allogeneic bone powder, its combination with TCP, bovine collagen, regardless of the form applied, and its combinations with either TCP or HA do not result in an increase in osteostimulation after 21 and 42 days compared to unimplanted controls. Even after 150 days the so called `multicentric` bone formation, supposedly elicitable by the collagen/HA combination, results only in a minute increase of the reparative processes.

Only in the combinations of BG either together with HA or TCP there is a significant increase in volume density bone and osteoid already after 21 days, lasting up to 150/180 days after implantation, compared to controls . The induction of on site or perhaps circulating pluripotent or progenitor cells via the bone gelatine with facilitation of the subsequent mineralisation of induced bone by the biodegradable TCP (rise in local Ca/P concentration) leads to a marked stimulation of the bone repair processes. In the BG/HA combination the lesser biodegradability of particulate HA with a smaller increase in local Ca/P concentration might be compensated by a larger active surface of the HA particles and an increase in mechanical stability at the implantation site, thus also facilitating bone formation compared to controls . Obviously collagen cannot induce proliferation and differentiation of potent bone forming cells at the same rate as BG (the same holds true for implantations of HA alone).

The combination of porous, particulate HA with an osteoinductive, osteostimulative agent like BG, preferably a higher extracted and purified growth factor, could be a promising bone replacement material for clinical application.

REFERENCES

1 H.W. Springorum, Adler, C.P. et al. Tierexperimentelle Untersuchung der Knochenregeneration am standardisierten Tibiadefekt des Kaninchens. Z.Orthop 115 (1977), 668-693.

2 J. Glowacki, Altobelli, D. et al. Fate of mineralised and demineralised osseous implants. Calcif Tissue Int 33, (1981), 71-76

3 M.R. Urist, Iwata, H. et al. Bone morphogenesis in implants of insoluble bone gelatine. Proc Nat Acad Sci USA Vol 70, No 12. Part 1. (1973), 3511-3515.
4 F.W. Thielemann, Spaeth, G. et al. Osteoinduction. Arch Orthop Trauma Surg 99 (1982) 217-222.
5 M.R. Urist, Huo, K.Y. et al. Purification of bovine bone morphogenetic protein by hydroxyapatite chromatography. Pro Nat Acad Sci USA Vol 81 (1984), 371-375.
6 T.K. Sampath, DeSimone, D.P. et al. Extracellular bone matrix derived growth factor. Exp Cell Res 142 (1982) 460-462.
7 J.R. Farley, Baylink, D,J. Purification of a sceletal growth factor from human bone. Biochemistry 21 (1982), 3502-3507.
8 S.N. Bhaskar, Brady, J.M. et al. Biodegradable ceramic implants in bone. Oral Surg 32 (1971), 336-346.
9 K. Koester, Karbe, E. et al. Experimenteller Knochenersatz durch resorbierbare Calziumphosphatkeramik. Langenbecks Arch Chir 341 (1976), 77-86.
10 J.F. Osborn. Implantatwerkstoff Hydroxylapatit. Quintessenzverlag Berlin (1985).
11 K. de Groot. Bioceramics consisting of calciumphosphate salts. Biomaterials Vol 1 (1980), 47-50.
12 H. Mittelmeier, Katthagen, B.D. Klinische Erfahrungen mit Kollagenapatitimplantationen zur lokalen Knochenregeneration. Z. Orthop 121 (1983), 115-123.
13 J.M. Rueger, Siebert, H.R. et al. Observation on bone formation sequence elicited by the implantation of bone gelatine together with calciumphosphate compounds. Biological and Biomechanical Performance of Biomaterials. ed. P. Christel, A. Meunier, A.J.C. Lee. Elsevier Science Publishers (1986) 45-50.
14 Bulletin Synthes. 4. Experimentelle Artikel zur Erprobung. Ceros 80 Granulat (1982).
15 G. Delling. Endokrine Osteopathien. Veröffentlichungen aus der Pathologie. Heft 98. Siegfried Fischer Verlag Stuttgart. (1975).
16 J.E. Lemmons. Inorganic-Organic combinations for bone repair. Biological and Biomechanical Performance of Biomaterials. ed. P. Christel, A, Meunier, A.J.C. Lee. Elsevier Science Publishers. (1986), 51-56.

Biomaterials and Clinical Applications,
edited by A. Pizzoferrato, P.G. Marchetti, A. Ravaglioli and A.J.C. Lee
Elsevier Science Publishers B.V., Amsterdam, 1987 — Printed in The Netherlands

STUDIES ON MECHANICAL PROPERTIES AND HYDROLYSIS BEHAVIOUR OF ABSORBABLE POLYMERS AND COMPOSITES

P. HELEVIRTA[1], J. LAIHO[1], J. KILPIKARI[2], S. VAINIONPÄÄ[3], P. ROKKANEN[3] and P. TÖRMÄLÄ[1]

[1]Tampere University of Technology, Institute of Plastics Technology, P.O.B. 527, SF-33101 Tampere, Finland

[2]A. Ahlström Oy, P.O.B. 46, SF-05821 Hyvinkää, Finland

[3]Department of Orthopaedics and Traumatology, Helsinki University Central Hospital, Topeliuksenkatu 5, SF-00260 Helsinki, Finland

SUMMARY

The mechanical properties and hydrolysis behaviour of different absorbable polymeric materials manufactured by injection moulding and compression moulding methods were examined. Polyhydroxybutyrate and polylactide based materials showed slow decrease of mechanical strength properties in hydrolytic conditions (in distilled water at 37°C) while polydioxanone, polyglycolide and polyglycolide/lactide copolymer based materials showed more rapid loss of mechanical strength.

INTRODUCTION

Polymeric materials, which are absorbable (resorbable) in tissue without causing harmful tissue reactions have aroused large interest during the last years because such materials can be applied to manufacture osteosynthesis devices or their components like plates, balks, rods, medullary nails, pins, screws or similar devices.

The manufacturing of osteosynthesis materials from absorbable polymers is known in the literature. There has been described the manufacturing of absorbable sutures and surgical elements of polyglycolide (PGA) (ref. 1, ref. 2), sutures manufactured of polylactide (PLA) (ref. 3), sutures manufactured of glycolide/lactide copolymers (PGA/PLA) (ref. 4), sutures and osteosynthesis devices manufactured of poly-β-hydroxybutyric acid (PHB) (ref. 5), sutures and osteosynthesis devices manufactured of polydioxanone (PDS) (ref. 6), absorbable surgical devices manufactured from polyesteramides (PEA) (ref. 7) and absorbable surgical sutures and surgical devices, which are manufactured of PGA/trimethylene carbonate (TMC) copolymer (ref. 8).

Certain prerequisities for success in the treatment of fractures by internal fixation may be defined (ref. 9). They include sufficient strength of the material to be used for fixation, good compatibility between bone tissue and material, good consolidation, and as little morbidity as possible. At a later stage the material should decompose gradually and the stress be transferred by steps to the healing bone, thus preventing a decrease in mineral content and strength of the bone tissue. If the need of a removal operation is eliminated, the human and economical gain is substantial. The ideal fixation method meets these criteria. PGA, PGA/PLA, PLA, PDS, PHB and PGA/TMC possess many of the above-mentioned properties.

Here we have studied mechanical properties and hydrolytic behaviour of rods manufactured by injection moulding and compression moulding of several of above materials and of their combinations (composites).

EXPERIMENTAL

Materials

The following absorbable materials were studied: PGA (Dexon® sutures of Davis + Geck, Great Britain), PGA/PLA (Vicryl® sutures of Ethicon of Johnson & Johnson, Sweden), poly-L-lactide PLLA fibers (M_v 100 000 - 300 000; of TNO, The Netherlands) and PHB flakes (M_w = 500 000; of Marlborough Biopolymers, United Kingdom).

Methods

Absorbable rods were manufactured by injection moulding of PDS and PHB melts by means of a self-made plunger-type injection moulding machine. Cylindrical moulds with inner diameters (Ø) 2.0 mm and 3.2 mm and with mould lengths between 40 - 70 mm were applied. The mould and polymer melt temperatures 5 or 10°C above the melting temperature of polymer were applied. The mould was cooled after injection rapidly with water or cooled air.

A hydraulic press was applied to manufacture reinforced and self-reinforced totally absorbable polymeric composite rods.

PDS/PGA (PDS-matrix, PGA fibre reinforcement) composite rods (length 50 mm, Ø 3.2 mm) were manufactured by compressing a mixture of parallel fibers of PDS (10 wt-%) and PGA (90 wt-%) in a cylindrical mould at 110°C with a pressure of 1000 bar for 6 minutes whereafter the mould was cooled rapidly.

The self-reinforced cylindrical PGA composite rods (length

70 - 50 mm and diameters of 4.5, 3.2 and 2.0 mm) were manufactured by a recently developed method by sintering the suture fibers partially together at an elevated temperature and pressure (ref. 10). The self-reinforced samples were materials with high content (> 60 wt-%) of biodegradable fibers in a matrix of the same polymer.

The flexural or shear strengths of three parallel test pieces were measured after production and after different hydrolysis periods under distilled water at 37°C. Strength values were measured at room temperature by the JJ T5003 tensile testing equipment. The bending test was done by the three-point method; the distance between the supports was 50 mm. The testing speed was 5 mm/min in both tests.

RESULTS AND DISCUSSION

Fig. 1 shows the shear strengths of PDS and PHB rods as a function of hydrolysis time at 37°C in distilled water.

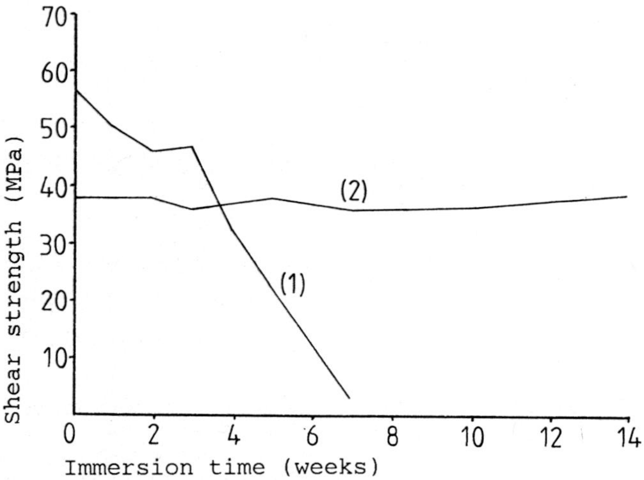

Fig. 1. Shear strength profile of injection moulded PDS (1) and PHB (2) rods (Ø of 2.0 and 3.2 mm, respectively) as a function of immersion time in distilled water at 37°C.

Fig. 1 shows the extremely slow degradation rate of PHB while during 14 weeks no decrease of shear strength was observed. PDS rods showed during the first three weeks only a slight decrease of shear strength whereafter an accelerated degradation led to the total loss of shear strength after 7 weeks. PDS rods had a clearly higher initial shear strength (58 MPa) than PHB rods (39 MPa). This was evidently a consequence of more strong longitudinal orientation of the thinner PDS rods because also PHB rods with Ø of 2.0 mm showed high initial shear strength values (max. 90 MPa).

Fig. 2 shows the shear strength profile of PDS/PGA rods (Ø of 3.2 mm).

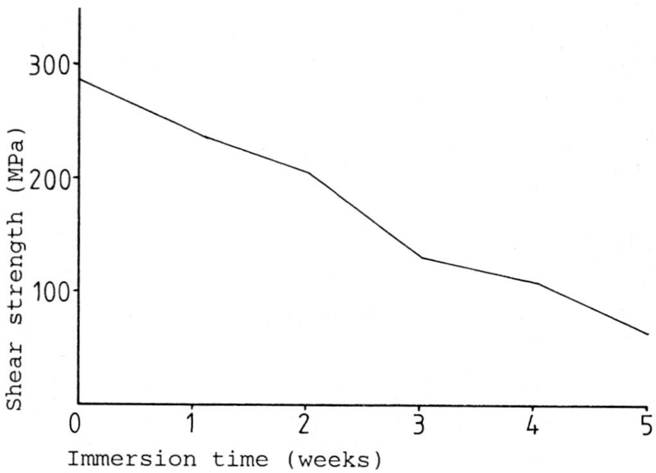

Fig. 2. Shear strength profile of compression moulded PDS matrix/ PGA fibre composite rods (Ø of 3.2 mm).

PDS/PGA composite rods showed a remarkably high shear strength value of 280 MPa. The loss rate of shear strength was moderate. Still after five weeks the shear strength had the value of 60 MPa.

Fig. 3 shows the shear force profiles of self-reinforced PGA rods of different diameters.

Also the self-reinforced PGA rods showed high initial strength values (210 - 280 MPa) which were inversely correlated to the diameters of rods. It is interesting to note that the thick rods lose their strength distinctly slower than the thin ones. This is evidently a consequence of the lower surface area/mass ratio of thick rods.

Fig. 4 shows the shear strength and flexural strength profiles of self-reinforced PLLA rods (Ø of 2.0 mm).

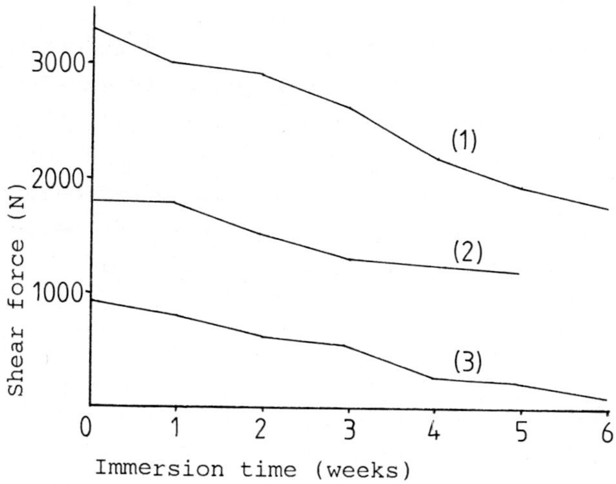

Fig. 3. Shear force profiles (shear load carrying capacity of self-reinforced PGA rods of diameters (1) 4.5 mm, (2) 3.2 mm and (3) 2.0 mm.

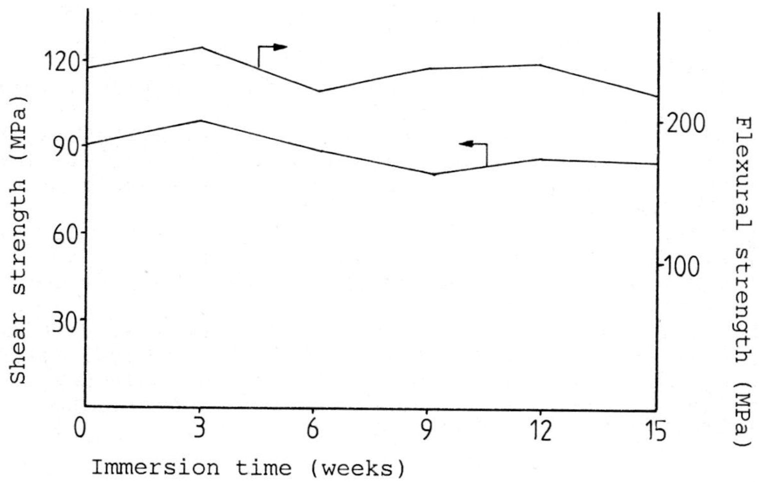

Fig. 4. Shear strength and bending strength profiles of self-reinforced PLLA-rods (Ø of 2.0 mm).

Self-reinforced PLLA rods showed good initial strength values taking into account the fact that the tensile strength of PLLA fibers was only ca. 200 MPa (the fibers were not high-tenacity fibers for mechanical applications). During the immersion time of 15 weeks no clear change of shear or bending strength of self-reinforced PLLA rods was observed. This is in agreement with earlier studies with PLLA fibers (ref. 11).

CONCLUSIONS

The results of this study have confirmed our earlier observations that self-reinforcing is an efficient method to manufacture strong absorbable polymeric materials (refs. 12 and 13). The strength and strength retention of these materials is so good that they are potential raw-materials of absorbable osteosynthesis devices. The first such device, the Biofix fixation device, was recently developed of self-reinforced PGA (ref. 14).

REFERENCES

1 U.S. Pat. No. 3 297 033.
2 U.S. Pat. No. 3 739 773.
3 U.S. Pat. No. 2 703 316.
4 U.S. Pat. No. 3 839 297.
5 G.B. Pat. No. 1 034 123.
6 U.S. Pat. No. 4 052 988.
7 U.S. Pat. No. 4 343 931.
8 U.S. Pat. No. 4 243 775.
9 S. Vainionpää, Biodegradation and fixation properties of biodegradable implants in bone tissue, Thesis, Helsinki University, Helsinki, 1986.
10 E.P. Pat. Appl. No. 86105465.8.
11 K. Jamshidi, Synthesis and properties of polylactides, Thesis, Kyoto University, Kyoto, Japan, 1984.
12 P. Törmälä, S. Vainionpää, J. Kilpikari and P. Rokkanen, The effects of fibre reinforcement and gold plating on the flexural and tensile strength of PGA/PLA copolymer materials in vitro, Biomaterials, in press.
13 S. Vainionpää, J. Kilpikari, J. Laiho, P. Helevirta, P. Rokkanen and P. Törmälä, Strength and strength retenrion in vitro, of absorbable self-reinforced polyglycolide (PGA rods for fracture fixation, Biomaterials, in press.
14 P. Törmälä, J. Laiho, P. Helevirta, P. Rokkanen, S. Vainionpää, O. Böstman and J. Kilpikari, Resorbable surgical devices, Proceedings of Vth International Conference of Polymers in Medicine and Surgery, Leeuwenhorst Congress Center, The Netherlands, 10-12 Sept. 1986, p. 16/1.

Biomaterials and Clinical Applications,
edited by A. Pizzoferrato, P.G. Marchetti, A. Ravaglioli and A.J.C. Lee
Elsevier Science Publishers B.V., Amsterdam, 1987 — Printed in The Netherlands

THE ROLE OF COMPUTERGRAPHICS IN THE DESIGN OF TOTAL JOINTS

Peter S. Walker, Ph.D.
Biomechanics Laboratory, Department of Orthopedic Surgery, Brigham and Women's Hospital, Boston, MA, VA Medical Center, West Roxbury, MA

ABSTRACT

The design of total joint replacement involves many considerations including anatomy, stability, motion, fixation and materials. Each aspect requires theoretical and experimental studies, as well as the results of clinical experience. Computergraphics is an extremely useful method whereby the designer can visualize many aspects of the design. It can be used not only for the anatomical displays and study of component fit, but also for motion studies and the presentation of stress analysis results. Finally, it is an excellent communciation method between surgeons and engineers.

METHODS

1. Average Bone Geometry

The primary goals of knee replacement are relief of pain and restoration of normal function. Precise control of motion is probably not an ideal aim for a total knee, because of the high stresses transmitted at the component-bone interfaces in a constrained design. Of the wide variety of design forms that can be used for knee replacement, the condylar replacement type is the most widely used because of its simplicity and general resemblance to the natural joint surfaces.

Most designs use geometrical descriptions obtained from planar projections of knee joints, with some modifications in specific areas to account for particular anatomical features. Methods to describe the natural knee in three dimensions are only now being applied. Our goal in the following laboratory procedure was to determine the "average knee geometry" as a basis for rational artificial joint design.

Intact knee specimens were embedded based on a reproducible axis system and sectioned in the sagittal plane. The section profiles were digitized, scaled to a selected linear dimension of the knee, and then averaged. When images of, say, 20 equivelent sctions form 20 knees were superimposed on the computer screen, the variations due to differences in shape were evident.

A contour averaging program was written where the user quickly drew transverse lines across the perpheries around the entire profile of superimposed images. These lines were perpendicular to the mean tangent of all profiles at that point. The mean intersections of the twenty profiles on these transverse lines defined a point on the mean profile. The user interaction was needed because, for example, the sections at each end of the joint varied considerably due to the irregular geomety at the sides of the main bearing areas. In another case, when sagittal sections were superimposed, the height of the intersection of a plane with the side of the shaft of the femur varied depending on the varus-valgus angle.

Once the sections on the main joint bearing surfaces were normalized for size, variations due to shape were quite small. The typical standard deviation from the mean profile of a group of profiles was only about one millimeter.

For more regularly shaped sections, an automated contour averaging program was possible. This was used for transverse section of the hip. Using computergraphics methods, an optimum fit total hip stem was designed from the average hip (fig 1, ref 1).

2. Mathematical Analogs of Anatomic Surfaces

Before designing a total artificial knee, a model of the knee was reconstructed with the average set of profiles. This was called "the average knee". A mathematically smoothed graphic model of the joint surfaces is primarily needed for design and machining, not for the more immediately apparent realistic image. Previous studies had shown that the posterior femoral condyles could be accurately modeled by spherical surfaces (2). It was likely that the remaining surfaces could be modeled by other geometrical solids. A program was written with which the sections of the femoral condyles could be defined interactively on the screen. Using printouts of various profiles, appropriate geometrical solids were identified.

The surfaces were defined by mathematical parameters of their various radii, centers of curvature, and linear dimensions. The distal and anterior condules were modeled as toroids and the patella groove was modeled as a conical surface with a toroidal base. Obtaining a series of sizes was simply a matter of increasing or decreasing the numerical dimensions. For design of a surface of a particular knee, key dimensions could be measured from the knee using CT scans, or more simply, from radiographs and keyed in to the surface-generating program. This opens up possiblities for individualized design.

3. Visualizing the fit

After the bearing surfaces were determined, the entire femoral component was designed by defining the back surface and the fixation pegs. The shape of the back represented the cuts made on the arthritic bone to accept the component. The present surgical method is to make square cuts using a sequence of spacing blocks and cutting guides. We added one more step with computer graphics: visualizing the component on the bone itself to assess the fit of the component. This was made easier by a series of optional transformations of the image data. The femur can be flexed on the tibia at any angle or where two viewing angles are specified and adjusted.

4. Design of the Tibial Surface

In the total artificial knee, the metal femoral component must work with a plastic tibial component, which presents its own set of problems. Were the artificial tibial surface the same as the cartilage surface, there would be considerable instability, especially in an artifical joint where all of the ligaments are not preserved and the remaining ones may be deficient. Some of the design considerations are: Should the femoral-tibial surfaces define and guide the motion? Which motions should be allowed? How much inherent instability should be built into the various degrees of freedom? In practice, there are many design solutions from one extreme to the other. The optimum solution requires data from experiments as well as long-term studies on patients, data which is at present incomplete.

Various tibial surfaces can be designed, inspected, and analytically evaluated with computer graphics techniques. Surfaces were generated by defining motion or stability criteria and forming the tibial surface in 3-D space by moving the femoral component through multiple of positions defined by these criteria (3). To get a surface for average knee motion, the femoral component was moved incrementally through the flexion range. To generate a surface with built-in laxity, for each angle of flexion the laxity characteristics were expressed as a polynomial and then the femur was moved in multiple positions at each of multiple flexion angles.

The surface coordinates were stored in data arrays. A gridwork was defined in the horizontal plane, and for each square on the grid, the point with the ininum y-value represented a point on the tibial surface. Sorting routines were developed for computing efficiency. A smooth surface was then obtained by extrapolation routines (fig 3). By reconstructing the positions of the femur on the tibia at different flexion angles, local contact points were defined and radii of curvature calculated. The contact stresses were then calculated from the elasticity theory.

Analytical computer graphics can be readily used to evaluate alternative designs. Force analysis of a model that includes ligaments reveals relative force distribution between ligaments and artificial surfaces. The effects of surgical misplacement of the femoral and tibial components can be determined and graphically displayed. Descriptions of the results by two or three dimensional models would be a great advantage in such a study.

SOLIDS, TRANSLUCENCIES, AND BEYOND

Simple computer pictures appear as "wireframe" models. This representation shows all the lines of the object, and the mind sorts out what which lines are in fron and behind. A more sophisticated feature, now common in mid-priced graphics softwhere, does not show the lines that it calculates to be unseen to the viewer, the hidden line feature. Modeling of surfaces, and of solids with shading provide further insights.

As a base for our custom solid modeling graphics the versatile program Movie.BYU, developed by H. H. Christiansen and colleagues at Brigham Young University has been used. Movie. BYU is made available at low cost as a testbed for many custom computer graphics projects. Gould De Anza Image Processor was used for display, a special-purpose graphics terminal, linked to a Digital Equipment minicomputer for the central processing. In Movie.BYU one or more objects can be displayed at any orientation with the effects of one or more simulated light sources.

Figure 3 shows a femur and tibia with the components at the artificial joint mounted on each bone. Everything in the images was created purely graphically and is not based on physical models. To learn more about the relationship between the various parts of the model, the user can make selected parts translucent. This advanced feature can be used to demonstrate contact regions, for example, the regions between the femoral and tibial surfaces. Overlap can be shown when the two surfaces are assigned different colors, but there has to be a small overlap between the surfaces, so that bleeding through one colour can be seen. The overlap is achieved by a small coordinate shift.

DISCUSSION

The possibilities of computer graphics go beyond what have been discussed in this article. Color intensity or shading can be used to quantitatively illustrate a variable, for example, the varying stress on portions of a bone would be a different shade (4). The roughness of a surface or the distribution of contact pressure can be displayed using contour lines or contour plots, graphical applications for which software is available. Ligaments and muscles can be included in joint models. For better graphics, multiple views can be included on the same image. Sequences of images can be produced to make video movies. Maximum clarity and distinction between different structures can be highlighted, literally, with effective schemes for color and lighting.

Communication across the medical and engineering disciplines has never been easy. Practical issues have often been inadequately defined by the orthopaedist and biological issues ignored by the engineer. Analytical data have often been applied to insufficiently realistic models, or the orthopedist has been unable to interpret the data presented to him. Graphical communication is a medium with both the engineer and the orthopaedist are more comfortable. Computer graphics is a new bridge to a much closer and more productive working relationship.

REFERENCES

1. Garg, Deland, Walker, Design of Intramedullary Femoral Stems Using Computer Graphics. Engineering in Medicine, 14: 89, 1985

2. Kurosawra, Walker, The Geometry of Motion of the Knee for Implant and Orthotic Design. J. Biomechanics, 18: 487, 1985
3. Walker, Zhou, The Dilemma of Surface Design in Total Knee Replacement Proc. Orthop. Res. Soc., San Francisco, Jan 1987, p291
4. Saejong, Hirano, Granholm, Walker, The influence of the Interface on Bone Strains and Stem-Bone Micromotion in Press-Fit Total Hip Stem Proc. Orthop. Rec Soc., San Francisco, JAN 1987, p484

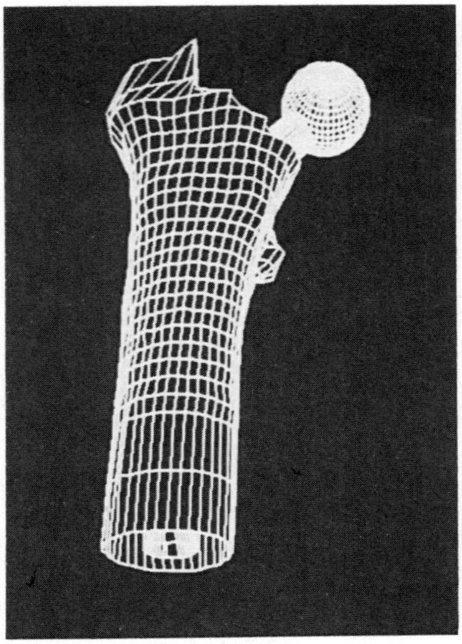

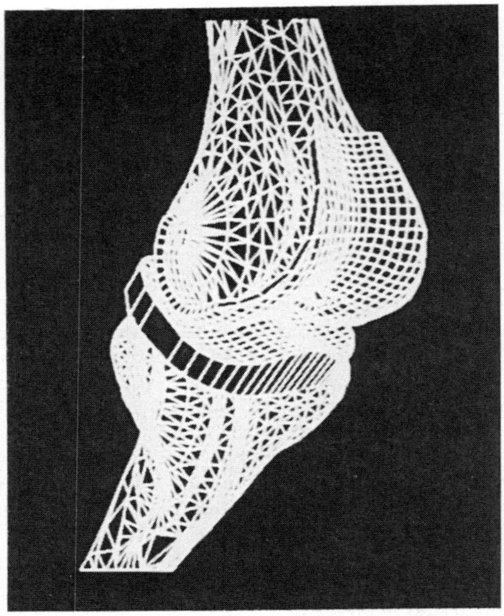

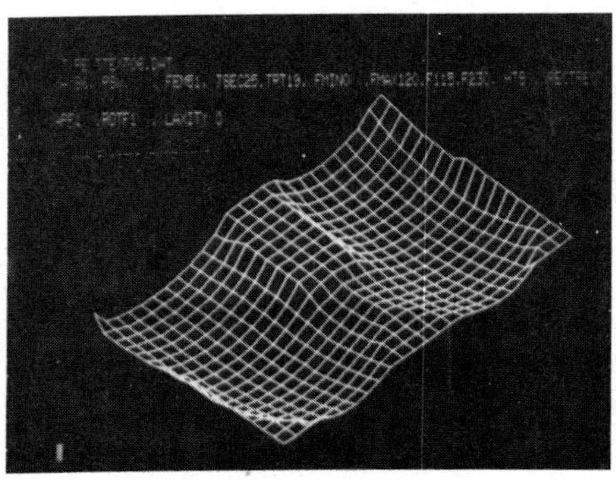

FIGURES

Figure 1. An outer view of a complete 3-D model of a hip stem in a femur. The stem and bone are stored in separate data files and combined for display.

Figure 2. Total knee components mounted on the bones.

Figure 3. The tibial surface is generated from the femoral surface by moving the femur through multiple positions describing a defined motion and laxity path.

Biomaterials and Clinical Applications,
edited by A. Pizzoferrato, P.G. Marchetti, A. Ravaglioli and A.J.C. Lee
Elsevier Science Publishers B.V., Amsterdam, 1987 — Printed in The Netherlands

PRESENTATION OF A NEW HIGHLY HYDROPHILIC POLYMER FOR EXTENDED WEAR CONTACT LENSES

G. OTTOLINI, M. DE GRANDIS, A. CALZAVARA
I.O.R./ GALILEO Industrie Ottiche Riunite S.p.A.
Via Fratelli Bandiera n. 9 - 30175 VENEZIA/MARGHERA ITALY

SUMMARY

The operational sequences used in the selection, control and impurities separation of every component, as well as in the polymerization process and inspection of the end-product, allowed us to obtain a balanced polymer with excellent optical and mechanical properties, high chemical - physical stability and resistance to degradation.

INTRODUCTION

The realization of a hydrophilic polymer, suitable for the production of a movable ocular prosthesis requires a reliable productive approach which is able to give a maximum guarantee of purity. It is difficult to specify the quality and quantity of the impurities and their presence can induce some undesired phenomena of tolerance in the finished product.

It is possible to describe the sequences which are adopted by the system of the quality control in the selection, control and purification of the single components and in the control of the various sequences of the production process.

METHODS

The general scheme (tables 1, 2 and 3) synthesizes the various phases and it points out the quality control filter activity which is carried out by physical, chemical-physical and chemical controls.

The fundamental parameters, settled by precise specifications for every phase, are fixed so as to guarantee the safety of the following phase.

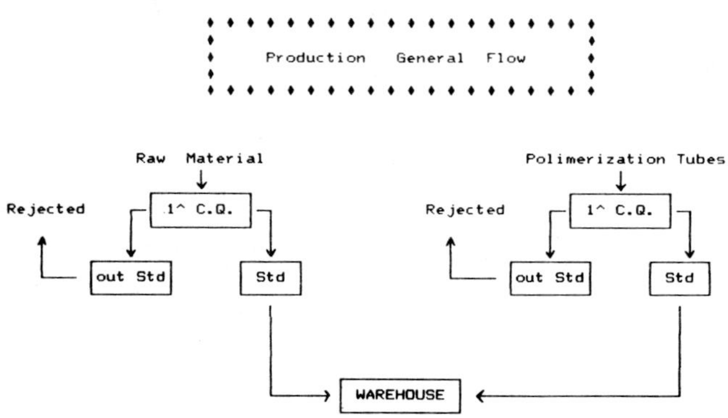

Fig. 1. Production General Flow - First step

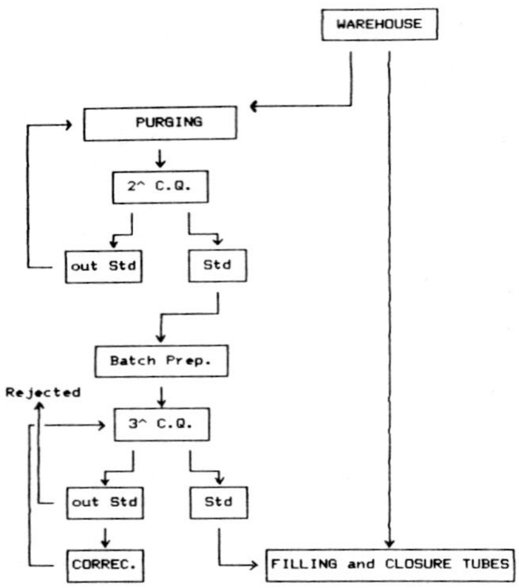

Fig. 2. Production General Flow - Second step

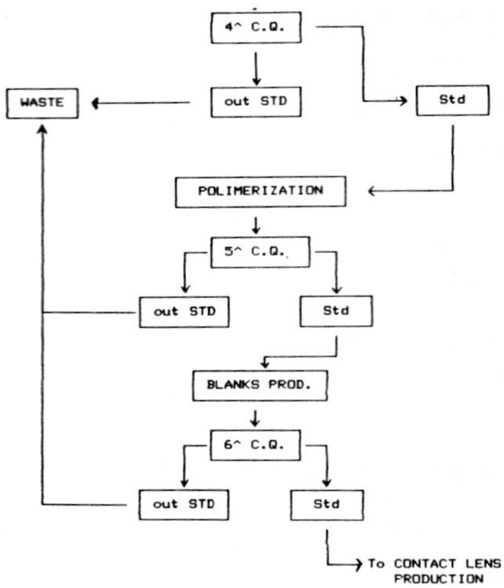

Fig. 3. Production General Flow - Third step

The single raw materials and the tubes of polymerization are checked on arrival and the acceptance depends on the correspondence of all parameters to the purchase specifications. The accepted materials are stocked according to suitable psychrometic conditions. The purification system of the raw materials are substantially of two kinds:

- distillation under high vacuum
- selective extraction of stabilizers and inhibitors

The purification treatment of the most important component of PT 70, the polyvinylpirrolidone, which is obtained by the polymerization of 2-N-vinylpyrrolidone, contained about 80% in the unhydrated polymer, is the high vacuum distillation.

The characteristics of the commercial 2 vinylpyrrolidone are:

2 VINYLPYRROLIDONE MONOMER

Aspect	Liquid
Odour	Typical
Apha Colour	200 max
Specific weight at 25% C	1,04
Boiling point at 14 mm Hg r.p.	96° C
Title (GLC)	97% min
Inhibitors	25 ppm max

Its use, as it is, is not possible and so we can proceed to distillation according to the the following conditions:

DISTILLATION CONDITIONS

Residual pressure	2 mm Hg max
Distillation range	65°C – 68°C
Theoretical plates	1
Production	1 Kg/H

The obtained distillate must fall within the following detailed specifications:

DISTILLED 2 VINYLPYRROLIDONE

Apha colour	10 max
Title (GLC)	99,5% min

The analyses GLC before and after the distillation point out the efficency of the distillation , the correspondences of the parameters to the specification and so the possibility of making use of the monomer in the following phases of production.

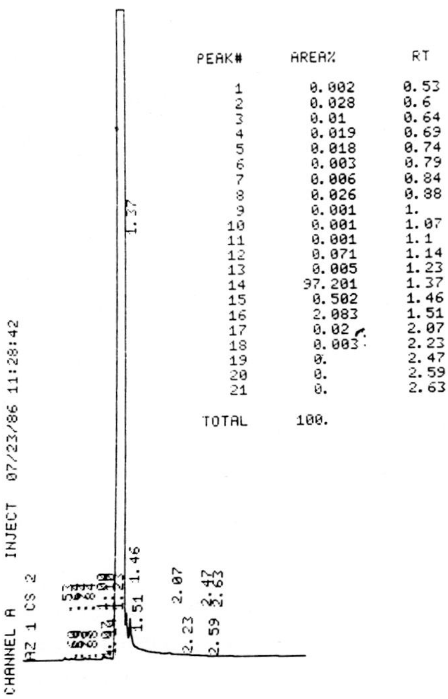

PEAK#	AREA%	RT
1	0.002	0.53
2	0.028	0.6
3	0.01	0.64
4	0.019	0.69
5	0.018	0.74
6	0.003	0.79
7	0.006	0.84
8	0.026	0.88
9	0.001	1.
10	0.001	1.07
11	0.001	1.1
12	0.071	1.14
13	0.005	1.23
14	97.201	1.37
15	0.502	1.46
16	2.083	1.51
17	0.02	2.07
18	0.003	2.23
19	0.	2.47
20	0.	2.59
21	0.	2.63
TOTAL	100.	

Fig. 4. Analysis GLC before distillation

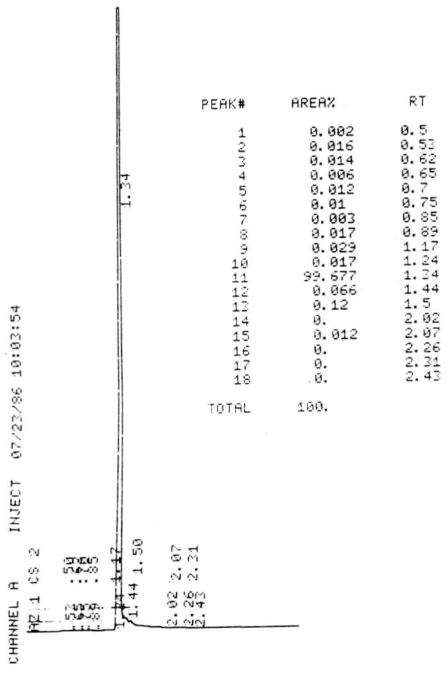

PEAK#	AREA%	RT
1	0.002	0.5
2	0.016	0.53
3	0.014	0.62
4	0.006	0.65
5	0.012	0.7
6	0.01	0.75
7	0.003	0.85
8	0.017	0.89
9	0.029	1.17
10	0.017	1.24
11	99.677	1.34
12	0.066	1.44
13	0.12	1.5
14	0.	2.02
15	0.012	2.07
16	0.	2.26
17	0.	2.31
18	0.	2.43
TOTAL	100.	

Fig. 5. Analysis GLC after distillation

The preparation of the batch consists in the mixing of the monomers, the catalysts and the cross-linking which are carefully pre-weighed in glass containers blown with nitrogen. When the homogenization is complete, a sample is taken so as to determine the correspondence to the following specifications:

PT 70 MONOMERS BATCH

GLC composition	+/- 2% in theoretical %
Inhibitors	Absent

The parameters out of the limits either induce correction or rejection. In the first case, the necessary adjustments are carried out and the step of control is repeated; in the second case, corresponding to incorrigible removals, the batch is rejected. The filling up and the closing of the tubes occurs automatically under nitrogen current after a preventive filtration.

The non-standard tubes are rejected, while those in specification are put into appropriate containers of the polymerization bath.

The thermic cycle of polymerization is controlled by a micro-processor and the temperature tolerances are more or less 0,5°C. The tank temperatures are registered for a constant control of the sequences of the thermic cycle of polymerization. At the end of the cycle, the tubes containing the polymer are passed to Q.C. according to the following parameters:

PT 70 NON HYDRATED POLYMER

Aspect	Transparent tube
Apha colour	20 max
Odour	Typical
Shore D hardness (at 20°C)	79,5 +/- 2,5
Refractive index (at 20°C)	1,530 +/- 0,01
Specific weight (at 20°C)	1,17 (medium)
Residual monomer	7% +/- 1%
Linear swell factor	1,500 +/- 0,01
DK at 35°C (hydrated product)	$30 \cdot 10^{-11}$

The minimum non-standard induces the rejection of the production. The accepted product passes to the automatic turning in a controlled environment (R.U. 40-50% and 20°C +/- 1°C) for the blank construction. Every lot of blanks is statistically controlled according to the MIL 105 D either in productive phase or concluded lot according to the following specific segments:

PT 70 BLANK

Aspect	as standard
Shore D Hardness (at 20°C)	79,5 +/- 2,5
Diameter	12,7 +/- 0,01 mm
Thickness	5 +/- 0,02 mm
Surface quality	Planar

The non-specific lots are rejected; the accepted blanks are kept in polythene tubes which are hermetically sealed at 20°C. The blank obtained can be utilized for the lens construction through a computered turning in conditioned environments: t. 21 +/- 1° and R.U. 45+/- 5% . The conditioning avoids dimensional variations which are due to the absorption of water surfaces.

The finished lens undergoes the treatment of hydration, of boiling and extraction of the remaining monomer in glass extractors. The controls on the extraction waters are the following:

PT 70 WATER EXTRACT FINISHED LENSES

pH t.q.	9 - 9,5
Residual monomers (potassium bicromate test)	traces max

Controls have been carried out on non-hydrated and hydrated lenses:

PT 70 FINISHED LENSES (Medium values)

Refractive index (at 20°C in NaCl sol. 0,9%)	1,390
Optical transmission	95%
Oxygen permeability (at 35°C DK)	$30 \cdot 10^{-11}$
Elongation to break (at 20°C in NaCl sol. 0,9%)	330 %
Water content (medium value) (at 20°C in NaCl sol. 0,9%)	68,5 %
Stability to boiling and autoclaving	Stable

by means of spectrometry Raman-Laser care off the Center of Biotechnological and Clinical Research in Ophthalmology "G. GALILEI" and the results

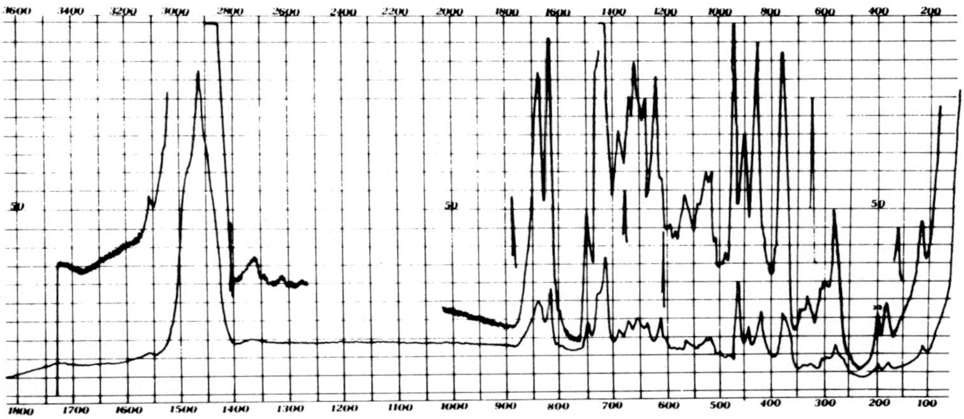

Fig. 6. Ràman-Laser spectra of the lens before hydration

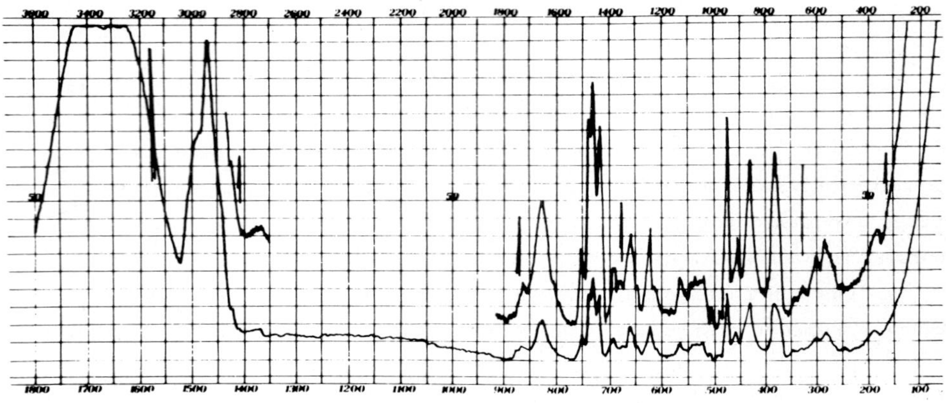

Fig. 7. Raman-Laser spectra of the lens after the residual monomer extraction

put in evidence the absence of residual monomer (R.M.) on the hydrated lens. The polymer PT 70 has given demonstrations of excellent bio-compatibility in chemical, physical, toxicological, morphostructural and clinical tests to which it has been submitted.

Biomaterials and Clinical Applications,
edited by A. Pizzoferrato, P.G. Marchetti, A. Ravaglioli and A.J.C. Lee
Elsevier Science Publishers B.V., Amsterdam, 1987 — Printed in The Netherlands

CHEMICO-PHYSICAL STRUCTURAL CHARACTERISTICS OF PT70 CONTACT LENSES BEFORE AND AFTER CONTINUOUS WEAR.

A.BERTOLUZZA,P.MONTI AND R.SIMONI

Istituto Chimico "G.Ciamician",Cattedra di Chimica e Propedeutica Biochimica, via Selmi 2, Bologna (Italy) ; Centro di Ricerche Biotecnologiche e Cliniche in Oftalmologia,Facolta' di Medicina e Chirurgia, Universita' di Bologna.

SUMMARY

Chemico-physical structural characteristics of highly hydrophilic contact lenses before and after continuous wear have been studied by different instrumental techniques,such as vibrational spectroscopy (Raman-laser and infrared) and thermal methods (thermogravimetric, differential scanning calorimetric and thermomechanical analyses).

The results are discussed in relation to the biocompatibility postulates of Wichterle and Lim regarding highly hydrophilic ocular biomaterials extending their applications to the lens after long periods of wear in aphakic patients.

INTRODUCTION

The use of highly hydrophilic soft contact lenses has recently undergone a number of developments.

As already established by Wichterle and Lim (ref. 1), a plastic material must possess four main properties in order to be used as ocular prosthetic material.In particular it must not contain reactive centres such as residual monomers due to low polymerization, impurities, etc. Moreover it must be hydrophilic and consequently permeable to metabolites. The finished material must possess a homogeneous stable structure and a water content which makes its elastic modulus similar to that of the surrounding tissues.Finally the lens must not undergo enzymatic degradation.

Our Center of research has been interested for many years in the applications of a non-destructive Raman-laser spectroscopy technique in the ophthalmological fields: intraocular lenses (ref. 2), soft contact lenses (ref. 3), cataract (ref. 4) .

In this work we present a chemico-physical and structural characterization of a new type of highly hydrophilic soft contact lens, Pt 70 Galileo, giving an instrumental response to Wichterle and Lim postulates extending their applications to the lens after long periods of wear in aphakic patients.

METHODS

Raman spectra of the components and of the material at different manufacturing stages (blank, dry lens, hydrated lens) were recorded using a Jasco R-300 spectrophotometer with a Lexel Ar^+ 4880 Å laser source. The hydrated lens was examined directly in its saline solution.

The spectra of the lens surfaces were collected with a Jasco FT/IR 3 Fourier Transform Infrared Spectrophotometer equipped with an ATR (Specac, 25 reflections) unit. A KRS5 crystal and a 45° incidence angle was used.

TG, DSC and TMA measurements were performed with a Mettler TA 3000 system with TG 50, DSC 20 and TMA 40 equipment. TMA measurements were made also on a human cornea sample. DSC measurements near 0°C were obtained using a Perkin Elmer DSC II, equipped with a scanning autozero and a liquid nitrogen subambient accessory.

RESULTS

PT 70 Galileo lenses are mainly made of N-vinylpyrrolidone crosslinked by di- and tri-ethyleneglycoldimethacrylate. Another component is n-butyl-methacrylate.

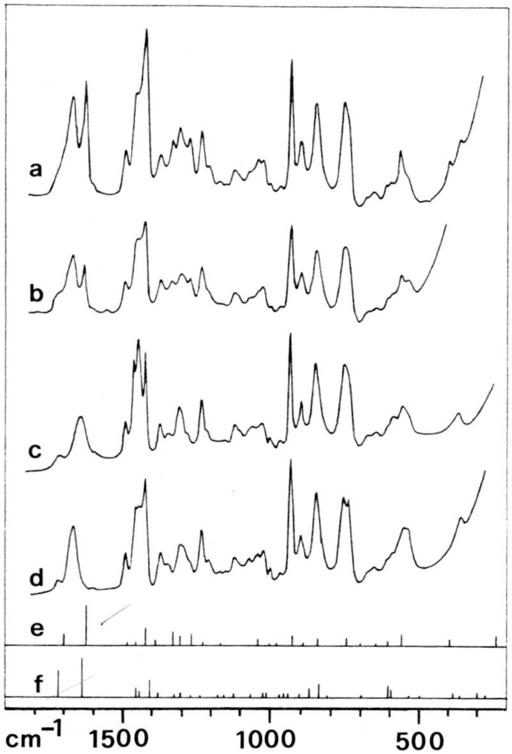

Fig. 1. Raman spectra of:
a) blank
b) non-hydrated lens
c) hydrated finished lens
d) air dried hydrated finished lens
e) N-vinylpyrrolidone
f) n-butylmethacrylate

Raman spectroscopic analysis shows that the finished lens possesses a homogeneous structure also due to the crosslinking structural homogeneity. Moreover the spectrum (Fig.1c and 1d) makes clear the absence of residual monomers or oligomers (as stated by Wichterle and Lim's requirements) since it lacks the strong C=C stretching bands which are located at 1628 cm^{-1} and at 1640 cm^{-1} in the Raman spectra of N-vinylpyrrolidone and n-butylmethacrylate respectively (Fig.1e and 1f). On the contrary, these bands are present in the Raman spectrum of the blank (fig. 1a).

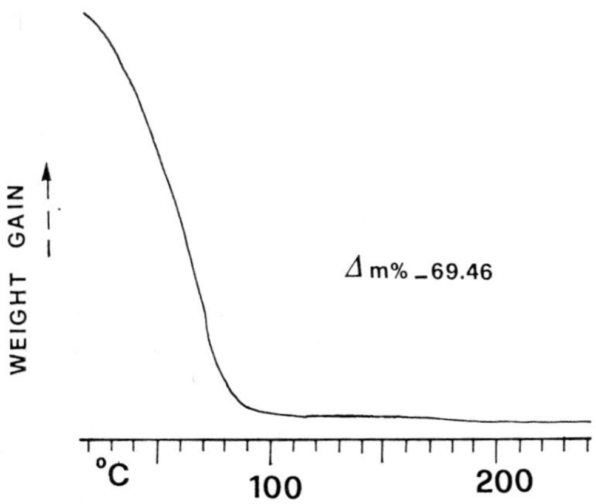

Fig. 2. TG curve of the hydrated lens.

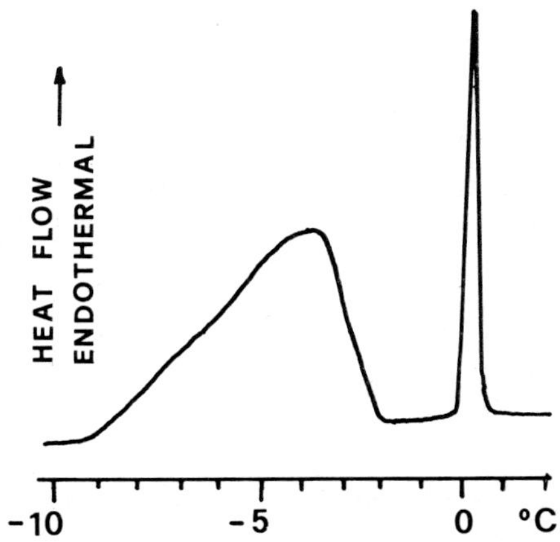

Fig. 3. DSC of the hydrated lens near 0°C.

Lens water content (∼70%) (Fig. 2) is higher than that of PT 64 Galileo (∼40%) which we examined in previous research (ref. 3) and which is made of poly- 2 -hydroxyethylmethacrylate. Differential scanning calorimetry in the vicinity of 0 °C shows the presence of at least two water states in the hydrated lens (Fig.3). The Raman spectra (Fig.1) reveal that not only the carbonylic bands at 1727 (methacrylate C=O group) and at 1671 (lactam C=O group), but also the bands between 1500 and 1400 cm^{-1} are affected by hydration. These spectroscopic modifications appearing between 1800 and 1400 cm^{-1} are attributable to the direct interaction of water with carbonylic oxygens by hydrogen bonds and to indirect conformational changes of CH_2 and CH_3 hydrophobic groups depending on their distance from the carbonylic groups. Thermoanalytical and spectroscopic measurements show that water closely interacts with the structural centres of the lens thus verifying the hydrophilicity of the material.

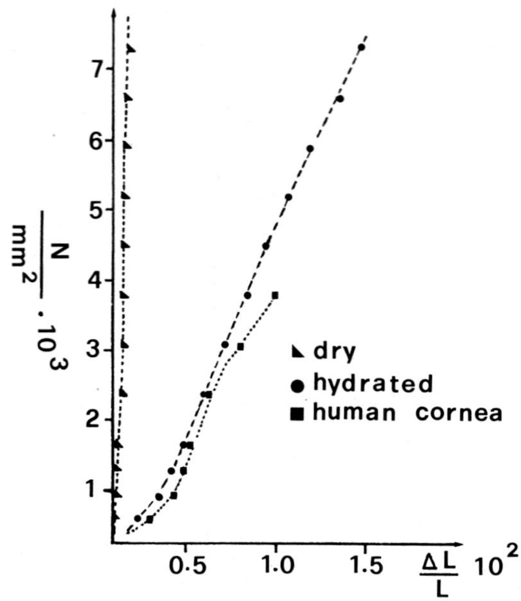

Fig. 4. Stress-strain curves of lens material and human cornea.

TABLE 1.

Water content of PT70 lenses after 4 months follow-up.

Sample	Water content weight %
1	63.4
2	64.7
3	64.9
4	65.1
5	65.7
6	66.4
7	67.2
8	68.3
9	69.7

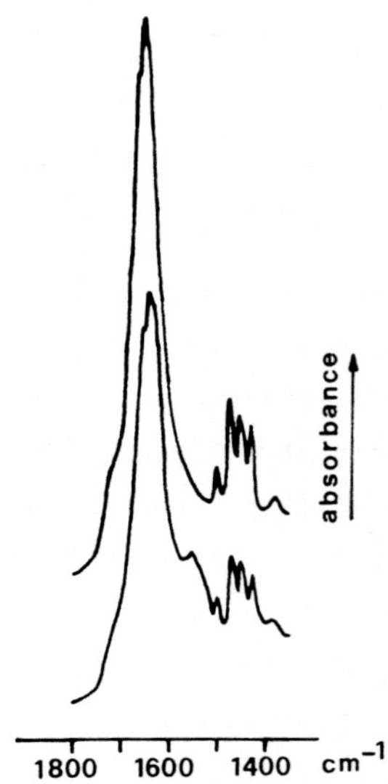

Fig. 5. ATR-FTIR spectra of a lens
a) before and
b) after application

In Fig. 4 the compressive stress strain curves for both hydrated and dry material are reported and compared with the curve obtained for the human cornea. As can be seen from the trends of the curves, water plays an important role in approaching the mechanical properties (in this case the modulus of elasticiy) of the material to those of the surrounding tissues.

As far as the chemico-physical and structural characterization of the lenses after application is concerned, Raman measurements do not show the presence of residual monomers or oligomers in any case. Consequently no biodegradation of the material has taken place.

The water amounts in the lenses after application are listed in Table 1. The values range from a minimum of 63.4% to a maximum of 69.7%. As can be seen there is a higher incidence of water intermediate content around 65%.

Quantities of water after lens application are affected by different factors which are related not only to the properties of the material but also to physiological and environmental elements. In this connection we could spectroscopically observe in a preliminary study on rabbit eye that a hydrophilic lens containing heavy water isotopically exchanges with the water present in the surrounding tissues in a short time. At the same time we observed that patient intolerance towards the lens increased in the case of lenses affected by considerable water loss.

The decrease in water content may be caused by the formation of deposits on the lens surfaces. With regard to this infrared ATR measurements were performed on the surfaces of the lenses after application. A typical spectrum is given in Fig. 5.

Spectroscopic analysis has shown the presence of different amounts of proteinic deposits both on cornea and tarsal surfaces. A preliminary qualitative evaluation is set out in Table 2.

TABLE 2.

Qualitative evaluation of surface deposits.

Sample	Corneal surface	Tarsal surface
1	+	++
3		+
5		+
6		
7		+
8		+
9	+	++

In conclusion we can say that Raman laser and ATR-IR spectroscopies have shown that the material is characterized by structural homogeneity, high hydrophilicity and absence of reaction to monomeric centres. These properties are still present after long wear in a 4-month follow-up.

Essentially, proteinic deposits have been shown and evaluated relative to the different lens surfaces (corneal and tarsal).

REFERENCES.

1 O. Wichterle and D. Lim, Hydrophilic gels for biological use, Nature, 185 (1960) 117-118.

2 A. Bertoluzza, P. Monti, R. Caramazza, M. Cellini and L. De Martino, Raman-laser spectroscopy in the study of polymethylmethacrylate IOL, Proc. of the XI Annual Meeting of the Society for Biomaterials, S. Diego, April 1985.

3 A. Bertoluzza, P. Monti, J.V. Garcia-Ramos, R. Simoni, R. Caramazza and A. Calzavara, Applications of Raman spectroscopy to the ophthalmological field: Raman spectra of soft contact lenses made of poly-2-hydroxyethyl methacrylate (PHEMA), J. Mol. Struct., 143 (1986) 469-472.

4 A. Bertoluzza, C. Fagnano, P. Monti, R. Caramazza and M. Cellini, Raman spectra of the human lens in relation to pathology and the anticataract effect of drugs, J. Raman Spectrosc., 17 (1986) 133-137.

Biomaterials and Clinical Applications,
edited by A. Pizzoferrato, P.G. Marchetti, A. Ravaglioli and A.J.C. Lee
Elsevier Science Publishers B.V., Amsterdam, 1987 — Printed in The Netherlands

NEW KIND OF KERATOPROSTHESIS

F. PINTUCCI and S. PINTUCCI

Roma (Italy)

SUMMARY

The Authors, to avoid the complications of commercially available keratoprosthesis (K) due to the organism's capability to encapsulate or extrude implants when they are only mechanically anchored, developed a K with the optic in PMMA and the aptic part in dacron tissue. This K is biologically integrated and not simply sutured to the eye. Our follow-up considers 4 patients 20, 14, 11, 10.5,& 5 months after surgery all with satisfactory results. The simplicity of the surgical technique and the anatomical and functional results encourage us to continue implanting this K.

INTRODUCTION

A keratoprosthesis (K) is indicated in cases of an opaque or otherwise severely damaged cornea, in which corneal transplants cannot be attemptedor have failed. The operation presupposes that the posterior segment of the eye is in good functional condition.

A K consists of an optical cylinder of PMMA which focuses the image on the retina and is anchored to eye tissues by means of an aptic part.

The optic of all K is made of PMMA, except for Polack's which is in corundum, but differ greatly in the choice of the aptic part in the attempt to find the ideal material capable of adhering the K to eye tissues permanently and without complications.

The main complications are due to the organism's capability to encapsulate or extrude alloplastic materials when they are partly included and are mechanically, and not biologically integrated, like most K that are simply sutured to eye tissues.

PMMA, Teflon and Dacron aptic parts, which are made of closed-cell foams cannot integrate biologically with eye tissues and do not adapt mechanically to eye deformations. These K break off the continous layers of the host bed and the contact inibition of the epithelial cells that are not anymore in close contact with each other, is stopped. The epithelial cells divide leading to complications such as an anterior epithelial overgrowth (encapsulation) or, if there is an empty space around the implant-eye interface, the epithelium downgrows along the shaft of the K leading to a retroimplant membrane with spontaneous extrusion, leakage and endophthalmitis.

Cardona states that inflammatory tissular erosion and melting begin around the optical cylinder favoured by eyelid movements, and mechanical stresses between eye tissues and rigid K.

In order to have a permanent biologically integrated K and in an effort to eliminate the implant-cornea interface, Strampelli placed a PMMA optical cylinder in tooth sections and implanted it covered by autologous oral mucosa (odontocheratoprotesi). The technical difficulty of the operation, the complications due to the mechanical stress, the small dimensions and the absence of integration of the dentin side have prevented its widespread use.

In our opinion the ideal aptic part should have the same mechanical characteristics as the surrounding eye tissues. Furthermore it should be porous in order to allow the ingrowth of fibroblasts and vessels incorporating it into host connective tissue with no degenerative changes.
The aptic part must remain soft and pliable, even after the ingrowth process is complete.

MATERIALS AND METHODS

We developed a new K with the aim to reduce the previous frequency of k extrusion (Fig. 1).

Our new K consists of a disk of 0.25 mm thick USCI Debakey woven dacron fabric with a central perforation used to anchor a 3,5-mm-diameter PMMA optical Cylinder. The cylinder is 5.5 mm long and its optical power is individually calculated with an ultrasound biometry of the eye axial length and with a personal formula. Since Dacron cannot be chemically glued, after several attempts in this direction, the PMMA-dacron anchorage is obtained with a PMMA solution that becames monolithic with the PMMA optical shaft and mechanically anchors the dacron felt fibres.
After removing PMMA monomers and impurities by boiling the prosthesis it is sterilized with ethylene oxide.

The choice of this dacron tissue was based on positive experiences in cardiovascular surgery; since 1954 vascular prostheses and trancutaneous connectors have remained in situ years after implantation, allowing the host tissues' ingrowth, remaining soft and pliable.

RESULTS

Our investigations on the long-term tolerance of Dacron tissues in the cornea, conjunctiva and oral mucosa of rabbits and men were satisfactory from the tolerance and fixation point of view.

Host fibroblasts and capillaries, as confirmed by Optical and Scanning Electronic Microscopy, migrate through the pores of the aptic part from the periphery of the implant to the center and deposit fibrin and collagen binding the implant to host tissues with little reaction. The aptic part remains soft and pliable and the epithelium can not proliferate along the implant-eye tissues interface being stopped by the connective tissue that ingrew the dacron felt aptic part.

Based on the conditions of the eyelids and conjunctiva, as well as the degree of tear production, candidates for keratoprostheses can be divided into a "wet eye group" and a "dry eye group". A through-the-lid procedure will be required for the latter and a trancorneal prosthesis with oral mucosa implant for the former.

To implant the K, a 360 degree peritomy of conjunctiva and Tenon with dissection toward the fornices is done. The lens should be removed if the patient is phakic. An anterior vitrectomy and resection of the iris are performed. The corneal center is marked for future reference. The cornea is trephined, Healon injected and the prosthesis inserted and sutured in the correct position. According to the surgical technique either the oral mucosa or the lids are sutured to cover the prosthesis.

After three months a slit is made in the central portion of the covering tissue so that the optical cylinder can be pushed through.

Our follow-up considers 5 patients 20, 14, 11, 10.5, 5 months after surgery all with satisfactory results.

The simplicity of the surgical technique and the anatomical and functional results we achieved encourage us to further continue to implant this K.

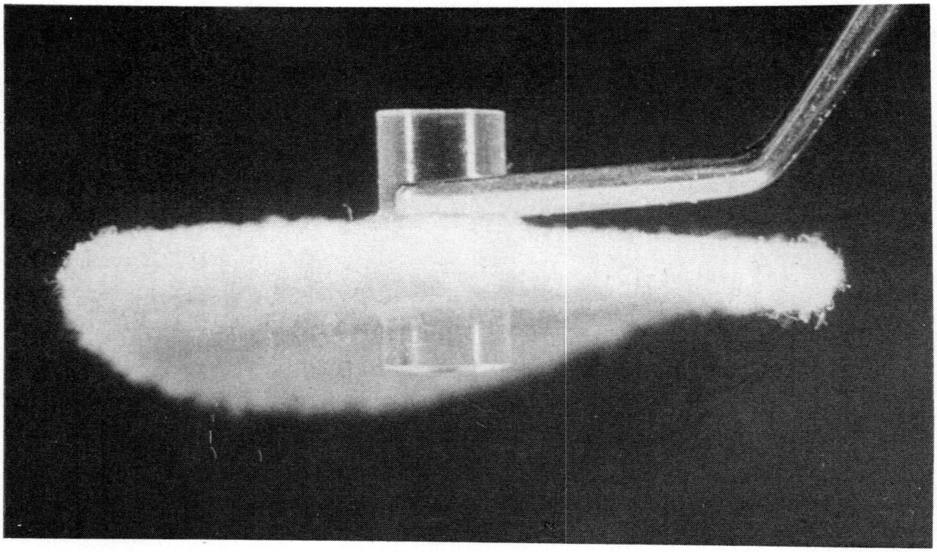

FIG.1 Keratoprosthesis (K) with the optic in PMMA and the aptic part in dacron tissue.

REFERENCES

1 H. Cardona, Prosthokeratoplasty, Cornea 2 (1983) 179-184.
D.P. Casey, Osteo-odonto-keratoprothesis and chondro-Keratoptothesis in: Proc. of the Royal Society of Medicine. Section of Ophtholomology, 63 (1970) 313-315
2 M.E. De Bakey, E.S. Crawford, G.C. Morris, D.A. Cooley, Patch graft angioplasty in vascular surgery, J. Cadiovasc. Surg. 3 (1962) 106-141.
3 C.H. Dohlman, Biology of Complications following Keratoprothesis, Cornea. 2 (1983) 175-176.
4 L.J. Girard, Keratoprothesis, Cornea 2 (1983) 207-224.
5 G. Heimke, F.M. Polack, Ceramic Keratoprothesis: Biomechanics of Extrusion in Through-the-lid Implantation, Cornea 2 (1983) 197-202.
6 F. Pintucci, S. Pintucci, Pemfigoide oculare in paziente adentula. Nuovo tipo di cheratoprotesi, in: Proc 65 Congresso Nazionale della Societa' Oftalmologica Italiana. 5-8 Dec. 1985 (in Press).
7 F. Pintucci, S. Pintucci, I materiali alloplastici nella chirurgia della cornea, in: Proc Congresso annuale 1985 della S. O. L. (in Press)
8 F.M. Polack, Clinical results with a Ceramic Keratoprothesis 2 (1983) 185-196.
9 W.Schraut, I. Kiso, P. Freed, C. Baechler, M. Barnhart, J. Riddle, E. Mammen, G. Mandell, A. Kantrowitz, Permanent in series cardiac assistance with the dynamic aortic patch: blood prosthesis interaction in long term canine experiments, Surgery 79(2) (1976)193-201.
10 B. Strampelli, M.L. Restivo, Studi istologici di radice dentaria nella palpebra di Macacus Rhesus (II parte), Ann. Oft. Clin. Ocul. 1969.
11 B Strampelli, Intervento per osteo-odonto-cheratoprotesi, in:Trattato di Tecnica chirurgica: Chirurgia Oculistica., UTET, Milano, (1984) pp 362-370.

Biomaterials and Clinical Applications,
edited by A. Pizzoferrato, P.G. Marchetti, A. Ravaglioli and A.J.C. Lee
Elsevier Science Publishers B.V., Amsterdam, 1987 — Printed in The Netherlands

MESOKERATOPROSTHESES:AN EXPERIMENTAL STUDY WITH A 5 YEAR FOLLOW-UP

R.CARAMAZZA,A.BERTOLUZZA, R.LASCHI, P.PUDDU, M.CELLINI, C.FAGNANO, P.MONTI,
P.VERSURA, M.C.MALTARELLO.

Centre of biotechnological and clinical research in Ophthalmology,Institutes of Ophthalmology, Clinical Electron Microscopy and Department of Chemistry and Biochemical Propedeutics, University of Bologna and IOR-Galileo, Italy.

SUMMARY
The Authors refer the data of hydrogel PT70 intrastromal implant in baboon eyes,with a five year follow up.They discuss the results of a correlative study carried out from a chemical-physical-structural, morphological and immunohistochemical point of view.

INTRODUCTION

The first approaches to correct ocular refraction by alloplastic implant utilized hydrophobic material (PMMA,Teflon) (1,2,3,4).Their failure was due to corneal ulceration and consequent lens extrusion, probably due to changes in the corneal metabolism.Recently, intracorneal implants of a high refractive index material (polysulfone) have been attempted (5).Since 1970,we have been using a new hydrophilic material,poly-hydroxi-ethil-methacrylate (poly-Hema), especially used for contact lens manufacturing.At that time we employed a 35% hydrophilic rate poly-Hema, but with poor results (6).At the beginning of the 80's we began a new series of experiments,using a 70% hydrophilic rate poly-Hema (namely PT 70 GALILEO) implanted in rabbit and non-human primate eyes. In the present study we discuss the results of a five year follow up.

MATERIALS AND METHODS

An hydrogel lens (70 hydrophilic rate, 6 mms.diameter) was implanted in the corneal stroma of an adult baboon.

Surgical procedure.(fig.1).A 3 mms.depth corneal incision was made from and parallel to the limbus.A lamellar dissector was used to open a pocket large enough to contain the implant.The incision was closed with a continue suture after draining puncture of the anterior chamber.Gentamicyne and midricayn were subconjunctively injected. 6 months after the surgery, the suture was removed.

Chemical techniques. The Raman spectra of the lens before and after implantation have been obtained using a Jasco R-300 spectrophotometer with a Lexel Ar^{+} 4880 A laser source.Thermogravimetric (TG) measurements were performed in a Mettler TA 3000 system with TG 50 equipment.

Morphological techniques.Fragments of cornea, iris and ciliary body were processed as follows: a) immersed in frozen isopenthane cooled in liquid nitrogen. Cryostatic sections (5 μm thick) were incubated for 30' in FITC conjugated anti IgG,IgM,IgA,C_{3c} antisera(supplied by Behringwerke, AG,Marburg).Sections were observed in a Zeiss III photomicroscope equipped with an epifluorescence condenser III RS. b) fixed in 2.5% glutaraldehyde in 0.1M phosphate buffer pH 7.4,postfixed in 1% OsO_4 in Veronal buffer, embedded in Araldite.Ultrathin sections were observed with a Zeiss Transmission Electron Microscope.c)fixed and dehydrated as for group b, critical point dried.The specimens were mounted on aluminium stubs, sputtered with gold (20 nm) and observed with a Philips 505 Scanning Electron Microscope.

A corneal piece containing the pocket was processed by fixation in 10% buffered formalin and embedding in Paraplast. Sections were stained with Alcian Blue pH 1 and 2.5.The lens was gently removed from the pocket,divided into two halves. One half was chemically analyzed, the other half was briefly fixed in 2.5% glutaraldehyde, washed in 0.15M phosphate buffer, allowed to dry at 37°C, sputtered with gold and observed in the Philips 505 SEM.

RESULTS

Clinical results. At 5 years follow up cornea appeared clear (fig.2) and the eyeglobe showed no inflammation signs.

Chemical results. The Raman spectra of the lens after (fig.3a) and before (fig. 3b) implantation are not different. In fact the stretching C=C bands due to residual monomers (N-vinylpyrrolidone and n-butylmethacrylate) or oligomers are not present. In addition, the bands sensitive to hydration (7), i.e. the carbonylic bands between 1800 and 1600 cm^{-1} and those between 1500 and 1400 cm^{-1} have the same trend, thus suggesting similar water content in the lens before and after implantation. This result is also confirmed by TG analysis (fig.4) which shows even after 5 years follow up a 70% water content.

Morphological results.Corneal epithelium had normal appearance (fig.5). Corneal endothelial cells were damaged in various areas (fig.6).Stroma showed disorganized lamellae anterior to the pocket (fig.7),very few and small blood

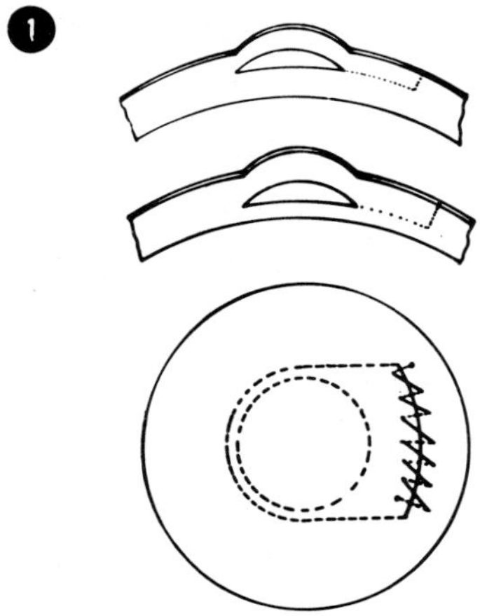

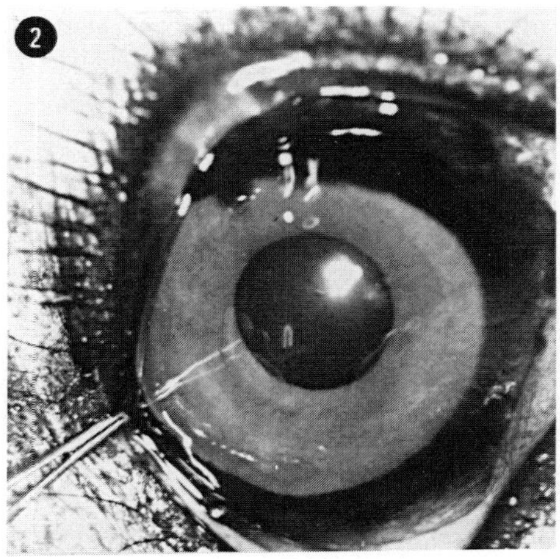

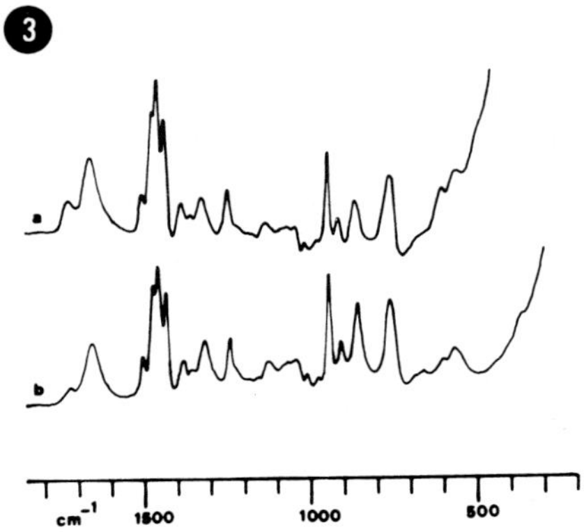

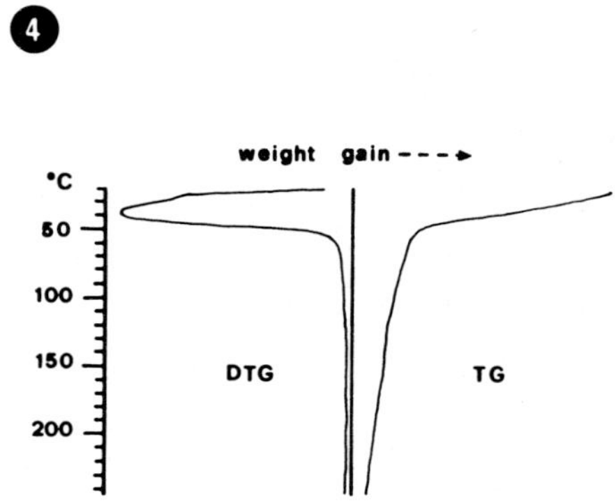

Fig.1. Surgical procedure. See explanation in the text.

Fig.2. Baboon's eye at 5 year follow up.Cornea appears clear, the implant is evident in transparency.

Fig.3. Raman spectra of: a) PT 70 lens after implantation b) before implantation.

Fig.4. Thermogravimetric (TG) and differential thermogravimetric (DTG) curves of PT70 lens after 5 year follow up.

vessels, no inflammatory cells, keratocytes in normal number and morphology were observed. Alcian blue staining did not reveal differences between the stroma outside & inside the pocket. Iris and ciliary body appeared normal, only a slight hyperemia and positivity for IgG and C_{3c} presence were detected in the ciliary body stroma. SEM observation of the lens surfaces did not show evidence of cell encapsulation, only small fragments of organic material were observed.(fig.8).

DISCUSSION

The chemical stability of the lens has been directly confirmed by Raman-laser spectroscopy which revealed the absence of monomers or oligomers due to biodegradation. Moreover, Raman spectroscopy has shown the persistency of the lens hydrophilicity and of the related properties. In particular, the water content, determined by TG analysis, is 70% $\frac{W}{W}$. This percentage is the same for the lens before and after implantation.

The acceptance of the PT 70 lens in the corneal stroma is confirmed from a clinical point of view by the corneal clearness even after 5 year follow up. However, our study evidenced tissue alterations, especially at the corneal endothelium level. We think that a subclinic dynamic equilibrium exists and as time goes by it could evolve to a clinically evident pathological event. We did not detect either corneal epithelial cell alterations or differences in glycoprotein composition in the stroma out- and insidethe implant bed. These findings suggest that the implant does not represent a barrier to energy suppliers from the aqueous; the alterations may be due to cytotoxic or mechanical action of the material. We have seen an immunological involvement of the choroid. This could be explained with the presence of "immunological messengers" from the cornea to the choroid through the perilimbar vessles. The endothelial alterations, so, could be due to some factors released in the aqueous directly by ciliary body and not primarily caused by the presence of the implant in the stroma.

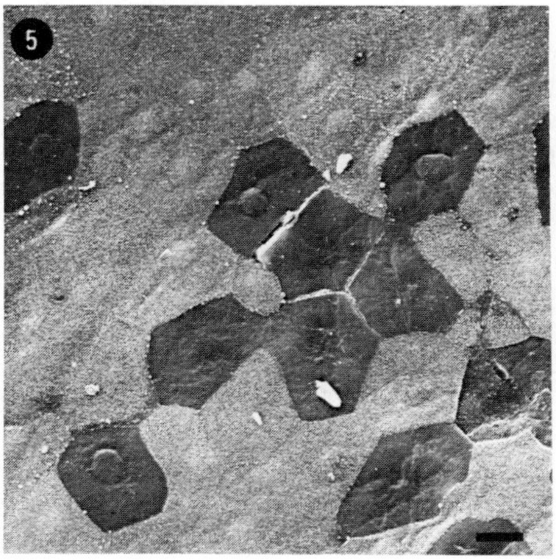

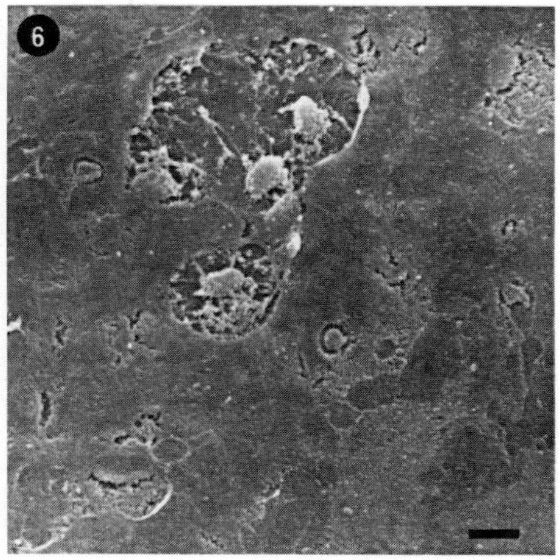

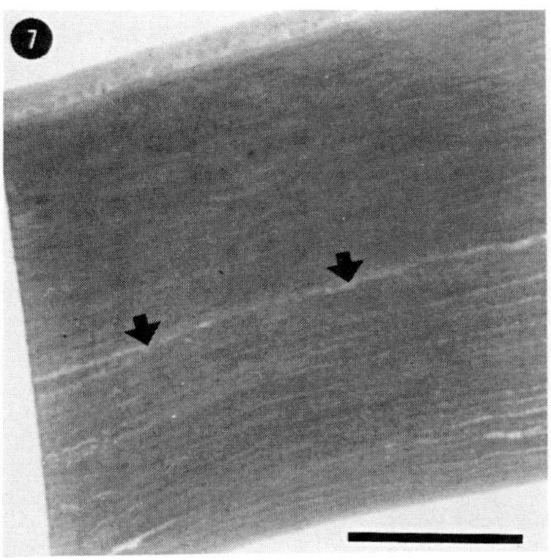

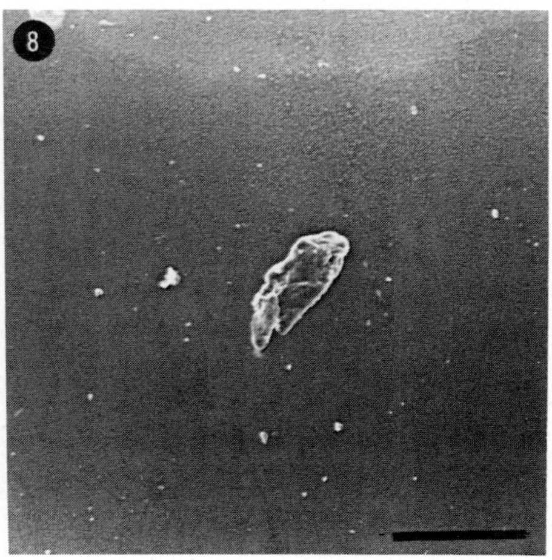

Fig.5.Corneal epithelial cells appear of normal morphology. SEM, Bar = 10 μm

Fig.6.Corneal endothelial cells appear severely damaged.SEM, Bar = 10 μm

Fig.7.Section of the cornea. The implant bed is evidenced by arrows. The anterior stroma display disorganized lamellae. SEM,Bar = 100 μm

Fig.8.Small debris of organic material on the lens surface.SEM,Bar = 100 μm

REFERENCES

1.Stone W.:Alloplastry in surgery of the eye. Reprinted from the:New England Journal of Medicine 258:486-490,533-540,596-602;1958.

2.Cardona H.:Keratoprosthesis. Am.J.Ophthalmology,54,284,1962.

3.Polack F.M.: Corneal Optical Prosthesis. Brit.J.Ophthal.,55,838,1971.

4.Barraquer J.(1960). Ann. Inst. Barraquer, I, 243.

5.Choyce P.: The correction of refractive error with polysulfone corneal inlays. A new frontier to be explored. Trans.Ophthalmol.Soc.UK 1958; 104, 332-342.

6.R.Caramazza et al.: Primi rilievi sperimentali di impianti alloplastici corneali con polimeri idrofilici biocompatibili. Atti dell'XI Convegno della Soc.Oftalmol.Meridionale, Palermo, 17-18-19 Giugno 1977.

7.A.Bertoluzza,P.Monti,R.Simoni, J.V.Garcia Ramos,R.Caramazza, M.Cellini,L.De Martino, A.Calzavara : Applications of Raman Spectroscopy to the ophthalmological field.Raman spectra of soft contact lenses made of polyvinylpyrrolidone (PVP). Proc.Laser Scattering Spectroscopy of Biological Objects,Praga July 6-10, 1986.

Biomaterials and Clinical Applications,
edited by A. Pizzoferrato, P.G. Marchetti, A. Ravaglioli and A.J.C. Lee
Elsevier Science Publishers B.V., Amsterdam, 1987 — Printed in The Netherlands

EXPERIMENTAL STUDY ON THE PROGRESSION OF FOREIGN BODY REACTION AFTER PMMA IOLs IMPLANT IN ANTERIOR CHAMBER

P.VERSURA,P.PUDDU,R.CARAMAZZA and R.LASCHI

Centre of biotechnological and clinical research in Ophthalmology, Institutes of Ophthalmology and of Clinical Electron Microscopy, University of Bologna and IOR-Galileo, Italy.

SUMMARY

PMMA IOLs were implanted in the anterior chamber of rabbit eyes.Eyeglobes were removed at 1,2,3,4 weeks.Corneal endothelial cell damage was largely found.The cells attached on the lens surface were typical for a foreign-body reaction.At 4 weeks follow up a reactive membrane developed encapsulating the lens. Immunoglobulins on the lens surface were also detected.

We can conclude that IOL and ocular tissues are in a subclinical dynamic equilibrium which, normally, does not interfere with the acceptance of the lens.When this situation breaks down, a clinically evident pathology occurs.

INTRODUCTION

In the last few years much progress has been made in the manufacturing of IOLs. Improved surgical procedures and care have been developed at the same time.Nevertheless, the fact is that IOL still represents a foreign-body for ocular tissues. An IOL is to be considered an inflammatory stimulus against which the biological organism reacts. For many years prosthetic materials,such as PMMA,poly-propylene and poly-Hema, were wrongly believed to be biologically inert and this has greatly delayed the introduction of a correct method of thinking and studying these problems.

In the present investigation we have analyzed the very first reactions of the host tissues against the IOL, both from an ultrastructural and immunohistochemical point of view.

MATERIALS AND METHODS

12 PMMA IOLs were implanted in the anterior chamber of albino rabbit eyes.

The animals were enucleated after 1,2,3,4 weeks.The eyeglobes were briefly washed in saline, corneas were excised by trephine,fragments of ciliary body and iris were cut by a razor blade.The specimens were prepared as follows:
-for SEM observation: fixed in 2,5% glutaraldehyde in 0.1M phosphate buffer pH

7.4 at 4°C for 3 hours,washed overnight in 0.15M phosphate buffer, post-fixed in 1% OsO_4 in Veronal buffer for 1 hour, dehydrated through a graded series of ethanol, critical point dried, sputtered with gold (20 nm),observed in a Philips 505 SEM operating in a range of 10-30 kV.

- for LM and immunohistochemistry: fixed in PLP (periodate-lisine-paraformaldehyde) following McLean and Nakane (1), washed overnight in 0.1M cacodyalate buffer containing 7% saccarose, abruptly dehydrated in absolute acetone(3 changes, 40 minutes each), embedded in JB_4 (glycol methacrylate,Polysciences Inc.,Warrington, Pa.,USA).Sections 4 µm thick were digested with 0.5 pronase in HCl M HCl pH 7.5 at 37°C for 30 minutes as suggested by Casanova et al.(2), overnight washed in 0.01M PBS at 4°C, incubated in fluorescein-isothiocyanate (FITC) conjugated anti-rabbit plasma protein antiserum (purchased by Behring, Scoppito,L'Aquila) diluted 1:30 in a phosphate buffered saline solution,pH 7.2 (0.15M NaCl;0.5M $Na_2HPO_4.2H_2O$; 0.2M KH_2PO_4),coverslipped with a drop of glycerol. Sections were observed in a ZEISS III RS photomicroscope equipped with an epifluorescence condenser.

The lenses at 1,2,3 weeks follow up were observed in LM whitin 10 minutes from the removal,by using the phase contrast mode; then were processed for SEM by fixation in 2.5% glutaraldehyde,washing in 0.15M phosphate buffer and then in double distilled water, air drying at 37°C for at least 72 hours. Lenses were observed in a Philips 505 SEM operating in a range of 10-15 kV.The lenses with 4 weeks follow up were processed for LM as described for tissues,except the step of dehydration.Sections 5 µm thick were incubated in the FITC -anti - rabbit plasma protein antiserum as described above.

RESULTS

Lenses.At 1,2,3 weeks follow up we observed by LM, strands and membranes (fig.1) on which cells (probably inflammatory lymphocytes and poly-morphonuclear leukocytes) were attached.At 4 weeks follow up by SEM (fig.2)we found fibroblast-like cells,macrophages and epithelioid-like cells. Large areas of the surface were covered by a cellular membranous coating.No endothelial cells were observed. Immunohistochemical analysis of the lens showed evidence of immunoglobulins (fig.3,4).

Tissues.In all the cases we studied, the tissue mostly involved by PMMA IOL implantation was corneal endothelium. Increased number of microprojections

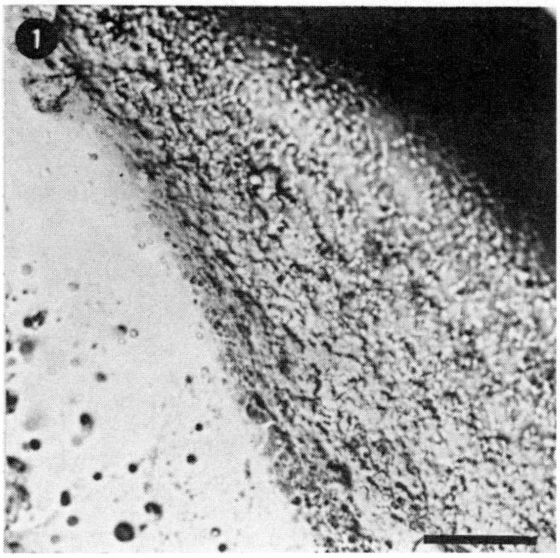

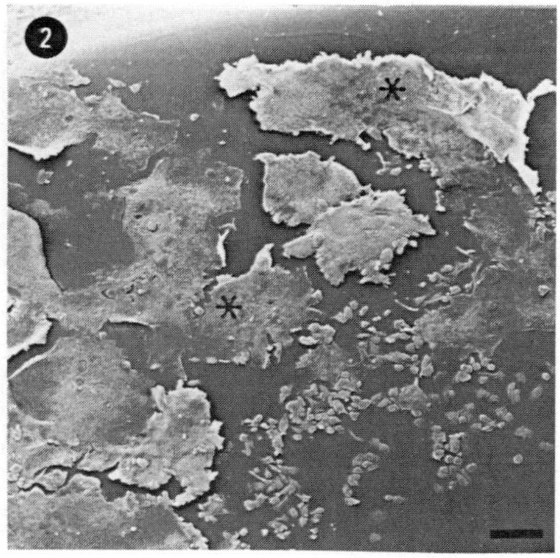

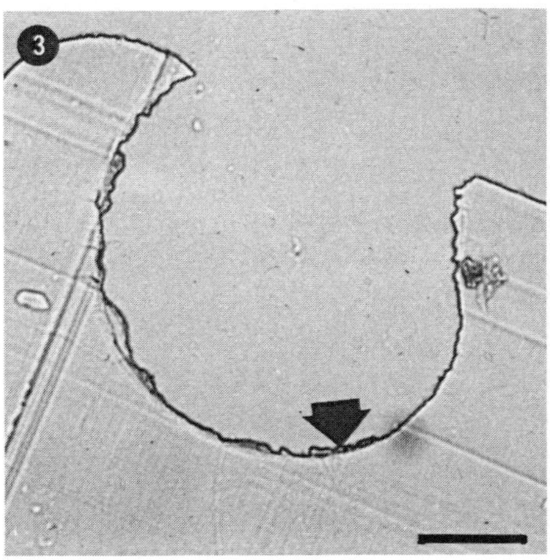

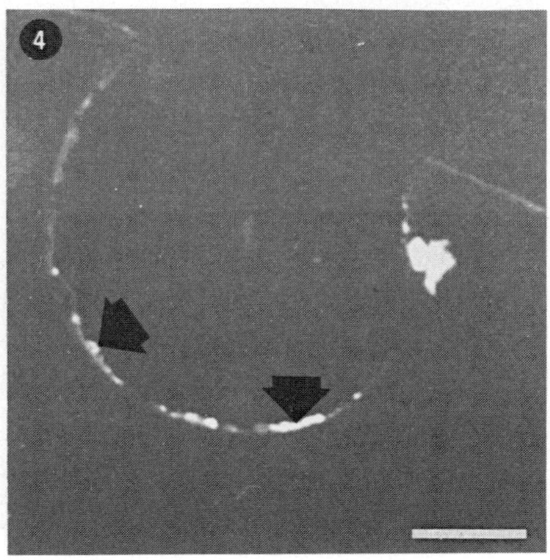

Fig.1.IOL at 2 weeks follow up.A strand of fibrin with inflammatory cells on it is shown. LM, Bar = 100 µm.
Fig.2.IOL at 4 weeks follow up.The surface of the implant is largely covered by a membranous coating (*).SEM, Bar = 100 µm.
Fig.3.IOL at 4 weeks follow up.A section of the lens shows the presence of the membranous coating (arrow). LM, Bar =100 µm.
Fig.4.IOL at 4 weeks follow up.Presence of IgG on the lens surface as detected by fluorescence microscopy(arrows)Same field offig.3. LM, Bar = 100 µm

(fig.5),presence of plasmalemmal blebs (fig.6),lacking of plasma membrane towards the aqueous (fig.7),large areas of bare Descemet's devoid of cells

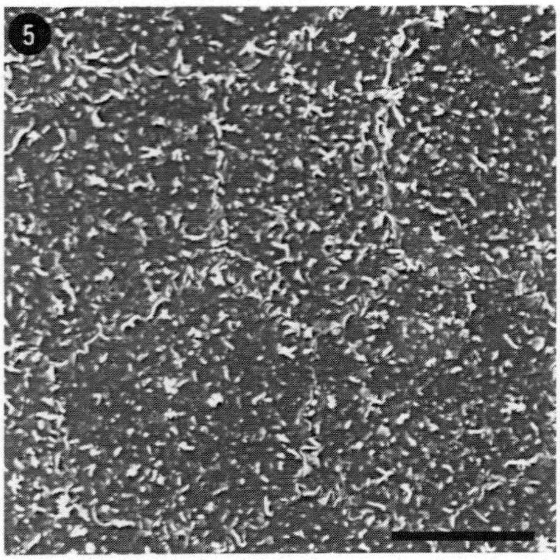

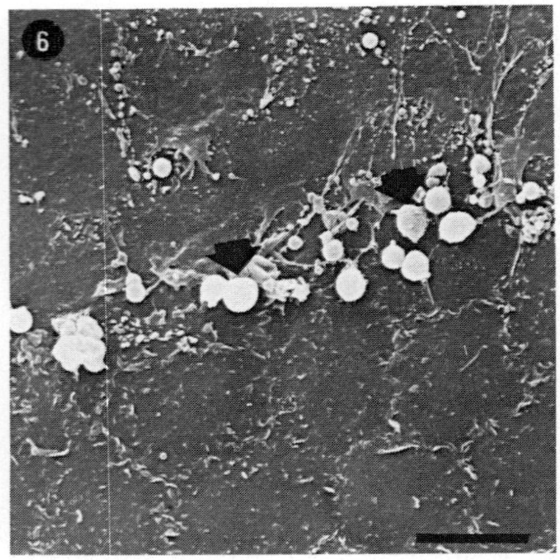

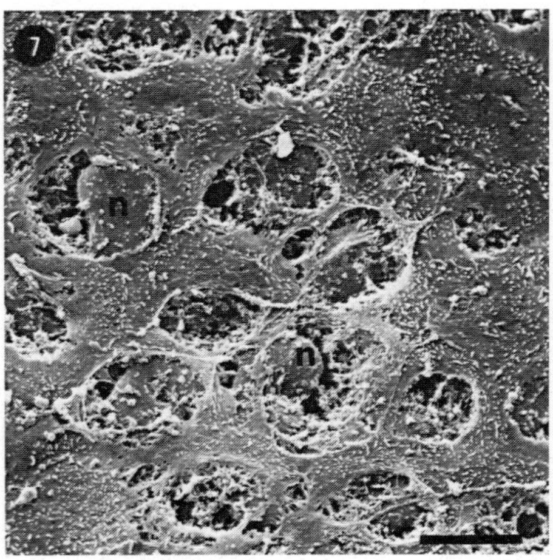

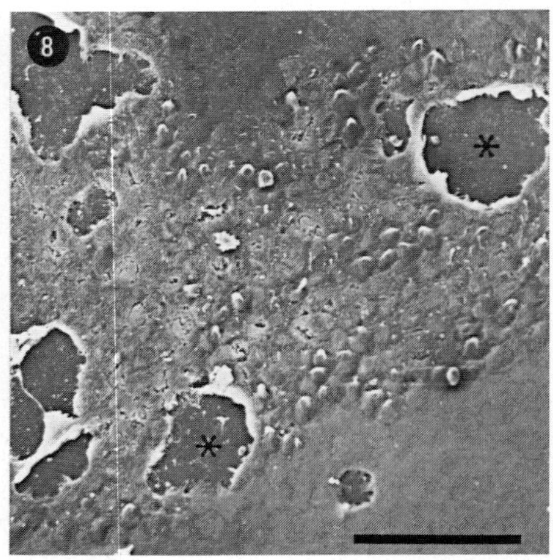

Fig.5.Corneal endothelium at 2 weeks follow up.The microvilli have greatly increased in number. SEM, Bar = 10 μm.
Fig.6.Corneal endothelium at 2 weeks follow up. Blebs(arrows) are present at the level of cell plasmamembrane. SEM, Bar 10 μm.
Fig.7.Corneal endothelium at 3 weeks follow up.Cell plasmamembranes have been torn off, thus exposing the inner cytoplasmic organelles and nucleus (N). SEM, Bar = 10 μm.
Fig.8.Corneal endothelium at 4 weeks follow up.Areas devoid of cells (*)show bare Descemet's membrane. SEM, Bar = 100 μm.

(fig.8) were observed.Strands of fibrin firmly attached to corneal endothelium showed small clusters positive for immunoglobulin presence (fig.9).Corneal

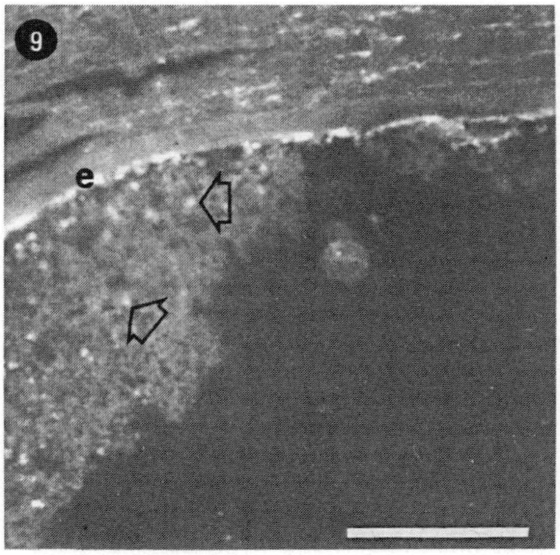

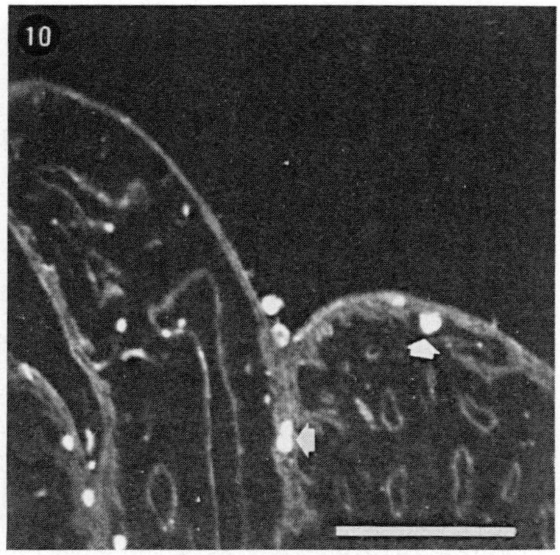

Fig.9.Corneal endothelium at 2 weeks follow up.A fibrin membrane adherent to corneal endothelium (e) shows small fluorescent clusters positive for Ig presence (arrows).LM,Bar = 100 μm.

Fig.10.Iris stroma at 3 weeks follow up.Plasmacells positive for Ig presence are observed (arrows).LM, Bar = 100 μm.

thickness was unaltered, stroma and epithelium were unaffected.At the limbus, an infiltration of inflammatory cells was found, probably due to the limbal scar not yet healed.In 3 cases we found in iris stroma inflammatory cells and plasmacells, with positivity for immunoglobulin presence (fig.10). In 1 case ciliary body stroma was infiltrated by eosinophilic leukocytes and plasmacells, in 3 cases large macrophages were found.Positivity of stroma for immunoglobulin presence was detected in 2 cases.

DISCUSSION

Our results are in agreement with the literature appearing in the very last few years.

The cell population of the lens surface was typical for a foreign body reaction. It seems that this reaction normally occurs, not interfering with the acceptance of the lens, as many successful implants do not show clinical pathological evidence even after long term follow up.On the contrary , the foreign body reaction can increase the success by encapsulating the implant with a membrane which renders the interface IOL-host tissues more compatible. Already at 4 weeks follow up we found the reactive membrane on the lens implant, whose composition is yet unknown.Wolter (5) speculated that this structure may be quite similar to the basal lamina of the lens capsule. It is probably composed of a proteinaceous exudate precipitated on the lens,as previous investigations failed to demonstrate it as a specific product of fibroblast-like or epithelioid-like cells (5).

We have detected the presence of immunoglobulins on the lens surface at 4 weeks follow up.Recently, Mondino at al. (6) found that PMMA IOLs generate C_{3a} and C_{5a} by activation of the alternative complement pathway. These important findings state that IOLs evoke an immunological response. An IOL is to be considered biocompatible when it is able to induce a biological reaction not leading to a clinically evident pathological situation.

Methacrylate surfaces adhere to corneal endothelial cell plasmamembranes, leading to massive cell damage. In our study we found an increase in number of microvilli and presence of blebs at the plasmalemmal level.These findings do reflect a reaction to the lens material, as reported also by Blumenthal and Yalon (4).

In other words, besides the role of surgical traumatism in causing endothelial damage, the necessity for a new material with higher biocompatibility is still to be stressed.

REFERENCES

1. McLean I.W. and Nakane P.K.,Periodate-lysine-paraformaldehyde fixative. A new fixative for immunoelectron microscopy. J.Histochem Cytochem 22 (1974), 1077.
2. Casanova S.,Donini U.,Zini N.,Morelli R. and Zucchelli P. Immunohistochem. staining on Hydroxyethyl-Methacrylate-embedded tissues. J. Histochem. Cytochem, 31 (1983): 1000-1004.
3. Wolter J.R. Lens implant cytology. Ophthalmic surgery 13 (1982):939-942.
4. Wolter J.R. Reactive membrane on a lens implant:three months after implantation. Albrecht von Graefe's Arch.Klin.Exp.Ophthalmol.219(1982):103-111.
5. Wolter J.R. Morphology of the capsule-like portion of the reactive membranes on intraocular lens implant.Albrecht von Graefe's Arch.Klin.Exp. Ophthalmol.,220(1983):58.
6. Mondino B.J., Nagata S. and Glovsky M.M. Activation of the alternative complement pathway by intraocular lenses. Invest.Ophthalmol.Vis.Sci., 26 (1985):905-908.

Biomaterials and Clinical Applications,
edited by A. Pizzoferrato, P.G. Marchetti, A. Ravaglioli and A.J.C. Lee
Elsevier Science Publishers B.V., Amsterdam, 1987 — Printed in The Netherlands

SILICONE OIL: BIOCHEMICAL CHARACTERISTICS, TECHNIQUES AND INDICATION IN COMPLICATED RETINAL DETACHMENT.

R. TITTARELLI[1], S. BENEDETTI[1] and C. MARIOTTI[1]
[1]Ancona University, Eye Clinic, Hosp. Reg. Torrette Italy

SUMMARY

This paper documents silicone oil physico-chemical characteristics like radiotrasparency, viscosity, density, refractive index , electric and volumetric resistence etc. pointing out the correlations between silicone oil properties and its clinical use.
The Authors describe their clinical and surgical experience in managing 54 P.V.R. retinal detachment operated during this last year. Emphasising their recent modifications, they recommend silicone oil use in particularly severe retinal detachment cases in order to flat mechanically the retina because this substance does not intervene in the biological P.V.R. process which can continue.

INTRODUCTION

Till few years ago silicone oil (S.O.) characteristics were unknown and its clinical use was doubtful since its toxicological effect on the retina was unknown.

Nowadays the knowledge of its chemical and physical properties and more codified surgical techniques including vitrectomy, membrane peeling have opened new horizons for the use of SO and defined its limits.

The empirical approach has became now a specific and more appropriate one, and for this reason S.O. is the substance of first choice for permanent internal tamponing in severe retinal detachment (R.D.).

CHEMICAL CHARACTERISTICS

S.O. is a polymer formed by molecules of silicone charged with oxygen and by organic groups such as methyl, ethyl, phenyl.

S.O. is colourless and transparent, it does not modify the luminous wave transmission of the visible spectrum.It is radiotransparent to conventional radiography but it shows a marked tomodensitometry hyperdensity. The S.O. normally used has a viscosity value ranging from 1000 to 5000 centistokes (1 stokes = $1cm^2/sec^{-2}$).

Variations in viscosity do not modify the physical oil characteristics but those regarding its use. The density varies only from 0,973 to 0,975 between 1000 and 5000 centistokes: the surface tension is 21,2 for viscosity 1000 and 2000 and 21,3 for viscosity 3000 and 5000 centistokes. The thermal expansion coefficient (0,59) the refractive index (1,404), the electric and volumetric resistence (10 Ohm/cm^2) are the same for S.O. from 1000 to 5000 centistokes.

However it must be remembered that there is a larger possibility of oil emulsion if viscosity is lower.(13) The sterilization is quite easy: it is dry sterilized for two hours at a temperature not higher than 160° to avoid release of toxic factor, recently it as been proved that S.O. is toxic when sterilized with ethylene oxide.

(23) S.O. in general has a specific weight lower than 1(0,975): only some fluorine-siliconics have a density higher than 1, but are toxic for eye structures. The surface tension in the air is 21,3 ERG/cm^2, and 40 ERG/cm^2 in the water. Surface tension is one of the most important characteristics for substances used as internal tamponade:it has been proved that the higher surface tension occurs between gas and water (70 ERG/cm) whereas between oil and water is 50 ERG/cm. (3) The refraction index of S.O. is 1,4035 and it is higher than that of the vitreous (1,3925) and 50% higher than that of the water. S.O. is a very good insulating material, its electric resistence being 10 Ohm/cm^2. For this reason electroretinographic response is absent if the silicone bubble is complete; it is not a question of toxic action on the retina but only due to its insulating characteristic. If S.O. is removed and if retina is flattened ERG becomes normal.(6-7-13-19) Long-term complications are well known to everybody (cataract, cornea decompensation, glaucoma) but they are not due directly to toxic, but to mechanical action. These complications do not limit the use of S.O. when it is strictly

indispensable especially considering the fact that is possible to remove it if there is no evidence of residual proliferation.

S.O. is not completely chemically inert; with gelcromatography it was possible to divide oil compounds having a low molecular weight (ciclosiloxanus with 4 or more siloxanus unit for ring) (octametil-ciclotetrasiloxanus). These are indicated as toxic compounds. The low molecular weight of a liquid is a characteristic which goes together with high volatility and determines easiness to evaporate and therefore to spread in surrounding tissues. On the other hand a substance of low molecular weight can easily emulsify. Emulsification is higher when viscosity is lower and this is in direct ratio to the molecular weight and the length of polymers. A toxic role seems to be played also by catalizers which are normally used to produce S.O. Their characteristics determine the chemical structure and therefore the kind of oil (diviniltetrametildixiloxano, polivinilmetilcicloxano, polidimetilxiloxano, this last is commonly used as inner tamponade) conditioning the electric specific resistance. The toxic action of catalizers may be linked with a possible interaction between unactivated residues and biological structures. The volume resistivity indicates ionic impurities which are present in the oil and are represented by these residues.(8)

The above mentioned characteristics make S.O. the only substance which can be safely used today as permanent internal tamponade, even though with reservation; we think that it is indicated in very severes cases as:

- Complicated detachments with P.V.R.
- Giant tears
- Traumatic detachments
- "Florid" diabetic retinopathy
- Iatrogenc retinal complication during vitrectomy

But we have to underline that the use of this substance necessitates a great experience in vitreo-retinal surgery.

For instance a primary R.D. with P.V.R. atsuch stages. A traumatic detachment, immediately after trauma, may lead to a S.O. vitrectomy even without the presence of P.V.R. On the contrary a traumatic detachment occurring some time after trauma can be managed conventionally because of the fact that we can consider primary detachment. In giant tears, vitrectomy and S.O. seem to be the only approach. This pathology is thought to be a prestage of P.V.R., but surgeon experience is essential in evaluating also these severe R.D. that is because, for example, in a superior giant tear without detachment a vitrectomy and gas can be successfully attempted. In diabetic patients with proliferating retinopathy and detachments due to traction, presenting vascoularized membranes, it is advisable to carry out vitrectomy and exchange with oil. Other indicatios, in the group of patients with diabetics can be: complete detachment, subtotal detachment, posterior breaks, florid retinopathy with or without detachment (high-risk pathology).Today a problem which assumes technical importance is that the retina can be detached even without the presence of a hole or break; it is assumed that this is possible because of the phenomenon of retina shortening which, on the contrary seems due to pre and subretinal proliferation. In these cases it is essential to remove any traction on the retina, carrying out a radical vitrectomy, a careful peeling of membranes a total removal of the "anterior scoffolds" in order to reduce reproliferation.The retina must be mobilized as possible, and if remains shortened, a retinotomy should immediately carried out.Infact a rigid retina will never be able to became flat and during the exchange there is increasing risk that has S.O. behind the retina, complicating the situation.

RESULTS

We selected 54 patients with complicated P.V.R. R.D. ; they had an average follow up of 6 months. All of them have been operated during this last year since we have partially modified our surgical approach. Infact we have used SO for about 7 years and of course we changed continuously techniques and indications in relation to our experience and new concepts in this kind of surgery.(31)

Therefore it is difficult to consider an homogeneous group of P.V.R. patients and decide to examine those one operated during the last year because our approach is partially changed. Nowadays the goal of our surgical technique is:

- lens removal to avoid late reproliferation after cataract extraction
- vitreous base, all anterior membranes and zonule removal
- radical vitrectomy and peeling
- retinotomy if necessary to avoid retina schortening.

Collecting our results in this paper we did not take care about visual acuity because we experienced that, most of the times, when we got surgical success there was functional success, even if it was not possible to quantify visual acuity, because so often it is limited to "navigation vision". So we decided to consider only surgical success on the table(46=85,1%) and failures (8=14,8%).

Examining success we had to underline what we consider partial success (10=18,5%), infact in these cases we found visible membranes reproliferation with or without localized R.D.; consequently many of this patients must be reoperated.

CONCLUSION

S.O. must not be considered a resolutive mean for P.V.R., infact it works only mechanically offering a resistence to retina retraction, but it does not intrude on the biological process of proliferation which may continue its course. Nowadays it is the only means available which could temporarily limit damages by so severe R.D. looking forward the day of further technical and pharmacological solution.

REFERENCES

1 Barthelemy F., Chauvaud D., Frota A. Utilisation de l'huile de silicone en tamponnement transitoire dans le traitement des decollements de rètine avec rètraction vitrèo-retinienne. Jour. Fr. Ophthalmol., 1984, 7, 273-277.

2 Beekhuis W. H., Van Rij G., Zivojnovic R. Silicone oil keratopathy indication for keratoplasty. Brit. J. Ophthalmol. 1985, 69, 4, 247-253.

3 De Juan E. Jr., Mccuen B., Tiedeman J. Intraocular tamponade and surface tension. Surv. Ophthalmol. 1985, 30, 1, 47-51.
4 De Molfetta V., Ardizzone F., Vinciguerra P., Zenoni S. Cataract after pars plana vitrectomy and silicone oil injection. Boll. Men. Soc. Fr. Ophthalmol. 1985, 96, 164-166.
5 Eckardt C., Marin H., Utermann D. Surgical management of subretinal strands in proliferative vitreoretinopathy. Klin. Monastbl. Augenheilkd. 1985, 187, 1, 21-24.
6 Foerster M. H., Esser J., Laqua H. Silicone oil and its influence on electrophysiologic findings. Am. J. Ophthalmol. 1985, 99, 2, 201-206.
7 Fraumar K. D., Gregor Z. J.,Carter R. M., Arden G. Electrophysiological responses after vitrectomy and intraocular tamponade. Proceedings of annual congress of the ophthalmological.Society of the United Kingdom, April 11-13, 1984. Trans. Ophthalmol. Soc. UK. 1985, 104, 2, 129-132.
8 Gabel P., Kampik A., Gabel CH., Spiegel D. Silicone oil with high gravity for intraocular use. In Press.
9 Glaser B. M., Debustros S., Michels R.G. Postoperative retinal breaks occuring after intravitreal silicone oil injection. Retina 1984, 4, 4, 246-248.
10 Gonvers M. Temporary silicone oil tamponade in the management of retinal detachment with proliferative vitreoretinopathy. Am. J. Ophthalmol. 1985, 100, 2, 239-245.
11 Gonvers M. Temporary use of silicone oil in the treatment of special cases of retinal detachment. Ophthalmological, Basel 187: 202-209, 1983.
12 Haut J., Larricart J. P., Van Effenterre G., Pinon- Pignero F. Some of the most important properties of silicone oil to explain its action. Ophthalmologica 1985, 191, 3, 150-153.
13 Haut J. L'intervention vitrectomie-silicone. A propos de 1000 cas. Masson 1984 p. 11-39.
14 Haut J., SeigleP., Larricart P., Flamand M., Vachet J.M. Circular subtotal retinectomy and inferior semicircular retinotomy: preliminary report. Ophthalmologica, Basel 1985, 191, 2, 65-74.
15 Leaver P.K. Principi di tamponamento intraoculare nel trattamento del distacco di retina. Boll. di Ocul.-Suppl. Anno 59-1980, Anno 60-1981, p. 155-157.
16 Leaver P.K. Indicazioni e trattamenti con olio di silicone nella retrazione massiva preretinica. Boll. di Ocul.-Suppl. Anno 59-1980, Anno 60-1981, p. 273-275.
17 Leaver P.K., Len J.S. Management of giant retinal tears using vitrectomy and silicone oil fluid exchange. A preliminary report. Trans. Ophthal. Soc. U.K. 1981, 101, 189.
18 Mccuen II B.W., Landers III M.B., Machemer R. The use of silicone oil following failed vitrectomy for retinal detachment with advances proliferative vitreoretinopathy. Ophthalmology 1985, 92, 8, 1029-1034.
19 Meredith T.A., Lindsey D.T., Edelhauser H.F., Goldman A.I. Elettroretinogramhic studies following vitrectomy and intraocular silicone oil injection. Brit. J. Ophthalmol. 1985, 69, 4, 254-260.

20 Michels R.G. Surgery of retinal detachment with proliferative vitreoretinopathy. Retina 1984, 4, 2, 63-83.
21 Miyamoto K., Refojo M.F., Tolentino F.I., Fournier G.A., Albert D.M. Perfluoroether liquid as a long-term vitreous substitute. An experimental study. Retina 1984, 4, 264-268.
22 Roussat B., Ruellan Y.M. Traitment du dècollement de rètine par vitrectomie et injection d'huile de silicone. Rèsultats ä long terme et complications dans 105 cas. J. Fr. Ophthalmol. 1984, 7, 1, 11-18.
23 Roy D., Tost M. Assessment of the compatinility of gassterilised silicone by implatation in experimental animals. Contactologia 1985, 7, 1, 10-13.
24 Ruellan Y.M., Roussat B. Dècollement de rètine: tamponnement interne provisoire par huile de silicone aprės vitrectomie. Rèsultats anatomiques et fonctionnels. J. Fr. Ophthalmol. 1985, 8, 2, 117-124.
25 Stenderberg P. Jr., Hatchell D.L., Foulks G.N., Landers M.B. The effect of silicone oil on the cornea . Arch. of Ophthalmol. 1985, 103, 1, 90-94.
26 Tavakolian U., Wollensak J. Results after silicone oil injection at different stages of proliferative vitreous retinopathy. 25, Tagung .Osterreich.Ophtalmol.Ges.Wien.,31, 5-2-6, 1984. Klin. Monasbl. Augenheilkd. 1985, 1986, 4, 268-271.
27 Tittarelli R., Benedetti S., Molino N., Attorresi L., Valazzi C.M. Considerazioni sui mezzi di tamponamento interno nella chirurgia vitreo-retinica. Boll. di Ocul. 1985, 64, 5-6, 583-591.
28 Tittarelli R., Benedetti S., Valazzi C.M. L'olio di silicone nel distacco di retina da massiva proliferazione periretinica: indicazioni, tecnica e risultati. Atti Congresso S.O.I., Roma 1982, p. 477-482.
29 Tittarelli R., Benedetti S., Renzulli E. Il ruolo della vitrectomia nei traumi del segmento posteriore. Boll. di Ocul. Anno 65, n.5-6, 1986, p.523-532.
30 Yoshizumi M.O., Dunn B., Ligh J.K., Allman II R.M. Physical properties of vitamin-e oil and silicone oil. Retina 1985, 5, 3, 163-167.
31 Zivojnovic R., Mertens D., Pepenkamp E. Das flussige silikon in der amotiochirurgie. II. Berickt uber 280 falle,weitere entwicklung der. Technik Klin Monatsbl Augenheilkd 1982;181:444 — 452.

Biomaterials and Clinical Applications,
edited by A. Pizzoferrato, P.G. Marchetti, A. Ravaglioli and A.J.C. Lee
Elsevier Science Publishers B.V., Amsterdam, 1987 — Printed in The Netherlands

CROSS LINKED HYALURONATE GELS FOR USE IN VITREOUS SURGERY

T. MÄLSON[a]*, P. ALGVERE[b], L. IVERT[a], B. LINDQVIST[a], G. SELEN[a], S. STENKULA[c]
[a]Pharmacia AB, S-751 82 Uppsala (Sweden)
[b]Dept. of Ophthalmology, Karolinska Hospital, S-104 01 Stockholm (Sweden)
[c]Dept. Ophthalmology, Örebro Region Hospital, S-701 85 Örebro (Sweden)

SUMMARY

Hyaluronic acid can be cross linked with di- or polyfunctional epoxides under alkaline conditions, to form stable ether linked hydrogels. These gels in their swollen state are clear and have a high liquid content (>99%). Their refractive indices are close to that of the swelling medium.

A crushed form of block polymerized gel forms an optically homogeneous mass that can be injected through an injection needle. By altering the synthetic procedure the rheological properties (viscosity, yield point) of these crushed gels can be influenced to differ considerably from those of hyaluronate solutions of similar concentrations. The gels show structural similarities with the natural vitreous.

These gels were injected into the vitreous cavity of vitrectomized rabbits or monkeys and were found to be well tolerated. Clinical evaluation showed no increased postoperative inflammation as compared to sham operated eyes. Intraocular pressure was reduced postoperatively and normalized within a week. The gel remained optically clear and seemed to fill the vitreous cavity. Histology showed signs of slight inflammation in some eyes but there was no difference between eyes injected with gel or salt solution. After six months the gels were still present in the vitreous cavity.

INTRODUCTION

Retinal detachment is the result of fluid accumulation between the photo receptor and the pigment epithelial layers of the retina. Most cases of retinal detachment are caused by the formation of holes in the retina in combination with vitreous tractions. The most common surgical procedure is a local scleral buckling combined with cryopexi. Extraocular surgery is however often insufficient. For example in cases of proliferative vitreoretinopathy (PVR) an intraocular approach with vitrectomy and vitreous injections is often necessary.

A lot of different materials have been tried as vitreous substitutes, to maneouver the retina into position and to support the retina until a firm retino-choroidal adhesion has been achieved. Air has been used for many years but has the disadvantage of being rapidly adsorbed. More recently expanding gases such as SF_6 or C_3F_8 (ref. 1) have proved to be more useful since they last

*To whom all correspondence should be addressed.

longer in the eye. Increased intraocular pressure and formation of posterior capsular cataract are not uncommon after the use of expanding gases. Injection of silicon oil gives a permanent retinal tamponade and the anatomical results are often good. However, since the complication rate is very high (cataract formation, glaucoma and keratopathy) silicon oil is used only in extremely severe cases (ref. 2).

Hyaluronic acid is a major component of the extracellular matrix of the vitreous. Sodium hyaluronate solutions (Healon®) have been shown to be a valuable tool in posterior segment operations (ref. 3). Soluble hyaluronate is however eliminated from the eye and the retinal supporting effect is not longstanding enough in the most severe cases. A rise in intraocular pressure is sometimes seen especially when large amounts of the substance have been used.

Insoluble cross linked hyaluronate gels for gelfiltration were first synthesized by Laurent et al (ref. 4). We have found that cross linked hyaluronate gels have many properties of an ideal vitreous substitute (ref. 5).

RESULTS AND DISCUSSION

The hyaluronate gels are prepared by block polymerization of high molecular weight hyaluronate with di- or polyfunctional epoxides as cross linking agents. The reaction is performed in alkaline solution giving stable ether linkages. Mild conditions have to be used since hyaluronic acid is sensitive both to alkali and heat degradation.

After the cross linking reaction the gels are washed and swollen in an isotonic buffer. The negative charge of the hyaluronate carboxylic groups causes large swelling of the gels, giving them a very high liquid content (>99%). The gel is completely transparent and the refractive index (~1.3350) is very close to that of the swelling medium and to that of the natural vitreous (1.3345-1.3348 (ref. 6)). The gels are thermostable and by heat treatment, they can be liberated completely from all traces of unreacted epoxy groups. They can be sterilized by autoclaving.

The gels in a crushed form can easily be injected through a 0.9 mm needle tip. The crushed gel consisting of irregularly shaped very soft particles, will fill out the space into which it has been injected, forming therein a clear, optically homogenous mass. Under low shear rate the gels have a very high viscosity which means that the gel does not flow out of the compartment into which it has been injected.

The completely swollen gels have a negligible colloid osmotic pressure. Gels with a controllable degree of swelling, can however be made by dehydration of the material. The dehydrated gels might have the advantage of being able to further push the retina back after implantation.

Cell growth experiments on the hyaluronate gels in the form of plates, have been performed with human fibroblasts, primary heart fibroblasts and epithelial cells. Some cells did attach to the gels but the cells were unable to spread out/proliferate or divide. This property of the gels may be important since secondary intravitreal cell proliferation is a common complication in retinal detachement surgery.

We have injected the gels into the vitreous cavity of vitrectomized phakic rabbits, cynomolgus and owl monkeys. More than half the vitreous volume has been exchanged for the gels. The animals have been observed for up to 14 months. No harmful effects of the gels to the eye have been seen.

The intraocular pressure was somewhat reduced postoperatively but normalized within a week. The pattern was the same as in the control BSS injected eyes. The gels remains clear through the whole period and the fundus could be examined with indirect ophthalmoscopy. Clinical evaluation of inflammation showed no difference between gel injected and sham operated eyes. This was also confirmed by white blood cell counts of the aqueous humour of the cynomolgus monkeys. Analysis of remaining gel in the rabbit eyes after six months showed that the injected gel amount was still present in the vitreous cavity.

Histology of the cynomolgus eyes after 14 months showed no damage of the neuroretinal cells, the pigment epithelial cells of pars plana, the ciliary body or the trabecular meshwork.

EXPERIMENTAL

Preparation of hyaluronate gels

Ex. 1. Sodium hyaluronate (molecular weight about 3×10^6, 400 mg) was dissolved in 0.25M sodium hydroxide solution (3 ml) in a centrifuge tube. 1,4-Butandiol diglycidyl ether (BDDE, 25 µl) was added. The tube was centrifuged and heated at $50^{o}C$ for two hours, whereupon it was left standing overnight at room temperature. The gel formed was cut into small pieces and washed thoroughly during a 24 hour period with distilled water to which acetic acid (150 µl) had been added. After heat treatment for 8 hours in boiling phosphate buffered physiological saline (0.276 g $Na_2HPO_4 \cdot 2H_2O$; 0.0395 g $NaH_2PO_4 \cdot H_2O$; 8.476 g NaCl per 1000 ml pH 7.3) the gel was drained and crushed through a 0.5 mm mesh size steel net. The gel was filled into syringes and autoclaved. The total gel yield was 58 g. The refractive index of the gel was 1.3350 and the colloid osmotic pressure 0.1 mm Hg.

The hyaluronate content of the gel was 0.38% measured with the specific hyaluronate method of Jourdian et al (ref. 7).

The amount of BDDE compared to hyaluronate was 3.5% w/w. This analysis was done with ^1H-NMR on an acid degraded gel sample by comparison of the BDDE methylene butane hydrogen atom signals around 1.65 ppm with the hyaluronate N-acetyl methyl hydrogen atom signals around 2.05 ppm.

The epoxide content was <1 ppm (BDDE std.) determined on hyaluronidase degraded gel by the procedure of Nelis and Sinsheimer (ref. 8).

Ex. 2. A somewhat harder gel was prepared in the same way as in 1. but 40 µl BDDE was used as cross linker. Yield: 40 g; Refractive index: 1.3352; Colloid osmotic pressure: 0.9 mm Hg; Hyaluronate content: 0.69%; BDDE/Hyaluronate: 5.0%; Epoxide content: <1 ppm.

REFERENCES

1 S. Chang, H.A. Lincoff, D.J. Coleman, W.J. Fuchs and M.E. Farber, Perfluorocarbon gases in vitreous surgery, Ophthalmology, 92 (1985) 651-656.
2 R. Zivojnovic, D.A.E. Mertens, E. Peperkamp, Das flüssige Silikon in der Amotiochirurgie, Klin. Mbl. Augenheilk. 181 (1982) 444-452.
3 S. Stenkula, L. Ivert, Sodium hyaluronate (Healon®) as an intravitreal aid in retinal and vitreous surgery, J. Ocular Therapy & Surgery 3 (1984) 109-114.
4 T.C. Laurent, K. Hellsing, B. Gelotte, Cross-linked gels of Hyaluronic acid, Acta Chem. Scand. 18 (1964) 274.
5 T. Mälson, B. Lindqvist, Gel av tvärbunden hyaluronsyra för användning som glaskroppssubstitut, Swedish Patent 442820.
6 B.P. Gloor, The vitreous, in: F.H. Adler (ed.), Adler's Physiology of the eye, Mosby, S:t Louis, 1975, p. 255.
7 G. Jourdian, M. Walfman, R. Sarber and J. Distler, A specific, sensitive method for the determination of hyaluronate, Anal. Biochem. 96 (1979) 474-480.
8 H.J. Nelis, J.E. Sinsheimer, A sensitive procedure for the determination of aliphatic epoxides under physiological conditions, Anal. Biochem. 115 (1981) 151-157.

Biomaterials and Clinical Applications,
edited by A. Pizzoferrato, P.G. Marchetti, A. Ravaglioli and A.J.C. Lee
Elsevier Science Publishers B.V., Amsterdam, 1987 — Printed in The Netherlands

CORRELATIVE STUDY OF 1.000 AND 3.000 Cts. SILICONE OILS INJECTED IN RABBIT VITREOUS CHAMBER: MORPHOLOGICAL AND IMMUNOHISTOCHEMICAL ASPECTS.

P.VERSURA, M.C.MALTARELLO, M.CELLINI, R.CARAMAZZA, R.LASCHI

Centre of biotechnological and clinical research in Ophthalmology, Institutes of Ophthalmology and Clinical Electron Microscopy, University of Bologna and IOR-Galileo, Italy.

SUMMARY

Two types of silicone oil at different viscosity (1000 and 3000 centistokes) were injected in the vitreous chamber of albino rabbit eyes. The animals were followed up to two months. Ocular tissues were studied by light microscopy (LM), transmission (TEM) and scanning electron microscopy (SEM); in addition, immuno-histochemical reactions were carried out.

Retina, choroid, ciliary body and iris were less severely involved when silicone oil 3000 cts was used. An immunologic response of the tissues against both materials was present after only one month from the injection.

INTRODUCTION

Liquid silicone oil is a material, usually inert, widely used in various areas of human medicine. Even if all ophthalmologists know the frequent and serious complications induced by the use of silicone oil in the retino-vitreal surgery it is still utilized as it allows positive results, otherwise not achievable.

In our study we have injected two types of silicone oil (1000 and 3000 cts) in the vitreous chamber of rabbit eyes. Retina, choroid, ciliary body, iris and corneal endothelium were studied in light microscopy (LM), transmission (TEM) and scanning electron microscopy (SEM). In addition, immunohistochemical reactions were performed to detect IgG, IgM, IgA and C_{3c} presence.

MATERIALS AND METHODS

16 albino rabbits with an average body weight of 2 kg. were used. The animals were divided into two groups:

1) 8 animals were injected with Dow-Corning silicone oil at a viscosity of 1000 centistokes.

2) 8 animals were injected with Dow-Corning silicone oil at a viscosity of 3000 centistokes.

The silicone (0.75 ml) was injected into the vitreous chamber using the pars-plana vitrectomy following the method of Mukai et al.(1).At the time of surgery 0.2 cc DEPO-MEDROL 40 mg. were sub-conjunctivalyinjected.Twice a day a cortisonic ointment was given topically. The animals were enucleated after 1 and 2 months. Eyeglobes were briefly washed in saline, corneas were excised by threphine to avoid mechanical trauma. The other ocular tissues were cut in small fragments by a razor blade.All the specimens collected were processed as follows:

1) fixed in PLP (periodate-lysine-paraformaldehyde) following (2) for 3 hours at 4°C, overnight washed in 0.1M cacodyalate buffer containing 7% saccarose, abruptly dehydrated in absolute aceton (3 changes, 40 minutes each),embedded in JB_4 (glycol methacrylate, Polysciences,Warrington PA.,USA).Sections 4 um thick were cut by Leitz microtome.We utilized anti-sera anti-rabbit IgG,IgA, IgM from goat, purchased by Miles Laboratories,Inc.,Elkhart, Ind. USA. The reactions were carried out by previous digestion of the section in a specific protease,as suggested by Casanova et al.(3).Sections were incubated following an indirect method in the first specific antiserum diluted 1:30 in PBS. The second fluoresceinated anti-goat IgG antiserum was diluted 1:10 in PBS. The anti-rabbit C_{3c} antiserum was purchased conjugated with FITC (from Nordic Immunological Lab.,Tilburg,The Netherlands) and thus a direct procedure was applied, the antiserum was used diluted 1:10 in PBS. All the labelled sections were observed at the ZEISS III photomicroscope equipped with an epifluorescence condenser.

2) fixed in 2.5% glutaraldehyde in 0.1M phosphate buffer for 3 h at 4°C,post-fixed in 1% OsO_4, embedded in Araldite. Ultrathin sections were observed at the ZEISS EM9 TEM.

Fig.1.Group 1 ---1 month follow up.The retina shows an enlargement of the inter cellular spaces among Mueller cells (arrows).LM,Bar = 100 μm.

Fig.2.Group 1 -- 1 month follow up.An electron dense encrustation is located in an enlarged intercellular space in the retina.TEM, Bar = 1 μm.

Fig.3.Group 1 -- 1 month follow up.Large macrophages (arrows)are observed in the ciliary body stroma. LM, Bar = 100 μm.

Fig.4.Group 1 -- 1 month follow up.IgG presence is evidenced in the ciliary body stroma by immunofluorescence.LM, Bar = 100 μm.

Fig.5.Group 1 -- 1 month follow up.An electron dense encrustation is located in the enlarged spaces among iris epithelial cells. TEM, Bar = 1 μm.

Fig.6.Group 1 -- 2 months follow up. Retina is focally infiltrated by inflammatory cells. LM, Bar = 100 μm.

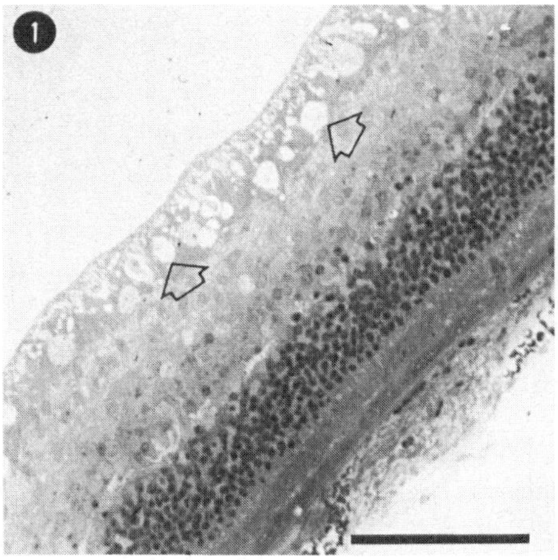
1

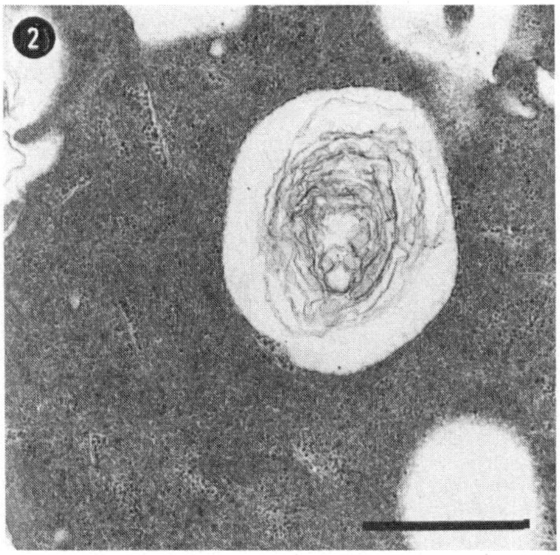
2

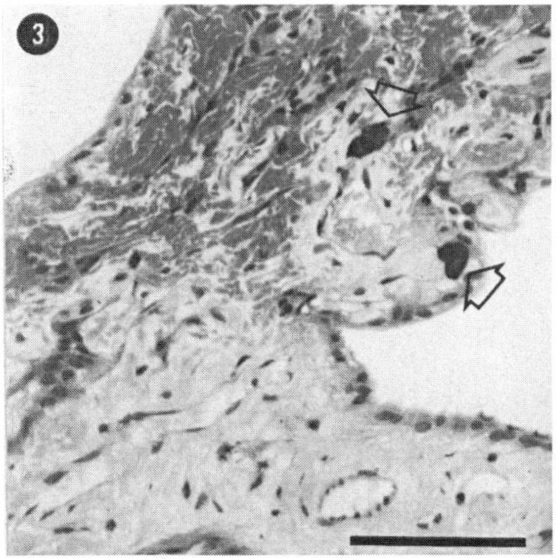
3

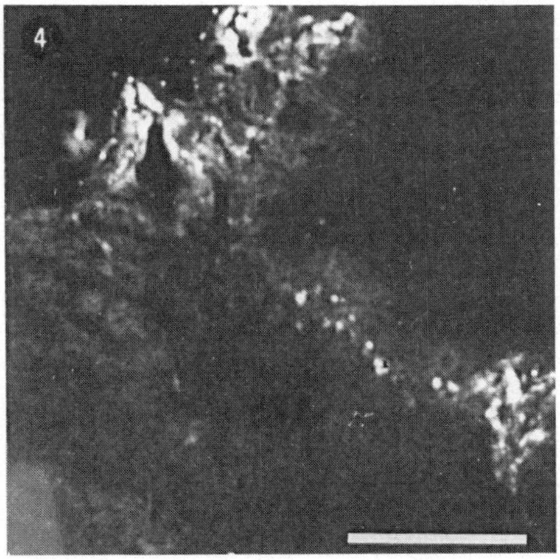
4

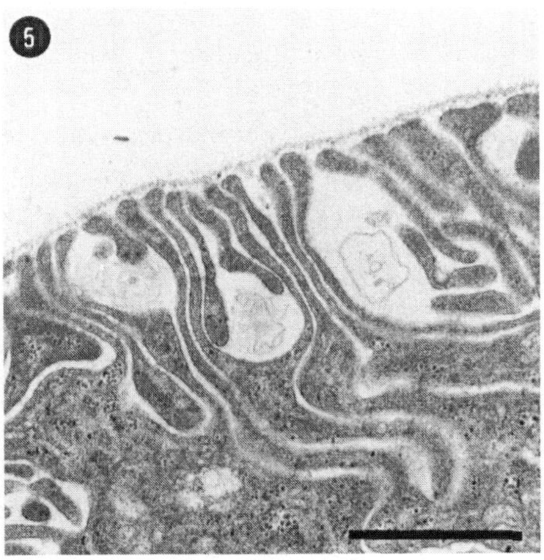
5

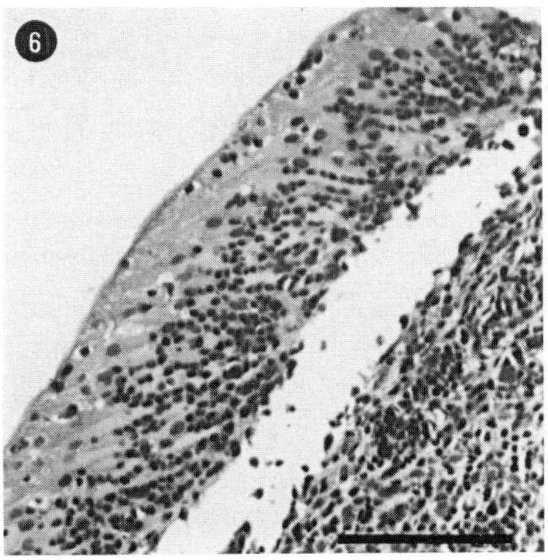
6

3) fixed and postfixed as described in the point 2.,critical point dried, mounted on aluminium stubs, sputtered with gold (20 nm), observed with a Philips 505 SEM.

RESULTS

CLINICAL RESULTS

We have followed up daily the retina by indirect ophthalmoscopy and weekly the anterior segment by slit-lamp examination.

group 1 eyes. In 3 cases, after 2 weeks from the injection, we observed the appearance of an inflammation process along with corneal oedema,Tyndall,shallow of the anterior chamber and finally iris rubeosis. In 1 case silicone oil bubbles were found after 1 week in the anterior chamber. No clinical difference was detected between 1 and 2 months follow up.

group 2 eyes. In this group we never observed inflammatory reactions in both the anterior and posterior segment. One rabbit, after 2 weeks from the injection developed an inverted hypopion which clinically disappeared after one week.

HISTOLOGICAL RESULTS

When the enucleated eyes were cut,the liquid silicone left the vitreous chamber free of any evidence of encapsulation or reaction.

group 1 eyes

1 month follow up. In the retina, we found an enlargement of the intercellular spaces among Mueller cells (fig.1). Numerous spaces contained electron - opaque encrustations (fig.2). In the ciliary body stroma we observed very large phagocitic cells (fig.3).Ciliary body stroma showed a positivity for IgG presence (fig.4). In the iris we did not detect any inflammatory reaction. At the epithelial cell level, we found encrustation figures located in the

Fig.7. Group 2.- 1 month follow up. Retina appears of normal morphology. LM, Bar = 100 µm.

Fig.8. Group 2.- 1 month follow up.IgG located at the iris epithelium level are evidenced by a fluorescent layer (arrow). LM, Bar = 100 µm.

Fig.9. Group 2.- 1 month follow up. C_{3c} in the ciliary body stroma.LM,Bar = 100 µm.

Fig.10.Group 2.- 1 month follow up.Corneal endothelium damage due to a previous hypopion. SEM, Bar = 10 µm.

Fig.11.Group 2.- 2 months follow up.A large macrophage (arrow)in the ciliary body stroma is shown. LM,Bar = 10 µm.

Fig.12.Group 2.- 2 months follow up.Iris morphology appears normal. LM, Bar = 100 µm.

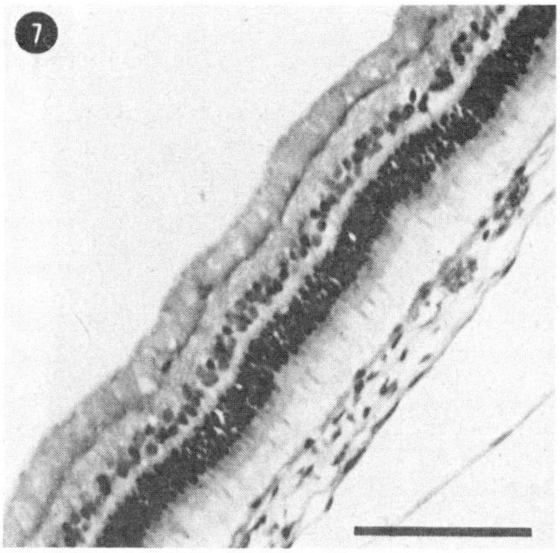
7

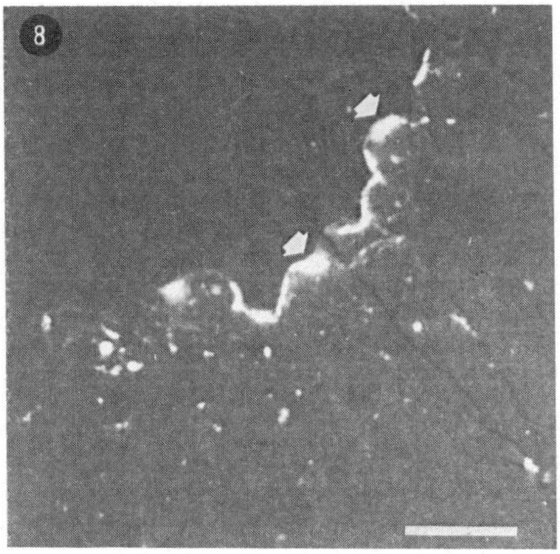
8

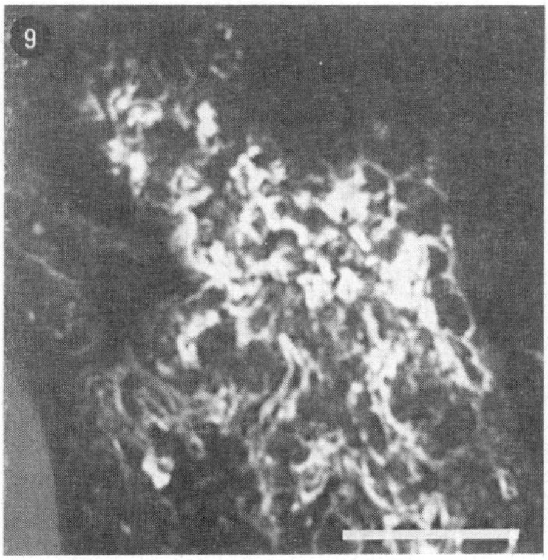
9

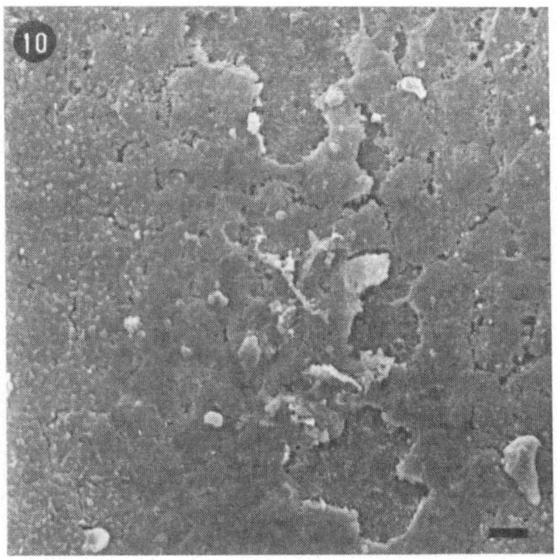
10

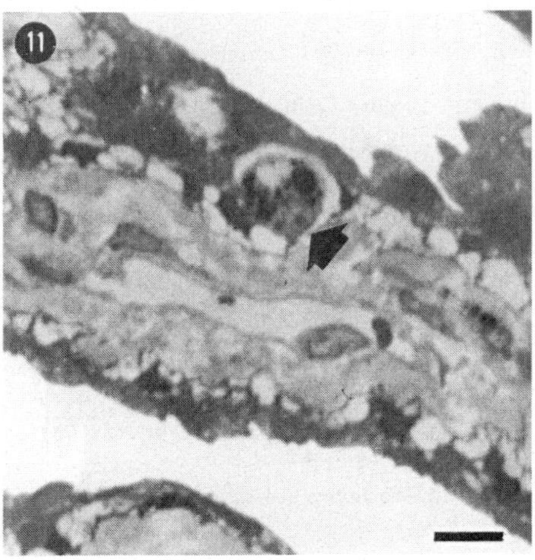
11

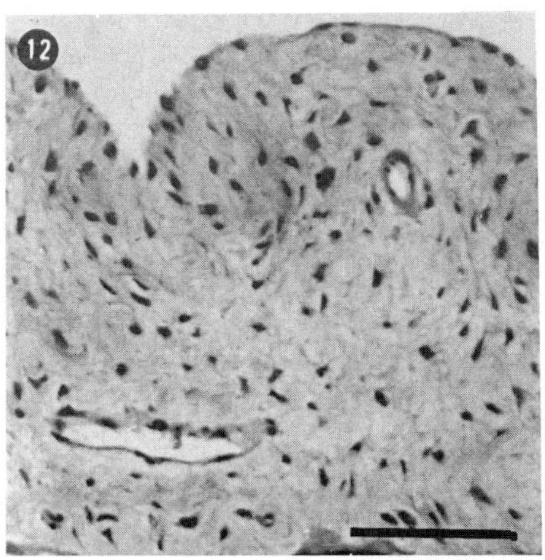
12

enlarged intracellular spaces,similar to those detected in the retina (fig.5).

2 months follow up.We found more severe alterations especially at the retinal and choroidal level.Focally the structure of the retina was almost completely altered as a consequence of a deep inflammatory reaction(fig.6).As to corneal endothelium, small areas devoid of cells were observed.

group 2 eyes

1 month follow up.The retina structure was unaltered(fig.7).Choroid,iris and ciliary body normal morphology was entirely preserved too.No encrustation figures were found as well as no inflammatory cells.IgG and IgM were detected at the iris epithelium level (fig.8) and C_{3c} positivity was shown in the ciliary body stroma (fig.9).In the case with previous hypopion,a severe corneal endothelium change was observed (fig.10).

2 months follow up.In the retina,rare encrustation figures were detected.In the ciliary body,large macrophages(fig.11)were observed.Iris was always of normal appearance (fig.12),only very rare plasmacells were evidenced.Ciliary body stroma was positive for both IgG and C_{3c} presence,iris stroma for IgG only.

DISCUSSION

Clinically,few differences between silicone oil 1000 and 3000 cts injected eyes were observed.According to Mukai et al.(4)the encrustation figures are the expression of a chemical interaction between the silicone oil and the retina cell plasmamembrane phospholipides.In the group 2 eyes we found very few of these figures.This probably because the higher viscosity of the material avoids a clinically evident emulsion of the oil.This characteristic leads to a less severe involvement of the retina,also up to two months follow up.An immunological reaction is present in both groups of eyes,even after only 1 month follow up. Ciliary body and iris epithelium have evidence of production of IgG.We conclude that,even if clinically tolerated, silicone oil (both 1000 and 3000 cts)evokes an immunological response and this fact has to be considered when evaluating the long-term permanence of the material in the human eye.

REFERENCES

1. Mukai N. et al. Intravitreous injection of silicone:an experimental study II Histochemistry and electron microscopy.Ann.Ophthalmol. 4(1972):273.
2. McLean at al. Periodate-lysine-paraformaldehyde fixative.A new fixative for immunoelectron microscopy. J.Histochem.Cytochem. 22 (1974):1077.
3. Casanova et al. Immunohistochemical staining on Hydroxyethyl-Methacrylate-embedded tissues. J.Histochem.Cytochem.31 (1983)1000-1004.
4. Mukai N.et al.A long term evaluation of silicone retinopathy in monkeys.Canad.J.Opht.10(75)391-402.

Biomaterials and Clinical Applications,
edited by A. Pizzoferrato, P.G. Marchetti, A. Ravaglioli and A.J.C. Lee
Elsevier Science Publishers B.V., Amsterdam, 1987 — Printed in The Netherlands

A COMPOSITE HYDROGEL FOR TREATMENT OF SKIN WOUNDS: SKIN GRAFT DONOR SITES IN PIGS AND HUMAN PATIENTS

M. SPECTOR[1], L. RHINELANDER[1] and F. NAHAI[2]

[1]Department of Orthopaedics
Emory University School of Medicine, Atlanta, GA, 30322, USA

[2]Division of Plastic Surgery
Emory University School of Medicine, Atlanta, GA, 30322, USA

SUMMARY

The objective of these studies was to evaluate the healing of partial-thickness skin graft donor sites treated with a polyacrylamide-agar composite hydrogel, Geliperm, in miniature pigs and human patients. Multiple donor sites on four miniature pigs were treated with Geliperm or fine mesh gauze (air-dried). Animals were sacrificed after five days and the thickness of the epithelium evaluated histomorphometrically. Human patients treated with Geliperm or Xeroform (air-exposed, dry control) were evaluated with respect to healing time and pain. The epithelium at Geliperm-treated donor sites on the pigs was thicker (89 vs. 55 µm) and more continous than at the air-exposed (dry) sites. Geliperm could be removed from the donor site during the treatment period without disrupting the regenerating epithelium. Human donor sites treated with Geliperm were judged to require no further treatment 5-7 days postoperatively. The Xeroform required 14-21 days to slough from the wound. Patients generally reported less pain with the moist treatment. These results demonstrate the beneficial effects of treating donor sites with a polyacrylamide-agar composite hydrogel.

INTRODUCTION

Over 20 years ago investigators demonstrated in animals (ref. 1) and in human patients (ref. 2) that a moist environment enhances epithelialization of partial-thickness excision wounds. However, dry dressing for skin graft donor sites is still widespread. The initial studies on moist wound healing and several current clinical investigations have employed occlusive (refs. 3-5) and semi-occlusive (refs. 6-9) films. An undesireable feature of these occlusive films is the excessive fluid accummulation that develops. This condition may potentiate infection; for it generally leads to leakage of fluid from the wound site contaminating surrounding areas.

The objective of this investigation was to determine the efficacy of a composite hydrogel (providing moist healing) for the treatment of skin graft donor sites in miniature pigs and human patients. Controls were sites covered with gauze and allowed to air dry. Previous investigations have demonstrated some of the potential advantages of hydrogel materials (refs. 10-13). These substances can maintain a moist environment at the wound site while absorbing some of the excess fluid exudate. Since the sheets are nonadherent to the skin surface, dressing changes can be accomplished without disturbing the epithelium. Moreover, these materials can be impregnated with selected agents for delivery to the wound site. One hydrogel that appears particularly promising is a polyacrylamide-agar composite (Geliperm, Geistlich-Pharma, Wolhusen, Switzerland). This substance is approximately 97% water. It is available in sheets 3.3 mm thick. Geliperm is impermeable to bacteria but permeable to molecules of 1 million dalton. It is nonadherent and transparent, plus has sufficient strength for the handling required when treating skin wounds. Previous studies have reported its performance in animal studies (ref. 14) and human trials (refs. 15,16). Its chemical and physical properties (ref. 17) and biocompatibility (ref. 18) have also been addressed in prior publications.

METHODS

Animal Studies

Four miniature pigs were employed in this investigation. Four to six partial-thickness skin graft donor sites were produced on each animal. The test sites were treated with Geliperm sheets. Control sites on the same animal were covered with a fine mesh gauze and allowed to dry with exposure to air. All animals were sacrificed five days postoperatively. Tissues from test and control sites were fixed in formalin, embedded in glycol methacrylate, and cut with glass knives on a Sorvall JB-4 microtome. Because removal of the fine mesh gauze disrupted the regenerating epithelium, histological sections were made with the gauze in place. The thickness of the regenerating epithelium at several different test and control sites was obtained with a computerized image analysis system.

Human Trial

A pilot trial of the Geliperm for treatment of donor sites was undertaken in 10 patients. Four of these patients had a second donor site employed as a control. The control sites were treated with Xeroform (gauze impregnated with a petrolatum blend) and allowed to air dry. The evaluation involved recording healing time (time at which treatment could be discontinued and the surface was judged to be reepithelialized). Estimates of site pain and fluid accumulation were also noted.

RESULTS

The hydrogel dressing could be removed from the donor sites without disrupting the underlying tissue. In contrast the fine mesh gauze was always found to be incorporated into the donor sites in the animals and human patients. Rarely was fluid accumulation found under the hydrogel sheets on the pigs. In the human patients, accumulation of some fluid exudate was found on the first two days postoperatively. The amount of fluid appeared to be related to the depth of graft harvested. For grafts of normal thickness minimal accumulation was noted.

After five days a milky substance was found under the Geliperm sheets at the moist donor sites in the pigs. At this stage, rarely had sloughing of the dried mesh gauze begun on the control wounds which were red and crusty. Histological evaluation revealed that the milky substance under the Geliperm comprised hydrated necrotic cells and proteinaceous exudate which were overlying the reepithelialized surface of the wound. The epithelial layer at the Geliperm treated sites was significantly thicker and more continous than that seen at the dry, air exposed controls (Fig. 1-Table 1). Moreover, more keratination was seen in the epithelium at the Geliperm treated sites than at the dry controls (Fig. 1a). Histologically, fibers of the fine mesh gauze

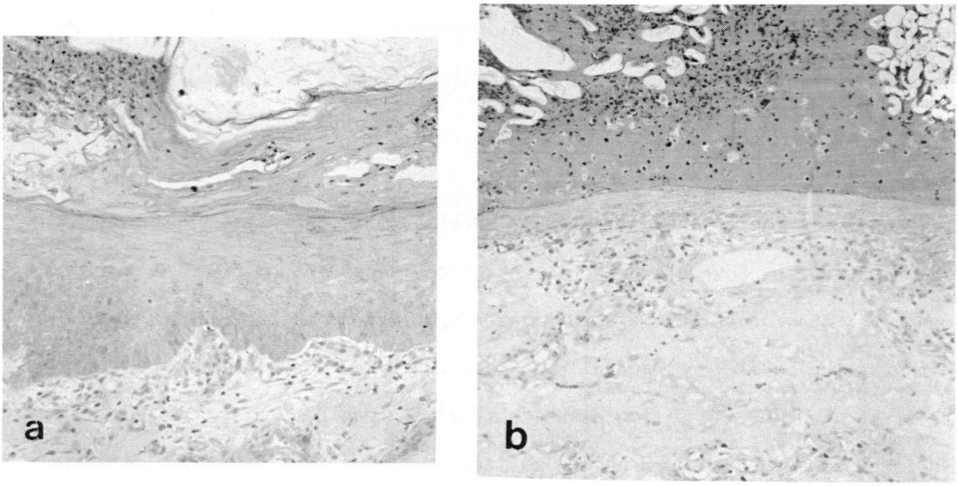

Fig. 1. Histology of Geliperm treated (a) and dry (b) donor sites (5 days).

TABLE 1

Thickness of the epithelium, 5 days postoperatively

	n	Thickness (μm)
Geliperm treated sites	6	89 ± 25
Dry, control	8	55 ± 22
$p < 0.01$		

were noted to be adjacent to epithelial cells, potentially interfering with reepithelialization (Fig. 1b). Histology also confirmed previous findings that the epithelial lining of the hair follicles was the source of the regenerating surface epithelium (ref. 19).

Geliperm treatment of 11 donor sites on 10 patients resulted in a mean healing time of 6.5 days. In a few patients extended times for healing (greater than 7 days) were due to slippage of the hydrogel from the wound with subsequent drying. Four control donor sites in this group, treated with Xeroform, required more than 12.5 days for the dressing to slough. These results are consistent with historical experience with Xeroform in which 14-21 days are required for the dressing to be removed from the wound without disrupting the epithelium. The patients generally experienced less pain at the moist sites than at those allowed to dry with exposure to air.

DISCUSSION

These results demonstrate that the moist environment provided by a hydrogel can accelerate the reepithelialization of skin graft donor sites. In the miniature pigs after five days the Geliperm treated sites displayed epithelium which was thicker and more continous than that seen at the air dried mesh gauze sites. In the human patients the healing time was on the order of five to seven days. These results are comparable to previous investigations evaluating the healing time at donor sites with moist treatment afforded by an occlusive, adhesive film (ref. 5). Donor sites treated with an adhesive polyurethane film were found to heal after seven days whereas sites treated with Scarlet Red impregnated gauze and porcine xenograft were found to heal after 10 and 12 days, respectively. However, potential drawbacks of treatment with the occlusive film were the considerable fluid accummulation and adherence of the dressing to the bordering skin.

In the current study one of the benefits seen with the hydrogel was the absorption of some of the excess fluid exudate. To further enhance the absorption of fluid from the wound site perforated sheets of Geliperm were investigated in a few patients. In the first two days postoperatively the exudate was found to pass through the perforations in the hydrogel sheet to be absorbed by the secondary gauze dressing overlying the Geliperm. Absorption of this transudate from the wound surfaces also facilitated stabilization of the sheets on the donor sites. In a preliminary series of three patients treated with the perforated sheets the healing time was found to be seven days.

These studies demonstrate the efficacy of a polyacrylamide-agar composite hydrogel for the treatment of skin graft donor sites.

REFERENCES

1 G.D. Winter, Formation of the scab and rate of epithelialization of superficial wounds in the skin of the young domestic pig, Nature, 193 (1962) 293-294.

2 C.D. Hinman and H. Maibach, Effect of air exposure and occlusion on experimental human skin wounds, Nature (London), 200 (1963) 377.

3 J.H. James and A.C.H. Watson, The use of Op-site, a vapour permeable dressing, on skin graft donor sites, Br. J. Plastic Surg., 28 (1975) 107-10.

4 M.J. Tavis, J.W. Thornton, R.H. Bartlett, J.C. Roth and E.A. Woodroof, A new composite skin prosthesis, Burns, 7(2) (1980) 123-30.

5 S.R. May, Physiology, immunology, and clinical efficacy of an adherent polyurethane wound dressing: Op-site, in: D.L. Wise (Ed.), Burn Wound, Volume II, CRC Press, Inc., 1984, pp. 53-78.

6 J.W. Alexander, L.M. Wheeler, R.C. Rooney, J.J. McDonald and B.G. MacMillan, ClinicaL evaluation of epigard, a new synthetic substitute for homograft and heterograft skin, 13(4) (1973) 374-83.

7 G.D. Winter, Epidermal wound healing under a new polyurethane foam dressing, Plast. Reconstr. Surg., 56 (1975) pp. 531-537.

8 M.I. Dinner, C.R. Peters, and J. Sherer, Use of a semipermeable polyurethane membrane as a dressing for split-skin graft donor sites, Plast. Reconstr. Surg., 64(1) (1979) pp. 112-114.

9 L. Norton and M. Chvapil, Comparison of newer synthetic and biological wound dressings, J. Trauma, 21(6) (1981), 463-8.

10 D.P. Dressler, W.K. Barber and R. Sprenger, The effect of hydron burn wound dressing on burned rat and rabbit ear wound healing, J. Trauma, 20(12) (1980) 1024-8.

11 R.J. Warren and C.F.T. Snelling, Clinical evaluation of the hydron burn dressing, Plastic and Reconstructive Surgery, 66 (3)(1980) 361-8.

12 S.H. Mandy, A new primary wound dressing made of polyethylene oxide gel, J. Dermatol. Surg. Oncol. 9(2) (1983) 153-5.

13 C. Migliaresi, A poly-2-hydroxyethylmethacrylate based laminate as potential burn wound covering, in: D.L. Wise (Ed.), Burn Wound, Volume II, CRC Press, Inc., 1984, pp. 137-146.

14 M. Spector, P. Weissgerber, N. Reese and S.L. Harmon, A polyacrylamide - agar hydrogel material for the treatment of burns, Trans. 8th. Ann. Mtg. Soc. for Biomat'l., 5 (1982) p. 68.

15 H. Wokalek, E. Schopf, E. Vaubel, B. Kickhofen, and H. Fischer, First experiences with a transparent liquid gel in the treatment of fresh operation wounds and chronic epithelial defects of the skin, Aktuelle Dermatologie, 5 (1979) 3-13.

16 U. Knapp, H.D. Rahn, and F. Schauwecker, Clinical experience with a new gel-like wound dressing after skin graft, Modern Trauma, 14(6), (1984) pp. 237-286.

17 B. Kickhofen, H. Wokalek, D. Scheel, and H. Ruh, Chemical and physical properties of a hydrogel wound dressing, Biomaterials, 7 (1986) 67-72.

18 D.E. Taylor and J.E. Penhollow, Comparative Biotolerance of polyacrylamide-agarose gel, silicone rubber and microporous PTEF as soft tissue implants, Biomaterials, 7 (1986) 277-82.

19 G.D. Winter, Epidermal regeneration studied in the domestic pig, in: H.I. Maibach and D.T. Rovee (Eds.), Epidermal Wound Healing, Year Book Medical Publishers, Inc., 1972, pp. 71-112.

Biomaterials and Clinical Applications,
edited by A. Pizzoferrato, P.G. Marchetti, A. Ravaglioli and A.J.C. Lee
Elsevier Science Publishers B.V., Amsterdam, 1987 — Printed in The Netherlands

A NEW PERMEABLE POLYETHERURETHANE WOUND COVERING: A PRELIMINARY STUDY OF WATER VAPOUR PERMEABILITY AND WOUND HEALING

M.F. JONKMAN[1], H.J. MEIJER[3], J.W. LEENSLAG[3], A.J. PENNINGS[3], P. NIEUWENHUIS[2] and I. MOLENAAR[1]

[1]Centre for Medical Electron Microscopy, [2]Department of Histology and [3]Department of Polymer Chemistry, State University of Groningen, Oostersingel 69/2, 9713 EZ Groningen, The Netherlands.

SUMMARY

An environment-independent method is described for assessment of water vapour permeability of membranes. A polyetherurethane (PEU) wound covering was compared with Op-Site for water vapour permeability. The in vitro permeability assessment correlated to the in vivo evaporative water loss in superficial wounds in rats. The permeable PEU wound covering promptly absorbs the wound exudate, forming a jelly-like clot underneath, that prevents further dermal desiccation. On the contrary, the more occlusive Op-Site adheres poorly to the wound surface. The epithelialization took 3 days for both coverings, while 5 days for uncovered wounds. Keratinization of the new epidermis was earlier found under PEU wound covering than under Op-Site.

INTRODUCTION

It is commonly accepted that the ideal wound covering should mimic many properties of human skin, that is, it should be adhesive, elastic, durable, impermeable to bacteria and occlusive (ref. 1). An occlusive wound covering limits evaporative water loss and thus prevents body heat loss. It also maintains a high humidity at the wound site, promoting cell migration across the wound surface (ref. 2).

However, an occlusive wound covering retaining too much wound exudate, gives rise to undesirable effects of poor adherence, bullae, tissue maceration and the risk of infection (ref. 3).

Preliminary results are presented of a study into the effect of evaporative water loss on wound healing, using a permeable and an occlusive wound covering in superficial wounds in rats. For this, we had to develop a new in vitro method for water vapour permeability assessment of membranes, which is also described.

MATERIALS AND METHODS

Material characteristics. Two wound coverings were compared: a polyetherurethane (PEU) film made by one of the authors and Op-Site^{R}, a

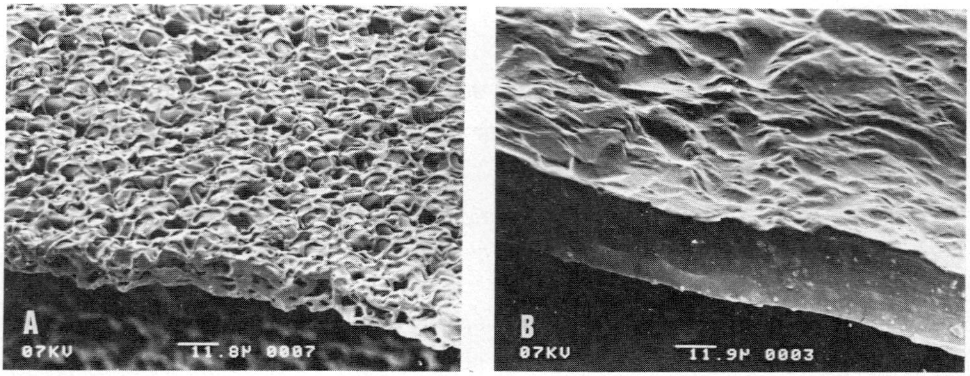

Fig. 1. Scanning electron microscopy of the PEU film showes a rough surface with microscopic holes underneath (a). Op-Site showes a smoother surface and lacks the cavernous structure (b).

commercially available product (T.J.Smith & Nephew Ltd., Hull, UK). Both wound coverings are photographed in dry state with the scanning electron microscope, therefore not showing the swollen state in water.

The material characteristics are summarized in Table 1.

TABLE 1

Material characteristics of two wound coverings in dry state.

	PEU wound covering	Op-Site
chemical composition		
- film	polyetherurethane	polyetherurethane
- adhesive layer	-	vinyl ether
thickness (μm)		
- dry	10	30
- wet	140	30
water absorbance (% dry wt)	2900	190
porosity (%)	50	0
hole size (μm)	15	-
Youngs modulus (10^6.N.m^{-2})	2.08	4.17
elongation (%)	1150	750
surface free energy (erg.cm^{-2})		
- wound side	53	26
- air exposed side	53	44

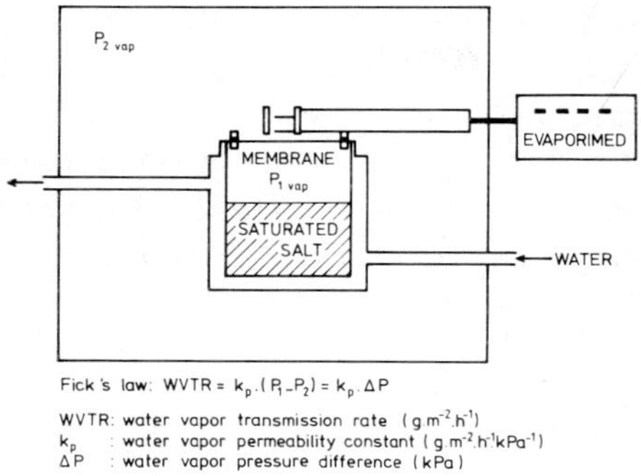

Fig. 2. Design for assessing water vapor permeability of membranes.

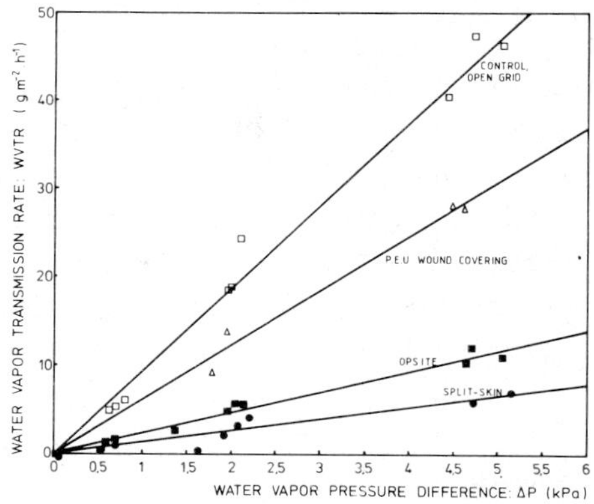

Fig. 3. Water vapor permeability of wound coverings in vitro.

<u>Evaporimetry in vitro</u>. The film is stretched over a glass vial (Fig. 2). The temperature can be controlled by flushing water through the double wall of the vial. The vapour pressure under the film is saturated and can be controlled by using different salt solutions ($Mg(NO_3)_2$, K_2SO_4) and temperatures (25°, 37° C).

The vial is housed in a climatebox. The vapour pressure P_{2vap} is measured with the evaporimeter EP1 (Evaporimed, Stockholm). By choosing $P_{1vap} > P_{2vap}$, a water vapour diffusion is generated upwards through the film, simulating the state of the moist wound. The water vapour transmission rate (WVTR) of the film is measured according to Nilsson (ref. 4), by placing the probe of the evaporimeter directly above the film. The WVTR is registered when the value has stabilized.

According to Fick's law of diffusion the WVTR through the film is linearly proportional to ΔP (Fig. 2).

This experiment was executed with PEU covering, Op-Site, human split skin and an open metal grid (porosity 64%) as reference at various P.

<u>Evaporative water loss in vivo</u>. Rats were anaesthetized with chloralhydrate and their backs clipped. A 2 x 5 cm dermabrasive wound was made with a scalpel by repeated scraping with the sharp edge until punctated bleeding was seen. The wound coverings were applied and protected by hydrophile bandage during the first two days.

The WVTRs of the applied wound coverings were measured with the evaporimeter after removal of the bandage under standard room conditions (P ~ 5 kPa) for 15 days.

Histology. Half of the wounds were covered with dry PEU wound covering, the other half with Op-Site. Of each wound a part was left uncovered as a control. The wound coverings were not replaced. A 2 mm punch biopsy was taken after 1, 2, 3, 5 and 7 days from the covered and uncovered part of each wound under ether aneasthesia.

The specimens were fixed in 2% glutaraldehyde in 0.1 M phosphate buffer (pH = 7.4) for 24 hours. The specimens were embedded in glycol methacrylate (GMA), cut in 2 um sections, stained in toluidine blue - basic fuchsine and observed with the light microscope.

RESULTS

Evaporimetry. The relationship between WVTR and ΔP for all 4 membranes (Fig. 3) is linearly proportional according to Fick's law. The permeability constants for water vapour are presented in tabel 2. The permeability of Op-Site most resembles the occlusive human split-skin. The permeability of PEU wound covering is relatively high: 70% of the permeability of an open metal grid.

TABLE 2
Water vapor permeablity constants of wound coverings

Wound covering	Permeability constant K_p ($g.m^{-2}.h^{-1}.kPa^{-1}$)
Control, open grid	9.1
PEU film	6.3
Op-Site	2.2
Split-skin	1.2

During the first day the WVTR in the covered wounds remained constant and declined in 7 days to normal values. Till day 4, PEU wound covering loose 3 times more water than Op-Site (Fig. 4). In the uncovered wound the high WVTR continued for 2 days and normal values were reached only after 15 days.

Wound healing. The depth of the standard wounds was subepidermal, leaving the hair follicles intact.

The PEU wound covering was easier to handle than Op-Site, because PEU had no sticky adhesive layer. The dry PEU wound covering promptly adhered to the wet wound surface and swells. In contrast, Op-Site only adhered to the dry intact skin surrounding the wound.

In the uncovered wounds the exudate had concentrated into a dry clot

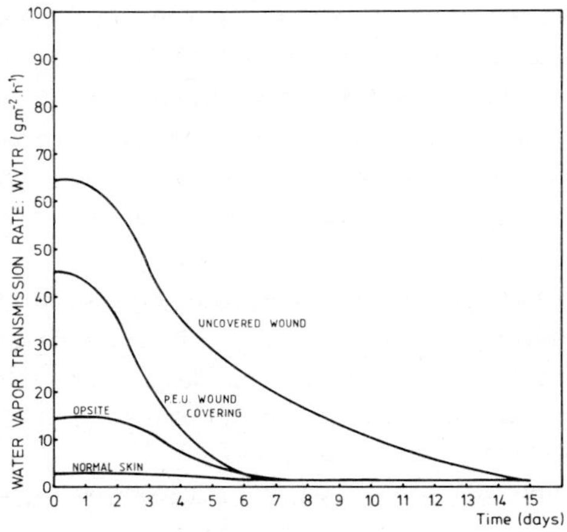

Fig. 4. Evaporative water loss in covered superficial wounds.

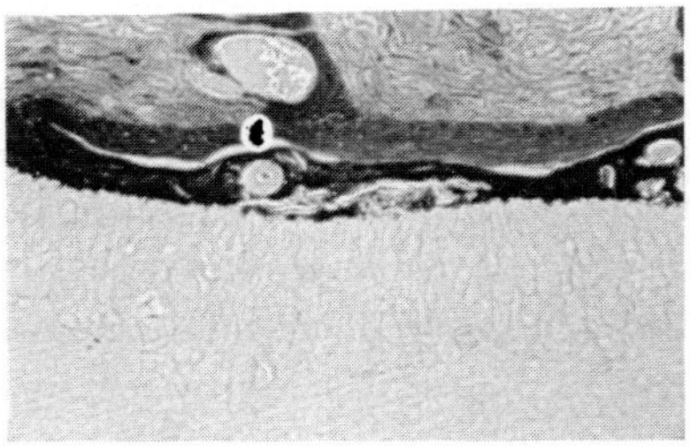

Fig. 5. PEU film adheres to the clot covering the new epidermis.

by **24 hours**; under the PEU wound covering a jelly-like clot had formed, while under Op-Site the exudate remained liquid.

In all wounds keratinocytes started to proliferate at the hair follicles after **2 days.** Under both wound coverings the keratinocytes used the dermal wound surface as a functional substrate for migration. Under PEU covering the migration took place under the clot, while under Op-Site migration was directly under the film. The PEU film firmly adhered to the clot (Fig. 5). In the uncovered wounds the top of the dermis dried out and formed, together with the clot, a dry scab that covered the underlying viable part of the dermis. The keratinocytes migrated under the scab thus separating viable and non-viable tissue.

After **3 days** all PEU- and Op-Site-covered wounds were completely reepithelialized. The control wounds did not yet show complete epithelialization. The starting keratinization of new epidermis under the PEU wound covering was more pronounced than under Op-Site.

By **7 days** Op-Site prematurely detached from half of the wounds. The PEU wound covering still remained adhering to the clot.

By **10 days** the PEU wound covering with the clot came off spontaneously, as did the scabs in the uncovered wounds. No infection was seen in any wound.

DISCUSSION

A new method was developed to determine permeability constants of films. This constant (K_p: $g.m^{-2}.h^{-1}.kPa^{-1}$) enables us to express water vapor permeability independent of environmental conditions.

The high permeability constant of the PEU wound covering is explained by the special cavernous structure of the material. Each hole becomes an extra force for water diffusion. The effective path for diffusion through PEU material is considerably shorter than the total film thickness, because water molecules have to pass only through approximately 15 PEU walls of 0.5 µm: the net polymer diffusion path is 7.5 µm instead of 20 µm in Op-Site.

The PEU covering adhered well to the wound surface, due to exudate absorption. The initial high evaporative water loss in PEU-covered wounds induces clot formation by concentration of the exudate. The PEU film and clot together are impermeable enough to prevent dermal desiccation, thus preserving the viabilility of the dermis.

The high absorbance capacity of PEU wound covering is probably due to the hydrophilic material in combination with the cavernous structure. The microscopic holes are not interconnected, so the PEU covering most probably will form a barrier to bacteria. Bacterial penetration studies are in progress.

A possible explanation for the early keratinization under PEU wound covering is the beneficial effect of the clot proteins on wound healing and exposure to air through the PEU membrane (ref. 5). The exudate is not totally dried out as in the uncovered wound, nor is it fluid as in Op-Site, but it remains in a jelly-like state.

In **conclusion**, our results demonstrate that PEU wound covering exhibits those properties that are considered ideal: it combines elasticity with high water absorbance capacity and good adherence to the wound surface. The relatively high water vapour permeability of PEU wound covering prevents infection of a fluid exudate, but concentrates the exudate to a jelly-like clot that apparently stimulates epidermal wound healing.

Acknowledgements: We gratefully wish to thank Bert Blauw for preparing the histological sections, Freark Dijk for preparing the scanning electron microscopy and Ietse Stokroos for designing the figures. This study was supported by grants from Science Park Foundation and the Prevention Fund.

REFERENCES

1 B. Alsbjörn, In search of an ideal skin substitute, Scan. J. Plast. Reconstr. Surg. 18 (1984) 127-133.
2 G.D. Winter, Formation of the scab and the rate of epithelialization of superficial wounds in the skin of the young pig, Nature, 193 (1962) 431.
3 K.J. Quinn, J.M. Courtney, J.H. Evans, J.D.S. Gaylor, W.H. Reid, Principles of burn dressings, Biomaterials, 6 (1985) 369-377.
4 G.E. Nilsson, Measurement of water exchange through skin, Med. & Biol. Eng. & Compat., 15 (1977) 209-218.
5 L.B. Fisher, H.I. Maibach, The effect of occlusive and semipermeable derssings on the mitotic activity of normal and wounded human epidermis, Br. J. Derm. 86 (1972) 593-600.

Biomaterials and Clinical Applications,
edited by A. Pizzoferrato, P.G. Marchetti, A. Ravaglioli and A.J.C. Lee
Elsevier Science Publishers B.V., Amsterdam, 1987 — Printed in The Netherlands

EFFECT OF FIBRIN SEALS ON HUMAN FIBROBLAST ATTACHMENT AND MULTIPLICATION.

M.F. HARMAND[1], D. MICHEL[1], M. BAGOT d'ARC[2], and D. DUCASSOU[1]

[1]INSERM SC 31 - Université de Bordeaux II, Rue Léo Saignat, F33076 BORDEAUX
[2]Service ORL - Hôpital Cochin, 27, rue du Faubourg St-Jacques,F75674 PARIS

SUMMARY

Growth of both dermal and gingival human fibroblasts was studied onto fibrin seal (FS) substrata, using varying thrombin, Ca^{++} and aprotinin concentrations. Final concentration of 50 UI thrombin per ml, 150-1500 KIU aprotinin per ml and 2-10 mM Ca^{++} allowed maximum mitogenic activity of thrombin. Three fibrin seals, commercially available, were compared using cell viability, attachment and proliferation as parameters of cytocompatibility : our study demonstrates the excellent biocompatibility of "FS I" when compared with both "FS II" and "FS III".

INTRODUCTION

Blood clot has been long proved effective in tissue adhesion and stimulation of normal healing, partly through a network of polymerized fibrin. Fibrin seals (FS) are two component seals : the first component, the fibrin seal proper, contains highly concentrated fibrinogen and factor XIII together with fibronectin, plasminogen and aprotinin, a protease inhibitor ; the second component, consists of thrombin and calcium chloride. Upon mixing the two components, coagulation occurs and the fibrin formed is progressively crosslinked by activated factor XIII. The purpose of the present work was to study the growth of both dermal and gingival human fibroblasts onto and within such reconstituted clots, particularly investigating the effect of thrombin.

METHODS

Cell cultures

Fibroblast cultures are obtained by subculturing of cells arising by outgrowth from biopsies of normal human skin (35 years - strain HSF 35) or healthy human gingiva (35 years - strain HGF 35). Cells are grown in a medium consisting of NCTC 109 Vitamin D_2 and A-free/RPMI 1640 (v/v) supplemented with 10 % (v/v) fetal calf serum, in an humidified atmosphere of 95 % air/5 % CO_2, at 37°C. Growth medium is changed every 3 days. Cells are used between the 2nd and fifth passage.

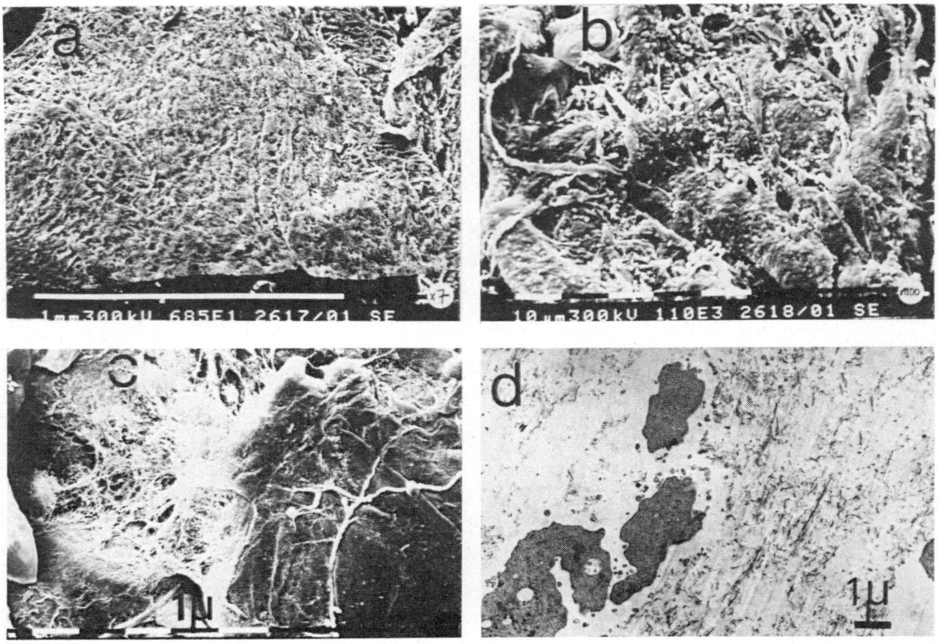

Fig. 1. Human skin fibroblasts cultivated onto "FS I" : (a) (b) (c) scanning electron microscopy, (d) transmission electron microscopy.

Preparation of fibrin-seal coated wells

Three fibrin sealants are studied : "FS I" (Tisseal® -Immuno-Vienne - Austria), "FS II" (Transglutine - CRTS-Strasbourg - France), "FS III" (Colle biologique - CRTS-Lille - France). The bottom of multiwell plates (15.5 mm in diameter - Nunc) is coated with 50 µl of the reconstituted seal, giving rise to a 200 µm polymerized fibrin layer. After 12 hour incubation in an humidified atmosphere at 37°C, cells are inoculated onto at a starting density of 5000 cells/cm^2 (Co).

Cell Proliferation

After the cells had grown on both negative control substratum (culture well plastic : Nunclon® Delta) and fibrin seal for 0 up to 15 days (logarithmic growth phase), medium is removed and 300 µl trypsin (0.25 % (w/v) in PBS Mg^{++}– and Ca^{++}– free) is added in order to detach cells and liberate fibrin entrapped cells. The resulting cell suspension is counted in triplicate. Each value given is the average cell number of 4 culture wells. The standard deviation was calculated and shown in the figures by vertical bars.

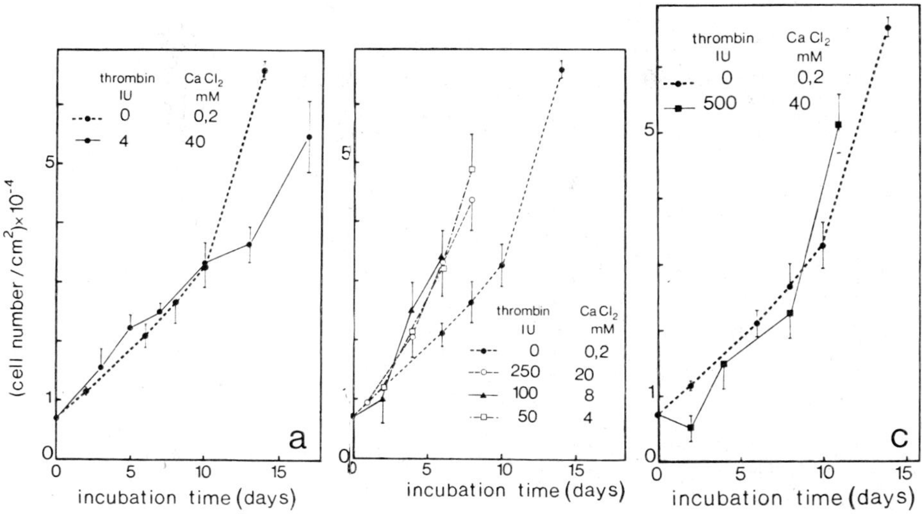

Fig. 2. Effect of thrombin and Ca^{++} concentrations of "FS I" on human skin fibroblast growth.

RESULTS

Electron microscopy

This study was performed using HSF 35 strain (skin fibroblasts), and wells coated with "FS I" (thrombin : 500 UI/ml, Ca^{++} : 40 mM). On day 11 following seeding, scanning electron microscopy (SEM) shows a dense layer of cells (35000 cells/cm^2) covering the surface of the fibrin (Fig. 1a). Cells exhibit long intermingled cytoplasmic extensions (Fig. 1b). One can observe a fine network of fibrils, possibly collagen fibrils, within the intercellular spaces (Fig. 1c). On the other hand transmission electron microscopy (TEM) shows that fibroblasts are able to invade and colonize the fibrin layer (Fig. 1d).

Effect of thrombin concentration on human skin fibroblast proliferation

A first experiment is conducted using "FS I" and the following thrombin concentrations : 4 UI/ml (Ca^{++} : 40 mM), 500 UI/ml (Ca^{++} : 40 mM) and 3 dilutions of the later, 250 UI/ml (Ca^{++} : 20 mM), 100 UI/ml (Ca^{++} : 8 mM), 50 UI/ml (Ca^{++} : 4 mM). The lowest concentration, 4 UI/ml, is ineffective on both cell attachment (day 2) and proliferation : doubling time is 4 days in both "treated" and control cultures (Fig. 2a). The highest concentration (500 UI/ml), significantly inhibits cell attachment (day 2 : 70 % Co and 45 % of control value, $P < 0.001$) whereas cell division is unchanged (doubling time 4

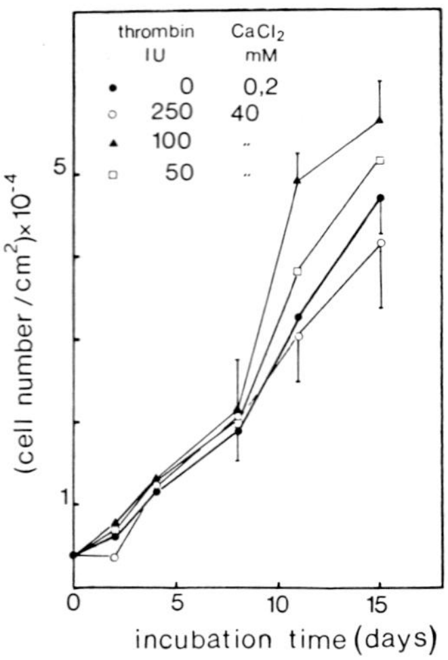

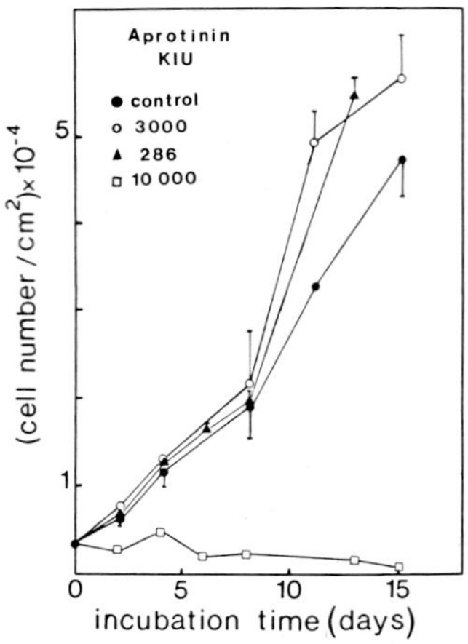

Fig. 3. Effect of thrombin concentration (Ca^{++}:40 mM) on human skin fibroblast growth
Fig. 4. Effect of aprotinin concentration (Ca^{++} : 40 mM) on human skin fibroblast growth.

days) (Fig. 2c). On the other hand, cell proliferation is significantly enhanced between 250 and 50 UI/ml (doubling time 3 days) ; at day 9, cell density was 143 % ($P < 0.001$) of the control (Fig. 2b). In order to evaluate the effect of Ca^{++} concentration, a second experiment was carried out using three thrombin concentrations (50, 100, 250 UI/ml) and constant Ca^{++} concentration (40 mM). Thrombin still enhances cell mitosis, but to a lesser extent (Fig. 2a, 2c, 3) : 4, 50, 250, 500 UI/ml were ineffective ; 100 UI/ml enhances cell proliferation (doubling time : 3 days), but the effect begins later than in the first experiment : 8 days instead of 2 days.

Effect of aprotinin level on human skin fibroblast proliferation

The sealant solution ("FS I" first component) is reconstituted with a solution containing various aprotinin concentrations : 286 KIU/ml ("FS II" concentration), 3000 KIU/ml ("FS I" concentration), 10000 KIU/ml ("FS III" concentration). Thrombin concentration is 100 UI/ml and Ca^{++}, 40 mM. Highest concentration of aprotinin studied exerts a strong toxic effect on cell attachment and consequently on cell proliferation (Fig. 4). Many dead cells and debris are found in the medium. Aprotinin levels between 300 and 3000 KIU/ml have no stimulating effect : the stimulatory effect (Fig. 4) observed

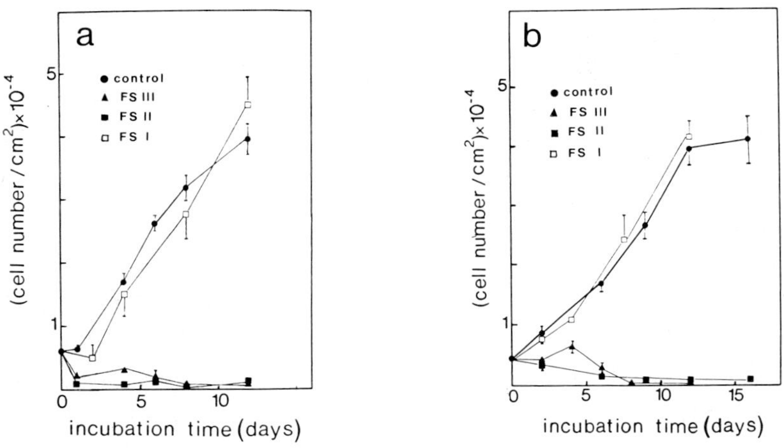

Fig. 5. Comparison of 3 fibrin sealants : effect on both human skin fibroblast (a) and human gingival fibroblast (b) growth.

is that of maximum effect thrombin concentration i.e. 100 UI/ml (Fig. 2b).

Comparison of 3 fibrin seals commercially available

Identical results were obtained with both skin (HSF 35 - Fig. 5a) and gingival (HGF 35 - Fig. 5b) fibroblasts. "FS I" (thrombin : 500 UI/ml, aprotinin : 3000 KIU/ml, Ca^{++} : 40 mM) inhibits slightly HSF attachment, as shown before, whereas cell growth is not affected. Both "FS II" (thrombin : 1000 UI/ml, aprotinin : 286 KIU/ml, Ca^{++} : 40 mM) and "FS III" (thrombin : 1000 UI/ml, aprotinin : 10000 KIU/ml, Ca^{++} : 40 mM) exert a strong inhibitory effect on cell attachment : few cells remain attached and many dead cells are found floating in the medium whereas cell proliferation is not detectable. An explanation could be that both sealants contain high thrombin levels. Moreover aprotinin concentration of "FS III" was shown to be highly cytotoxic.

DISCUSSION

Thrombin is able to stimulate "in vitro" growth rate of human fibroblasts cultivated onto "FS" substratum, which confirms the mitogenic activity of thrombin observed by several authors (refs.1, 2). Maximum effect is noted at 100 UI/ml (final concentration in the sealant : 50 UI/ml). Low concentrations are ineffective, and concentrations higher than 250 UI/ml (125 UI/ml sealant) seem to partly inhibit cell attachment to the seal. However proliferation rate was unchanged. Moreover our results suggest that high [Ca^{++}] (40 mM) inhibits thrombin mitogenic activity : Ca^{++} is slowly released into the growth medium thus delaying the effect of thrombin, until the first two medium changes eliminate excess of Ca^{++}, and allow thrombin action to begin. What is the mechanism involved ? Could it be a long lasting "growth-factor"-like effect ?

Comparison of "FS I", "FS II" and "FS III" clearly demonstrates the excellent cytocompatibility of "FS I".

CONCLUSION

This study shows that thrombin, Ca^{++}, aprotinin content of fibrin seals exert "in vitro" considerable effect on viability, attachment and growth rate of both dermal and gingival human fibroblasts. This results lead us to think therefore that some fibrin sealants are able to promote "in vivo" growth of repairing cells. Therefore, the question arises whether the observed promotion of growth rate by thrombin is correlated or not to cell phenotype stimulation ?

REFERENCES

1 Zetter B.R., Sun T.T., Chen L.B., Buchanan J.M., Thrombin potentiates the mitogenic response of cultured fibroblasts to serum and other growth promoting agents, J. Cell Physiol., 92, (1977), 233.
2 Pohl J., Bruhn H.D., Christophers E., Thrombin and fibrin-induced growth of fibroblasts : role in wound repair and thrombus organization, Klin. Wochenschr., 57, (1979), 273-277.

* * *

*

Biomaterials and Clinical Applications,
edited by A. Pizzoferrato, P.G. Marchetti, A. Ravaglioli and A.J.C. Lee
Elsevier Science Publishers B.V., Amsterdam, 1987 — Printed in The Netherlands

PURIFIED BOVINE TENDON COLLAGEN AS A WOUND DRESSING IN ORAL SURGERY

Mannai, C., Leake, D.L., Moore, L.J.[1]; Pizzoferrato, A., Ciapetti, G., Stea, S.[2]

[1]Oral and Maxillofacial Surgery
Harbor-UCLA Medical Center
Torrance, California 90509

[2]Rizzoli Institute
40136 Bologna, Italy

SUMMARY

This paper presents our observations on the clinical use of collagen in oral and maxillofacial surgery as a wound dressing for tooth extraction sites and as a wound dressing for split thickness skin graft donor sites from the lateral aspect of the thigh.

The histology of collagen sponges placed in extraction sites in dogs were evaluated at three days, one week, and six months after tooth extraction. In none of the collagen filled extraction sites was any foreign body reaction observed. Fibroblasts and osteoblasts were seen in the bony walls following the formation of the initial clot composed of red cells and fibrin. At one week, a nidus of newly formed calcified osteoid trabeculae could be seen. By six months, the bone histology is normal and no distinction between those extraction sites filled with collagen and those that were left to be filled in only by the clot could be made.

The second part of this paper addresses the observations on 12 patients who had split thickness skin grafts taken from the lateral aspect of the thigh as part of a preprosthetic surgical procedure. These grafts measured 5 x 14 centimeters. Half of each donor site was covered with Helistat[R] brand collagen sponge used as a skin wound dressing and the other half was covered with Xeroform gauze. The collagen was shed from the donor site several days (13th to 17th day postoperatively) before the Xeroform gauze (17th to 21st day postoperatively). Both dressings became quite stiff and as the patient moves about the dressing tends to tug at the skin surface, thus early shedding of the dressing improves patient comfort.

INTRODUCTION

Collagen is used widely as a biomaterial in such applications as dialysis membranes and for sutures. Because collagen initiates hemostasis, it is also useful in treating wounds to help prevent or control bleeding.

(CollaPlug[TM] and Helistat[R] are manufactured by American Biomaterials Corporation, Plainsboro, New Jersey.)

One of the theories of the pathogenesis of localized osteitis following tooth extraction is that the clot is dislodged, perhaps due to enhanced plasmin-mediated fibrinolysis. This suggested that placing a degradable biomaterial in extraction sites might create an artificial clot and prevent early loss of the protective covering that clots provide.

In the work presented here, one study was designed to evaluate the histologic response of bone and surrounding soft tissues to purified bovine tendon collagen sponges (Collaplug™) in fresh tooth extraction sites in dogs.

The other clinical application of collagen as a wound dressing was for split thickness skin graft donor sites which was evaluated by comparing its use with that of Xeroform gauze.

Materials and Methods: Tooth Extraction Dressings

Four mongrel dogs weighing approximately 10 kilograms each were used in this study. Under general anesthesia, four teeth were extracted on each side of the mandible in each dog. Collagen sponges measuring 0.5 x 1 centimeter were placed deep into two sockets on each side of the mandible. The bone containing the sockets was resected, at intervals of three days, seven days and six months, and placed in 10 percent formalin. Following fixation, the sections were prepared and stained with hemotoxylin and eosin or Paragon. (Fig. 1)

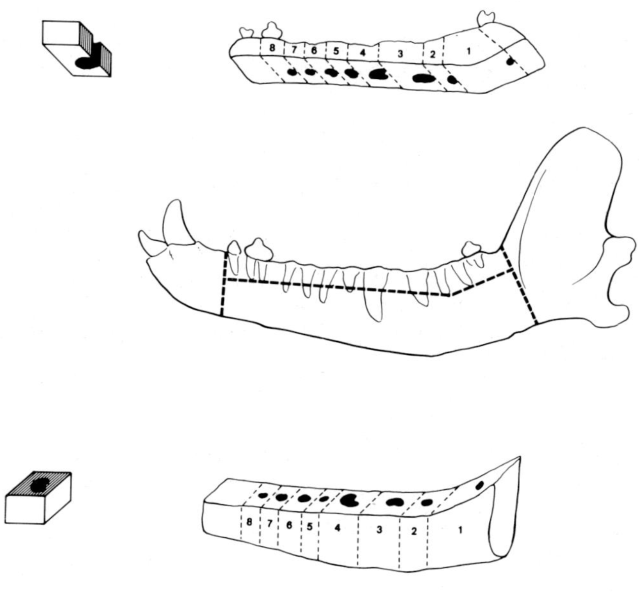

Fig. 1. Sections were cut from blocks of the mandible. The alveolar ridge was cut horizontally through the extraction sites. Transverse cuts were also made through each extraction site.

Results with Collagen

In the collagen filled extraction sites at three days after tooth extraction, the extraction site was filled with red cells. Fibrin turned into connective tissue and there was an invasion of fibroblasts. The layer of connective tissue adjacent to the alveolar wall underwent osteoblastic transformation. (Fig. 2)

At seven days after tooth extraction, the horizontal sections of these alveolar cavities were filled with dense connective tissue. The preexisting mandibular bone clearly circumscribed a nidus of newly formed osteoid trabeculae which underwent calcification. Also observed were some multinucleated cells indicating osteoblastic formation. Small bone ridges branched off from the alveolar wall and joined to form an interlacing of new trabeculae. (Figs. 3 & 4)

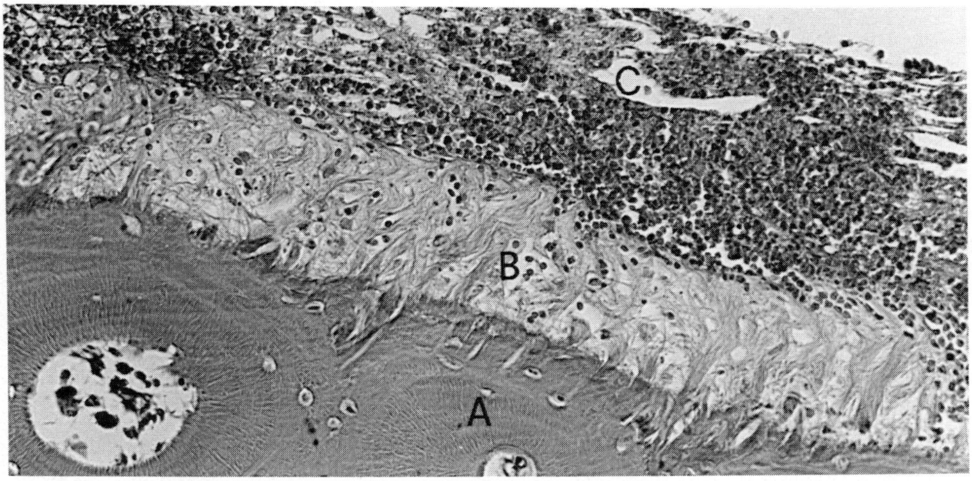

Fig. 2. Three days after extraction and placement of collagen in the alveolar cavity, a connective tissue layer can be seen adhering to the alveolar wall and osteoblasts are forming. A. Cortical bone B. Connective tissue C. Blood clot (Magnified x 25).

The control extraction sites presented essentially the same phenomenon. Ossification was lacking in the central area and, compared to the sockets containing collagen, the trabecular net seemed less dense.

Six months after tooth extraction, no evidence of any collagen was found in the bone or in the medullary tissue. There were no inflammatory cells. Histologically, the bone was normal and demonstrated a normal medullary cavity.

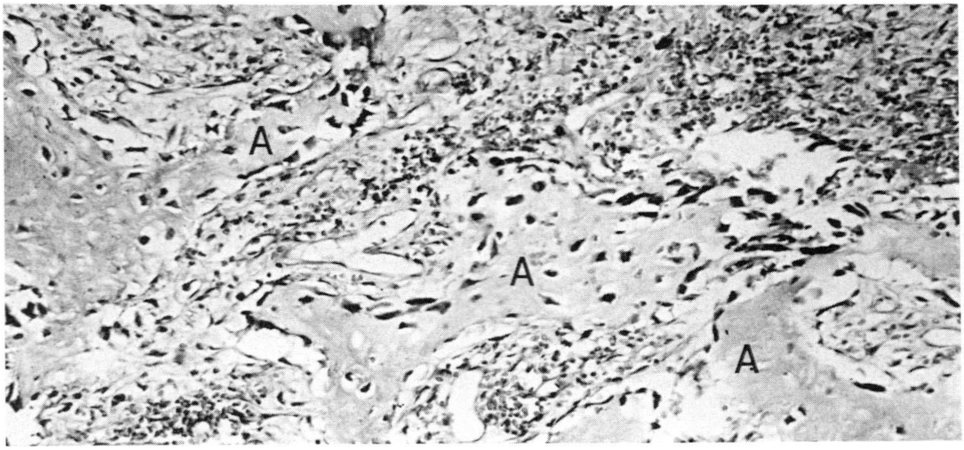

Fig. 3. At seven days after extraction, this horizontal section through the alveolus, filled with collagen at the time of extraction, shows a net of newly formed trabeculae with spinnerets of osteoblasts (Labeled A). (Magnified x 25).

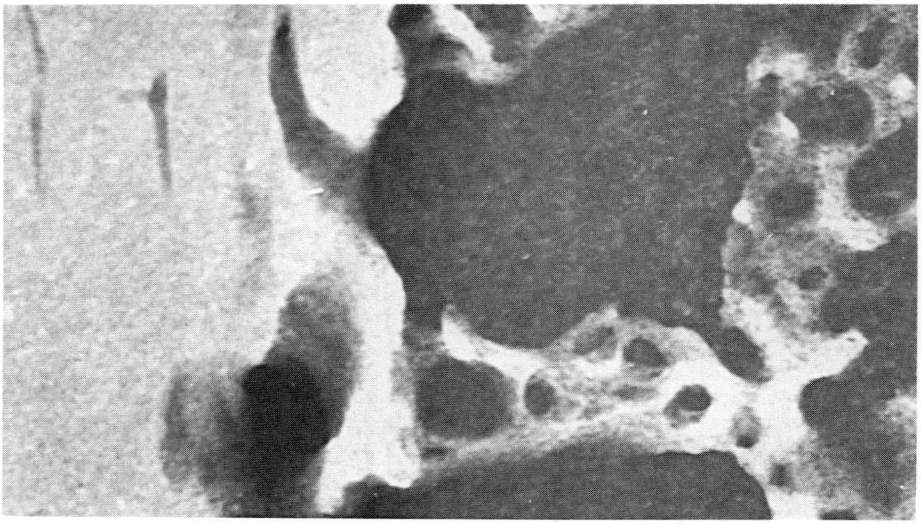

Fig. 4. Microphotograph of new bony trabeculae found in the alveolar cavity. (Magnified x 10).

Controls

At three days, no differences could be noted between the healing process of the collagen filled alveoli and in the control alveoli. Both sockets were coated with a connective tissue layer.

At seven days, the osteoid trabeculae were branching from the alveolar wall and the cavities within the trabeculae were invaded by connective tissue and blood vessels. The control extraction sites were comparable except that the trabeculae were dense. The collagen material was invaded by connective cells and there was an intense capillary vascular invasion. The histologic sections showed normal appearing connective tissue and collagen was indistinguishable from the surrounding tissue. There was only a slight lymphocytic reaction but no foreign body reaction as has been described with some other materials such as Gelfoam, Surgicel or polylactic acid.

This collagen material is marketed under the name Collaplug^{TM} and has been used in dental extraction sites for a period of 3 months. Thusfar, no adverse reactions have been reported in patients receiving this material and clinicians have observed that hemostasis is enhanced by the presence of collagen.

Skin Graft Donor Site Dressings

The other study presented here describes the use of collagen as a split thickness skin graft donor site dressing. A common oral surgical procedure is a split thickness skin graft over a supraperiosteal dissection of the mandible or maxilla to provide a vestibule after alveolar ridge augmentation, or, in some patients, where the alveolar bone is adequate but the mucosal attachment is high.

The split thickness skin graft donor site is comparable to an abrasion. The epidermis and a portion of the dermis are removed but epithelial remnants including the rete pegs and skin appendages remain in the epidermis for re-epithelialization.

Epithelialization occurs more rapidly on a moist, occluded surface than on dry, open surfaces. The disadvantage of a wet dressing, particularly in donor sites from the lateral aspect of the thigh, is a greater risk of wound infection and the resultant destruction of epithelial remnants.

Epithelial cells from the margins of the wound, sweat glands, sebaceous glands, hair follicles and rete pegs are potential sources for new epithelium. The rate of the healing is affected by the thickness of the split graft. A thin graft leaves more epithelial appendages and less dermis is exposed in the donor site and thus heals somewhat sooner than thicker grafts. It is well known that the healing donor site is also affected by the type of dressing, thus very thin graft donor sites covered with wet dressings may heal in three to four days. Very thick graft donor sites treated as a dry open wound may require three to four weeks of healing.

The donor site for these skin grafts is the lateral aspect of the thigh and the grafts measure approximately 5 x 14 centimeters. In the study reported here, half of each donor site was covered with Helistat^{R} brand collagen sponge wound dressing, and the other half was covered with Xeroform gauze. The patients were observed at weekly intervals. Hemostasis was better with the collagen dressing than with the Xeroform gauze. The collagen was shed from the donor site several days (13th to 17th day postoperatively) before the Xeroform gauze (17th to 21st day postoperatively).

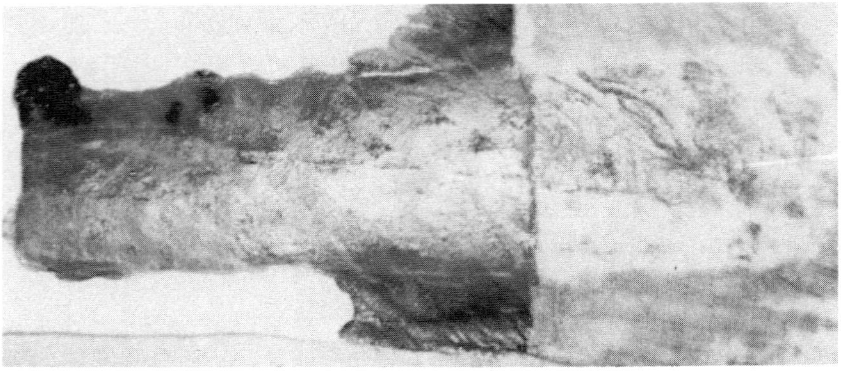

Fig. 5. First Postoperative Day. The collagen dressing is on the left, Xeroform is on the right.

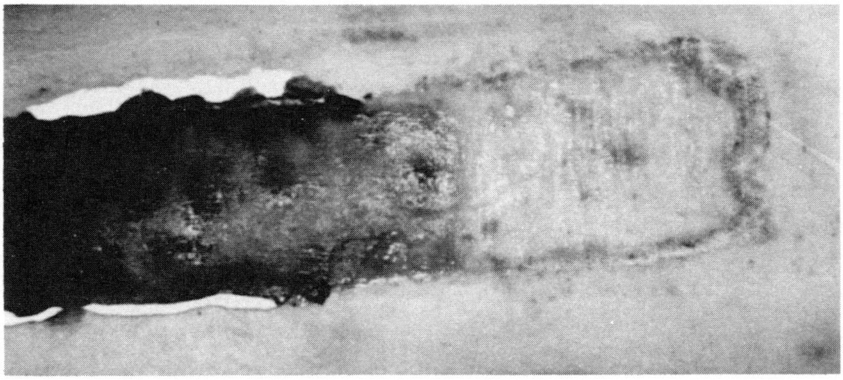

Fig. 6. 4th Postoperative Day. The collagen donor site dressing is on the left and Xeroform is on the right.

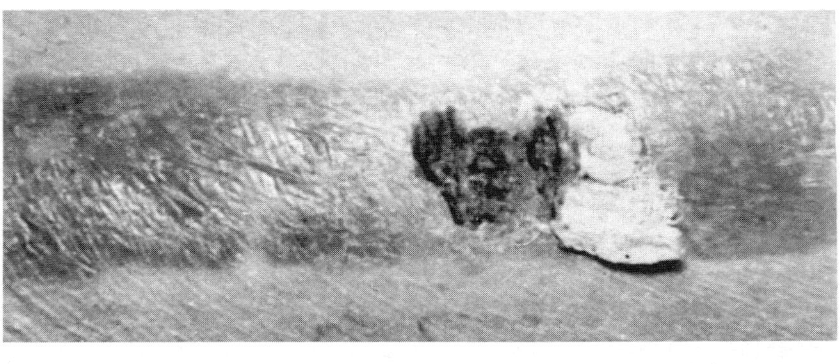

Fig. 7. 18th Postoperative Day. The skin graft donor site initially covered by collagen is now bare on the left side of the photograph and a remnant of Xeroform remains on the right side of the skin graft donor site. The collagen skin dressing fell off the wound on the 14th postoperative day.

Biomaterials and Clinical Applications,
edited by A. Pizzoferrato, P.G. Marchetti, A. Ravaglioli and A.J.C. Lee
Elsevier Science Publishers B.V., Amsterdam, 1987 — Printed in The Netherlands

ARTERIAL WALL REPLACEMENT WITH A DEGRADABLE VASCULAR PROSTHESIS

S. GOGOLEWSKI[1], G. GALLETTI[2] and G. USSIA[2]

[1]R & D Department of Biomaterials, Medinvent SA, P.O. Box 549, CH-1001 Lausanne (Switzerland)

[2]Institute of Experimental Surgery, University of Bologna, I-40138 Bologna (Italy)

SUMMARY

Microporous, compliant vascular prostheses have been constructed from fractionated segmented polyurethanes of various hydrolitic stabilities.

Prostheses were implanted in pigs, as a substitute for 5-7 cm long sections of the abdominal aorta.

Implanted prostheses degraded gradually with time, inducing a growth of a functional neo-conduit.

INTRODUCTION

The concept of partially degradable and/or completely degradable vascular prostheses has attracted increasing interest during the last decade (1-8).

It is believed that a degradable vascular substitute when ingrown and finally replaced with functional tissue, may diminish the chances of aneurysm formation and reduce the long term foreign body response (2,3).

The presence of a degradable matrix in the vascular graft also seem to stimulate the formation of neointima (4).

Compliance mismatch between the host vessel and a vascular prosthesis is also claimed to be one of the main reasons for early thrombosis of small-caliber grafts (9).

Thus a degradable yet compliant vascular graft might eventually become a solution to this problem.

It has recently been reported that use of a degradable vascular prosthesis prepared from a mixture of polylactide and polyurethane, induced a growth of biologically and mechanically functional neo-artery in rats (2,3).

The same results were obtained when vascular prostheses produced exclusively from degradable polyurethane, were implanted in the abdominal aorta of the rat (5,6) and the pig (7,8).

In this paper the data on implantation of polyurethane vascular prostheses in pigs are presented. It will be shown that the performance of the graft *in vivo* is to a great extent dependent on the hydrolytic stability of the polyurethane used for preparation of the vascular prostheses.

MATERIALS AND METHODS

Two types of segmented polyurethanes were used for preparation of vascular grafts:

a) Commercial, medical grade aliphatic polyurethane (CAP) claimed by the producer to be hydrolytically stable.

b) Proprietary fast degrading aliphatic polyurethane (PAP).

Type I vascular grafts were produced from (CAP) polyurethane.

Type II vascular grafts were constructed in such a way that the lumen side of the graft was made from a fast degrading (PAP) polymer while the rest of the graft wall was made from (CAP) polymer.

Type III was produced exclusively from a fast degrading (PAP) polymer. Except for an early design, all the prostheses used in the present study had a conical conformation to match the shape of the pig abdominal aorta.

Prostheses with an average diameter of 8 mm and wall thickness of 0.7-1.0 mm were prepared according to the method reported elsewhere (10).

The structure of the grafts was studied with a Cambridge scanning electron microscope, while their mechanical characteristics were determined using an Instron 1211 tensile tester (20 N load cell, 10 $mm\text{-}min^{-1}$ crosshead speed).

Grafts with a length of 6 cm were implanted in pigs as a substitute for a section of the infrarenal aorta for a period of time from 1 to 12 months. Extirpated grafts were evaluated histologically. Animals received aspirin 8 days prior to surgery and daily up to 180 days.

RESULTS AND DISCUSSION

Structure of grafts

The typical porous structure of the grafts is presented in Fig. 1. The lumen side has a porosity in the range of 5-15 µm, while the wall of the graft has a porosity of 30-60 µm. It was found in a previous study, that this type of pore configuration facilitates fast tissue ingrowth in the polymeric substrate and enhances formation of neointima.

Mechanical characteristics

Vascular grafts used in the present study were highly compliant. Grafts with an adequate wall thickness of 0.7-1.0 mm, showed elongation at break of 800-1200 %. Subjected to a hydraulic pressure (glycerin-water) they could withstand pressures up to 3 bar.

Grafts with the wall thinner than 0.5 mm underwent an extensive dilatation and fracture at pressures of 0.5-1 bar. Fracture of the grafts in this case resulted in a crack propagating through several pores to form an extensive opening.

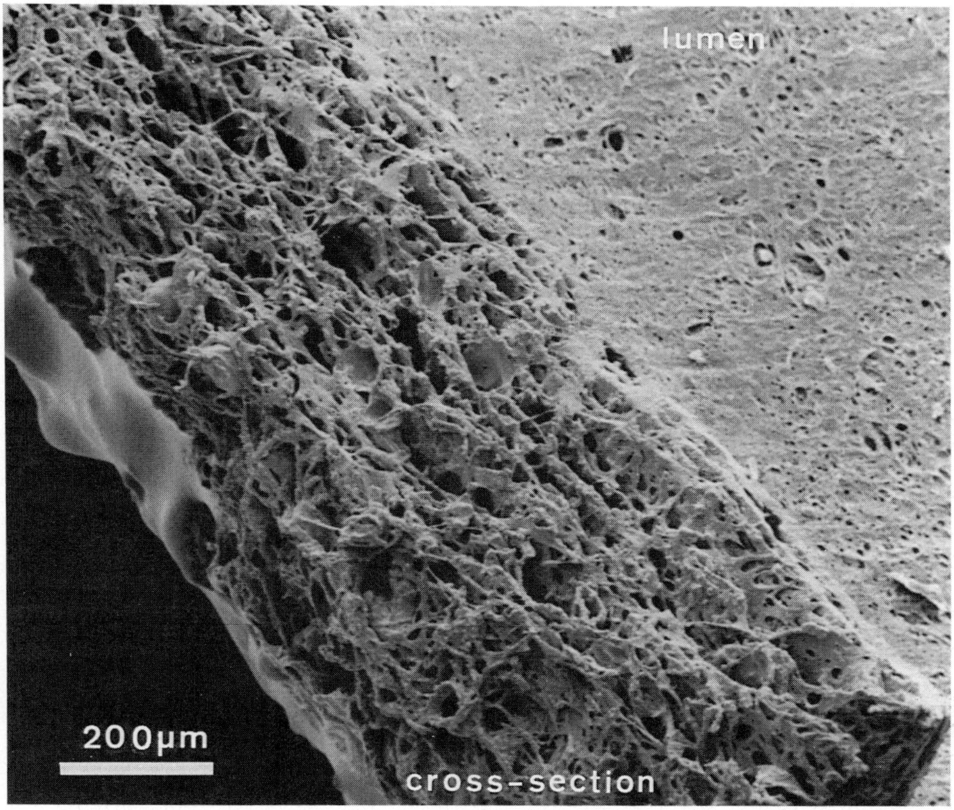

Fig. 1. Cross-section of degradable polyurethane vascular prosthesis.

In vivo stability of polyurethane grafts

In general the *in vivo* stability of polyurethane implants is strongly affected by the chemistry of the polyurethane, the structure of the implant and the site of implantation.

It has been proved experimentally that implants from aromatic polyetherurethaneureas are hydrolitically more stable than those from aliphatic polyesterurethanes.

Porous polyurethane implants are much more suspectible to degradation than the nonporous ones.

The presence of cell enzymes significantly affects the stability of polyurethane.

Polyurethane implants subjected *in vivo* to a permanent stress, usually degrade faster than those non-stressed.

Preparation of the elastomeric, degradable vascular prosthesis, requires a polymer with well-balanced chemical and physical properties. As a consequence of the definition of a degradable graft, the implant is finally degraded, although the degradation process should not take place before the tissue ingrowing the implant takes over the function of the graft.

On the other hand, too slow a degradation of the graft may affect the quality of the tissue grown on the polymeric substitute and thus finally the biological and mechanical performance of the conduit.

Prostheses type I used in the present study were made from a hydrolytically stable or rather, very slowly degrading polyurethane. *In vitro* tests with microporous membranes produced with this polymer, carried out at pH-7 and 37°C in sodium phosphate buffer, showed neither a drop in the absolute weight of the sample nor its molecular weight and only 10 % reduction in the tensile strength up to one year period.

In vivo tests in rats with the same membrane resulted, however, in about 5-10 % drop in the weight of the sample, 10 % drop in the viscosity average molecular weight and 10 % reduction in the tensile strength for each 2-3 months of implantation.

Prostheses type II were prepared from the polyurethane used in the prostheses type I (about 95 % of the prosthesis wall), and the fast degrading polyurethane to be described below.

These prostheses showed the hydrolytic stability similar to that described for the prostheses type I except for the lumen side the prosthesis, which degraded within about 4 months.

Prostheses type III were constructed from the fast degrading polyurethane.

In *in vitro* tests (pH-7.5, 37°C, sodium phosphate buffer) the polymer did not show evident degradation up to 6 month period.

Test microporous membranes prepared from this polymer, when wrapped against the abdominal aorta degraded almost completely within 120 days.

Results of implantation

Vascular prostheses of series I prepared from slowly degrading polyurethane, showed limited patency up to 4 weeks of implantation. Administration of aspirin did not improve the patency.

Vascular prostheses of series II having the lumen side made from fast degrading polyurethane, were patent up to sacrifice at 285 days.

The neointima which completely covered the surface of the graft, was composed of endothelial-like cells. Elastic fibres with elastin, myocytes and collagen fibres were identified under transmission electron microscopy. In the median layer there were large cell aggregates, composed predominently of macrophages and giant cells which diminished in number upon time of implantation.

Vascular prostheses of type III showed similar performance to the prostheses type II, although the prosthetic material was completely gone at 120-140 days of implantation. In statistically comparable series of implantation, the completely degradable vascular prostheses showed the highest patency rate up to 3 month period (this was the longest implantation time for the type III prostheses at the moment this paper was written).

The main reason of failure of the degradable prostheses were premature degradation or fracture of the prostheses due to a lack of uniformity in thickness of the prosthesis wall and/or infection.

CONCLUSIONS

Degradable polyurethane vascular prostheses implanted in the aorta of pigs induce a growth of a functional neo-conduit, composed of cells typical to those of healthy native artery.

ACKNOWLEDGEMENT

The authors acknowledge the assistance of Miss M. Nawrocka, M.Sc. in the preparation of the vascular prostheses.

REFERENCES

1. R.J. Ruderman, A.F. Hegyeli, B.G. Hattler and F. Leonard, Trans. Amer. Soc. Artif. Intern. Organs, 18 (1972), 30-33
2. S. Gogolewski, A.J. Pennings, E. Lommen and Ch.R.H. Wildevuur, Makromol. Chem. Rapid Commun. 4 (1983), 213-219
3. S. Gogolewski and A.J. Pennings, Progress in Artif. Organs-1983, 1 (1984), 294-297, ISAO Press, N° 204, Cleveland 1984
4. S. Bowald, C. Busch and I. Erikson, Surgery, 86 (1979), 722-729, Acta Chir. Scand. 146 (1980), 391-395
5. S. Gogolewski and G. Galletti, Life Support Systems, Suppl. 1(2) (1984), 324-328
6. S. Gogolewski and G. Galletti, Colloid & Polymer Sci., 264 (1986), in press
7. S. Gogolewski, G. Galletti and G. Ussia, Trans. Amer. Soc. Biomat., 8 (1985), 187
8. G. Galletti, G. Ussia and S. Gogolewski, Eur. Surg. Res. 17(S1) (1985), 16
9. C.E. Kinley and A.E. Marble, J. Cardiovas. Surg. 21 (1980), 163-170
10. S. Gogolewski, Medinvent SA, proprietary

Biomaterials and Clinical Applications,
edited by A. Pizzoferrato, P.G. Marchetti, A. Ravaglioli and A.J.C. Lee
Elsevier Science Publishers B.V., Amsterdam, 1987 — Printed in The Netherlands

ANASTOMOTIC INTIMAL HYPERPLASIA

T. CURTI[1], O. PARAGONA[1], P. BACCHINI[2], A. STELLA[1], L. PERDRINI[1],
F. BERTONI[2], M. D'ADDATO[1]
[1]Chair of Vascular Surgery. Policlinico S. Orsola - Bologna
[2]Department of Pathology - M. Malpighi Hospital - Bologna

SUMMARY

The intimal hyperplasia occurring at the anastomoses is an important cause of late graft failure in vascular surgery.

The authors report their experience based on the retrospective study of three groups of patients (aorto-iliac occlusive disease, vascular access for haemodialysis and leg tumor) in which a vascular prostatic graft was inserted.

They discuss the pathogenesis of the anastomotic intimal hyperplasia (A.I.H.), based on haemodynamic, mechanical, immunological factors and suggest that research into vascular grafting must be directed toward materials having mechanical properties close to those of the host artery.

INTRODUCTION

The late thrombosis of a vascular graft may be caused by various pathological events. The process that develops on the anastomotic side, anastomotic intimal hyperplasia (A.I.H.), seems very interesting to us. In some cases, it is shown that early anastomotic stenosis is the cause of acute thrombosis of the graft. The aims of our work are two: 1) to analyse our experience, pointing out aetiology and pathogenesis, 2) to collect useful ideas in the actual and future choice of prosthetic materials and anastomotic surgical techniques.

METHODS

We examined, in a retrospective study, a <u>first group</u> of 900 patients operated for aorto-iliac occlusive disease, with an aorto mono- or bi-femoral Dacron by-pass graft. The incidence of late thrombosis was 7.2% (follow-up 6 months to 7 years). In about 30% of late thrombosis in this series, the cause was an A.I.H. in the groin; in 41.5% it was a progression of the atherosclerotic disease and a worsening of the run-off.

The difference between these two conditions was established by these criteria: 1) Angiographic aspect 2) early manifestation (< 2 years) 3) histological characterisitics.

A <u>second group</u> of 55 patients, in which a prosthetic P.T.F.E. vascular access for haemodialysis was inserted, was examined. We observed an incidence of 30% in late thrombosis in PTFE grafts during the follow-up (6 months to 3 yaers). A.I.H. at the venous anastomosis was one the major causes of thrombosis (12%).

In a <u>third group</u> of patients, operated for bone tumor in a leg, a vascular graft was inserted in femoro-femoral or femoro-popliteal position. At the angiographic post-operative control generally performed within 6 months, we observed anastomotic stenosis in some cases.

The second and third group of patients may be useful to understand the pathogenesis of A.I.H., histologically very similar in atherosclerotic and non-atherosclerotic patients.

DISCUSSION

The true incidence of this pathological evolution of the vascular anastomosis is difficult to determine. Szilagyi et al. (1) performed a series of angiographic controls in 561 by-pass grafts and observed a 2.6 percent incidence of anastomotic stenosis; the majority of the lesions appeared within the first year of operation.

Rosemberg et al. (2) observed A.I.H. in 30% of late thrombosis of femoro-popliteal bovine grafts.

Similar lesions have been described in autologous vein by-pass grafts in femoro-popliteal (3) and aorto-coronaric (4) position, but with a very low incidence.

Imparato et al. (5) observed numerous A.I.H. in many sectors of arterial revascularization, and he found very similar histologic characterisitics.

Very important are hemodynamic factors in the genesis of A.I.H. Imparato et al. (6) proved that in a high flow end-to-side anastomosis, a continous stripping of endothelial cells occurred, a fragmentation of the intimal elastic lamella and a migration of smooth muscle cells from media to intima, where they look endothelial-like in the surface and fibroblast-like in the depth. These phenomena explain the continued proliferations.

Some authors have questioned whether a difference in the kind of anastomosis (end-to-side or end-to-end) may contribute to reduction of the lesion: in reality, in the presence of a synthetic graft (i.c. Dacron) A.I.H. develops in the same percentage (7).

Many other important factors are the mechanical and biophysical properties of arteries and graft. We must remember some basic concepts of the pulsatile flow.

The compliance is a measure of the distensibility of an artery (i.e. % diameter change for mmHg).

The impedance is the opposition to flow in a pulsatile system.

A low compliance means a stiff vessel, with high pulse wave velocity and high impedance (8). When we insert a stiff graft in an artery, we realise a sudden change in mechanical properties: the compliance increases, the impedance decreases, pulse wave velocity decreases, pressure pulse wave velocity decreases. These phenomena produce, at the anastomoses, local haemodynamic discontinuity resulting in a high local turbulence and vibrations, damaging the arterial wall. These effects cause endothelial damage, deposition of thrombus and fibrin and neo-intimal proliferation. The compliance of the graft is modified by the fibrous tissue reaction due to thrombus deposition. In vivo measurements demonstrate a decrease in compliance two hours after implantation (9): this evolution causes a worsening of the difference between graft and host artery.

Operative reaction due to the handling of tissue and the passage of sutures through the tissue, must be considered in pathogenesis of A.I.H. Generally, in the anastomotic line, there is a primary deposition of platelet and fibrin, replaced by fibrous tissue. We have no controlled study to demonstrate a relation between early thrombus deposition and A.I.H. The dissection of tissue near the vessels causes an interruption of "vasa vasorum" and a change in smooth miocells, developing an A.I.H. (10).

There is indirect evidence of immunologic response initiated by graft material or by reaction of the host arteries to the graft. The use of immunosuppression affects long term patency in Dacron-velour by-pass grafts and seems to condition a thinner A.I.H. (11).

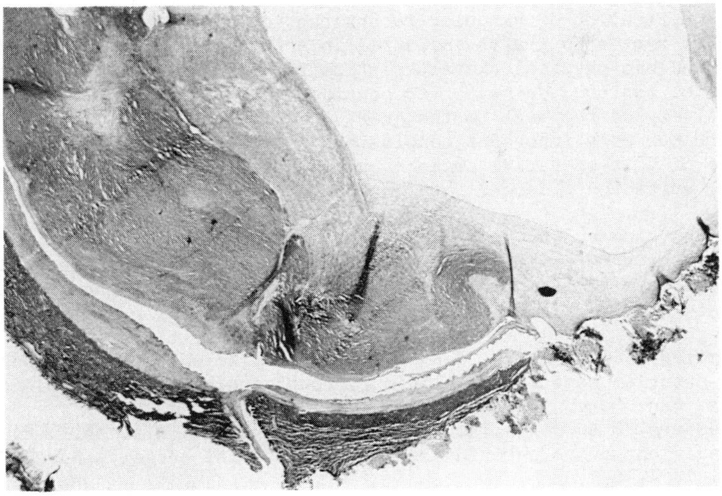

Fig. 1. Anastomotic Intimal Hyperplasia in end-to-side anastomosis.

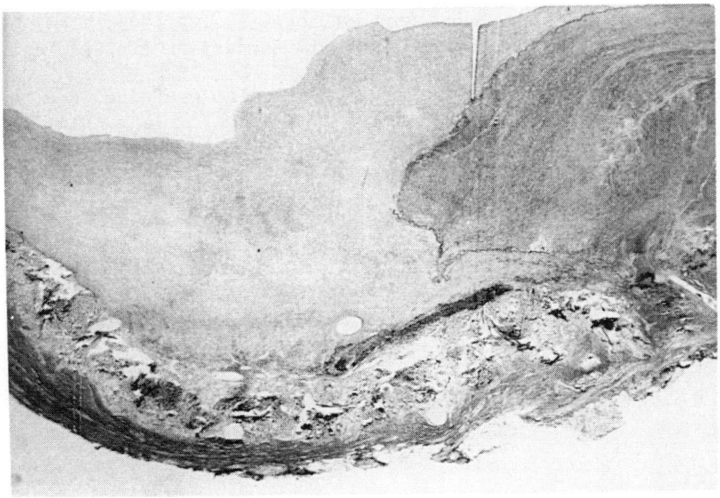

Fig. 2. Anastomotic Intimal Hyperplasia in end-to-end anastomosis.

CONCLUSIONS

Our experience and a wide review of the literature confirm that A.I.H. is an important complication of vascular reconstructions.

Certainly, synthetic grafts implanted in a relatively healthy artery, have mechanical and bio-physical characteristics that are the main cause in the evolution of the lesions. We must also consider hemodynamic factors and a lively local reactivity of the host to the graft.

These are our more important conclusions:

1) Make use of post-operative angiographic control and non-invasive vascular techniques, suitable to demonstrate an anastomotic stenosis before the final thrombosis.

2) Correct the stenosis by an angioplasty.

3) Work out, through research into vascular grafts, materials whose structure and texture most closely match the mechanical properties of the host artery.

REFERENCES

1. D.E. Szilagyi, R.F. Smith, J.P. Elliott, H.M. Allen, Long-term behavior of Dacron arterial substitute: clinical, roentgenologic and histologic correlations, Ann. Surg. 162 (1965), 453-477.
2. D. Rosemberg, B.A. Glass, N. Rosemberg, N.R. Levis, W.A. Dall, Experiences with modified bovine carotid arteries in arterial surgery, Surgery, 68 (1970), 1064-1073.
3. C. Breslan, J.A. De Weese, Successful endophlebectomy of autogenous vein by-pass graft, Ann. Surg. 162 (1965), 251-254.
4. L. Campean, D. Grochet, J. Lesperance, M.G. Bourassa, G.M. Grodin, Post-operative changes in aortocoronary saphenous vein graft revisited circulation, 52 (1975), 369-373.
5. A.N. Imparato, A. Bracco, G.E. Kim, R. Zoff, Intimal and neointimal fibrous proliferation causing failure of arterial reconstructions, Surgery 72 (1972), 1007-1017.
6. A.N. Imparato, F.G. Baumann, J. Pearson, G.E. Kim, T. Davison, I. Ibrahim, I. Nathan, Electron microscopic studies of experimentally produced fibromuscolar arterial lesions, Surg. Gynecol. Obstet. 139 (1974), 497-504.
7. C.E. Phillips, J.A. De Weese, L. Campeti, Comparison of peripheral arterial grafts, Arch. Surg. 82 (1961), 38-42.
8. A.N. Nicolaides, Haemodynamic aspect of vascular grafting, Rec. Adv. Vasc. Graft, System 4 Ass. (1985), 43-57.
9. E.J. Santiago, R.N. Miller, D.E.M. Taylor, Effects of intramural thrombus or haemodynamic performance of 5-6 mm. vascular prostheses, Proc. European Soc. Art. Organs XII (1983).
10. J.A. De Weese, Anastomotic Intimal Hyperplasia - Vascular Grafts - Appleton Century Crofts, New York (1977), 147-152.
11. L.N. Hoepp, J.A. De Weese, A. Elbadawi, Effects of steroids and immunosuppression on anastomotic intimal hyperplasia in femoral arterial by-pass graft, Surg. Forum 27 (1927), 215-219.

Biomaterials and Clinical Applications,
edited by A. Pizzoferrato, P.G. Marchetti, A. Ravaglioli and A.J.C. Lee
Elsevier Science Publishers B.V., Amsterdam, 1987 — Printed in The Netherlands

ULTRASTRUCTURAL INVESTIGATION ON DACRON GELSEAL GRAFTS IMPLANTED IN SHEEP CAROTID

R. LASCHI[1], T. CURTI[2], G. PASQUINELLI[3], P. PREDA[1], R. ANGELINI[2], M. D'ADDATO[2]

[1]Institute of Clinical Electron Microscopy, University of Bologna (Italy)

[2]Department of Vascular Surgery, University of Bologna (Italy)

[3]Institute of Normal and Pathological Cytomorphology, CNR, Bologna (Italy)

SUMMARY

A new prosthetic graft, Dacron Gelseal Triaxial, has been implanted into the common carotid of sheep. The animals were sacrificed after varying periods of time (7-120 days). Multiple specimens, collected from graft and anastomoses, have been studied by light microscopy, transmission and scanning electron microscopy. At the same time, an immunocytochemical analysis has been performed for the ultrastructural detection of actin, desmin and vimentin.

The submicroscopic features of cells and extracellular matrix involved in the graft incorporation are described in detail.

A complete endothelialization occurs in all Dacron Gelseal Triaxial grafts four months after surgery. Our results show that both the anastomotic regions and the central portion of the graft appear to be involved in the morphogenesis of the neointimal coverage.

INTRODUCTION

A morphological and immunocytochemical investigation was performed on a new Dacron Triaxial graft implanted in sheep carotid. Dacron Gelseal Triaxial (D.G.T.) is a warp knitted Dacron graft impregnated with a biodegradable modified mammalian gelatin of low thrombogenicity. It presents a porosity of zero requiring no preclotting or pre-treatment prior to implantation. The early clinical application of this graft appears very encouraging.

The aim of our study was to point out:

- the evolution of the cellular response both at the prostheses and at the anastomoses;
- the mechanisms involved in the production of a stable graft coverage able to prevent graft failure.

METHODS

D.G.T. grafts (6 cm. in length , 6 mm. in diameter) have been implanted with end to end anastomoses into the common carotids of sheep (8 animals, weighing $\simeq$ 90 kg). The vessels containing the grafts were carefully resected en bloc from the sacrificed animals after periods varying from 7 to 120 days. Specimens (artery next to anastomoses, proximal and distal anastomoses, grafts) were immediately collected and processed both for light and electron microscopy as suggested by M. Durand et al. (ref. 1) in order to minimize tissue artifacts. The morphological analysis was performed by light microscopy (LM), scanning electron microscopy (SEM) and transmission electron microscopy (TEM). Moreover, some tissue fragments, fixed in periodate-lysine-paraformaldehyde and embedded in araldite, were subjected to the immuno-gold technique for the ultrastructural detection of actin, desmin and vimentin.

RESULTS

Seven days after implantation

Our data, as for the early deposition of fibrin and blood cells on Dacron surfaces, agree with others from literature (refs. 2-4) . Seven days after implantation, the graft lumen was covered by a fibrin lining of medium thrombogenicity whereas a layer of granulation tissue surrounded the tubular prosthesis. Gelatin was still present among the interstices of Gelseal Triaxial fabric. Foreign body giant cells were not detected.

Worthy of attention was the occurrence of numerous rounded and spindle-shaped cells migrating from the artery media to the adjacent fibrin coverage, at anastomoses. By TEM, the rounded cells showed features of activated smooth muscle cells: large rounded nuclei with dispersed chromatin and prominent nucleoli. Their cytoplasm contained free polyribosomes, cisternae of rough endoplasmatic reticulum (RER) and myofilaments. A basal lamina coated most of the cell body. The spindle cells showed characteristics of both fibroblasts (well developed RER) and smooth muscle cells (myofilaments, pinocytotic vesicles and basal lamina). Thus, they seemed to be smooth muscle cells transformed to myofibroblasts.

Typical fibroblasts were focally present.

Fifteen days after implantation

The fibrin lining, next to the anastomoses, was replaced by a multiple layering of spindle-shaped cells of less thrombogenicity (pseudointima), which were arranged parallel to the blood flow. These cells, engaged in the synthesis of extracellular matrix, were characterized as myofibroblasts and fibroblasts by TEM and appeared as flat, elongated and loosely interconnected cells with very smooth surfaces at SEM (Fig. 1).

On the contrary, the central portion of the graft displayed a poorly developed pseudointimal coverage. Monocytes, activated macrophages as well as resting foam cells were easily recognized by LM and TEM. Clusters of elements of the monocyte-macrophage-system (MMS) were also present near the spindle cells.

By LM, no trace of gelatin was detected on the D.G.T. graft. Scattered foreign body giant cells were seen adhered to the Dacron fibrils.

Two months after implantation

The graft was completely covered by the pseudointima whose inner layer was, in part, lined by endothelial cells. At the anastomoses, a continuous advancing front of endothelial cells was observed by SEM (Fig. 2). Islands of endothelium were also evidenced in the central zone of the prosthesis.

Four months after implantation

At this time, D.G.T. graft displayed a continuous neointimal coverage. Neointima was composed of a single lining of endothelial cells placed on a multiple layering of spindle-shaped cells (mainly myofibroblasts and young smooth muscle cells).

Endothelial cells were characterized according to ultrastructural and immunocytochemical criteria.

By SEM, the endothelial cells appeared well oriented with bulging nuclei and few surface projections. At TEM, they showed large and oval nuclei whereas the cytoplasm contained a fair amount of intermediate filaments as well as pinocytotic vesicles (Fig. 3). Tight junctions were also present.

The intermediate filaments were located throughout the cytoplasm as loosely packed bundles . They were immunocytochemically characterized as vimentin

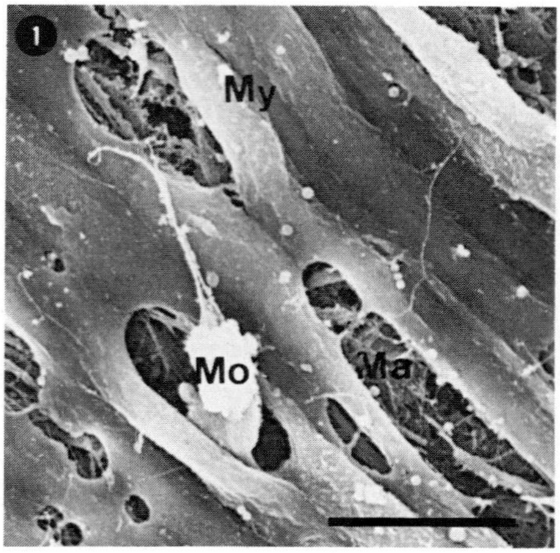

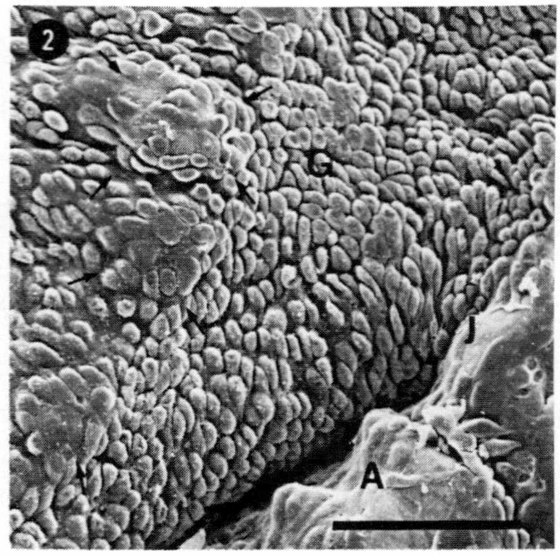

Fig. 1. Fifteen days after implantation. SEM view of pseudointima. My: myofibroblasts; Mo: mononuclear cell; Ma: intercellular matrix. Bar = 10 μm.
Fig. 2. Two months after implantation. SEM image of graft endothelialization. A: artery lumen; J: junction between artery and graft; G: graft lumen; arrows: foci of proliferating endothelial cells. Bar = 50 μm.

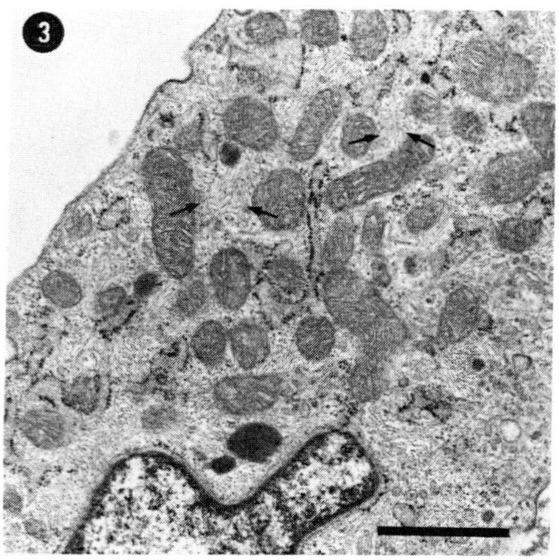

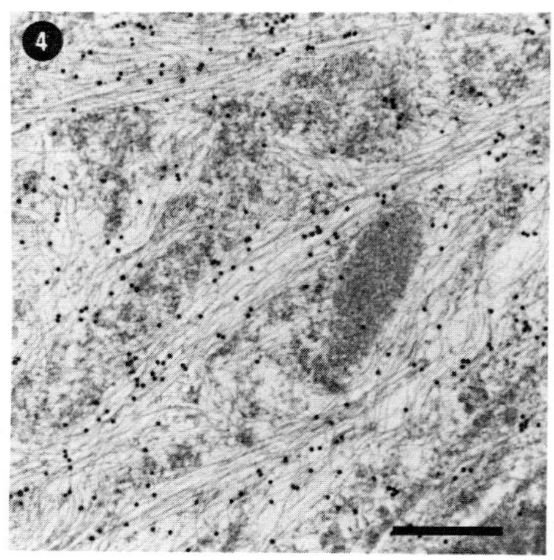

Fig. 3. Four months after implantation. TEM image of an endothelial cell. Arrows: intermediate filaments. Bar = 1 μm.
Fig. 4. Four months after implantation. Immuno-gold localization of vimentin. Bar = 0.5 μm.

filaments (Fig. 4). Immunostaining for desmin was always negative. Characteristic peripheral bundles of actin microfilaments, comparable to the stress fibers of cultured endothelial cells, were also seen.

DISCUSSION

These results suggest that a true endothelial lining develops on D.G.T. graft in our experimental model, four months after implantation.

The endothelial colonization most likely requires:
i) the activation of medial smooth muscle cells, which could represent the major source of myofibroblasts; ii) the recruitment of the MMS, which is involved in the remodelling of the early fibrinous lining both by clearing fibrin and cellular debris and by modulating myofibroblast proliferation; iii) the synthesis of a suitable intercellular matrix by myofibroblasts.

These processes, which immediately arise after surgery, seem to be critical for the subsequent graft endothelialization.
Aggressive factors, such as mechanical stresses, could modify this pattern of healing thus predisposing graft to failure.
In this respect, the gelatin impregnation seems to promote the prosthesis healing.

REFERENCES

1 M. Durand, C. Arrouvel, P. Banzet, An improved method for electron microscopic study (SEM and TEM) of vessel prosthesis anastomoses in microsurgery, J. Submicrosc. Cytol., 17 (1985) 429-434.
2 V.S. Sottiurai, J.S.T. Yao, W.R. Flinn, R.C. Batson, Intimal hyperplasia and neointima: an ultrastructural analysis of thrombosed grafts in humans, Surgery, 93 (1983) 809-817.
3 G. Nightingale, I. Fodgestam, B. O'Brien, Scanning electron microscope study of experimental microvascular anastomoses in the rabbit, Br. J. Plast. Surg., 33 (1980) 282-298.
4 H.M. Mehodorn, J.J. Townsend, P.R. Weinstein, N.L. Chater, R. Meyermann, H.J. Buncke Jr., Endothelialization of a new arterial microvascular graft material, Scanning Electron Microsc., III (1979) 851-856.

Biomaterials and Clinical Applications,
edited by A. Pizzoferrato, P.G. Marchetti, A. Ravaglioli and A.J.C. Lee
Elsevier Science Publishers B.V., Amsterdam, 1987 — Printed in The Netherlands

PATENCY FACTORS OF PROSTHESES EMPLOYED IN THE RECONSTRUCTION OF THE FEMORO-POPLITEO-TIBIAL DISTRICT

TEALDI D.G., ODERO A., BORGNA M., and RUBERTI U.

II° Clinica Chirurgica, University of Milan

SUMMARY

Factors conditioning the long-term patency of the femoro-popliteo-tibial reconstructions are numerous. Some of them are of biologic nature and other of hemodynamic etiology. Biologic factors are bound to the state of the peripheral vascular bed and the evolution of the atherosclerotic disease. Among the hemodynamic factors, we mention the requirement of overcoming angulations, the size and length of the prosthesis, which favour the formation of subintimal hyperplasia in the seat of distal anastomosis and activate the platelet aggregation, in relationship with their biophysical characteristics.

Autologous saphenous vein is the first-choice prosthesis, even though it is not devoid of negative features.

The best results, apart from saphenous vein, were obtained with the umbilical vein and PTFE, whereas the use of dacron and bovine carotid has been relinquished.

In conclusion, the employ of various types of prostheses applied as alternate to autologus saphenous vein, is dictated more by personal considerations rather than by objective data. Indeed, the different opinions attest the deficiency of the prostheses presently marketed concerning the compliance and intimal surface.

The long-term patency rate of small-caliber grafts (less than 6 mm) has been constantly rather disappointing and has conditioned the management of occlusions of the peripheral arterial district.

Employment of biologic and synthetic grafts of new concept, which integrate the autologous saphenous vein graft, seems to have improved the long-term prognosis in this population of patients which is becoming always more numerous (more than one hundred thousand interventions per year).[1].

The factors conditioning the patency of grafts employed in the peripheral district are of biologic and physical nature. Among the first ones, we mention the following:

- presence of an inadequate runoff

- evolution of the arteriosclerotic disease
- biologic response of the host to the graft.

The term "runoff", universally accepted, according to Strandness is of not univocal interpretation and results from two elements: the conditions of vessels providing egress of blood flow, and the ability to sustain flow from graft. [2]

The angiographic classification based on the number of arteries patent, the measurement of the pressure gradient existing between the popliteal artery and the peripheral vessels and the recording of the input resistance of the vascular bed, were found to be not suitable for the prognostic assessment of the graft survival.

Vascular surgeons ascribe a real importance to the runoff conditions and this is evidenced by the attempt of increasing its receptivity by technical measures [13-8]. This is basically true and meets a need which appeared in the clinico-diagnostic stage.

The advancement of the arteriosclerotic disease is the main factor.

The reduction of the inflow or of increasingly larger sections of the peripheral area, the involvement of the coronary circulation with changes of the heart activity, along with changes in the fat turnover, diabetes mellitus, hypertension, tabagism and scarcely hygienic life style, have a direct or indirect influence on the graft life [3-4-5-6].

The response of the host depends on several factors and is able to modify the graft flow through an action on purely theoretical hemodynamic parameters present at the time of the implantation.

These factors are mainly the physico-chemical properties of grafts, their size and length and the resulting flow hemodynamic features.

We deem not necessary to describe the healing process of the graft, but we only want to point out some fundamental aspects. The formation of the pseudo-intima, whose thickness ranges from 0.5 to 1.5 mm, assures on one hand a sliding surface enough suitable for the flow, but it changes its diameter especially in grafts of a lower section.

This involves a remarkable increase in resistance after the Pouiseuille equation, namely: in view of a pseudo-intima of 1 mm thickness in a graft of 6 mm of caliber, a 56% reduction of the true caliber is obtained and a 406%

increase in resistance with resulting energy losses. [7].

Moreover, the pseudo-intima meets the requirement of having a non-thrombogenic surface available. This requirement is partially not-met, since at the flow contact an activation of platelets and Factor XII occurs, from which the mechanism of thrombosis is triggered. [8].

The more properly physical factors are bound to the molecular structure of the tissue, the type of prosthesis (biologic or synthetic), the method of its manufacturing and the mix of measures applied by the vascular surgeon during surgery.

These latter are: caliber and length of prosthesis site of the anastomosis and mode of its manufacturing.

The diameter of the prosthesis is more important than its length, since it, along with blood viscosity, increases the flow resistance.

The prosthesis diameter should be equal or slightly greater than the one of the recipient artery. Anastomosis should be manufactured so as to make the passage of flow between the two structures gradual.

This is accomplished by minimizing the angle of anastomosis and performing an arteriotomy, whose length is three times the prosthesis diameter.

In the opposite case, turbulence and stagnation areas are forming in the point of passage of the flow, with further energy losses, deterioration of the tightness of anastomosis and increased thickness of psudo-intima, with the obvious hemodynamic consequences. [11-12].

The above and below knee site of the anastomosis is scarcely important, if the anastomosis is manufactured in the popliteal artery [5].

Angiographic examinations performed with different types of prosthesis (saphenous vein, umbilical vein, PTFE, external supported PTFE) with progressive flexion of the knee, never showed the presence of stenoses or angulations at the level of the joint.

On the contrary, prostheses anastomized on more peripheral vessels have a shorter life. This difference should be related rather to the poor runoff and hemodynamic problems depending on this anastomosis than to the length of prosthesis. Our experience in the treatment of distal femoral injuries covers more than 300 arterial reconstruction followed-up for a maximum of 7 years. Surgical indication has been always extremely selective with a preference for the necessary interventions (limb salvage) to the others.

This clinical premise, in our opinion, is indispensable for the global evaluation of the long-term results, as the 85% of interventions have been performed as an alternate to the amputation, with all the resulting problems related to the limb pathology.

By-pass has been performed in most cases (95%) and the preferential site of the anastomosis was the subgenual popliteal artery (91%).

The autologous saphenous vein is the first-choice material; it is employed reversed or in situ.

Its negative features are the following: uneven caliber, need of using it inverted, relative reliability since it can exhibit aneurysmatic dilations and segmentary lesions depending on wall thickenings.

Among the most interesting characteristics we mention: the inner surface biologically more similar to the one of the artery, the ability of defending from the platelets activated by the secretion of endothelial prostaglandins. (10)

This biologic defence could appear to be important, especially because the prosthesis patency depends ultimately on the ratio of flow to activation of platelet and factor XII. Below a critical T.T.V. (thrombotic threshold velocity) which cannot be quantized and is different for each prosthesis, the mechanism of thrombosis triggers. [8].

The autologous saphenous vein has a compliance more similar to the one of the artery. Several data suggest a direct relationship between compliance and long-term patency of prosthesis even though it has not yet been demonstrated [1].

Therefore, compliance and non-thrombogenic inner surface are the base features conditioning the vein patency. However, this is not always available (12 to 30% of cases) [9].

We employed the saphenous vein in 44% of cases. This is not in accordance with literature [2-3-4] and is due to the fact that the veins having a caliber lower than 4 mm have been discarded preferring a good prosthesis of an adequate caliber to a bad saphenous vein. As an alternate, the homologous human umbilical vein, PTFE with or without an external support, were employed. Dacron and modified bovine grafts have been relinquished long since, owing to the disappointing results.

The early patency for the salvage interventions is 80% and decreases to 59% after 3 years.

The maximum frequency of acute graft obliterations occurred in the first 6 months. The exploration of the proximal and distal anastomoses (in 22 patients) showed in about half of cases the advancement of arteriosclerotic disease in the recipient artery and in the peripheral district, so that it was not possible to perform a new operation. In 25% of patients a sub-intimal thickening appeared involving the anastomotic area with secondary graft thrombosis.

The best results were achieved by the use of the inverted autologous saphenous vein, then of the umbilical vein and PTFE. However, the rate differences are non-significant. The evaluation of the different behaviour of the various types of graft is extremely critical: it should view a series of variables appearing in time and capable to change the fate of the graft, even though basing on clinically homogeneous groups of patients (at least theoretically).

The use of prosthesis other than the autologous saphenous vein is dictated (in our opinion) by personal considerations and preferences rather than by objective findings.

Autologous saphenous vein is the material of choice as it is used in coronary surgery.

Therefore, in our opinion, it is mandatory to evaluate its reliability in the single patient before adopting an alternate material.

The investigations on the endothelization of synthetic grafts, in order to obtain a non-thrombogenic surface, and on some of their physical properties (compliance, transmission of the flow wave), along with the synthesis of pharmacologic principles capable to act on the coagulation mechanism, are the goals of vascular surgery of the 90's, to improve the fate of the small-size grafts.

REFERENCES

1 J. Megerman, W.M. Abbott, Compliance in vascular grafts. Vascular grafting, Ed. C.B. Wright Boston 1983.

2 Stradness D.E., Summer D.S., Haemo-dynamics for surgeons, Ed. Grune and Stratton, New York 1975.

3 Darling R.L., Linton R.R., Durability of femoro-popliteal reconstructions: Endarterectomy versus vein by-pass grafts, Am. J. Surg. 123, (1972), 472-479.

4 De Weese J.A., Rob L.G., Autogenous venous grafts ten years later, Surgery 82, (1977), 775-784.

5 Szilagyl D.E., Hageman J.H., Smith R.F., Autogenous vein grafting in femoro-popliteal atherosclerosis: The limit of it effectiveness Surgery 86, (1979), 836-851.

6 Lynch T.G., Hobson R.W., An overview of femoro-popliteal and femoro-infrapopliteal reconstruction. Vascular grafting, Ed. L.B. Wright, Boston.1983.

7 Nicolaides A.N., Haemodynamic aspects of vascular grafting. Int. Symposium on vascular prosthesis. Nijmegen April 28-28, 1984.

8 L.R. Savage, External supported prostheses for axillo-femoral and femoropopliteal by-pass vascular grafting, Ed. C.B. Wright, Boston 1983.

9 Bosher L.P., Deck J.D., Thubrikarm, Role of the venous valve in late segmental occlusion of vein grafts. J. Surg. Res. 26, (1979), 437-440.

10 Tealdi D.G., Signorelli M., Gaeta A., Problemi inerenti la scelta dei materiali protesici. Atti del IX Congresso della Soc. Ric. Chirurgia. Milano 28-29 Ottobre 1983.

11 Wesolowski S.A., Performance of material prosthetic bloodvessels bull N.V. Ac. Med. 48, (1972), 33-335.

12 Malan E., Noseda G., Longo T., Approach to fluid dynamic problems in reconstructive vascular surgery. Surgery 66, (1969), 994-999.

13 Ibrahim I.M., Sussman B., Dardik I., Adjunctive arteriovenous fistula with tibial and peroneal reconstruction for limb salvage. Am. J. Surg. 140, (1980), 246-252.

Biomaterials and Clinical Applications,
edited by A. Pizzoferrato, P.G. Marchetti, A. Ravaglioli and A.J.C. Lee
Elsevier Science Publishers B.V., Amsterdam, 1987 — Printed in The Netherlands

UMBILICAL VEIN GRAFTS IN ARTERIAL RECONSTRUCTIONS

G. VERCELLIO, M. COLETTI, R. CARLESI and G. AGRIFOGLIO

Institute of Vascular Surgery, University of Milan, Via Commenda I2, 20I22 Milan (Italy)

SUMMARY

The Authors report their experience with umbilical vein,adopted in absence of suitable saphenous vein.

Between November I980 to March I986,28 human umbilical veins were employed in the revascularization of the popliteal, tibial or peroneal artery.

The distal anastomoses were performed in I0 patient on the popliteal artery (4 above knee, 6 below knee), in I0 on the anterior tibial, in 5 on the posterior tibial and in 3 patient on the peroneal artery.

In II patients an adjunctive AV fistula at the level of the distal anastomosis was performed.

The life table method shows a cumulative patency rate of 67,0% at 48 months and a limb salvage rate of 80,3% at the same period.

Our results encourage to consider the umbilical vein as a substitute of choice to the autogenous saphenous vein in reconstructive procedures of the lower limb.

INTRODUCTION

Femoro-popliteal grafting could be considered an important field for testing any new vascular substitute.

Selective revascularization of the tibial or peroneal vessels represents even more an important and critical field to evaluate a vascular prosthesis as reliable alternative to the autogenous saphenous vein.

The umbilical vein graft developed by Dardik was employed in our Institute as alternative to our technique of choice, the "in situ" saphenous graft (69 procedures), for femoro-distal bypass grafting.

The umbilical grafts available consist of prepared umbilical veins stabilized with glutaraldehyde and covered with a netlike polyester mesh.

Immunologic studies confirmed that the small glutaraldehyde moleculescan effectively establish crosslinks and result in a stabilized graft that resist biodegradation (refs. I-2) .

METHODS

In the Institute of Vascular Surgery of the University of Milan, from November I980 to March I986, 28 biografts were implanted for imminent limb loss in 25 patients to revascularize popliteal, tibial and peroneal arteries.

We used umbilical vein biografts as alternative, in case of unsuitable saphenous vein; in 4 (I4,2%) cases the biograft was employed after failure of a previous saphenous graft.

The age range was 36 to 82 years (mean 62,8 years). There were I4 men and II women.

Associated diseases included hypertension in 3 (I0,7%), coronary artery disease in II (39,2%), abnormal lipid level in 7 (25,0%), diabetes in 4 (I4,2%) and a history of smoking in I0 patients (35,7%).

Indication for surgery was rest pain in 9 (32,I%), ischemic ulcer or gangrene in I4 (50,0%), including one case of Bürger disease, acute ischemia in 5 cases (I7,9%).

The site of proximal anastomosis was in I5 (53,7%) the common femoral artery, in 9 (32,I%) a prostheses at inguinal level, in 3 (I0,7) the common iliac artery and in I (3,5%) case the popliteal artery above knee.

The distal anastomosis was in I0 (35,7%) the popliteal (4 above knee, 6 below knee), in I0 (35,7%) the anterior tibial, in 5 (I7,9%) the posterior tibial and in 3 (I0,7%) cases the peroneal artery.

In 11 (39,2%) cases an adjunctive distal arteriovenous fistula was performed in order to reduce the caliber incongruence between the graft and the artery, mostly in presence of very high peripheral resistences and poor run-off, (loss of the plantar arch and diameter of the recipient artery less than 1,5 mm.).

Heparin (1 mg/kg) was intravenously given in all cases during surgery.

After having the proximal anastomosis the grafts were systematically placed in a subcutaneous, extraanatomic route. This position offers several advantages: easer and quicker procedure, no kinking in knee flexion, better control of the graft pulsatility and easer access for thrombectomy by a simple skin incision in local anesthesia. In addition in some instances the extraanatomic route is mandatory to avoid infected areas (ref. 3) .

Postoperatively the operated limb is kept flexed for a few days in order to avoid any mechanical trauma at the level of the anastomoses and to obtain a better healing of the graft.

RESULTS

No patient died during the operation or in the post-operative period.

There were 8 (28,5%) early thrombosis: 6 were restored by successful thrombectomy, 2 required primary amputation (1 after two months for the infection of the graft).

There were II (39,2%) late thrombosis in 9 patients, 6 cases of these required thrombectomy successfully performed in 3; out of 3 unsuccessfully thrombectomies 2 patients required amputation. Three cases of late thrombosis treated by thrombectomy associated with intraarterial infusion of urokinasi allowed the limb salvage in 2 cases. Two patients with thrombosed graft at 43 and 47 months could save the limb without operation.

The life table method shows a cumulative patency rate of 67,0% at 48 months and a limb salvage rate of 80,3% at the same period.

In our series the early and late results in patients with gangrenous lesions and patients submitted to surgery for rest pain are similar (ref. 4) .

CONCLUSIONS

These results seem to encourage the use of the umbilical vein as alternative to saphenous vein in femoro-distal bypass procedures, when the vein is not available.

Complications relating to the use of the umbilical vein graft are similar to those following any other graft material, including saphenous vein.

Early thrombosis is of course the most common complication and is usually due to faulty technique, lack of familiarity with the umbilical vein graft, or to the degree of run-off. Perioperative thrombosis due to technical errors can be minimized by performing routine intraoperative arteriography.

The umbilical vein is not immune from infection (one case in our series), there is some evidence that the use of glutaraldehyde as the tanning agent imparts some degree of increased resistance of infection.

True aneurysms of the umbilical vein grafts are uncommon (no case in our series).

We found in the umbilical veins some changes in early and late angiographic controls, as intraluminal segmentation and lightening but these findings did not appear responsible for the failure of the grafts.

Properties of compliance and smooth inner surface represent in our opinion an important advantage of biografts for small artery reconstructions.

Some disadvantages of this arterial substitute, as a very frail and rather thick wall can be surmounted if an exquisite surgical technique is employed.

REFERENCES

I H. Dardik, R.E. Baier, M. Meenaghan, J. Natiella, S. Weinberg, R. Turner, B. Sussman, B. Kahn, I.M. Ibrahim, I. Dardik, Morphologic and biophysical assessment of long term human umbilical cord vein implants used as a vascular conduits, Surg. Gynecol. Obstet., I54 (I982 I7-26.
2 H. Dardik, Clinical status of the umbilical vein as a vascular graft, in: S.H. Skotnicki, F.G.M. Buskens, H.H.M. Reinaerts (Ed.), Proc. Int. Symposium on Recent Advances in Vascular Grafting, Nijmegen, Netherlands, April 26-28, I984, Redwood Burn LTD, Trowbridge, Wiltshire, I985, pp. I34-I42.
3 H. Dardik, I.M. Ibrahim, B.C. Sussman, M. Kahn, I. Dardik, Indications and critical factors for thesuccess of lower extremity bypass in the subcutaneous position, in: R.M. Greenhalgh (Ed.), Extra-anatomic and Secondary Arterial Reconstruction, Pitman, Marshfield, I982, pp. 368-379.
4 G. Vercellio, M. Coletti, R. Carlesi and G. Agrifoglio, Femoro-distal bypass, debridment, and skin grafting as principles of treatment of extensive lower gangrene, in: P.C. Maurer (Ed.), Proc. I4th World Congress International Union of Angiology, Munich, W-Germany, July 6-II, I986, W. Zuckschwerdt Verlag, München, I986, pp. 432-433.

Biomaterials and Clinical Applications,
edited by A. Pizzoferrato, P.G. Marchetti, A. Ravaglioli and A.J.C. Lee
Elsevier Science Publishers B.V., Amsterdam, 1987 — Printed in The Netherlands

CLOSURE OF ATRIAL DEFECTS WITH RESORBABLE PATCH MATERIALS

K.H.LEITZ[1], N. TSILIMINGAS[1], J.HOLSTE[2], H. OSTER[1]

[1]Department of Thoracic and Cardiovascular Surgery,
Krankenhaus "Links der Weser", D-2800 Bremen (F.R.G.)

[2]Ethikon, 2000 Hamburg-Norderstedt (F.R.G.)

SUMMARY

In 10 young minipigs resorbable patch materials were evaluated, 6 had a PDS- and 4 a Vicryl-patch. After doubling their body weight the PDS animals were sacrified 184 days after operation, two Vicryl animals after 90 days and the other two Vicryl pigs after 180 days, too. Macroscopically there were 10 mm large elliptical grey-white areas in all pigs with smooth covering. Microscopically the excised tissue was replaced by scar tissue. Heart muscle fibers were only seen in the marginal zone of the scar. In both groups islands of non resorbed PDS and Vicryl material could be found. In the PDS group these non resorbed areas were larger and had a tendency to calcification. Because of the calcification tendency we would prefer Vicryl for human application. Until now 9 patients had closure of their atrial septum defect by Vicryl patches.

INTRODUCTION

The direct suture is very often impossible for closing intracardiac defects. Therefore the patch principle was introduced by Carrel (ref. 1) in the beginning of this century. A variety of patch materials have been used so far: Woven or knitted Dacron, PTFE and heterologous or autologous pericard. The ideal material for the various clinical situations has not been defined yet. An absorbable material would be of interest for the following reasons: it is weakly reacting and does not provoke an excessive foreign body reaction, it allows tissue regeneration with replacement of the original material by autologous tissue and as an autologous tissue it allows growth in a growing organism.

In the following our results are presented with resorbable patch materials. We used Polydioxamon and Polyglactin experimentally and started with Polyglactin patches in patients to close atrial septal defects.

METHODS

The experiments were done with 10 young female Göttinger minipigs. The right atrium was exposed through a small right sided thoracotomy. The free anterior wall of the atrium was partially excluded with a Satinsky clamp and resected. The resected area mostly as large as a penny was replaced by a PDS patch in 6 and by a Vicryl patch in 4 minipigs. In the PDS group the patches were attached to the atrial wall by PDS suture, in the Vicryl group by Vicryl suture. After the operation the pigs were freely mobile in cages and fed a standard diet. The animals showed an ordinary development, doubled their bodyweight from operation to autopsy (15,5 kg to 33,1 kg), which took place in the PDS group 184 days postoperatively. Two animals of the Vicryl group had autopsy after 91 days and two after 180 days. The patches were investigated by lightmicroscopy and rasterelectromicroscopy.

So far 9 patients, 2 male and 7 female, with an age rage from 4 - 63 years were operated. They all had secundum type of atrial septum defects, the left to right shunt was 50 % - 85 %, the pressures in the pulmonary artery were almost normal. The operation was done via a sternotomy incision with standard heart-lung-machine equipment. For the cardiac arrest Bretschneider cardioplegic solution was used.

The patches were woven material supplied sterile 3 times 5 cm large. The suitable size was produced by a minicauter to seal the fibers and to prevent the fibers from splitting off. The patches were preclotted by unheparinazed blood in the usual way. An intraoperative picture of an implanted Vicryl patch in a patient shows Fig. 1. The fixation of the patch was achieved by 5/0 Vicryl suture. Even the atrial closure was done by Vicryl suture, too.

RESULTS

All animals survived the operation. There was no pneumonia or wound infection. Elevated temperatures were not observed during the whole time. At autopsy of both groups of animals the heart weight with 120 g was normal. The implantation area at the right auricle was a 10 mm large elliptical white scar visible from out- and inside (see Fig. 2). There was some degree of adhesions between epi- and pericard. In 1 animal of the PDS group we found a little thrombus over the tricuspidal valve beyound the patch area. The pulmonary vessels showed no thrombotic material in both groups. Histologically the excised tissue was replaced by scar tissue with fibrocytic-fibroplastic cellular elements and collagen fibers in both groups (see Fig. 3). There took place no regenaration of cardiac muscle cells. Cardiac muscle was only seen in the marginal zones of the scar. In the Masson Goldner staining the collagen fibers are green and you realize a green picture all over.

Partly giant cell elements were found, which help in the absorption of the PDS and Vicryl material. The luminal aspect of the grafted area was covered by an endothel like cellular layer (see Fig. 4), which was smooth, if you look at the material through rasterelectromicroscope (see Fig. 5). In both groups islands of non resorbed PDS and Vicryl material could be found. In the PDS

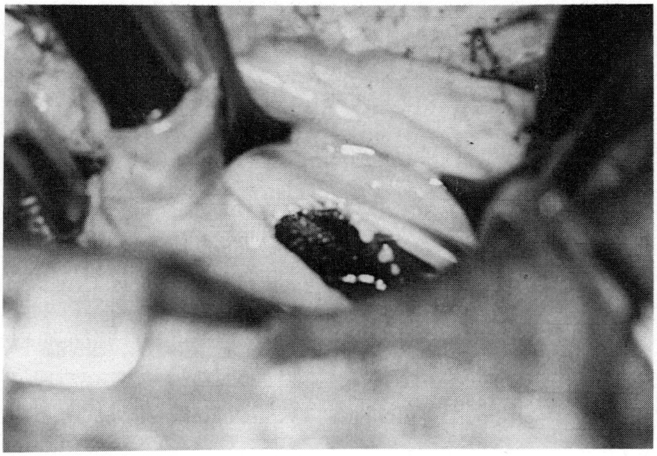

Fig. 1. Closure of an atrial septum defect in a patient,

group these non resorbed areas were larger and showed a tendency to calcification. In the PDS group the calcified islands were bigger, while the Vicryl animals showed only little fragments of calcification in the specific Kossa staining. This difference of calcification between the two groups was so striking for us, that we decided to use Polyglactin in humans.

All the patients survived the operation. There were no complications. Three patients were restudied by our cardiologists. From clinical and radiological standpoint the patch works well. In all three patients you could listen to a respiration dependent splitting of the second heart sound, which excludes a

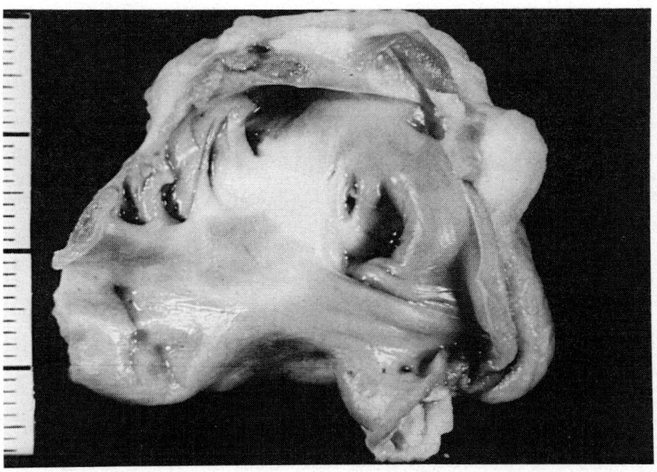

Fig. 2. The patch material is resorbed. Macroscopically a white scar is visible.

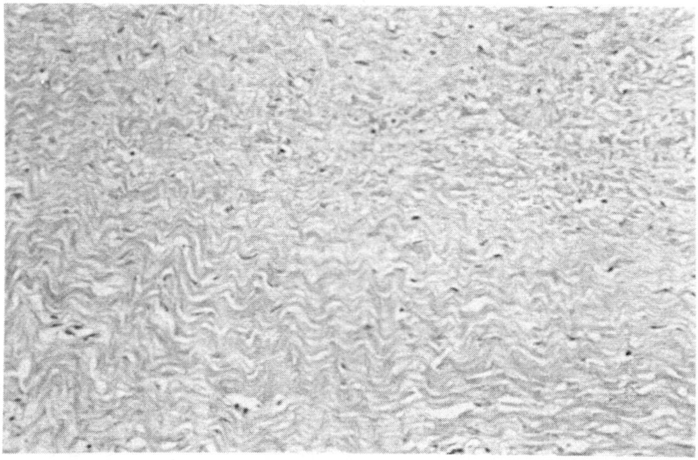

Fig. 3. The PDS and Vicryl material is replaced by scar tissue with fibrocytic-fibroplastic cellular elements and collagen fibers, Masson Goldner staining.

shunt vitium. The typical radiological sign of pulmonary overflow was absent in all postoperative control chest x-ray pictures. The right ventricle dimensions diminished according to echocardiography (from a mean valve of 39,3 mm to 26,3 mm). The normal range of 23 mm was not yet reached, but the positive tendency speaks for a good working patch.

All three patients had normal dye dilution curves without signs of a remaining shunt (see Fig. 6). The remaining 6 patients will have cardiological evaluation in the next weeks after complete resorption of their patch material.

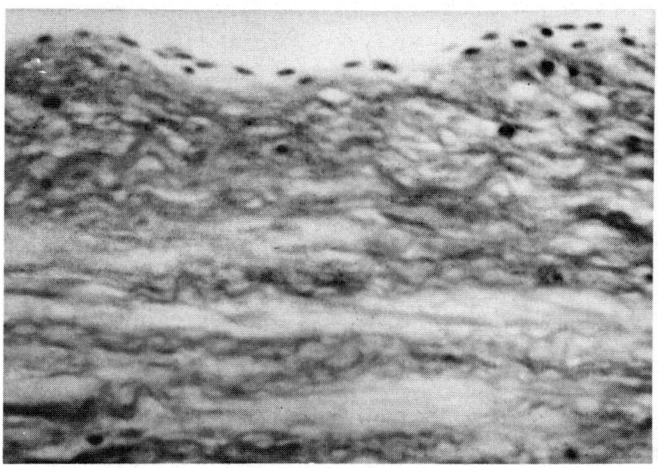

Fig. 4. The inner lining of the scar tissue was built up by an endothel like layer, Elastica v. Gieson staining.

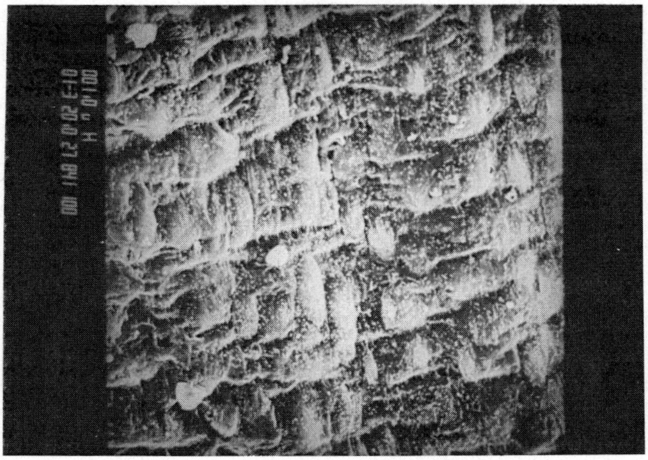

Fig. 5. Rasterelectromicroscopic picture of the inner lining of an Vicryl patch, 1.000 time magnification.

DISCUSSION

The ideal material for closing intracardiac defects should be inert, durable, flexible, easy to suture, ready available and inexpensive. In most instances autologous pericardium is available in the first operation. However when the patient has had previous palliative operation, pericardium may not be available for subsequent operations. Therefore one has to look for artificial materials. Dacron, Teflon, PTFE, preserved dura mater and bovine pericardium have been used with different clinical results (refs. 2-4).

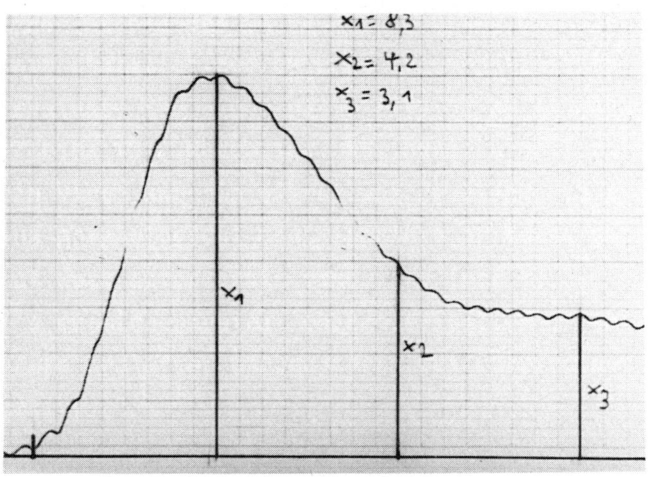

Fig. 6. Postoperative normal dye dilution curve 6 month after closure of an atrial septum defect by a Vicryl patch.

The disadvantage of all these materials is summarised as follows: Bad endothelial covering and degeneration of the inner lining with peeling off, thrombus formation and peripheral embolisation.

Resorbable materials have the advantages, that they serve as scaffold. They were replaced by body own tissue. The resorption time of PDS seems prolonged in heart tissue. The above mentioned calcification tendency seems to be disadvantageous especially in the growing organism, because in young patients the calcium metabolism is exaggerated. Therefore we decided to use Vicryl patches in humans, because the resorption time is only 60 days and the calification tendency is less.

Till now 9 patients had closure of their atrial septum defects by Vicryl patches. The first cardiological control studies show almost normal values. Further evaluation is urgently needed and is going on.

IN CONCLUSION

Resorbable patch material can work in the atrial position. We would recommend Polyglactin, because the calcification tendency is less compared to PDS. The first clinical results are encouraging.

REFERENCES

1 A. Carrel and C. C. Guthrie, Uniterminal and biterminal venous transplantation, Surg. Gynec. Olestet 2 (1906) 266-271.
2 F. A. Crawford, R. M. Sade and F. Spinale, Bovine pericardium for correction of congenital heart defects, Ann. Thorac. Surg. 41 (1986) 602-605.
3 O. Osinowo, J. L. Monro and J. K. Ross, The use of glycerol-preserved homologous dura mater grafts in cardiac surgery: the Southampton experience, Ann. Thorac. Surg. 39 (1985) 367-374.
4 H. Mohri, R. W. Barnes, E. A. Rittenhouse, D. D. Reichenbach, D. H. Dillhard and K. A. Merendino, Fate of autologous pericardium and dacron fabric used as substitutes for total atrial septum in growing animals, J. Thorac. Cardiovasc. Surg. 59 (1970) 501-508.

Biomaterials and Clinical Applications, 411
edited by A. Pizzoferrato, P.G. Marchetti, A. Ravaglioli and A.J.C. Lee
Elsevier Science Publishers B.V., Amsterdam, 1987 — Printed in The Netherlands

SYNTHETIC VASCULAR PROSTHESES - THE EVOLUTION OF AN INTERNATIONAL STANDARD

E.G. Brown[1], J.K. Drury[2], R. Maini[1], J.G. Pollock[2]

[1]Vascutek Limited, Newmains Avenue, Inchinnan, Renfrewshire, PA4 9RR, Scotland

[2]Peripheral Vascular Unit, Ward 63, Glasgow Royal Infirmary, 16 Alexandra Parade, Glasgow, G31 2ER, Scotland

SUMMARY

The development of an international standard for synthetic vascular prosthesis is discussed with comments on problem areas.

INTRODUCTION

The aim of all manufacturers of vascular prostheses is to supply surgeons with perfect prostheses every time. However there is an immediate need for standardised procedures in the evaluation of the performance, safety, and efficacy of vascular prostheses. A high quality product, be it a vascular prosthesis or any other critical product, does not merely attain a high quality by frequent and repeated testing; quality must be designed in, from research right through to the planning of manufacturing controls.

National regulatory bodies, such as the American FDA or National Ministries of Health oversee the vascular prostheses manufacturer, either by vetting the design and clinical testing of the product and/or by insisting on a rigid system of manufacturer control known as good manufacturing practice. In addition the manufacturer himself will establish a series of in process quality controls to monitor critical parameters such as length and diameter, strength, porosity etc., as well as exercising strict control over the details of labelling and product traceability.

An attempt is currently being made to standardise many of these tests in the work of the International Standards Organisation on the draft standard for synthetic vascular prostheses which should shortly be ready for international approval. Two of the authors are members of the British Standards Institution established in 1901 and which was the first National Standards body in the world. Over 80 countries now have similar organisations, most of which are members of the International Organisation for Standardisation (ISO).

The proposed standard looks into many aspects of graft manufacture and testing. However, because of variances in graft testing between manufacturers, several test methods for various parameters are accepted by the ISO although it would be better if there were universal agreement about the use of single test methods. This paper describes the main content of the proposed standard and outlines where there are important areas of difference between manufacturers.

SPECIFICIATION FOR SYNTHETIC VASCULAR PROSTHESES

The specification for synthetic vascular prostheses includes their biological and biocompatibility properties, sterility controls, physical properties and the labelling and packaging of the product.

Biocompatibility and Biological Properties

These are concerned with the acceptance of the prosthesis into living tissue and ensuring that it is non toxic. This is potentially controversial since few standards exist for such criteria as biostability and haemocompatibility. Also the current generation of vascular prostheses do not meet the ideal. For example Dacron, one of the commonest materials of construction and with 30 years of clinical history is considered more thrombogenic than would be ideal. An ISO statement emphasises the difficulty of definition consequent on a lack of consensus on the above properties or what constitutes the ideal. Concerning biostability, the ISO writes: "the types of materials of which the prostheses are made shall have been tested by means of appropriate published test methods to determine the physical and chemical effects on the material of body fluids and tissue, and suture and other materials for stitching the prostheses and also to determine the effects of the methods of sterilisation that are employed or recommended by the manufacturer of the prostheses. The details of the test methods and the results shall be made available by the manufacturer of the prostheses upon request. Appropriate data shall be made available whenever the types of materials used to make the prostheses are changed."

Sterility

The main methods of prosthesis sterilisation are by means of heat, radiation and gas. Standardisation of sterility is, however, difficult as there is no international consensus. Many countries have in existence or in preparation regulations covering the sterility of implantable medical products. For example some countries insist on carrying out sterility testing on representative samples whilst others, including the United Kingdom, disapprove of sterility testing on the basis that the rate of experimental error is much greater than the incidence of non sterile units from an approved manufacturer.

The current trend is away from extensive testing and much more towards assessing individual manufacturers on the basis of GMP (Good Manufacturing Practice). This relies on the system of validation and process control to yield the desired result.

Physical Properties

Defining physical properties such as porosity, strength, dimensions and surface characteristics would appear to be one of the easier areas to standardise. However, the specification of strength and water porosity highlight the difficulties.

Strength is currently expressed in 2 ways - tensile strength and bursting strength. There are 2 different ways of measuring and expressing tensile strength and 3 ways for burst strength. The results of these methods are not comparable although a categorisation of different grafts by one method will usually be similar to that produced by another method. Because of entrenched opinions within existing manufacturers all 5 methods have meantime been retained.

The probe test method seems to be the most acceptable method for measuring burst strength. The equipment required is a Lloyd tensile tester with an SKN load cell, a compression cage with probe and sample holder and a sample tensioning device. The fabric is burst by the probe at 70mm/min. Using this method the burst strength in KPa can be recorded with reliability and comparisons can be readily made between various graft types.

Water porosity attempts to indicate to the surgeon how much leakage there will be from the woven or knitted graft supplied by the manufacturer. It is essentially measured by recording the amount of pure water at a given temperature and pressure which will flow through 1 square centimetre of graft material in 1 minute. To allow settling times for flow to be established the original draft DP7198 specified that only once a steady flow of water was recorded should the actual measurement period of 1 minute commence. This approach was ideal for the woven grafts and first generation knitted grafts. However, it has been shown by Dr. Guidoin and by Vascutek Ltd., that modern knitted grafts have the characteristics of slowly reducing in water porosity over the first 5-10 minutes of flow. This effect is due to small movements in the individual Dacron fibres making up the knitted structure. Since the surgeon will normally be interested in potential leakage over the first few minutes the specification has been amended to require the reading to be taken within the first 5 minutes of the test.

Using the above test method on a Buxton and Cooley test rig (ref. 1) satisfactory reproducibility of the order of 1% can be obtained. However, different laboratories will achieve very different levels of porosity. It is essential, therefore, to compare grafts by measurements in one laboratory, or by relating figures obtained to the known published figure for one particular graft.

Other physical parameters can readily be obtained. The relaxed internal diameter of the graft is measured using cones. A simple frame and weights measure usable length. Grafts of knitted construction are stretched with a 125gm weight, wovens are stretched with weights from 250gms to 1000gms.

Labelling and Packaging

The proposed standard defines correct labelling and packaging with the main aims of safety and lack of confusion. There should be a sterile unit container enclosed in an outer container with instructions inserted. The labelling should be clear and precise.

CONCLUSION

An international standard on synthetic vascular prostheses is about to be produced. However, the document currently available in draft form still allows individual manufacturers to utilise a range of different tests. Therefore comparison between data from different manufacturers can be difficult.

REFERENCES

1 Brian F. Buxton, Don C. Wukasch, Carlos Martin, William J. Liebig, Grady L. Hallman, Denton A. Cooley, Practical Considerations in Fabric Vascular Grafts, The American Journal of Surgery, Vol. 125 (1983).

Biomaterials and Clinical Applications,
edited by A. Pizzoferrato, P.G. Marchetti, A. Ravaglioli and A.J.C. Lee
Elsevier Science Publishers B.V., Amsterdam, 1987 — Printed in The Netherlands

ACTIVATION OF BLOOD COAGULATION FACTORS AFTER CONTACT WITH BIOMATERIALS

L. PRATELLI, E. CENNI, G. CIAPETTI, S. STEA, C. TARABUSI, G. PROSPERI

Centro di Ricerca per la Biocompatibilità dei Materiali da Impianto
Istituto Rizzoli, Bologna, Italy

SUMMARY

In vitro test methods are widely used to assess blood-material interactions when candidate vascular materials are to be evaluated.

In this study a number of methods aimed to explore both blood coagulation processes and platelet performance when plasma is exposed to different materials was performed.

The results obtained by using such assays are presented and their significance is briefly discussed.

INTRODUCTION

Initial testing for host response to blood contact materials is usually done in vitro. Since it is not conceivable to expect a single evaluation method to describe the performance of blood when in contact with biomaterials, a number of tests to assess blood-material interactions has been developed(Ref. 1).

In vitro methods show several advantages, as they are quantifiable, they can be run with human blood, they are quite fast and relatively inexpensive to use for checking on the numerous materials under test.

The major limit of such methods is obviously the lack of the dynamic components of the in vivo blood flow, so that their relevance to in vivo events can not be taken for granted, but must be proved in each case (Ref. 2).

METHODS

Some vascular materials and orthopedic materials were tested. In addition, two kinds of Dacron-urethane composites and Copper were used as comparison. The materials were the following :

- Expanded polytetrafluoroethylene (PTFE), (Gore, Flagstaff, Arizona, U.S.A)
- Knitted Dacron (KD),(USCI, CR. Bard, Inc., Billerica, Massachusetts, U.S.A.)
- Woven Dacron (WD), (USCI, CR. Bard., Inc.)
- Straight Knitted Velour Dacron (SKVD), (USCI, CR. Bard, Inc.)
- Double Velour Dacron (DVD), (USCI, CR. Bard, Inc.)
- Dacron-urethane (DU), (D.L. Leake, Dept. of Dentistry and Surgery University of California, Los Angeles, CA, U.S.A.)
- Dacron-urethane coated with isotropic carbon (DU/C), (General Atomic Co., San Diego, California, U.S.A.)
- Alumina (Al_2O_3: 99.5% purity), (IRTEC, Faenza, Italy)
- Stainless steel 316 L,(Höganas, AB, Sweden)
- Epoxy-carbon,(Reglass SpA, Italy)
- Copper (99.9% purity), (Officine Ortopediche Rizzoli, Bologna, Italy).

The Aa. performed on one hand test procedures related to the coagulation process, that is the activation of the intrinsic and extrinsic pathways and the activity of the blood coagulation factors, as well as the antithrombin III activity. On the other hand, the platelet related phenomena, that is platelet retention following contact with the materials and platelet activation through the release of three platelet-specific factors (Ref. 3), were evaluated.

The first series of tests was performed on platelet-rich-plasma (PRP) samples, that is a pool of plasma taken from healthy donors was centrifuged at 120 x g at 4°C for 10 minutes. Then, 2.5 ml of plasma was kept at gentle rotation for 30' at room temperature in a siliconized tube which contained a 1.5 cm-sided square of the material under test. Following the 30 min. period of contact a platelet count was performed on an aliquot of the rotated plasma.

Another 1 ml-aliquot of the samples was combined with a mixture to block platelet activation, then the sample was centrifuged at 2000 x g at 4°C for 30 minutes to obtain a platelet-poor-plasma and eventually frozen at -20°C. Radioimmunoassays to detect the different factors released from platelets following the contact with the materials were performed on such plasma samples after thawing.

RESULTS

The Activated Partial Thromboplastin Time (APTT) measures the amount of time for clot formation to occur in a siliconized glass tube once adequate phospholipid, activator and calcium mixture is added to citrated plasma. By using this assay, neither any of the vascular materials nor the Dacron-urethanes, as well as stainless steel and carbon-resin composite, showed any difference

from the control sample, as shown in fig. 1. Only in presence of alumina and copper the clotting time was indefinitely or strongly prolonged, respectively.

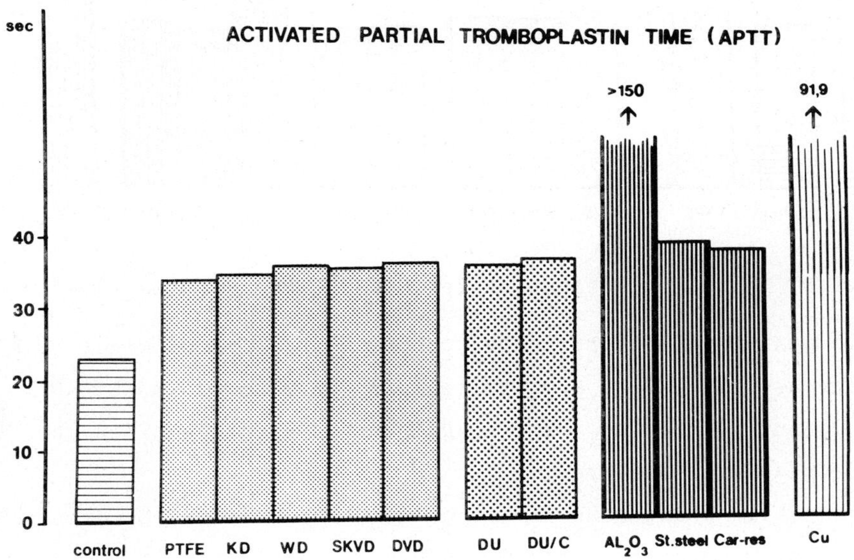

Fig. 1. APTT test.Each column represents the mean of six experiments

The Prothrombin Time (PT) measures the activation of the extrinsic pathway of coagulation, by recording the time for clot formation when tissue thromboplastin plus calcium reagent is added to the sample.

Fig. 2 shows that also the extrinsic pathway of the coagulation process was not altered by the presence of both vascular and orthopaedic materials when comparing the recorded times to the clotting time of unexposed plasma.

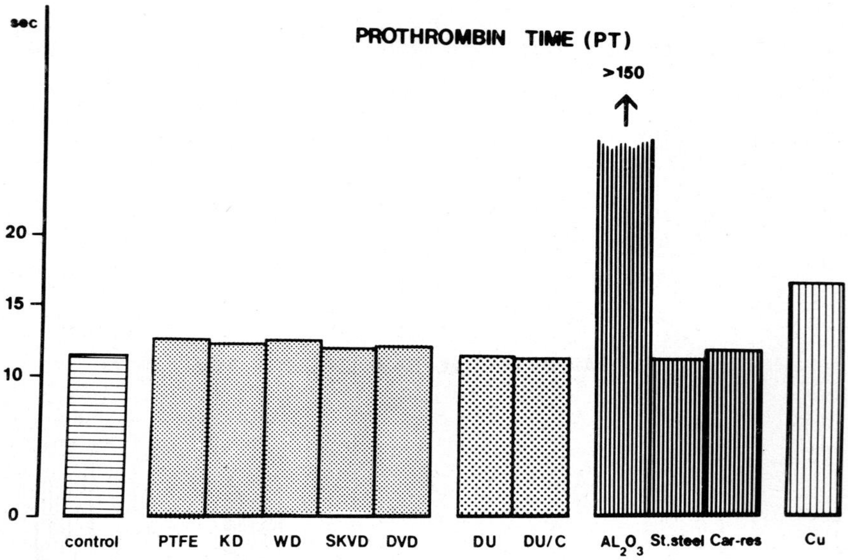

Fig. 2. PT test. Each column represents the mean of six experiments.

Once again, alumina strongly prolonged the time of clotting. This finding, as well as the similar behavior of alumina in the APTT test, is not surprising, since aluminum hydroxyde is often used to deplete plasma of factors.

More subtle changes in the coagulation process may be detected by assaying separately the various blood coagulation factors.

The test involves the addition of plasma samples to plasma deficient in the factor assayed and the recording of the clotting time.

When the factors of both the intrinsic and the extrinsic pathways are measured and their activity expressed as percent, there was no significant change induced by any material,but alumina, compared to the control sample.

To complete the exploration along the coagulation pathways, a test for detecting any changes in antithrombin III level was performed, and once again no significant alteration was induced by any materials.

Then the effect of the materials under test on platelets was evaluated.

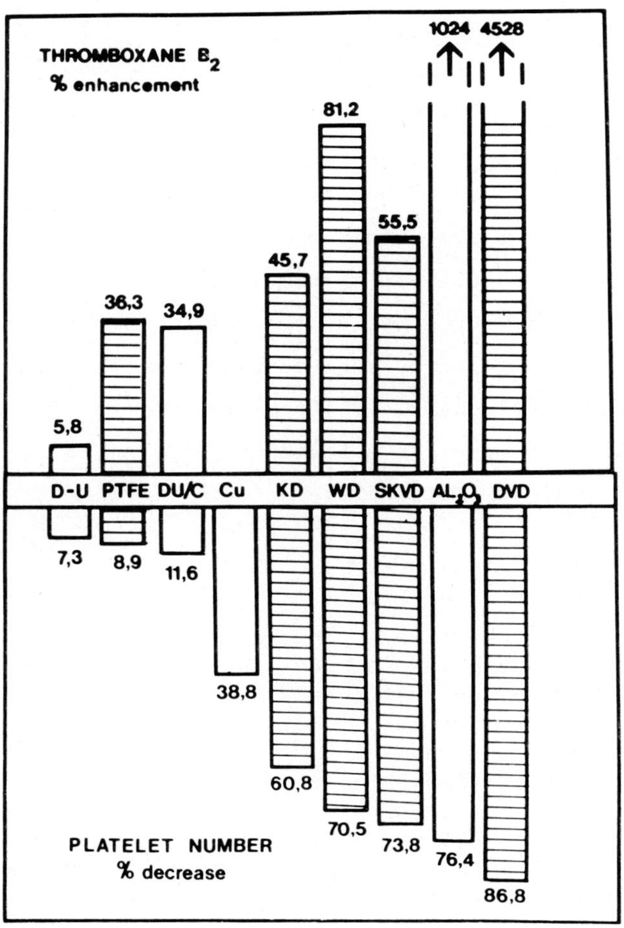

Fig. 3. TxB2 released by platelets and platelet counting.

The decrease of platelet number in plasma samples exposed to the different materials when compared to the unexposed sample was expressed as percent of the control (Fig. 3, bottom). It was found that some vascular materials, and in particular KD, WD, SKVD and DVD, caused a marked retention of platelets to their surfaces.

When this behavior was compared to the release of factors from the aggregated platelets, it was found (Fig. 3, top) that thromboxane B_2 was highly released from highly platelet-retenting materials, while the other two factors behave differently.

Thus, B-thromboglobulin was actively released when WD and DVD were present, while KD and SKVD were less active in this respect.

Finally, platelet factor 4 was highly released only by DVD, while the other materials were far less inducing.

DISCUSSION

This study demonstrates that in vitro examination of blood compatibility of biomaterials can predict the immediate undesirable interactions of materials with various blood components, such as activation of the coagulation systems or alterations of platelets.

In our hands the components of the coagulation processes were not significantly altered by the vascular materials tested, while they differently but remarkably affect the number of platelets and the factors they release, so allowing an evaluation of the possible thrombogenicity of the materials.

REFERENCES

1 Evaluation of blood-material interactions in vitro, in: Guidelines for blood-material interactions, Report of the National Heart, Lung and Blood Institute Working Group, NIH Publication no. 80-2185, September 1980, pp. 35-64.

2 S.D. Bruck, Problems and artefacts in the evaluation of polymeric materials for medical uses, Biomaterials, vol. 1 (1980) 103-107.

3 S.K. Bowry, J.M. Courtney, C.R.M. Prentice, J.T. Douglas, Utilization of the platelet release reaction in the blood compatibility assessment of polymers, Biomaterials, vol. 5 (1984) 289--292.

Biomaterials and Clinical Applications,
edited by A. Pizzoferrato, P.G. Marchetti, A. Ravaglioli and A.J.C. Lee
Elsevier Science Publishers B.V., Amsterdam, 1987 — Printed in The Netherlands

THE MECHANICAL PROPERTIES OF BOVINE PERICARDIUM

J C BARBENEL[1], P ZIOUPOS[1], J FISHER[2]

[1]Bioengineering Unit, University of Strathclyde, 106 Rottenrow, Glasgow (United Kingdom)

[2]Department of Cardiac Surgery, Royal Infirmary, Glasgow (UK)

SUMMARY

Bovine pericardium is used to manufacture heart valve substitutes. The load-extension behaviour of fresh pericardium was investigated using an inflation technique which indicated the presence of systematic variations in extensibility. The curvature of the pericardium, due to the shape of the heart, was insufficient to explain the anisotropy, and tensile tests were carried out on excised tissue strips. The load-extension response of these specimens indicated that the tissues were mechanically anisotropic.

INTRODUCTION

Chemically modified bovine pericardium has been used for the construction of substitute heart valves over fifteen years, (ref 1). When testing completed valves in flow simulators, mismatch between leaflets may be apparent, making them functionally unsuitable for clinical use. The mismatch is related to variations in the geometry and the mechanical properties of the tissues of the leaflets. The mechanical properties depend on the properties of the native bovine pericardium, the geometrical constraints induced during chemical treatment of the tissue, and the nature of the chemical treatment itself.

Pericardium shows non linear load-extension behaviour and time dependence which is typical of the fibrous soft connective tissues, (ref 2). Many such tissues, which, like pericardium, occur as sheets are also anisotropic. It is uncertain whether pericardium is anisotropic. Previous investigators who have carried out uniaxial tension tests report the tissues to be isotropic, (refs 3 and 4), nearly isotropic, (ref 5) or obviously anisotropic, (ref 6). The results obtained in biaxial extension all indicate that pericardium is anisotropic, (refs 7 to 10).

It is often difficult to investigate the anisotropy of body tissues, because there may be major intersite and inter subject differences between specimens. The orientations of the principal axes of anisotropy are not generally known and may be difficult to determine using strip specimens.

The work reported here utilised a non-destructive inflation method for detecting the direction of the axes of elastic symmetry. This was followed by uniaxial tests carried out on specimens cut from the pericardium and aligned in the directions of the axes of symmetry.

MATERIAL AND METHODS

Tests were carried out on samples of fresh bovine pericardium at a test site overlying the right ventricle.

Test material

The pericardium was obtained from cattle which were slaughtered at eighteen to thirty months of age. The pericardium was removed from the heart and transported from the abbatoir in 0.9% isotonic saline and stored at 4°C until tested. At the test site the tissue was relatively uniform, with the thickness of the specimens being between 0.3 and 0.4 mm.

The pericardium was defatted and a tissue specimen cut from the test site, the orientation of the specimen having been marked. The excised specimen of tissue was allowed to relax on a saline lubricated sheet of glass, with the epicardial surface downwards. The specimen was maintained in this relaxed configuration during subsequent handling and specimen preparation by placing a piece of light card on the tissue surface, to which it adhered. The glass was then gently removed by sliding the specimen along the glass surface. The shape of both the card and the specimen depended on the subsequent test.

Inflation

Circular specimens of pericardium 41.5 mm in diameter were clamped between a Perspex and an aluminium annulus, the specimen being supported from beneath by a perforated Perspex disc. The membrane was inflated to a pressure of 0.82 kPa (5mm Hg) and the shape of the deformed surface determined by using Moire fringes, which were formed between a grating and the shadow of the grating cast on to the membrane. The grating was a flat sheet of 50% transmission with parallel lines at a density of 2.5 lines per mm. For preparing the specimen, the card was cut as a disc slightly smaller than 90 mm in diameter and with a central hole of 41.5 mm diameter.

An additional insert with a square aperture having sides 26 mm could be placed within the aluminium disc to allow for the inflation of square specimens. Before use fiducial marks were printed on to the surface of the specimen, which were then inflated incrementally to a maximum pressure of 16 kPa.

Simple tension

Tensile tests were carried out on strips of tissue from the area which had been inflated. Between the biaxial and uniaxial tests the specimen was allowed to relax for twenty-four hours at 4°C. Two sets of three parallel strips were cut in orthogonal directions. Each set was cut using a template, which allowed all three to be prepared at the same time. The template and cutting blades produced strips which were 3 mm wide and 70 mm long. The specimen, and the adherent card, were mounted in spring loaded grips containing a gauge block which produced an intergrip specimen 15 mm long. The specimen and grips were mounted vertically in an Instron 1195 tensile test machine, the gauge block removed and the supporting card cut. At tests were carried out at 37°C in one quarter strength Ringer's solution.

The specimens were pre-conditioned by extending them repeatedly at a constant extension rate. When a stable and reproducible cycle had been obtained a final test response was obtained by stretching the specimen at 5 mm per minute until rupture occurred.

RESULTS

The Moire contour lines produced on all the inflated circular specimens were oval. indicating that the pericardial specimen showed systematic variations in extensibility. The orientation of the principal axis of the oval was consistent in all specimens, being within 10° of the circumferential direction. The ovals were symmetrical with the axis of the oval, and therefore of elastic symmetry, being at right angles.

Following the inflation of the circular disc the square aperture plate was inserted with the sides of the square aligned in the direction of maximum and minimum

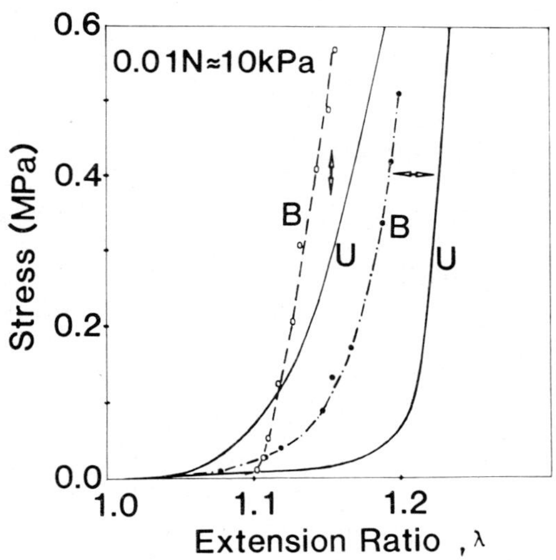

Fig. 1 Results of uniaxial (U) and biaxial inflation (B) tests carried out on the same specimen at the same site. The horizontal arrows (<—>) indicate the pair of circumferential results, the vertical arrow the axial results.

extensibility. The shape of the inflated square specimen was determined from orthogonal photographs, and the stresses and strains calculated from the inflation pressure and the shape and thickness of the specimen, on the assumption that it could be treated as a thin membrane. A typical pair of stress-strain curves obtained from a specimen is shown in Fig. 1, in which the inflation results are marked 'B'.

In uniaxial tension repeated load cycling stretched the specimen, and increased its unloaded length from the original 15 mm. Under these conditions it is difficult to define the stress free configuration and the point at which the smallest detectable load was transmitted by the specimen was taken as the strain origin. The reference load used was 0.01 N, which was equivalent to a stress of approximately 10 kPa. Results of uniaxial tension tests on two orthogonal strips are shown in Fig. 1 (marked "U").

Fig. 2 shows the results obtained when orthogonal strips were stretched until they failed. In this case the specimens were 5 mm wide, with the original gauge length being 25 mm.

DISCUSSION

The qualitative results obtained by inflating circular discs of pericardium showed that the inflated membrane was not axisymmetric. The contours were ovals, with the anatomical orientation of the principal axes of the ovals being relatively consistent between the different samples.

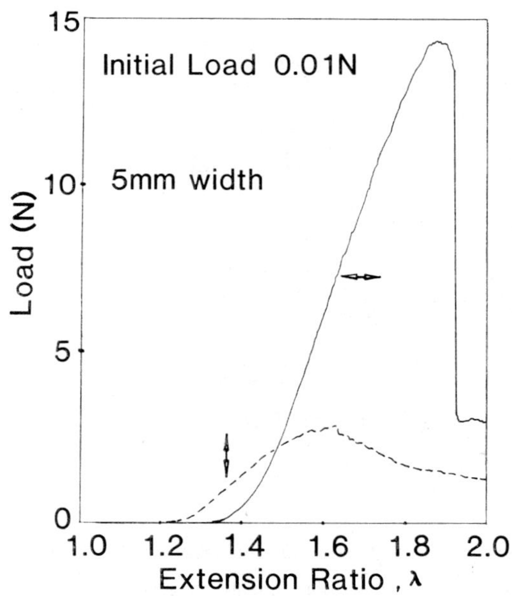

Fig. 2. Uniaxial tension tests till specimen failure. The orientation of the specimens indicated as in Fig. 1.

The quantitative biaxial results obtained from inflating square specimens confirmed that the tissues were anisotropic. This is clearly seen in Fig. 1, in which equal stresses produce a greater extension in the circumferential than in the axial direction. This directional variation in extensibility may have geometrical or mechanical causes. The heart, and the pericardium which clothes it, is curved, but the inflation specimen is initially constrained to be planar. Measurements of curvature at the test site were made on a plaster cast of a bovine heart and the circumferential curvature was found to be greater than the axial. Calculations suggested that this difference contributed to, but was too small to fully explain, the directional variation in extensibility.

The results obtained in the uniaxial tension tests confirmed the presence of the anisotropy shown biaxially. The difference of extension at the same stress is clearly apparent in Fig 1. The slope of the terminal part of the stress-strain curve was also found to be different, with the incremental modulus consistently being greater in the circumferential than in the axially orientated strips. Comparison of the results obtained on seven pericardia, using the Friedman non-parametric test, indicated that this difference was statistically significant. ($P < 0.01$).

Anisotropy was also apparent in the failure characteristics. The ultimate tensile strength was significantly greater in circumferential than in aixial strips, (Friedman test, $P < 0.01$). Failure is also more abrupt in the circumferential of specimens.

Results obtained from inflating square specimens are consistent with biaxial results reported by previous investigators (refs 7 to 11). Although these were obtained using different test methods, the general form of the stress-strain response, including the presence of anisotropy, and the magnitude of the stresses in extensions are similar. Comparisons with the previously reported uniaxial results are rather more problematical. Vito (ref 6) reported that pericardial specimens were anisotropic. Lee and Boghner (ref 3) concluded that canine pericardium was isotropic, but, nevertheless, suggested that the tissue showed slight but significant directional variations in tensile modulus and in ultimate tensile strength - a finding supported by the present study. More detailed comparisons are impossible because of differences in species, test site, specimen geometry and test method.

CONCLUSIONS

The results of the inflation of disc shaped specimens of pericardium indicate that the tissues show significant directional variation of extensibility. The method appears to be a useful non-destructive technique for locating the principal axes of anisotropy before further tests are made. Both the biaxial and uniaxial tests confirm that pericardium shows the anisotropy which is typical of many other soft connective tissue membranes. The anisotropy of load extension behaviour also occurs in the failure characteristic of the tissue.

REFERENCES

1 M. I. Ionescu, A. D. Tandom, N. R. Saunders, M. Chidambarem and D. R. Smith, Clinical experience of the pericardial xenograft, 11 year's experience. In L. H. Cohn and V. Galluci (Eds.), Cardiac Bioprostheses, Yorke Medical Books, New York, 1982, pp. 42-60

2 J. C. Barbenel, J. H. Evans, Soft connective tissues: Mechanical properties. In McAinsh (Ed.), Physics in Medicine Encyclopedia, Pergammon Press, Oxford, 1986, pp. 780-783

3 M. J. Lee and D. R. Boughner, Mechanical properties of human pericardium. Circ. Res., 57 (1985) 475-481

4 E. A. Trowbridge, M. M. Black and C. L. Daniel, The mechanical response of gluteraldehyde fixing bovine pericardium to uniaxial load. J. Mat. Sc., 20 (1985) 114-140

5 M.J. Lee and D. R. Boughner, Tissue mechanics of pericardium in different test environments. Circ. Res., 49 (1981) 533-544

6 A. W. Wiegner, O. H. L. Bing, T. K. Borg and J. B. Cauldfield, Mechanical and structural correlates of canine pericardium. Circ. Res., 49 (1981) 807-814

7 R. P. Vito, The mechanical properties of soft tissues - I: A mechanical system for biaxial testing, J. Biomech., 13 (1980) 947-950

8 M. C. Lee, M. M. LeWinter, G. Freeman, R. Shabetai and Y.C. Fung, Biaxial mechanical properties of the pericardium in normal and volume overloaded dogs. Am. J. Physiol., 249 (1985) (Heart Circ. Physiol., 18), H222-H230

9 F. C. P. Yin, P. H. Chew and S. L. Zeger, An approach to quantification of biaxial tissue stress-strain data, J. Biomech., 19 (1986) 27-37

10 P. H. Chew, S. L. Zeger and F. C. P. Yin, Determination of material properties of biological tissues: pericardium. In G. W. Schmid-Schonbern, S. L. - Y, Woo and B.W. Zweifach, (Eds.), Frontiers of Biomechanics, Springer-Verlag Inc., New York, 1986, pp. 86-97

Biomaterials and Clinical Applications, 427
edited by A. Pizzoferrato, P.G. Marchetti, A. Ravaglioli and A.J.C. Lee
Elsevier Science Publishers B.V., Amsterdam, 1987 — Printed in The Netherlands

PHYSICAL PROPERTIES AND BIOCOMPATIBILITY OF SOME POLY(ETHER-AMIDOAMINE-UREA-URETHANE) BLOCK COPOLYMERS

M.C.TANZI[1], M.LEVI[1], M.MUTTONI[1], G.TIEGHI[1] and R.FUMERO[2]

Dipartimenti di [1]Chimica Industriale e Ingegneria Chimica "Giulio Natta" e di [2]Energetica, Politecnico, Piazza L. da Vinci, 32 - 20133 Milano (Italy)

SUMMARY

Synthesis, physical and biological properties of new heparinizable segmented polyurethanes, namely poly(ether-amidoamine-urea-urethane)s (PEAUU), are described. The copolymers, prepared by coupling isocyanate-terminated macrodiols with amino-terminated poly-amidoamines (PAA), prove to retain the heparin complexing ability characteristic of pure PAAs, and show a considerable blood compatibility.

Among the synthesized PEAUUs, those derived by polytetramethylene oxide (PTMO) show better mechanical properties and stability in biological environments. New results of some relevant characterizations of these materials after blood exposition in closed circuit are reported, suggesting that the new PEAUU copolymers, when heparinized, exhibit an improved blood compatibility with respect to poly(ether-urethane-urea)s, that have been already introduced in the biomedical field.

INTRODUCTION

The preparation of copolymers molecularly including heparinizable segments has been considered by our research group, in order to obtain biomaterials with improved non-thrombogenic properties. As heparinizable segments, linear polymers with poly-amidoamine (PAA) structure were chosen (refs.1,2). The heparin complexing ability of PAAs was discovered some years ago, and has been related to the presence, in their structure, of tertiary amino groups which are able, when protonated, to electrostatically interact with the negatively charged groups present in the heparin molecule (ref. 3).

Since the mechanical properties of PAAs do not allow their direct use as biomaterials, the preparation of copolymers can be considered, in order to obtain materials in which an appropriate mechanical behaviour is joined to the heparin adsorbing ability. Following this way, polystyrene/PAA block copolymers, and polyethylene/PAA graft copolymers have been previously prepared (refs. 4-6). Moreover, PAA chains can be grafted onto the surface of pre-synthesized materials (refs.2,3).

More recently, our attention has been directed toward a new family of poly-(ether-amidoamine-urea-urethane)s (PEAUU), in which poly-ether-urethane segments are coupled with PAA segments. This paper gives an outline of the results so far obtained with these new materials, with regard to physico-chemical, heparin adsorption, and biocompatibility properties. In addition, new results on physico-mechanical and blood-compatibility properties of two PEAUUs after blood exposition in closed circuit are presented.

SYNTHESIS

At first, the synthesis of PEAUUs was carried out by reacting commercial macrodiols (like polypropylene oxide, PPO) with 4,4'-diphenylmethane diisocyanate (MDI), and coupling the resulting macrodiisocyanate with secondary- or primary-amino terminated PAAs, following the scheme:

1) HO- POLYETHER -OH + 2 MDI $\xrightarrow[N_2,\ 80°C]{DMSO,}$

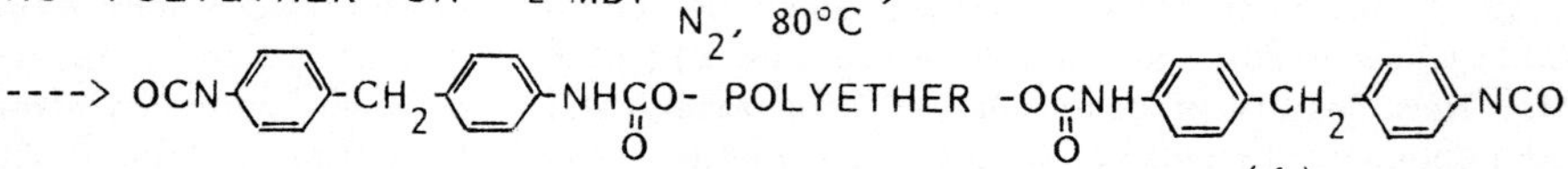

(A)

2) n (A) + n HN(R)--PAA--NH(R) $\xrightarrow[N_2,\ 80°C]{DMSO,}$ PEAUU

R = H, or CH_3

The structure of some PAAs used in the synthesis is reported in Table 1.

TABLE 1

Structure of poly-amidoamines utilized in the synthesis of PEAUUs

Type A, B, and D PAAs

$$Z\text{-}\left[CH_2CH_2\text{-}\underset{O}{\overset{\|}{C}}NHRHN\underset{O}{\overset{\|}{C}}CH_2CH_2\text{-}\underset{CH_3}{N}\text{-}(CH_2)_6\text{-}\underset{CH_3}{N}\text{-}\right]_x\text{-}CH_2CH_2\text{-}\underset{O}{\overset{\|}{C}}NHRHN\underset{O}{\overset{\|}{C}}CH_2CH_2\text{-}Z$$

HRH= $\left\langle\begin{matrix}CH_2\text{-}CH_2\\CH_2\text{-}CH_2\end{matrix}\right\rangle$: PAA A3; R= $-(CH_2)_{12}-$: PAA B3; R= $-CH_2-$: PAA D3

secondary amino terminated PAAs : $Z = \text{-}\underset{CH_3}{N}\text{-}(CH_2)_6\text{-}\underset{CH_3}{NH}$

primary amino terminated PAAs : $Z = -NH_2$

By this synthetic line, good results have been obtained, especially when type B PAAs, i.e. the lower molecular weight and the less hygroscopic ones, were utilized (refs.7,8).

Subsequently, a low molecular weight diamine, like propanediamine (PDA), was utilized in the second step as additional chain extender. By this way, higher molecular weight PEAUUs can be obtained, with higher yields, particularly in the case of PEAUUs containing polytetramethylene oxide (PTMO) and type A3 or D3 PAAs (ref.9).

For comparison, segmented polyurethanes (SPUs) without PAA segments were prepared following the same synthetic pathway, using PDA as chain extender.

Some synthesized segmented polyurethanes are listed in Table 2.

PROPERTIES

(i) Thermal properties. Differential Scanning Calorimetry (DSC) of PU_{725}-B3 and PU_{1000}-B3 showed melting effects attributable to the crystallizable PAA segments, whereas no noticeable crystallinity was detectable in all the other PEAUUs. The PEAUUs synthesized without PDA showed two different glass transition temperatures (Tg), attributable to polyurethane segments and PAA segments. PEAUUs containing PDA units, and reference SPUs, showed only one Tg: at about -30°C in the case of PPO-derived PEAUUs and SPUs, and at -50÷-66°C in the case of PTMO-derived PEAUUs.

(ii) Heparin adsorbing ability was evaluated after a 16h treatment of PEAUU sheets with 1% heparin in acetate buffered solution (pH = 4.8). The presence of heparin at the surfaces was investigated, and confirmed, by ATR/FT-IR spectroscopy (refs.7-9). The stability of the complex with heparin was analyzed after

TABLE 2

Formulation and characteristics of poly(ether-amidoamine-urea-urethane)s (PEAUUs) and reference polyurethanes (SPUs)

Name	Formulation	$[\eta]^{30°C}_{DMF}$	PAA content* (weight %)	Ref.
PU_{725}-B3	PPO(MW=725), MDI, PAA-B3	0.25	nd	7
PU_{1000}-B3	PPO(MW=1000), MDI, PAA-B3	0.35	nd	8
PP-A3-UU	PPO("),MDI, PAA-A3, PDA	0.31	20	9
PP-D3-UU	PPO("),MDI, PAA-D3, PDA	0.36	14	9
PP-UU	PPO("),MDI, PDA	0.28-0.38	--	8,9
PT-A3-UU	PTMO("),MDI, PAA-A3, PDA	0.69	15	9
PT-D3-UU	PTMO("),MDI, PAA-D3, PDA	0.55	6	9
PT-UU	PTMO("), MDI, PDA	0.75	--	9

(*) = by titration of the tertiary N atoms with 0.1N HCl in DMF/EtOH mixture treating the heparinized sheets with saline solution first, and then with aqueous 0.1N NaOH; the release of heparin in the solutions, evaluated by biological or chromogenic techniques (refs.7,9), resulted practically negligible in saline, whereas it was substantial in the NaOH solution, i.e. under strong hydrolytic conditions.

From the above tests, we concluded that heparin can be strongly adsorbed on PEAUUs, even when the PAA content is less than 10% by weight.

(iii) Mechanical properties. All the synthesized PEAUUs, and reference SPUs generally show a rubber-like behaviour. A much higher tensile strength and elongation at break were shown by PTMO-based materials compared with PPO ones (ref.9).

(iv) Hydrolytic stability and blood compatibility. The tests, carried out by exposing in vitro sheets of PPO-, and PTMO-based copolymers to various solutions (buffered saline, 0.1N NaOH, bovine plasma or blood) revealed a good stability, better in the case of PTMO-based PEAUUs. (More details can be found in ref.9).

In all the tests with blood, no clotting effects, and no noticeable changes of the specimens surfaces have been observed; moreover the blood elements deposition resulted much lower on the surface of the heparinized sheets.

BLOOD COMPATIBILITY IN CLOSED CIRCUIT OF PTMO-BASED COPOLYMERS

DMF-cast sheets of PT-A3-UU, PT-D3-UU, and PT-UU were dried under vacuo, then equilibrated in saline for 24 h. Some PEAUU sheets were heparinized, as described above, and then all the samples were immersed in the reservoir of a test apparatus, similar to the extracorporeal lines adopted during pediatric cardiopulmonary bypass, equipped with a section simulating the patient's resistance and compliance. Pulsatile flow (0.6 l/min) was delivered by a pump prototype.

The experiment was performed at 26°C, with 1 l of heparinized fresh bovine blood, and lasted 4 h. Before and after the test, hemogas analysis has been performed; no appreciable changes in the registered parameters were observed, as shown in Table 3. After the experiment, and before further characterizations, the sheets were fixed with 1% glutaraldehyde solution for 10 min.

(i) Mechanical tensile properties have been evaluated with an Instron Dynamometer 1121-10 KN, on 10x30x0.5 mm specimens. As reported in Table 4, the

TABLE 3

Parameters registered by gas analysis of the bovine blood before and after the experiment in closed circuit.

PARAMETERS	INITIAL	FINAL
pH	7.30	7.33
pCO_2 (mmHg)	55.8	45.7
pO_2 (")	18.3	27.4
HCO_3^- (mmol/l)	27.7	24.7
Total CO_2 (")	29.4	25.6

results were comparable to those obtained on the starting materials, thus confirming that blood exposition does not affect the tensile properties of these copolymers.

(ii) DSC traces, registered after the experiment with blood on both dried and not dried sheets, resulted fairly similar, Tg values included, to those of materials before the contact with blood.

(iii) Surface morphology and blood deposition were analyzed by optical and scanning electron microscopy (SEM). As already observed in previous experiments, the surface of the samples appeared almost unchanged after the contact with blood: the blood deposit, constituted by particles of 8-10 μm diameter, resulted much poorer on the heparinized sheets. Examples of S.E. Micrographs are shown in Figure 1.

TABLE 4

Tensile properties of PTMO-based copolymers

MATERIAL	CONDITIONS	STRENGTH (MPa)	ELONGATION AT BREAK (%)	MODULUS (MPa) (100% elongation)
PT-A3-UU	A	20.1	560	3.2
PT-D3-UU		20.3	600	4.4
PT-A3-UU	B	19.0	450	3.8
PT-D3-UU		20.9	530	4.9
PT-A3-UU	C	20.3	555	3.5
PT-D3-UU		20.5	545	4.4

A: after 16 h contact with saline solution;
B: after 4 h contact with bovine blood in closed circuit;
C: heparinized specimens, under B conditions.

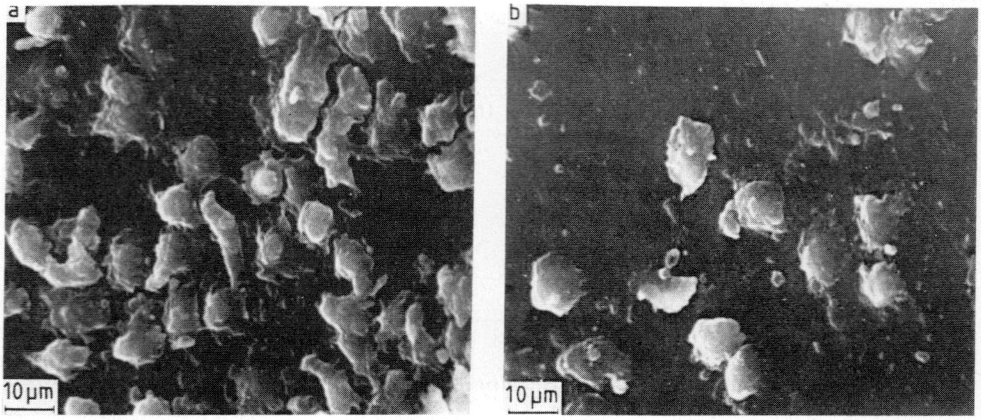

Fig.1. S.E. micrographs of not-heparinized (a) and heparinized (b) PT-D3-UU sheets after contact with blood in closed circuit.

REFERENCES

1 F.Danusso and P.Ferruti, Synthesis of tertiary amino polymers, Polymer, 11 (1970) 88-113.
2 P.Ferruti, M.A.Marchisio and R.Barbucci, Synthesis, physico-chemical properties and biomedical applications of poly(amido-amine)s, Polymer, 26 (1985) 1336-48.
3 R.Barbucci, G.Casini, P.Ferruti and F.Tempesti, Surface-grafted heparinizable materials, Polymer, 26 (1985) 1349-52.
4 P.Ferruti, D.Arnoldi, M.A.Marchisio, E.Martuscelli, M.Palma, F.Riva and L.Provenzale, Synthesis and properties of new potentially nonthrombogenic polymeric materials, J.of Polymer Sci.Pol.Chem.Ed., 15 (1977) 2151-62.
5. E.Martuscelli, L.Nicolais, F.Riva, P.Ferruti and L.Provenzale, Synthesis and characterization of a potentially non-thrombogenic poly-ethylene poly (amido-amine) graft copolymer, Polymer, 19 (1978) 1063-66.
6 M.C.Tanzi, C.Barozzi, G.Tieghi, R.Ferrara, G.Casini and F.Tempesti, Heparinizable graft copolymers from chlorosulphonated polyethylene with poly(amido-amine) segments, Biomaterials, 6 (1985) 273-276.
7 M.C.Tanzi, C.Barozzi, G.Tieghi, L.Grassi and R.Fumero, New poly(ether-amidoamine-urea-urethane) block copolymers for biomedical use, in: CNR (Ed.), Proc.Int.Workshop on future trends in polymer science and technology. Polymers: commodities or specialities?, Capri, Italy, October 8-13, 1984, Tipolito Teti, Napoli, Vol. 2, pp.265-269.
8 M.C.Tanzi, P.Albonico, C.Barozzi, A.Bolognesi, R.Fumero and G.Tieghi, Heparinizable segmented polyurethanes for cardio-vascular applications, in: Polymers in Medicine, E.Chiellini, P.Giusti, C.Migliaresi and L.Nicolais (Eds.), Plenum Press, New York, in press.
9 M.C.Tanzi, R.Fumero, M.Levi and G.Tieghi, New heparinizable, blood compatible segmented polyurethanes: properties and stability tests, in: Polyurethanes in biomedical engineering, Elsevier, Amsterdam, in press.

Biomaterials and Clinical Applications,
edited by A. Pizzoferrato, P.G. Marchetti, A. Ravaglioli and A.J.C. Lee
Elsevier Science Publishers B.V., Amsterdam, 1987 — Printed in The Netherlands

OSTEOMESH™, A DACRON POLYETHERURETHANE COMPOSITE FOR RECONSTRUCTIVE SURGERY

Leake, D.L.; Habal, M.B.; Pizzoferrato, A.; Schwartz, H.D.; Moore, L.J.; Mannai, C.

Oral and Maxillofacial Surgery
Harbor-UCLA Medical Center
Torrance, California 90509

SUMMARY

This paper presents our observations on the clinical applications of a composite material made of polyethyleneterephthlate (Dacron) mesh and a polyetherurethane elastomer (OsteoMesh™) for the restoration of bony contour defects. Work on this material dates from 1970 when our first studies were undertaken in dogs for the reconstruction of mandibular discontinuity defects using autologous cancellous bone (refs. 1-3). In the interim, various other defects of the skeleton have been restored using the material by itself, with bone grafted from the patient or from banked bone or with synthetic materials such as hydroxylapatite or HTR™ (porous methacrylates)(refs. 4-6).

Custom fabrication for restoration of large defects of the skull and other facial bones has been improved by using three dimensional imaging techniques. A precise model of the defect can be created from the three dimensional image ona computer screen by stacking a series of CT slices. A solid model of the defect can then be created in plastic using computer assisted milling and the restoration of the defect can be perfectly achieved by using the mirror image of the normal side to recreate the contour of the defective side. From this template, a precise implant can be made of the OsteoMesh™ material to achieve an anatomically symmetrical reconstruction.

Other applications have included the reconstruction of the anterior chest wall of an infant born with ectopia cordis and no sternum. The prosthesis provided ample chest wall stability to permit the generation of negative intrathoracic pressure by the infant who was subsequently weaned from mechanically assisted ventilation. A study using the Dacron urethane material for the prosthetic replacement of large defects of the cervical trachea in dogs has recently been published (ref. 7). Additional studies have included restoration of long bone defects in dogs (ref. 8) and most recently, at the Rizzoli Institute, a study of the comparative thromboresistance of Dacron combined with various urethanes as a potential material for a thromboresistant small diameter vascular prosthesis (ref. 9).

The Mandible

Large bony discontinuity defects of the mandible have been difficult to reconstruct because the mandible is highly contoured and because it is a stress bearing bone covered only by a thin layer of mucosa. Solid autologous bone grafts, usually from the iliac crest or from the rib, have commonly been employed but they are difficult to adapt to facial contours and they undergo unpredictable resorption. Consequently, reconstructive surgeons have sought other methods for restoring mandibular discontinuity defects. A number of metallic trays have been used but because of their rigidity, they are difficult to adapt at the time of surgery.

Importance of Postreconstruction Irradiation

The patient who undergoes irradiation for cancer therapy is generally a poor candidate for mandibular reconstruction. However, should the patient require irradiation postreconstruction, the Dacron urethane prosthesis does not alter radiation dosimetry in any clinically important way whereas the metallic prostheses produce an increase in the dose of irradiation which may lead to dehiscence secondary to excessive radiation. However, studies of bone grafts to mandibles irradiated preoperatively in laboratory animals, have resulted in soft tissue dehiscence in 60 to 100 percent of the animals studied (ref. 10). This complication results in the loss of the bone graft. When it is feasible, combined radical surgery with reconstruction and subsequent postoperative radiotherapy results in a decrease in surgical wound complications without diminishing the survival of the bone graft.

In a recently published study of postoperative irradiation of fresh autogenic cancellous bone grafts in surgical defects in dogs (ref. 11), 14 adult mongrel dogs had two centimeter discontinuity defects created in the horizontal ramus of the mandible. The periosteum was resected in half of the animals and defects were immediately grafted with fresh autologous cancellous bone taken from the ilium. The Dacron/urethane mandibular prosthesis stabilized the cancellous bone grafts. Twelve dogs subsequently achieved the equivalent dose of 5,750 rads of super voltage radiation. Radiotherapy was begun at intervals of 3, 4, 5, 6, 7, 8, and 9, 11 and 12 weeks after grafting. The two remaining dogs were not irradiated. Half of the animals were sacrificed at six months postoperatively and the other half at one year. Results showed complete incorporation of all bone grafts irrespective of whether the grafts have been irradiated or of the interval between surgery and radiotherapy. The contour was regular. Thin trabeculae tended to form centrally and heavier trabeculae aligned the periphery of the bone.

Based on the observations in animals, Dr. Schwartz has reconstructed a number of patients in whom radiotherapy began postoperatively. The results in humans have matched those of the laboratory animals.

Skull Reconstruction

Anatomically precise reconstruction of the skull begins with a CT scan capable of three dimensional imaging, with cuts made at one millimeter intervals. The scan requirements include the use of a flat beam filter, no gantry tilt, no recalibration of the table, minimum patient movement, and symmetry of patient positioning. The scanner reconstruction requirements include a normal reconstruction filter, high resolution reconstruction matrix, target or zoom reconstruction in the region of interest to increase resolution and, to achieve the image data, use of mag tape for data processing. The image data is interfaced with a computer assisted milling device to manufacture the anatomical model. With finely cut scan information, the models thus created can be produced with tolerances below one millimeter. A mirror image of the normal side is then used to reestablish the contour of the defective side. From this restored model of the defect, an OsteoMesh™ craniofairing can be fabricated that will have a margin of one centimeter overlap around the defect. Because of this method of custom fabrication, the implant fits perfectly on the skull.

The surgical technique is as follows:

A full thickness flap is elevated and reflected to expose the dura and the surrounding bone margin of the defect. The bone margins are freshened with a power driven burr under copious irrigation. Bone graft material is then placed in the defect. For small defects, cancellous bone will suffice but, for large defects, both cancellous bone and split ribs are used. The ribs are contoured with bone bending forceps and cut to fit the defect precisely. The OsteoMesh™ craniofairing is then placed over the bone graft overlapping the margin of the normal skull by about one centimeter. If there is any question of the stability of the implant, small diameter metal screws, five to seven millimeters in length, can be placed in the margin of the implant into the host bone to stabilize the implant during the healing phase.

Figs. 1-3

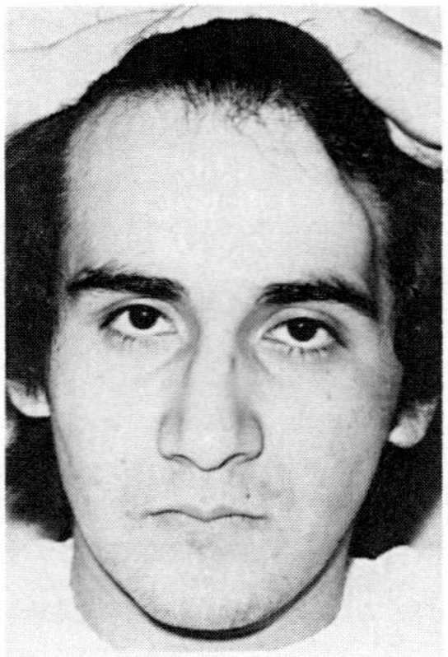

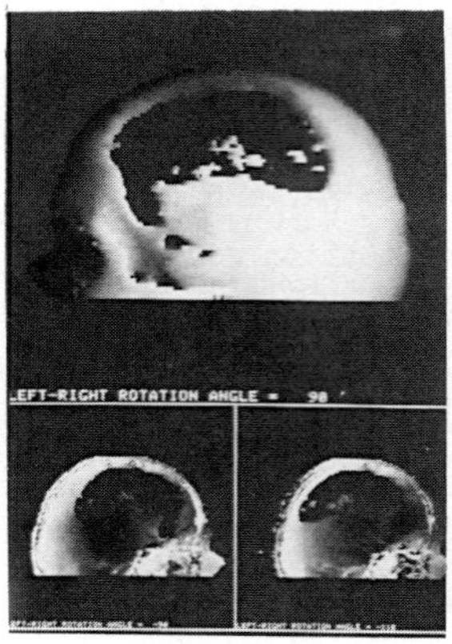

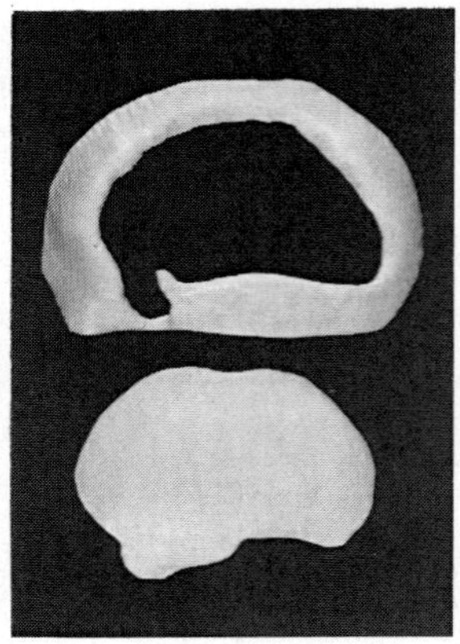

Figs. 4-5

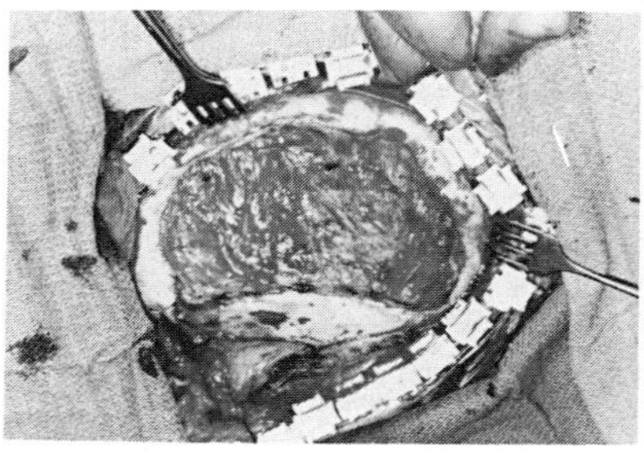

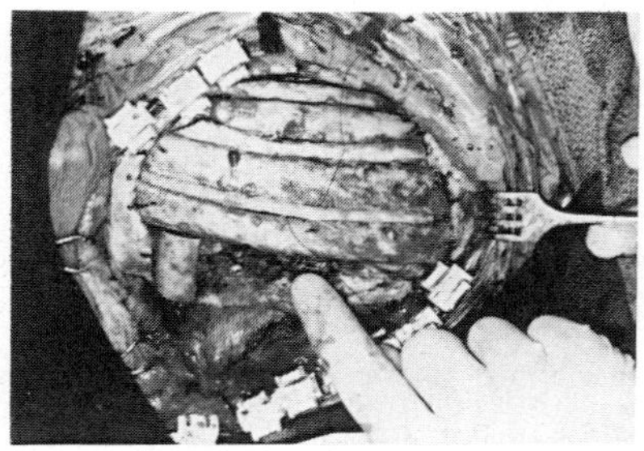

Figs. 6-7

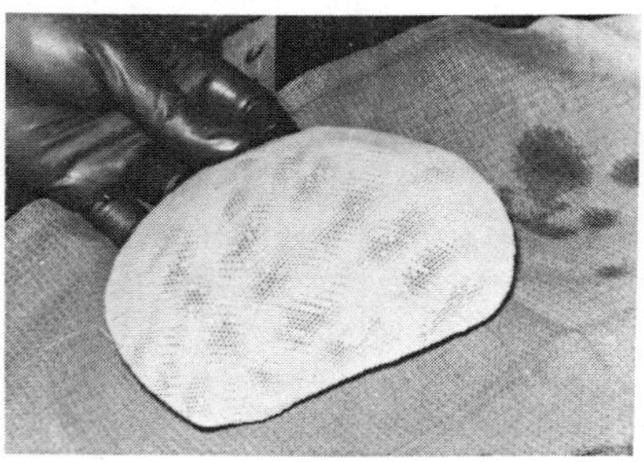

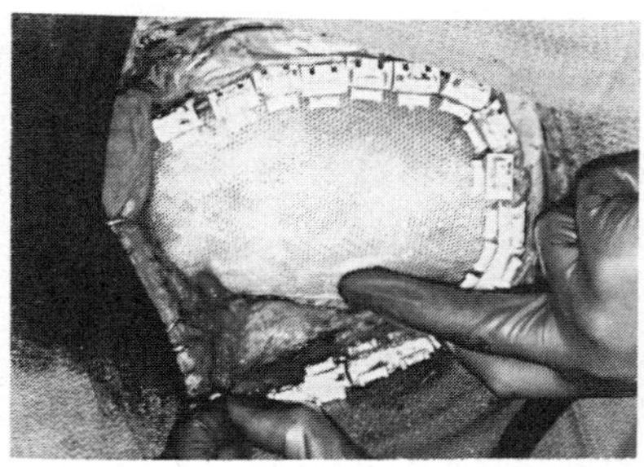

Fig. 8

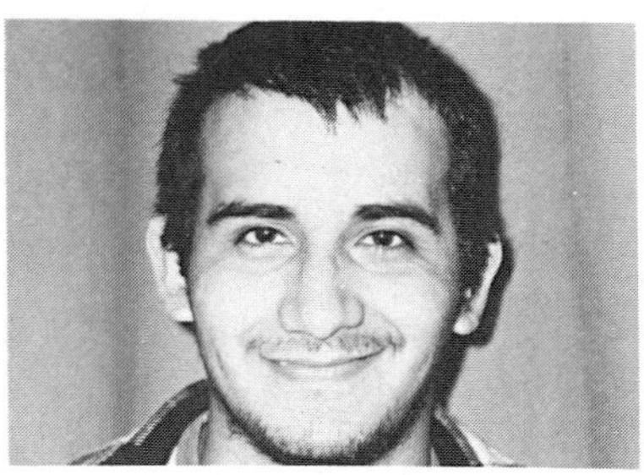

Fig. 1 - Preoperative left frontal parietal defect.
Fig. 2 - 3-D CT Scan.
Fig. 3 - A Model of the defect (above) with the mirror image of the normal side (below).
Fig. 4 - An intraoperative view of the defect.
Fig. 5 - The rib grafts in place.
Fig. 6 - The OsteoMesh implant.
Fig. 7 - The OsteoMesh in place.
Fig. 8 - The postoperative view.

Figs. 9-10

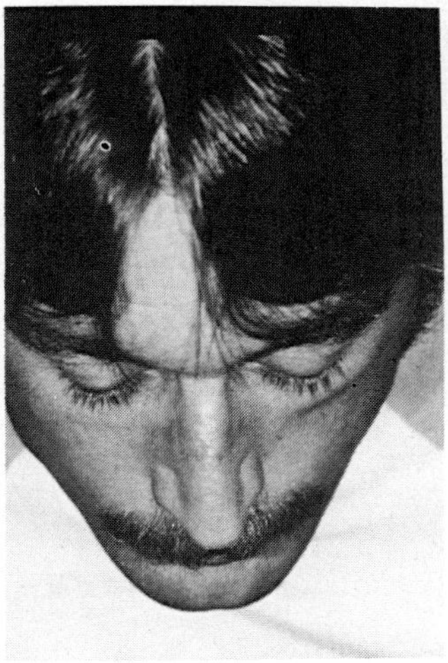

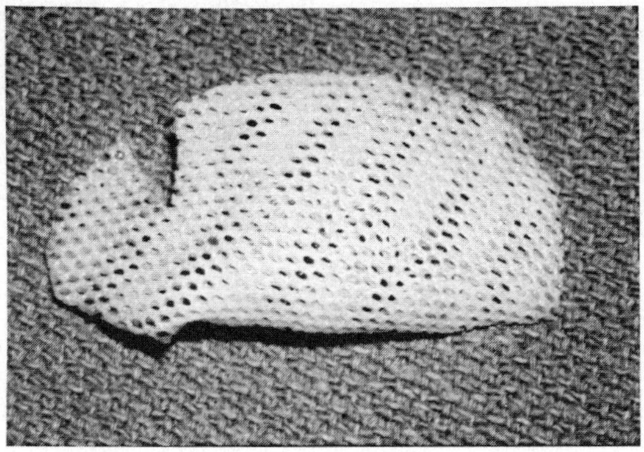

Figs. 11-12

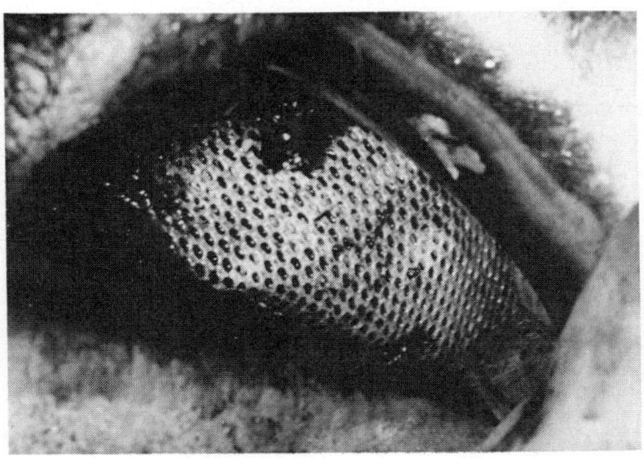

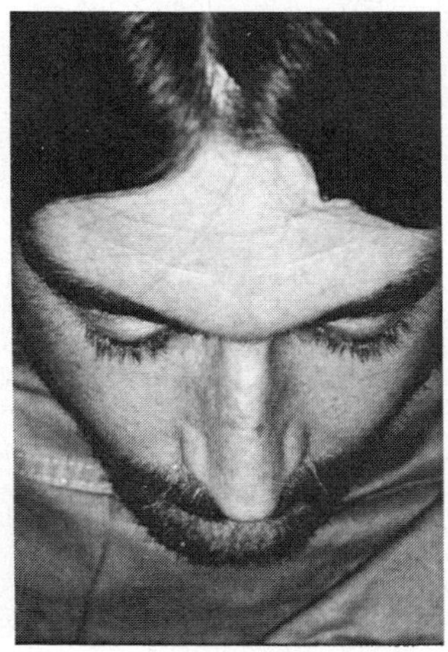

Fig. 9 - Defect of the left malar bone.
Fig. 10 - An OsteoMesh implant notched for the infraorbital nerve.
Fig. 11 - The OsteoMesh implant is secured in place with the notch widened, and has been filled with hydroxylapatite.
Fig. 12 - The postoperative view with facial asymmetry restored.

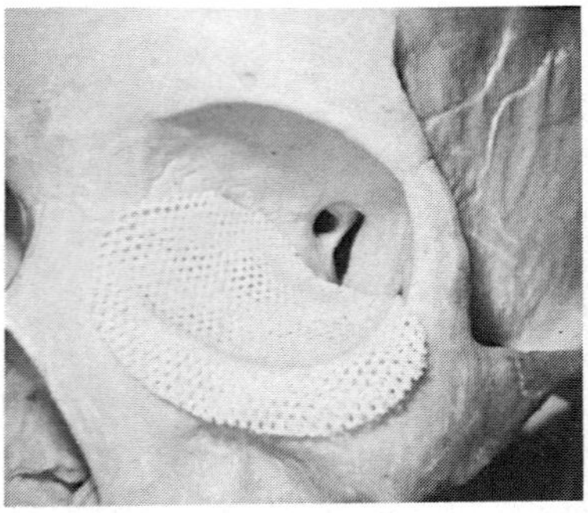

Fig. 13 - An OsteoMesh implant restores the orbital floor.

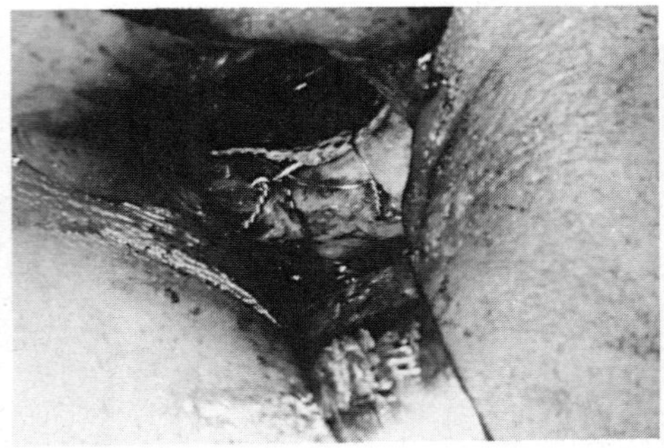

Fig. 14 - The implant has been trimmed and wired in position with stainless steel sutures.

REFERENCES

1 Leake, D. L. and Rappoport, M., Mandibular Reconstruction, Bone Induction in an Alloplastic Tray. Surg., 72:332-336, 1972.
2 Rappoport, M. and Leake, D. L., Current Experiments in Polymeric Mandibular Implants for Bone Induction. Brit. J. Oral Surg., 10:341-348, 1973.
3 Leake, D. L., Mandibular Reconstruction With a New Type of Alloplastic Tray, A Preliminary Report. J. Oral Surg., 32:23-26, 1974.
4 Habal, M. B. and Leake, D. L., a New Method for Reconstruction of Severe Craniofacial Deformities. Surg., Gyn & OB. 142:750-752, 1976.
5 Habal, M., Leake, D. L., Maniscalco, J., and Kim, J., Repair of Major Cranio-orbital Defects With an Elastomer Coated Mesh and Autogenous Bone Paste. Plastic and Reconstructive Surgery, 61:394-404, 1978.
6 Leake, D. L. and Habal, M. B., Mandibular Reconstruction and Craniofacial Fairing. Brit. J. Oral Surg., 16:198-206, 1978-79.
7 Leake, D., Habal, M., Pizzoferrato, A., and Vespucci, A., Prosthetic Replacement of Large Defects of the Cervical Trachea in Dogs. Biomaterials, 6:17-22, January, 1985.
8 Velasco, R. U., Habal, M. B., Spiegel, P. G., Lotz, M. and Leake, D. L., A Study of Autologous Cancellous Bone Particles in Long Bone Discontinuity Defects. Clinical Orthopaedics and Related Research, 177:272-281, 1983.
9 Leake, D. L., Lenni, E., Cavedagna, D., Stea, S., Pizzoferrato, A., Transactions 11th Annual Meeting of the Society for Biomaterials VIII, 114, April 24-28, 1985. San Diego, California.
10 Marciani, R. D., Gonty, A. A., Synhorst, J. B., and Page, L. R., Cancellous Bone Marrow Grafts in Irradiated Dog and Monkey Mandibles. Oral Surg. 47:17, 1979.
11 Schwartz, H. C., Leake, D. L., Kagan, A. R., and Snow, H., Pizzoferrato, A., Postoperative Irradiation of Fresh Autogenic Cancellous Bone Grafts. Plastic Reconst. Surg. 77:122-126, 1986.

Biomaterials and Clinical Applications,
edited by A. Pizzoferrato, P.G. Marchetti, A. Ravaglioli and A.J.C. Lee
Elsevier Science Publishers B.V., Amsterdam, 1987 — Printed in The Netherlands

IN VIVO EVALUATION OF 8 DIFFERENT POLYMERS FOR USE AS OSTEOSYNTHESIS MATERIAL IN MAXILLO-FACIAL SURGERY

K.L. GERLACH[1], J. EITENMÜLLER[2]

1 Department of Maxillofacial Surgery, University of Cologne,
Joseph- Stelzmann Straße 9, 5ooo Köln 41 (West Germany)
[2]Surg.University Hospital Bergmannsheil
4630 Bochum (West Germany)

SUMMARY

Eight different polymers and copolymers based on poly-l-, d,l- lactic and glycolic acid were evaluated in vivo in particular in view of mechanical strength, molecular weight changes and of their tissue response. Whereas all polymers showed a comparable tissue response only high molecular weight poly-l-lactide and the stereopolymer of them with 10% d,l-lactide had acceptable mechanical values in vivo for use as osteosynthesis material in maxillo-facial traumatology.

INTRODUCTION

Biodegradable devices for internal fixation of bone require materials which maintain high initial mechanical strength for the time of fracture healing and should have a degradation rate within an acceptable period of time. Furthermore the material used should be biocompatible. In order to produce biodegradable polymers for use as an osteosynthesis material in maxillo-facial traumatology different lactic and glycolic acid based polymers were examined. These polymers have already been shown to possess a very good biocompatibility (refs.1-3), different biodegradation rates (refs.2,3,6) and decrease of mechanical strength in vivo (refs.2,6). This study is concerned with the evaluation of 8 different polymers and copolymers in order to determine a feasible polymer for the idented range of indications.

MATERIALS AND METHODS

This study was carried out with poly-l-lactide (PLA) of molecular weight 500 000, 800 000 and with an admixture of 2% silverphosphate, as well as stereopolymers of PLA with 10%,25% and 50% d,l-lactide and copolymers of PLA with 10% and 2% glycolic acid. Test pieces (25 x 3 x 2mm) were prepared for strength measurement and for histological examination (2 x 3 x 3mm) and were implanted after sterilisation with ethylene oxide into the back muscles of 80 rats. 5 animals were sacrificed weekly up to two months and later once monthly up to two years. Flexural strength and Young´s modulus were measured according to DIN 53 452 and 53 457 and compared with determined values before implantation. The molecular weight changes of the PLA specimens were determined by the inherent viscosity (refs.3 u.7) and the rate of crystallinity was calculated comparing the melting endotherms of the PLA specimens with those of fully crystalline PLA (refs.8,9).

The experimental area including the specimens for histological examination was exised, fixed in formalin, imbedded in methylmethacrylate, sectioned at 20 microns and stained with toluidin blue.

RESULTS

Initial strength measurements: Relative high values of flexural strength between 113 N/mm² to 142 N/mm² and of Young´s modulus from 3565 to 5144 N/mm² were found only for specimens of PLA with high molecular weight and for the stereopolymer of them with 10% d,l-lactide. The other tested polymers had lower values (Fig, 1 and 2).

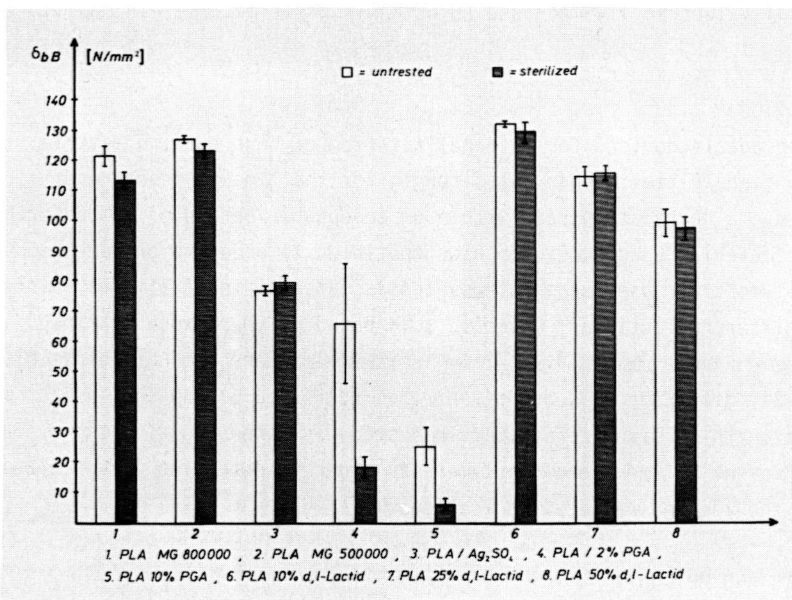

Fig. 1 Flexural strength of the different polymers and copolymers (white column untreated, black column after sterilisation with ethylene oxide)

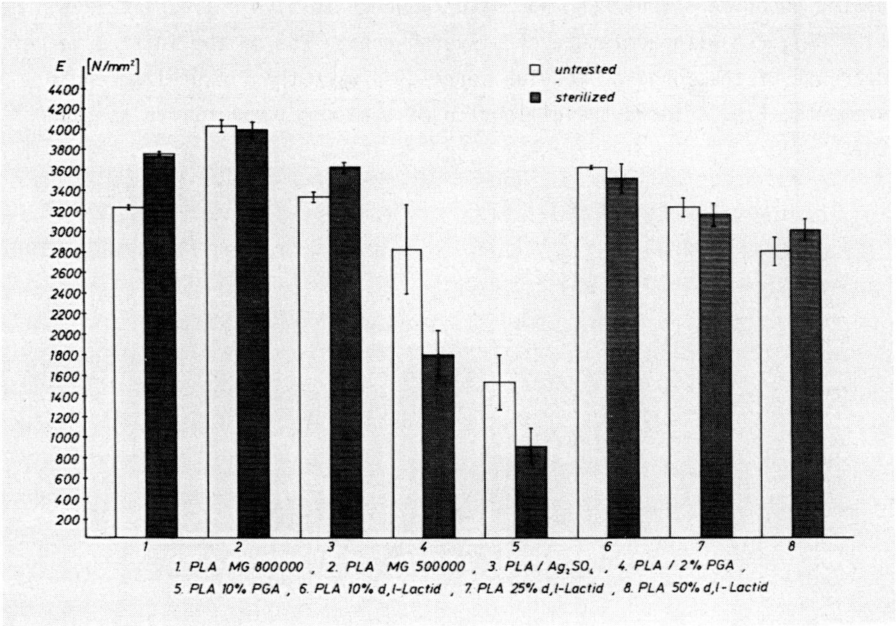

Fig. 2 Young´s module of the different polymers and copolymers before (white) and after sterilisation (black) with ethylene oxide

In vivo evaluations (strength measurements): 4 weeks after implantation the flexural strength of PLA indicated 50% and of the stereopolymer (PLA/10% d,l-lactide 73% of the initial values, after 8 weeks 24% and 35% respectively. All values decreased slowly until the end of 32 weeks. Fig. 3 typifies the effect of in vivo exposure for PLA with a molecular weight of 800 000.

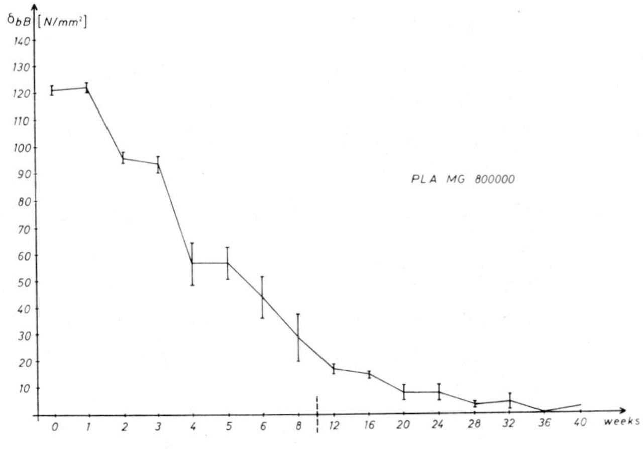

Fig. 3 Decrease of flexural strength in vivo (poly-l-lactide)

The tested copolymers (PLA/PGA) had after 4 weeks in vivo only 20% (2%PGA) and 10% (10%PGA), PLA with admixture of silverphosphate 25% of the initial values. The decrease of the Young´s modulus correlated with the flexural strength measurements, Fig. 4 shows the diminution of the Young's modulus for specimens of PLA.

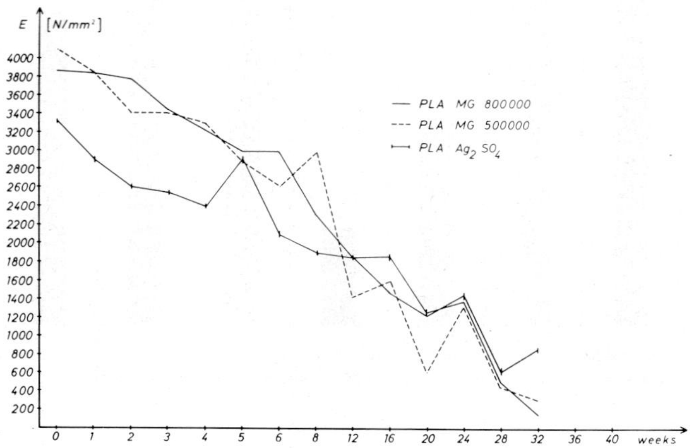

Fig. 4 Decrease of Young´s module in vivo (poly-l-Lactide)

The change of molecular weight was determined by inherent viscosity for PLA specimens only, e.g. PLA with molecular weight 800 000 decreased rapidly within the first 4 weeks to 90 000 and more slowly to 10 000 after 60 weeks (Fig. 5). No strength measurements were possible below a molecular weight of 32 000, we found a direct correlation between the molecular weight and flexural strength (r = 0,9846)

The initial rate of crystallinity of the PLA specimens amounted to 80%. In vivo we found no significant change, after 32 weeks the rate was determined as 85%. The degradation time of PLA/ 10% PGA amounted to one year, PLA/ 2% PGA less than 2 years, the stereopolymers less than 2 years and the degradation of the PLA was calculated to 2 years. Histology: All specimens produced a mild inflammatory response during the first week in that the reactive zone was limited to only a thin layer of polymorpho-nuclear leucocytes, occasional lymphocytes and only few eosinophiles (Fig. 6).After two weeks the material was enmeshed in the connective tissue comparatively to a surgical scar (Fig.7).

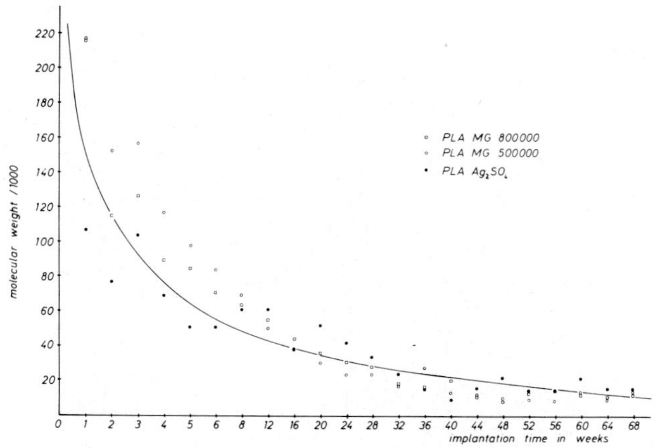

Fig. 5 Decrease of molecular weight (poly-l- Lactide)

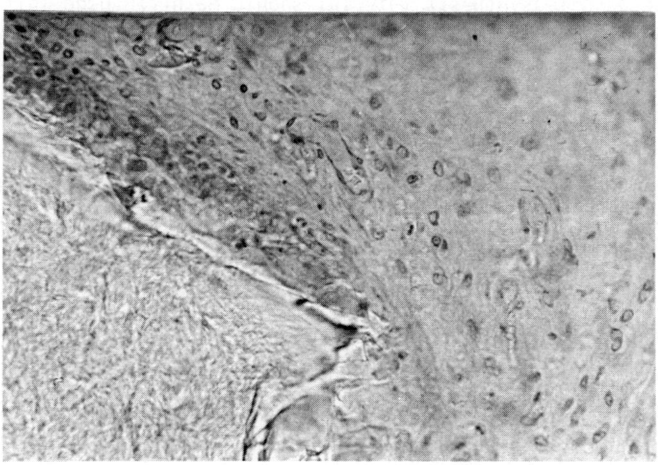

Fig. 6 Granulation tissue around poly-l- Lactide , 1 week after implantation, toluidin blue, 85 x

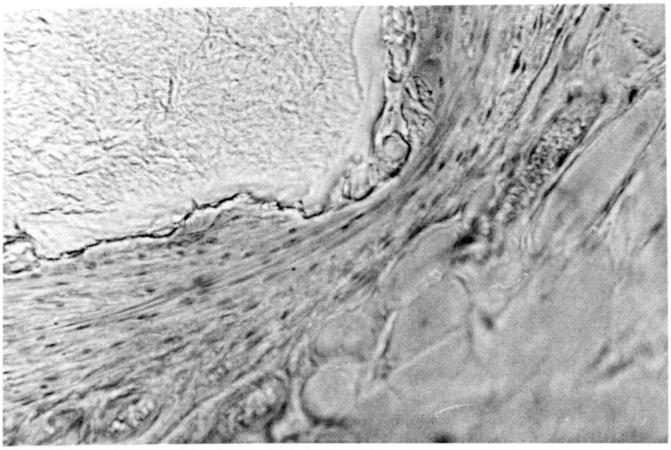

Fig. 7 Connective tissue around implant after 16 weeks, poly-l-lactide, toluidin blue, 80x

DISCUSSION

Besides the biodegradability and only minimal tissue reaction, absorbable polymers for use as osteosynthesis material should maintain high initial strength for the time of fracture healing. Among the evaluated polymers only high molecular weight poly-l-lactide and the stereopolymer with 10% d,l-lactide showed acceptable mechanical values comparable to results of another study in which implants of poly-l- lactide were used to stabilize tibial fractures of dogs (ref.6). The initial strength of these polymers and their loss of strength between 50% and 30% within 4 weeks after implantation seems to be sufficient for use in maxillo-facial traumatology, because former studies with an electric test procedure for evaluating the load resistence of patients with mandibular fractures who had undergone plate osteosynthesis showed that after 4 weeks in vivo only 51% of the test values of a control group were reached (ref.10). Possibly the increase of molecular weight and the preparation of composite materials (ref.11) will optimize mechanical properties. Work is currently under way to improve the strength of the polymers.

REFERENCES

1. D.E. Cutright, E.E. Hunsuck, Tissue reaction to the biodegradable polyactic acid suture. Oral Surg. 31,(1971) 134
2. M. Vert, P. Christel, F.Chabot, J. Leray, Bioresorbable plastic material for bone surgery. In: Macromolecular Biomaterials. Ed.: D. Hastings,, P.Ducheyne CRC Press Inc., Boca Raton, Florida, S. 119 (1984)

3. M. Reed, In vivo and in vitro studies of biodegradable polymers for use in medicine. Thesis,Liverpool 1978
4. R.K. Kulkarni,E.G.Moore,A.F.Hegyeli, F. Leonhard, Biodegradable polylactic acid polymers. J. Biomed. Mater.Res. 5, (1971) 169
5. J.M. Brady, D.E. Cutright, R.A. Miller, G.C. Battistone, E.E. Hunsuck, Resorption rate, route of elimination and ultrastructure of the implant site of polylactic acid in the abdominal wall of the rat. J. Biomed. Mater. Res. 7,(1973) 155
6. D.L. Tunc, W.B. Lehmann, A. Stronwater, F.Kummer, Evaluation of a high molecular weight polylactide osteosynthesis device. Transaction: The Society for Biomaterials, S. 214 (1985)
7. W. Dittrich, R.C. Schulz, Kinetik und Mechanismus der ringöffnenden Polymerisation von L-Lactid,Angew. Makromol.Chem. 15,(1971) 109
8. G. Menges, Werkstoffkunde der Kunststoffe, Carl Hanser Verlag, München-Wien (1984)
9. E.W. Fischer, H.J. Sterzel, G.Wegner, Investigation of the structure of solution grown crystals of lactide copolymers by means of chemical reactions. Kolloid- Z. u. Z. Polymere 251,(1973) 980
10. K.L. Gerlach,H.-D. Pape ,P. Nußbaum, Untersuchungen zur Belastbarkeit nach der Miniplattenosteosynthese von Unterkieferfrakturen. Dtsch. Z. Mund-, Kiefer-, Gesichts- Chir, 8 (1984) 363
11. M. Vert, F. Chabot, Stereoregular bioresorbable polyesters for orthopaedic surgery. Makromol. Chem. Suppl. 5,(1981) 30

Acknowledgments

This study was supported by the DFG (German investigation community)

Fa. Boehringer Ingelheim, KG, West Germany, offered the used polymers.

Biomaterials and Clinical Applications,
edited by A. Pizzoferrato, P.G. Marchetti, A. Ravaglioli and A.J.C. Lee
Elsevier Science Publishers B.V., Amsterdam, 1987 — Printed in The Netherlands

FIRST RESULTS OF COMPUTED TOMOGRAPHY FOLLOWING LOWER JAW AUGMENTATION WITH POROUS HYDROXYAPATITE CERAMIC GRANULES

J.F. OSBORN

Clinic of Maxillo-Facial Surgery, University of Bonn, D-5300 Bonn, West Germany

SUMMARY

Clinical experience with one-stage augmentation of the atrophic jaw by means of the so-called tunneling method shows that extra-mucosal splints are not capable of retaining implanted hydroxyapatite (HA) ceramic granules in the adequate form of a new alveolar process. Hence, ectopic hydroxyapatite ceramic granules in the perimandibular soft tissues are frequent complications. Particle dislocation is surely avoided by the two-stage augmentation method. Alveolar processes which had been restored in this way were examined by means of computer tomography (CT). Four phases are discernible for the time-related development of the HA-ceramic granulate augmentates: sedimentation, condensation, consolidation and compaction. Parts of the augmentate with absorption values greater than those of sedimented HA-ceramic granulate are rated as 'hyperdense'. Hyperdense zones are first observed in five month old augmentate. Dependent on the time-related form stability of the augmentate, the insertion of a temporary, unloaded prosthesis not sooner than six weeks post-operatively and the definitive insertion of a gradually more heavily loaded prosthesis nine weeks after implantation of the HA-ceramic granulate is recommended.

INTRODUCTION

Treatmentmodalities with respect to alveolar plasty have changed significantly during the last six years due to clinical application of new calciumphosphate materials, but in particular the hydroxyapatite ceramics (see overview (1)).

A completely new preprosthetic surgical technique is exhibited by the alveolar extension plasty (2, 3). During this technique, an interlamellar space is created through vertical osteotomy of the alveolar process as well as the mobilization of the vestibular cortical plate, which will in turn be filled with hydroxyapatite ceramic granules. The characteristic advantage of this technique is that the granules are placed rather intraosseously. Five years of experience indicate that this method most likely ensures an enduring and stable alveolar process, whose contours satisfy prosthetic requirements. However, this newly developed technique is only suitable for alveolar processes with knife edged involution, thus limiting its indication to a few patients.

In most cases requiring preprosthetic surgical treatment we are dealing with a lower jaw, whose surface is plane, or almost plane due to subtotal or total involution of the alveolar ridges. This type of anatomy forces us to reconstruct the lost jaw profile via epiosseous implantation, i.e. to implant the augmentation materials between the bony surface and the mucoperiosteum.

Brachmann was the first to prepare the subperiosteal tunnel as space for the application of augmentation materials in 1950 (4). In 1948, De Kleine (5) introduced a technique to particularize the implantation material - at that time still cartilage - and to apply it with a syringe. Employing HA-ceramic granules, in 1980 Kent et al. (6) described augmentation of deficient alveolar ridges via the tunneling technique which had evolved from the combination of the procedures from Brachmann and De Kleine. During this one-stage method, the implanted granules should be retained in the subperiosteal tunnel with the aid of an extramucosal splint, which must be held in place through circumferential wiring for 3 weeks. Clinical experience, however, shows that this technique is not sound, since ceramic particles frequently dislocate into the floor of the mouth as well as the vestibular tissue, especially at the penetration sites of the circumferential wirings. These dystopic particle conglomerations prevent the denture from marginal adhesion and have to be eliminated in subsequent troublesome operations.

THE TWO-STAGE AUGMENTATION METHOD

In order to achieve a reliable primary fixation of the HA-ceramic granulate in loco the two-stage augmentation method has been developed (7). Temporary augmentates were prepared on a plaster model (Fig. 1) from hot polymerizing soft silicon (Molloplast B^{TM}). A single vertical incision in the midline of the vestibulum is sufficient to prepare the epiosseous tunnel bilaterally avoiding injury to the mental nerve. Both silicon implants are inserted one after the other, and the wound is closed. Three weeks later the incision is reopened and the temporary augmentates are removed (Fig. 2). The tissue responds to the silicon by lining the inner wall of the tunnel with a fibrous membrane, which adheres lingually and vestibularly to the jaw so that the interior space is smooth and precisely defined. Therefore there are no fissures in the tissue, into which ceramic particles can dislocate and migrate beyond the denture bearing area. Delivered from the syringe HA-cera-

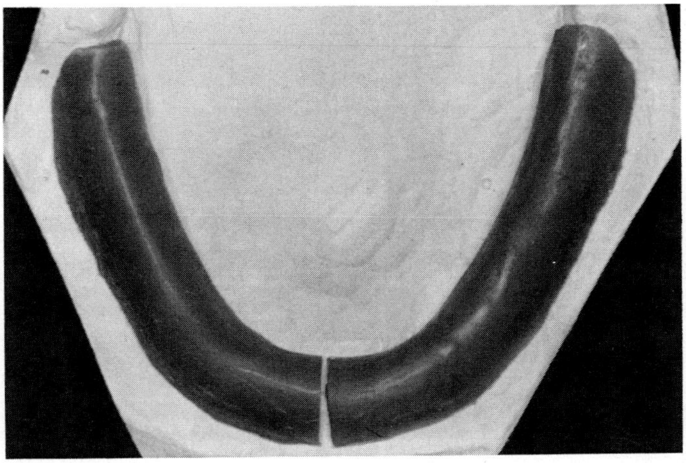

Fig. 1. On premade stone casts wax models are fabricated which function as a template for the temporary augmentate. After midline division the temporary augmentates made out of the heat polymerizing polydimethylsiloxane are ready to be implanted.

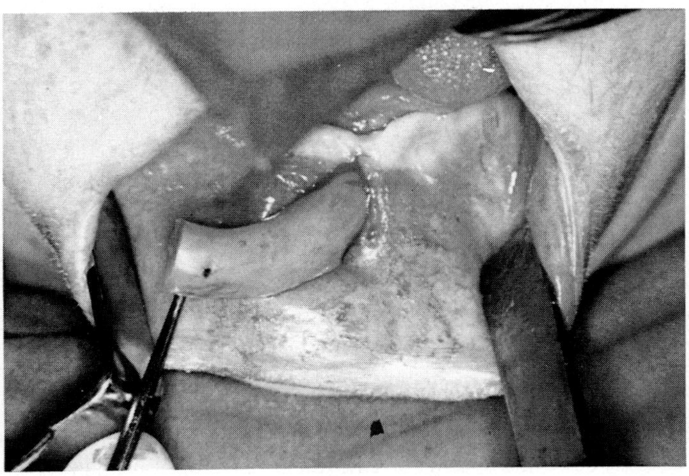

Fig. 2. Via a retractor the temporary augmentates are easily removed through the vertical midline incision;- remaining is the 'preformed epiosseous space'.

mic granules are then applied into this 'preformed epiosseous space'.

Performing histological evaluation much evidence has been found, that the connection of dense granules to the bone surface is fibrous, whereas porous granules are fused to the jaw by newforming bone. This is the reason why we use porous HA-ceramic granules for jaw augmentation, specifically the polygonal rounded Osprovit 1.2™, which has proved to be of sufficient resistance to biodegradation.

THE OBJECTIVE ASSESSMENT OF AUGMENTATES

An objective assessment of the true quality of these augmentates by clinical observation is inadequate, and conventional X-ray examination is inappropriate due to its inevitable superimpositions. Computed tomography however obtaining absorption profiles from different directions affords assessments in which

- overshadowing effects are eliminated
- specific local values can be obtained and
- data are quantified and suitable for secondary analysis.

One day after augmentation the reactive seroma increases extensively the volume of the preformed epiosseous space. In the fluid of this seroma we find the granules sedimented on to the surface of the jaw. The density of this sediment is measured to be 1477 X-ray absorption units. This sediment density represents the maximum value, that the Osprovit 1.2™ can attain on the basis of a purely physical stacking process in an aqueous medium (8). Density analysis, obtained in scanning a single jaw cross section, is computed up to 8100 absorption data. On the CT density scale, water is given the value 0, whereas cancellous bone lies within the range of 600 - 800, and cortical bone within 1600-1900. One month after augmentation the initial hyperhydration will have been decreased for a long time, and the granule complex has changed its form to that of the planned augmentate. This development of spatial arrangement is called condensation. Two months after augmentation spatial analysis firstly demonstrates small areas, in which the effective density exceeds the limit described for the sediment of the HA-ceramic (Fig. 3). This hyperdense state can only be the result of biological forces, because control experiments showed that granulate densities remained constant in vitro. This biologically mediated organisation of the augmentate is called consolidation.

Measurements support the hypothesis that under functional loading of the denture, rearrangement of the augmentate occurs following biomechanical criteria - resulting 5 months after augmentation in increased density values in nearly concentric zones, with lowest

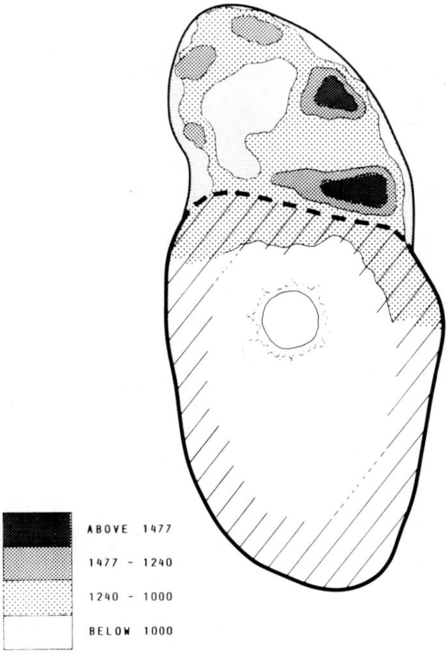

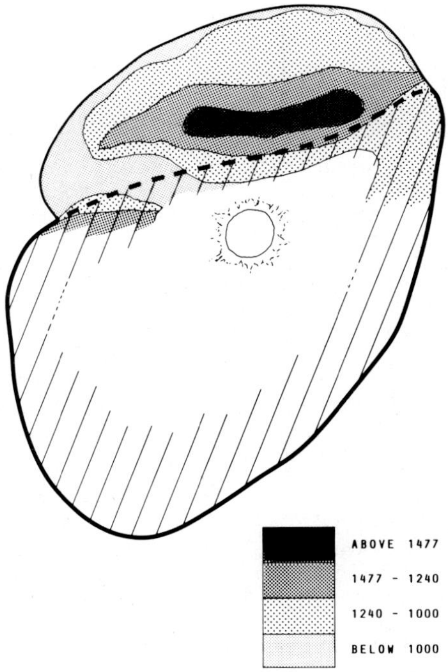

Fig. 3. (left) Coronal CT-section from the left lower jaw 2 months after augmentation. Absorption values are divided into four subdivisions and represented as a distribution diagram (picture consisting of 3024 single, measured data). The darkest areas represent hyperdense zones.

Fig. 4. (right) Coronal CT-section from the left lower jaw 5 months after augmentation (picture consisting of 4800 absorption values). The zone of hyperdensity,- darkest areas-, corresponds with the centre of the augmentate.

density in the submucosal area to a maximum density in the augmentation centre (Fig. 4). Under such functional loading the process of compaction finally seems to remodel the augmentate into a configuration similar to the cancellous-cortical architecture of the mandibula itself. Whether the consolidation and the compaction of the augmentate are due to ceramo-fibrous or ceramo-osseous regeneration processes cannot be answered yet (8).

For the clinical practice the conclusion is as follows: Dependent on the time-related form stability of the augmentate, the insertion of a temporary, unloaded prosthesis not sooner than 6 weeks post-operatively and the definitive insertion of a gradually more heavily loaded prosthesis 9 to 12 weeks after implantation of the HA-ceramic granules is recommended.

REFERENCES

1 J.F. Osborn, Implantatwerkstoff Hydroxylapatitkeramik - Grundlagen und klinische Anwendungen, Quintessenz, Berlin, 1985.

2 J.F. Osborn, Preservation and reconstruction of the alveolar bone using hydroxyapatite ceramic, In: Oral and Maxillofacial Surgery, Proceedings from the 8th International Conference on Oral and Maxillofacial Surgery, Quintessence Publishing, Chicago, 1985, pp. 552-556.

3 J.F. Osborn, Die Alveolar-Extensions-Plastik, Neue Operationsverfahren zur Behandlung des alveolären Kollapses und der gratartigen Alveolarfortsatzatrophie, Quintessenz 36 (1985) 9-16, 239-246.

4 G.B. Brachmann, Die plastische Wiederherstellung des zahnlosen unteren Alveolarfortsatzes durch frischen Leichenknorpel zwecks besserer prothetischer Versorgung (Russian), Stomatologija, Moskau, Number 1 (1950) 24, Abstract: Dtsch. Zahn-Mund-Kieferheilkunde 15 (1951) 395.

5 E.H. de Kleine, The chondrojet. A simplified method for handling of diced cartilage, Plast. Reconstr. Surg. 3 (1948) 95-102.

6 J. Kent, R. James, I. Finger, M. Jarcho, J. Taggert, S. Cook, Augmentation of deficient edentulous alveolar ridges with dense polycrystalline hydroxylapatite, 1st World Biomaterials Congress, Baden near Vienna, Austria, April 8-12, 1980.

7 J.F. Osborn, M. Kapovits, P. Karl, Die zweizeitige Augmentation des atrophischen Kiefers mit Hydroxylapatitkeramik-Granulat, Coll. med. dent. 30 (1986) 149-160.

8 J.F. Osborn, G. Brecht, M. Kapovits, C.A. Stuckenholz, Die computertomographische Analyse von Unterkieferaugmentaten aus Hydroxylapatitkeramik-Granulat, Coll. med. dent. 30 (1986) 165-178.

Biomaterials and Clinical Applications,
edited by A. Pizzoferrato, P.G. Marchetti, A. Ravaglioli and A.J.C. Lee
Elsevier Science Publishers B.V., Amsterdam, 1987 — Printed in The Netherlands

A NEW RECONSTITUTED CONNECTIVE TISSUE MATRIX : PROPERTIES AND APPLICATION IN DIGESTIVE SURGERY.

M. RABAUD[1], M. APRAHAMIAN[2], C. DAMGE[2], E. LOZA[2], M. WILHELM[2], R. SCHMITTHAEUSLER[3], J. MARESCAUX[2]

[1]INSERM U8 Avenue du Haut Lévêque, 33600 Pessac (France)

[2]INSERM U61 3, avenue Molière, 67200 Strasbourg (France)

[3]CRTS 10, rue Spielman, 67000 Strasbourg (France)

SUMMARY

Monomers of fibrin generated by thrombin reacted with elastin to give a new addition product or adduct, whose formation results from a covalent bond between both proteins. Addition of fibronectin together with fibrinogen and collagen did not inhibit the reaction but rather conferred to the product the qualities of an artificial connective tissue matrix. The biochemical, structural and biomechanical aspects of this biomaterial have been investigated. According to these properties, the biomaterial has been successfully used for experimental surgical obturation of coecal fistula in rats.

Collagen and elastin are major components of connective tissue matrices of the skin, the lungs, the arteries. Elastin is always degraded during pathological processes as in cutix laxa, emphysema and atherosclerosis. As we were trying to isolate plasmatic factors involved in elastin degradation, we observed that elastin, suspended in plasma dialysed against PO_4 buffer containing Ca^{++}, was modified by a chemical reaction yealding a stable addition product or adduct between a derivative of fibrin generated by thrombin and elastin (ref. 1). This derivative has been characterized as the fibrin monomers. The excess of insoluble fibrin could aggregate to each grain of adduct and gave a sort of connective matrix. The objectives of the present report were to improve the biomechanical qualities of the original matrix by adjunction of fibronectin, collagen, sulfure derivatives and γ rays. Together with fibrin and elastin, that made a new reconstituted connective tissue which can be investigated in a wide range of biological and surgical applications.

EXPERIMENTS

Preparation of adduct with elastin and pure human fibrinogen

Human fibrinogen lyophilised powder was dissolved in PO_4 buffer and dialysed for 30 min. to remove citrate. The concentration of clottable fibrinogen remaining in the dialysis bag was 10 mg/ml. An aliquot of ^{125}iodine fibrinogen was added in order to study the kinetic and the stoechiometry of the reaction with elastin. The reaction was initiated by adding 1 ml of fibrinogen solution (10 mg/ml) to 50mg of elastin suspended in 1 ml of PB 7.4 and mixed at room temperature. The suspension was heated at 37°C then stirred and thrombin (1.25 U/ml final conc.) was added. The insoluble adduct that was formed by the reaction of elastin and fibrin derivative was immediatly decanted and separated. The adduct was washed with PB 7.4 several times until no radioactivity (^{125}I) or 280 nm optical density could be measured in the supernatant.

Preparation of adduct with elastin and cold insoluble proteins (C.I.P.)

The lyophilised powder of C.I.P. was dissolved at 37°C in 6 ml of PB 7.4. The cryoprecipitate contains about 40 g/l fibrinogen and 7 g/l fibronectin. Again, the adduct was prepared by mixing gently at room temperature a suspension of elastin (50 mg/ml PB 7.4) and 0.1 ml of cryoprecipitate solution ; then thrombin (1.25 U/ml final conc.) was added. The adduct was immediatly formed and separated as described above.

Preparation of the Patch and test pieces

When adduct was formed, instead of a rapid decantation, it was let without stirring; the excess of fibrin could aggregate to each grain of adduct and gave a sort of connective matrix : the PATCH. Adjunction of other ingredients : collagen, thiourea, aprotinin... could be done before thrombin and carefully mixed. The yielded mixture was immediatly poured into a mould ; then, the test piece was withdrawn, and the excess of buffer removed. The biomaterial can be conserved in dried state and equilibrated with physiological serum before use.

Scanning electron microscopy study

Dessicated specimens were coated with gold and examined in a Philips 501 B SEM operated at 20 KV. Photomicrographs were taken at x 1250 magnification.

Mechanical tests

The mechanical resistance properties of these materials have been tested by measuring the breaking strength of the test pieces (6 samples) of various compositions until rupture occured. Load and strain were coupled to measuring bridges connected to an x, y recorder. The specimen was loaded until breaking and curves were continuously recorded giving directly the breaking strength, the lengthening and the elastin stiffness.

Experimental in vivo study

48 adult Wistar rats were anaesthetized with ether. After laparotomy, a hole of 1 cm in diameter has been performed in the anterior face of the caecum, in front of the

Bauhin valve. Then the hole has been obturated using a Patch of 1.4 cm, sticked with a fibrin sealant (Transglutine R, Centre de Transfusion, Strasbourg). Eight animals were sacrified every 5 days until 20 days then at the 30th and 40th post-operative day. The incriminated caecal tissue was removed, fixed in Susa solution, dehydrated and embedded in paraffin. Sections of 5 µm thickness were stained with orcein and examined in a photonic microscope.

RESULTS AND COMMENTS

Biochemical properties

The biomaterial results from the combination of two chemical reactions : the first one was a covalent bound between elastin and soluble fibrin monomers generated by thrombin ; the second resulted from the affinity of fibronectin for elastin (see Fig. 1). The excess of insoluble fibrin could aggregate to each grain of the resulting product and coat them to give a sort of matrix. The properties of this matrix were markedly improved by adding a little amount of collagen acting as a cement and aliquots of thiourea acting as a vulcanizing agent. Other parameters were γ-rays which generated a secondary reticulation - certainly between elastin fibers - and aprotinin (Zymofren, Specia - Paris) that allowed to protect the biomatrix against its specific biological degrading agents : elastase and plasmin.

Biological properties

Structural : There were clear morphological differences between the adduct (elastin - fibrin monomers) and the patch (elastin - fibrin monomer - collagen and the excess of insoluble fibrin), as illustrated in Fig. 2. The adduct exhibits the shape of a well reticulated network ; several links can be observed between elastin fibers. The patch shows

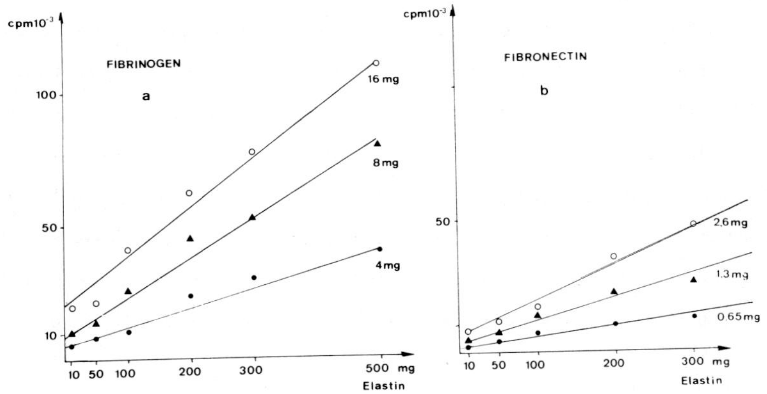

Fig. 1

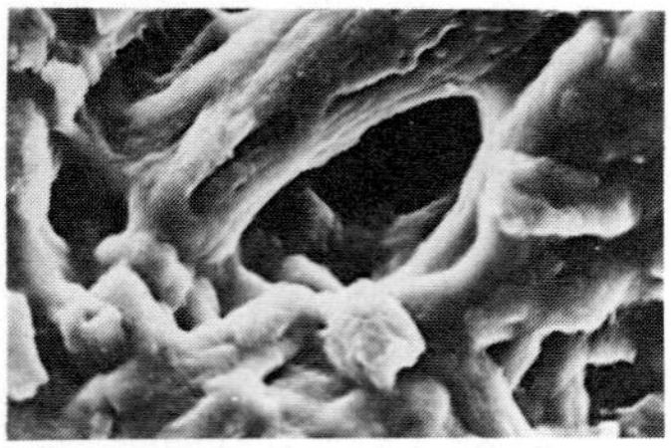

Fig. 2

adduct

Patch

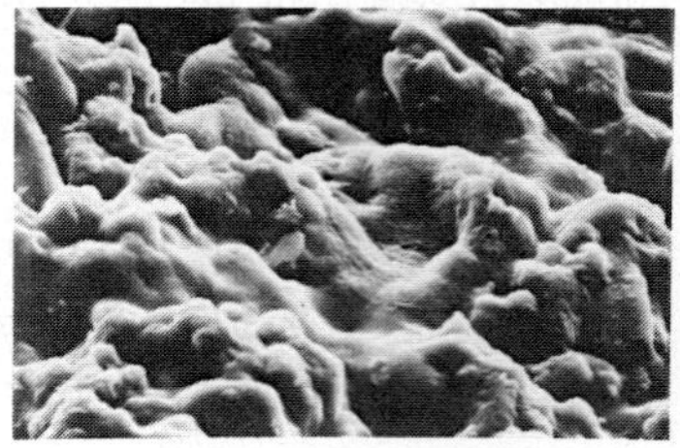

a more dense structure : the meshes of the primary network were filled with collagen and insoluble fibrin ; the surface of the yielded matrix was smoother and more compact.

Biomechanical : As shown in Fig. 3, the performances of the investigated patches, as test-pieces, were markedly different in correlation with their composition. Mainly, addition of collagen as well as thiourea, till an optimal concentration, increased the breaking strength or the lengthening that conferred to the biomaterial the better elastic stiffness.

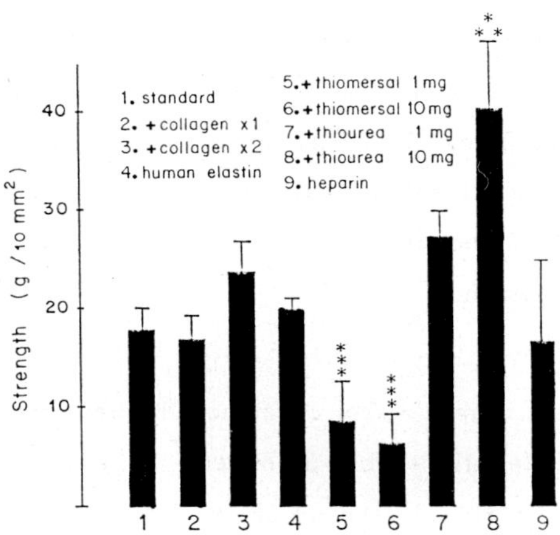

Fig. 3

Surgical : The macroscopic examination of the wound showed a progressive disappearance of the patch with time ; indeed, between the 30th and 40th post operative day, the patch was replaced by an intestinal wall. The microscopic observation of slices performed throughout the healing tissue exhibited at the 20th day a complete reconstitution of both mucosae and serosae while the muscular layer was only achieved at the 40th post-operative day (see Fig. 4). The patch disappeared progressively : at this time (40th day), only a small, encapsulated, orcein-positive material remained in the external layer of the serosa , suggesting that elastin may be degraded with time.

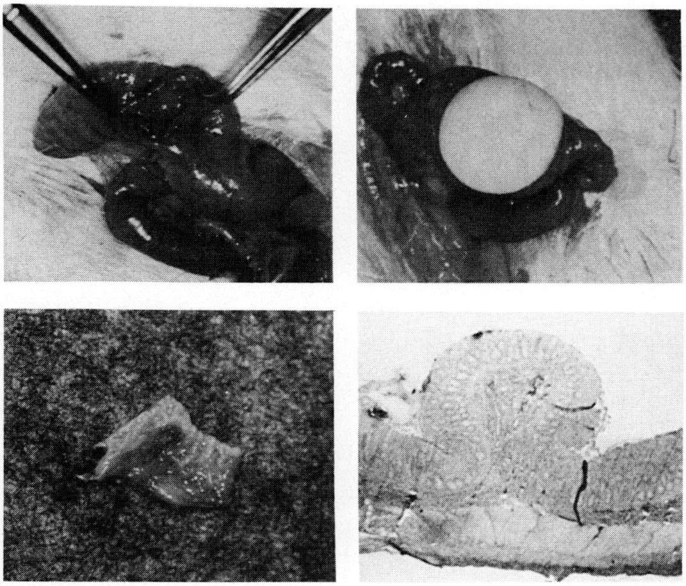

Fig. 4

To conclude, this new biomaterial results from a reaction between elastin, a normal component of connective tissues and a fibrinogen derivative generated by thrombin. This reaction, that occurs in biological conditions, appears to be very important since elastin reacts covalently with fibrin leading to a true new artificial connective matrix, as confirmed by our structural and in vivo studies. Well tolerated, this new biomaterial may be applied in surgical fields since it likely acts as an extracellular matrix which allowed and promoted epithelial and muscular gut wound healing.

REFERENCE

1 M. Rabaud, F. Lefebvre, Y. Piquet, F. Belloc, J. Chevaleyre, M.F. Roudaut and H. Bricaud, Soluble fibrinogen derivatives generated by thrombin : affinity for elastin, Thromb. Res., 43 (1986) 205-211.

Biomaterials and Clinical Applications,
edited by A. Pizzoferrato, P.G. Marchetti, A. Ravaglioli and A.J.C. Lee
Elsevier Science Publishers B.V., Amsterdam, 1987 — Printed in The Netherlands

USE OF ABSORBABLE OSTEOSYNTHESIS MATERIAL FOR MANDIBULAR FRACTURE TREATMENT OF DOGS

K.L. GERLACH[1], H.-R. KRAUSE[1] and J. EITENMÜLLER[2]

[1]Department of Maxillofacial Surgery, University of Cologne,
Joseph-Stelzmann Straße 9, 5ooo Köln 41 (West Germany)

[2]Surg. University Hospital Bergmannsheil
4630 Bochum (West Germany)

SUMMARY

15 mandibular fractures of 12 dogs were stabilized with resorbable plates and screws made of high molecular weight poly-l-lactide (PLA) and of a stereopolymer (PLA/ 10% d,l-lactide). The used plates showed a breaking load between 366 N and 536 N. The uncomplicated fracture healing was demonstrated by x-ray and histological examinations.

INTRODUCTION

During the past decades the operative treatment of mandibular fractures has been influenced and modified by a variety of experimental and clinical studies. Most osteosynthesis has been achieved using metallic devices, which permitted a stable fixation of the bony fragments and led to good clinical results (refs.1-6). However there are still disadvantages in discussion. Because of the different elastic modules of the metallic implants and of bone, metallic plates may cause cortical bone to atrophy as the healing process progresses (ref. 7 and 8). Furthermore these materials require surgical removal after fracture healing.

A biodegradable polymer with sufficient initial strength and acceptable degradation kinetics could provide the solution to these problems. First attempts using different poly-l-lactide plates and screws to stabilize experimental animal fractures had been made for mandibular fractures in dogs (ref.9), for tibia fractures in sheep (ref.10) and radii fractures in dogs (ref.11). and were finally used in the case of reconstructive facial surgery (ref.12).

After in vivo evaluations of different glycolic- and lactic acid based polymers (ref.13) the purpose of this study was to examine the efficiency of plates and screws of high molecular weight PLA in the reduction of mandibular fractures in dogs.

MATERIALS AND METHODS

To achieve osteosynthesis in the beagle´s mandible we used plates and screws made of poly-l-lactide with molecular weight 800 000 and comparably made of a stereopolymer (PLA/ 10% d,l-lactide). Flexural strength of these materials were determined to be 113 to 142 N/mm^2 and Young´s moduli between 3565 and 5144 N/mm^2. Four hole plates made of the Sherman type with a cross-section of 4x9/15 mm and a length of 45 mm. We used countersunk screws with a heart diameter of 3 mm (PLA) and 1.9 mm (PLA/ 10% d,l-lactide) and buttress threads with a pitch of 3°/30° (Fig. 1). The plates showed a breaking load of 536 N (PLA) and 366 N (PLA/ 10% d,l-lactide).

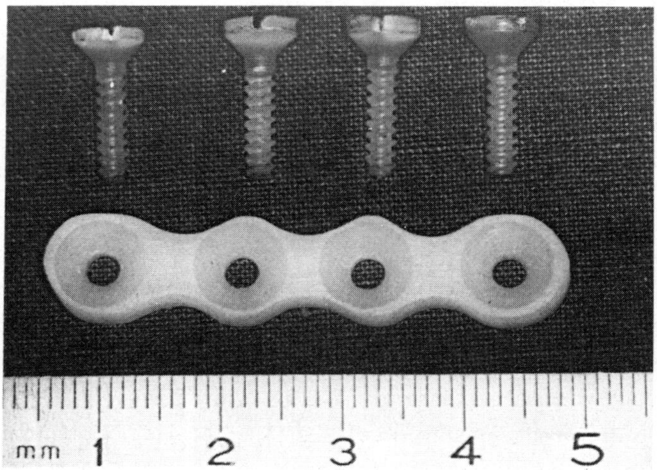

Fig. 1. Plates and screws made of PLA

12 adult beagle dogs were used for the study. The operation was performed under general anaesthesia. After a sterile surgical preparation, the mandible was exposed through a submandibular approach and a complete fracture was created between the third premolar and the first molar (Fig. 2). Following reduction the plates were adapted to the bony surface by grinding and holes correspondig to the diameter of the screws were drilled into the mandible. Finally the holes were enlarged to the screw size using a screw-tap. The screws then were placed through the holes in the plate to stabilize the fracture in position, wounds were closed in layers. Postoperatively the animals received normal food. 2 dogs respectively were sacrified 4,8 and 12 weeks post operatively and after 6, 8, 9, 10 and 12 months only one was sacrified. X-rays were taken and nondecalcified sections were prepared for histological examination.

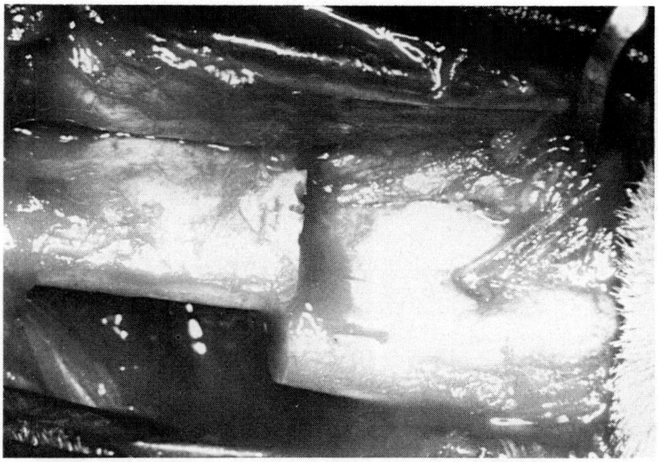

Fig. 2 Experimental mandibular fracture.

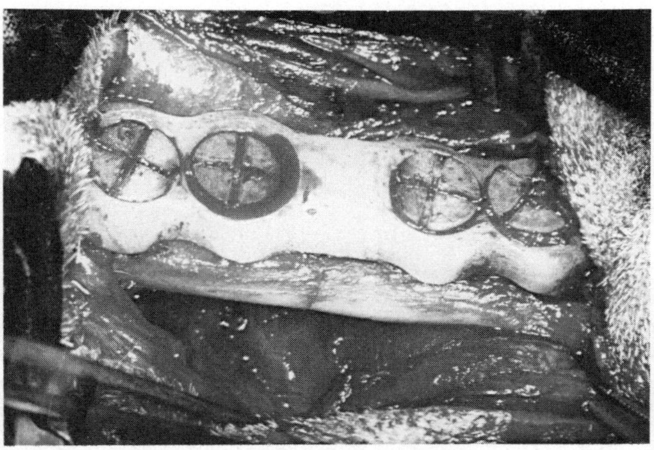

Fig. 3. PLA plate and screws in final position after reduction of fragments.

RESULTS

In all animals undisturbed wound healing and uncomplicated fracture healing was observed. After four weeks the fragments were already consolidated although some of the screws were found broken. The implants were covered by a firm sheet of connective tissue without inflammatory symptoms (Fig. 4).

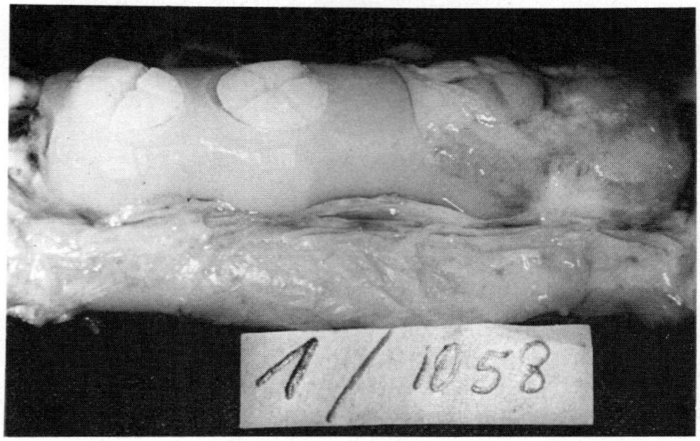

Fig. 4. Position of the osteosynthesis material 3 months postoperatively

Radiologically a small fracture gap and only little callus formation were detected (Fig. 5). At 8, 12 and more weeks postoperatively the x-ray pictures showed a normal undelayed fracture healing.

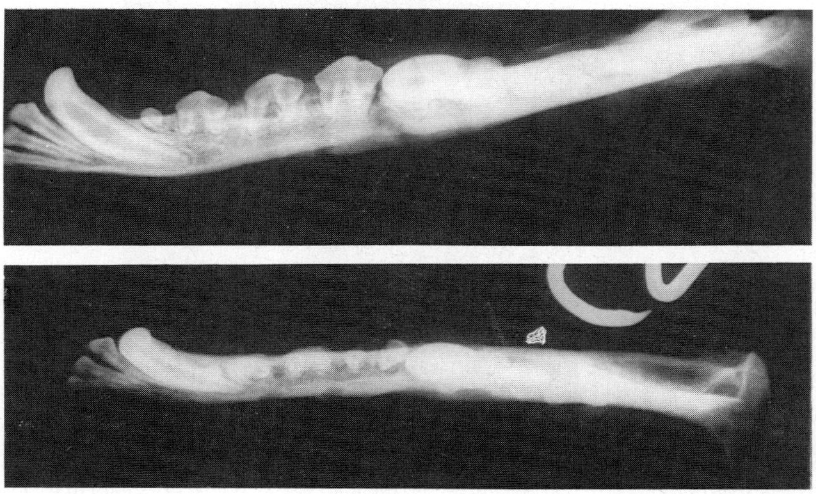

Fig. 5. X-ray pictures 1 month (above) and 3 months (below) postoperatively

Histologically after 4 weeks a small periosteal callus appeared beside network bone within the outer cortex and the spongiosa. No cartilage could be found (Fig. 6). After 8 and 12 weeks the fracture site was well healed without secondary callus formations.

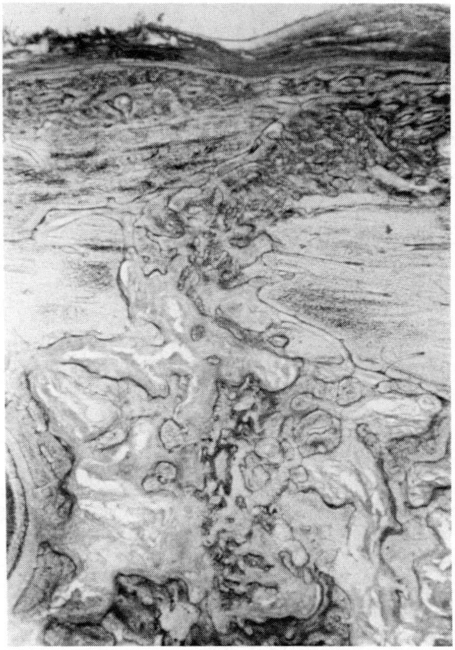

Fig. 8. Net-work bone within the outer cortex (above) and the spongiosa, basic fuchsine, 4x

DISCUSSION

The possibility of mandibular fracture treatment by use of plates and screws made of a composite material including PLA and polyglycolic acid has been previously shown in a clinical study (ref. 12). Our study confirmed the potential for using PLA with high molecular weight as an osteosynthesis material in maxillo-facial traumatology. Strength loss of the material between 50% and 30% within 4 weeks after implantation seems to be sufficient: former studies with an electric test procedure for evaluation of the load resistance of patients with mandibular fractures who had undergone plate osteosynthesis showed that after four weeks only 50% of the test values of a control group were reached (ref. 14). These clinical experiments encourage us to use such plates and screws for fracture treatment in maxillo-facial traumatology. Work is currently under way to optimize the strength of the used materials.

REFERENCES

1 H.G. Luhr, Zur stabilen Osteosynthese bei Unterkieferfrakturen, Dtsch. zahnärztl. Z. 23, (1968) 754.

2 B.Spiessl, G.Schargus, K.Schroll, Die stabile Osteosynthese bei Frakturen des unbezahnten Unterkiefers. Schweiz. Mschr. Zahnheilk. 81 (1971) 39.

3 H.Niederdellmann, W.Schilli, Funktionsstabile Osteosynthese im Unterkiefer Dtsch. zahnärztl. Z. 27, (1972) 138.

4 R.Becker, E. Machtens, Druckplattenosteosynthese zur Frakturbehandlung und bei orthopädisch-chirurgischen Maßnahmen am Gesichtsschädel. Osteo-News (Schweiz) 19 (1973) 2.

5 M.Champy,J.P. Loddé, R. Schmitt, J.H. Jaeger, D. Muster, Mandibular osteosynthesis by minature screwed plates via a buccal approach,J.max-fac.Surg. 6 (1978) 14.

6 E.W. Steinhäuser, Bone screws and plates in orthognathic surgery, Int. J. oral Surg. 11 (1982) 209.

7 H.K. Uhthoff, The use of Ti-6 Al-4V plates in the treatment of fractures an experimental study, Paper present. at the Soc.for biomater.Philadelphia, April 9-13 (1976).

8 K. Diehl, H. Mittelmeier, Biomechanische Untersuchungen zur Erklärung der Spongiosierung bei Plattenosteosynthese, Z. Orthop. 112 (1974) 235

9 L.Getter, D.E.Cutright, S.N.Bhaskar, J.K.Augsburg, A biodegradable intraosseous appliance in the treatment of mandibular fractures, J. Oral Surgery 30, (1972) 344 .

10 M.Vert, P.Christel, F.Chabot, L.Leray, Bioresorbable plastic material for bone surgery, In: Macromolecular Biomaterials. Ed.: D. Hastings, P.Ducheyne CRC Press Inc., Boca Raton, Florida, S.119 (1984).

11 D.L. Tunc, W.B.Lehmann, A. Stronwater, F.Kummer, Evaluation of high molecular weight polylactide osteosynthesis device, Transactions: The Society for Biomaterials, S. 214 (1985).

12 M.Audion, Preliminary clinical study in the application of bio-degradable osteosynthesis materials in maxillo-facial surgery, Transactions 5th European Conferenve on Biomaterials 1985, S. 39.

13 K.L. Gerlach, J.Eitenmüller, In vivo evaluation of glycolic and lactic acid-based polymers for implant devices used in management of maxillofacial traumatology, Transactions, 12th Annual Meeting Soc. Biomaterials 1986, S.18.

14 K.L. Gerlach, H.-D. Pape, P. Nußbaum, Untersuchungen zur Belastbarkeit nach der Miniplattenosteosynthese von Unterkieferfrakturen, Dtsch. Z. Mund-, Kiefer-, Gesichts-Chir. 8 (1984) 363.

Acknowledgments

This study was supported by the DFG (German investigation community)

Fa. Boehringer Ingelheim KG, West Germany offered the used polymers.

Biomaterials and Clinical Applications,
edited by A. Pizzoferrato, P.G. Marchetti, A. Ravaglioli and A.J.C. Lee
Elsevier Science Publishers B.V., Amsterdam, 1987 — Printed in The Netherlands

SURFACE MODIFICATION OF SILICONE FOR TISSUE ADHESION

T. OKADA, Y. TAMADA, AND Y. IKADA

Research Center for Medical Polymers and Biomaterials, Kyoto University
53 Kawahara-cho, Shogoin, Sakyo-ku, Kyoto 606 (Japan)

SUMMARY

To obtain a silicone with bioactive surface, proteins were covalently bound to a medical-grade silicone. When the silicone sheets to which collagen, gelatin, or fibronectin had been immobilized, were subcutaneously implanted in rabbits up to nine weeks, bioadhesion was observed to occur between the implant and the contacting living tissue. Among the three proteins collagen was the most effective for tissue adhesion.

INTRODUCTION

Silicone is a chemically-inert, hydrophobic elastomer and has been widely utilized as polymeric implants (ref.1). However, some problems appear, similar to other polymeric materials, when the silicone is implanted for a long term. The most crucial defect is a lack of adhesion with the living tissue in contact and formation of a thick fibrous tissue encapsulating the silicone. To overcome these disadvantages, attempts have been made, for instance, physically coating with collagen (ref. 2), plasma treatment (ref.3), and radiation-induced graft copolymerization (ref. 4). However, no successful results have been reported.

The aim of this work is to modify the silicone by covalent immobilization of cell-adhesive proteins. The protein immobilization will be achieved by covalent binding to poly(carboxylic acid) chains that have been grafted onto the silicone surface. The proteins employed are bovine collagen, gelatin (denatured collagen), and human fibronectin.

EXPERIMENTAL

Surface modifications of silicone

A silastic® silicone sheet with size of 12 x 50 mm^2 and thickness of 0.5 mm was exposed to corona discharge at 9 KV for 2 min to introduce peroxides onto the surface (ref. 5). Graft copolymerization of acrylic acid or acrylamide was conducted at 50 °C for 1 hr by immersing the corona-treated sheet in the deaerated aqueous solution of monomers at 10 wt% concentration. After removal of the homopolymers with water at 70 °C for 15 hr under stirring, the silicone sheet grafted with poly(acrylic acid)(PAA) was subjected to protein immobilization in the following manner. Following the reaction of the PAA-grafted silicone at 0-4 °C with 1-ethyl-3-(3-dimethyl aminopropyl) carbodiimide (WSC) at a concentration of 10 $mg \cdot ml^{-1}$ in PBS, the activated silicone was immersed in protein solutions at 4°C for 2 hr to bind the proteins to the PAA chains through amide linkage. The protein concentration and pH of each solution were 0.5 $mg \cdot ml^{-1}$ and pH 3 (collagen), 1 $mg \cdot ml^{-1}$ and pH 7.4 (gelatin), and 0.7 $mg \cdot ml^{-1}$ and pH 7.4 (fibronectin). The amount of immobilized proteins was determined by the Ninhydrin method (ref. 6).

Implantation and adhesion test

The virgin and surface-modified silicone sheets were subcutaneously implanted in the backs of Japanese rabbits, perpendicular to the spine, and fixed to the muscle layer with silk suture. After implantation for predetermined periods of time, the rabbits were sacrificed and the rabbit back was dissected to expose the implanted silicones. An end of the sheet was clamped with a clip that was connected to a load cell of a tensile test machine. The force to pull out the sheets was determined by moving the load cell at a speed of 10 $mm \cdot min^{-1}$.

Histological observation

The silicone sheets explanted from the rabbits together with the surrounding tissue were sectioned with a microtome after fixation with 10 % formalin and then stained with haematoxylin-eosin(H.E.). The sheets obtained after the tensile test were directly stained with H.E. to observe the cell attachment to the surface.

RESULTS

Protein immobilization

Fig.1 shows the amount of collagen immobilized on the PAA-grafted silicone as a function of the reaction time with WSC. The maximal amount of collagen immobilized is 13 $\mu g \cdot cm^{-2}$, which is approximately 10 times larger than the value presumed for a monolayer adsorption. The reason for definite immobilization of collagen even at the zero reaction time may be due to polyion complex formation between collagen and PAA molecules, whereas a decrease in the immobilized amount with time in the range of reaction duration longer than 30 min may be explained in terms of side reactions. Under a similar reaction condition, gelatin and fibronectin were also effectively immobilized on the PAA-grafted silicone.

Adhesion of implanted silicones

Adhesion between the modified silicone and the surrounding tissue was

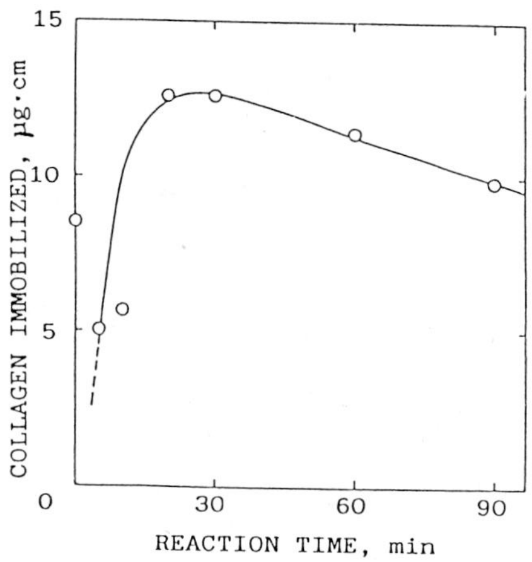

Fig.1. Effect of WSC reaction time on collagen immobilization onto the silicone surface having carboxylic groups.

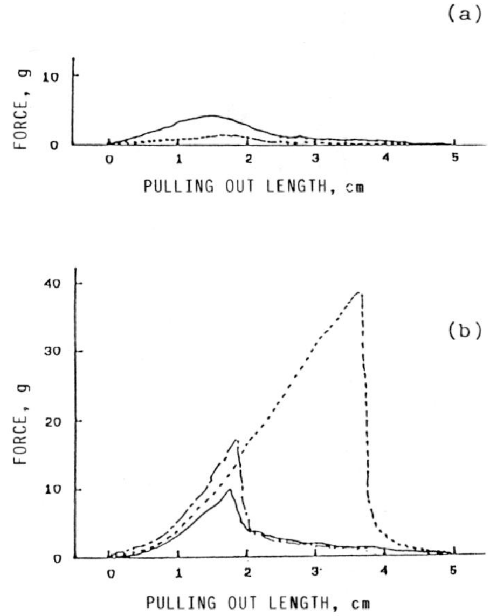

Fig.2. Forces required for pulling-out the surface-modified silicones subcutaneously implanted in rabbit for 3 weeks. (a) virgin and PAAm-grafted; ——:virgin, ---:PAAm-grafted, (b) protein-immobilized: ——:fibronectin, ---:collagen, —— · ——:gelatin

evaluated according to the method described in EXPERIMENTAL. In Fig.2(a) and 2(b), forces required to pull out the silicones from the implanted site are plotted against the pulling-out length for the specimen implanted for three weeks as an example. As is seen in Fig.2(a), where the results for the virgin silicone and the polyacrylamide(PAAm)-grafted silicone are given, these silicones could be smoothly pulled out with weak force. On the other hand, much higher forces were needed for pulling-out the silicones on which proteins had been immobilized, as shown in Fig.2(b). Comparison of Fig.2(b) with Fig.2(a) clearly indicates that the pulling-out curves for the protein-immobilized silicones have sharp peaks in contrast with those for the virgin and the PAAm-grafted silicone. This strongly suggests that the silicone surfaces possessing the immobilized proteins such as collagen, gelatin, and fibronectin represent positive adhesion with the subcutaneous tissue.

The maximal force achieved at the pulling-out test, which provides a measure of bioadhesion, is given as a function of implantation time in Fig.3(a) to 3(e). As can be seen, the pulling-out force does not increase in all cases any more after implantation approximately for two weeks. The silicone

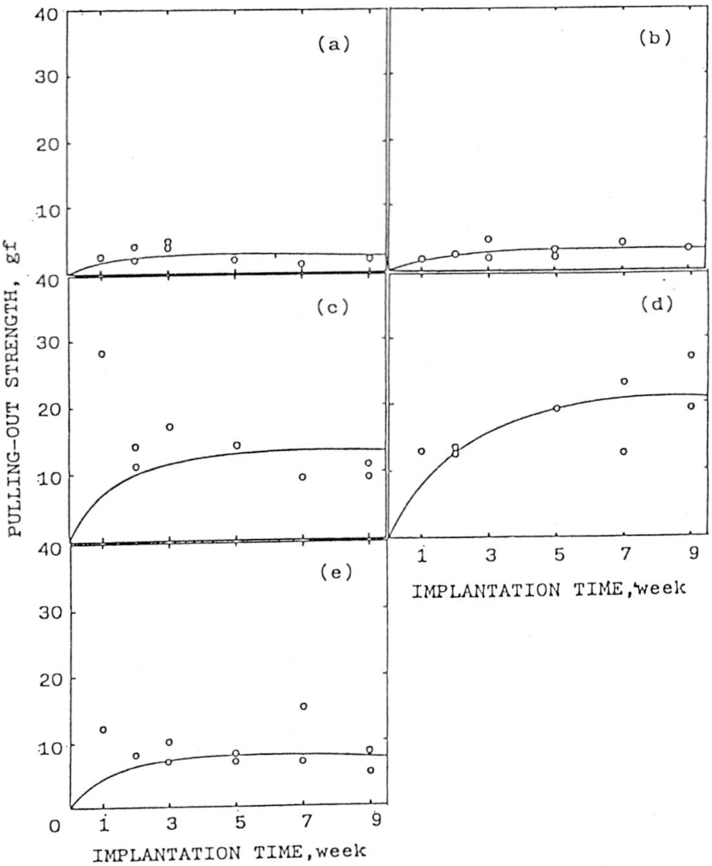

Fig.3. Maximal pulling-out strength plotted against the implantation time for surface-modified silicones. (a) virgin, (b) PAAm-grafted, (c) gelatin-immobilized, (d) collagen-immobilized, (e) fibronectin-immobilized

groups belonging to the lowest adhesion includes the virgin and the PAAm-grafted silicone, while the highest adhesion is achieved by immobilization of collagen. The gelatin- and fibronection-immobilized silicones are ranked in between.

Histological study

Fig.4(a) to 4(e) shows the light microphotographs of a cross-section of the silicones implanted for seven weeks. It is seen that the virgin silicone as well as the PAAm-grafted silicone undergo encapsulation by a thin fibrous tissue, but represent no attack by inflammatory cells. Protein immobilization onto silicone also does not invoke any severe tissue reactions and the surfaces

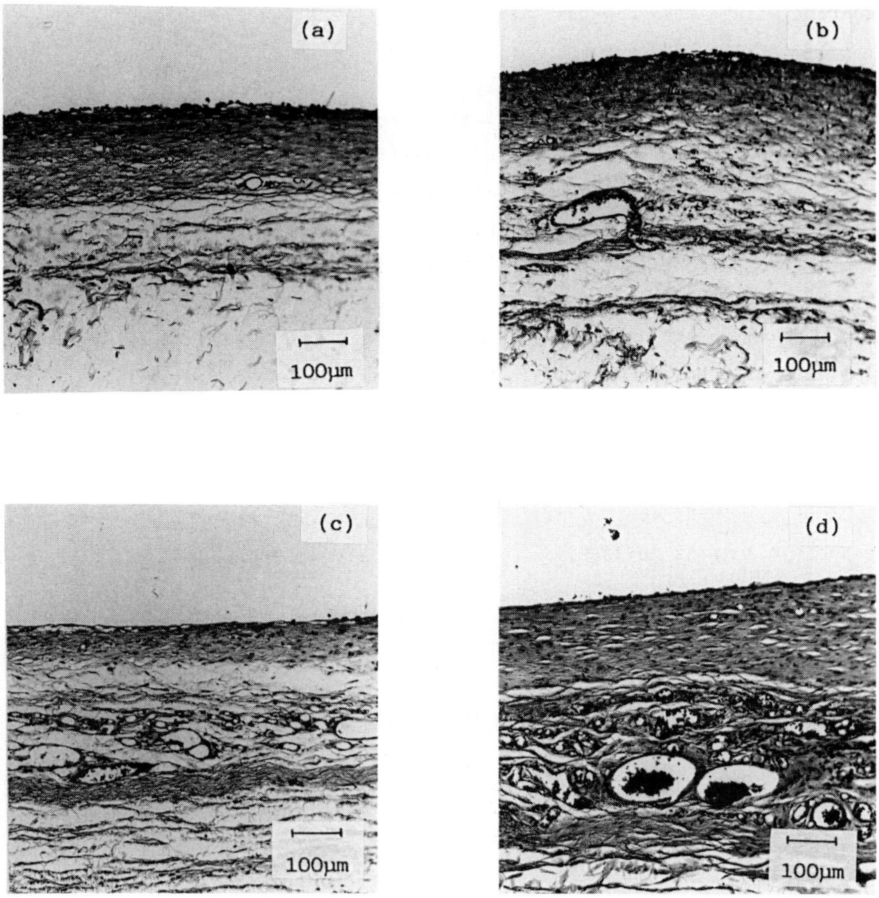

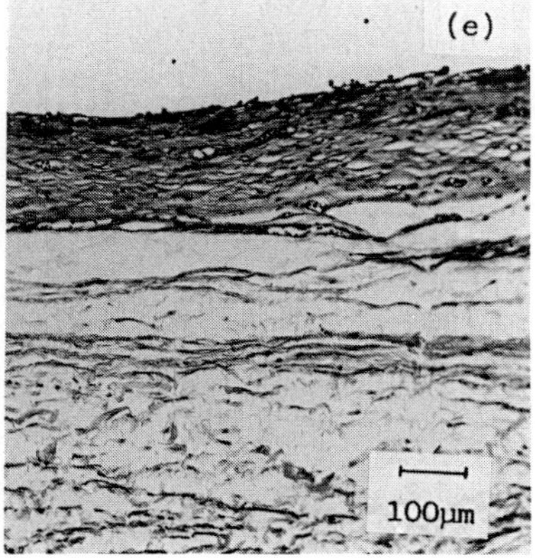

Fig.4. Light photomicrographs of subcutaneous tissues in direct contact with surface-modified silicones implanted in rabbit for 7 weeks (hematoxylin-eosin staining). (a) virgin, (b) PAAm-grafted, (c) gelatin-immobilized, (d) collagen-immobilized, (e) fibronectin-immobilized

are in contact with a thin fibrous tissue.

DISCUSSION

As previously reported (ref. 7), the material surface that is either extremely hydrophobic or extremely hydrophilic, strongly rejects the cell growth on it. This may be the major reason for the findings that insignificant bioadhesion took place for the virgin silicone (extremely hydrophobic) and the PAAm-grafted silicone (extremely hydrophilic).

There is no reason to suspect that the strong bioadhesion to the collagen-immobilized surface has occurred because of a high propensity of collagen to fibroblast attachment (ref. 8). The less bioadhesion of the gelatin-immobilized surface may be ascribed to higher enzymatic attack to gelatin than to the native collagen.

It may be concluded that good bioadhesion would be obtained between the living tissue and silicone if its surface is covalently covered by a cell-adhesive protein such as collagen.

REFERENCES

1 E.E. Frisch, Polymeric Materials and Artificial Organs: Silicones in Artificial organs, in: C.G. Gebelein (Ed.), ACS Symposium series 256, 1984, pp. 63-97.

2 Y. Shimizu, R. Abe, T. Teramatsu, S. Okamura, T. Hino, Studies on Copolymers of Collagen and a Synthetic Polymer, Biomat., Med. Dev., Art. Org., 5(1), (1977) 49-66.

3 P.M. Triolo, J.D. Andrade, Surface modification and evaluation of some commonly used catheter materials. I. Surface properties, J. Biomed. Mater. Res., 17 (1983) 129-147.

4 A Chapiro, D. Domurado, M. Foëx-Millequant A.-M. Jendrychowska-Bonamour, Radiation Grafting of N-Vinylpyrolidone into Silicone Tubes, Synthesis of Polymers with Improved Hemocompatibility and Implantation Tests in Lambs, Radiat. Phys. Chem., 18(5-6) (1981) 1203-1206.

5 T. Okada, Y. Tamada, Y. Ikada, Graft polymerization of Acryl Amide onto silicone surface pretreated with corona discharge, Preprint of the Society of Polymer Science, Japan, Kobe Meeting, Japan, July 5-6, 1984, p. 38.

6 R. McGrath, Protein Measurement by Ninhydrin determination of Amino Acids Released by Alkaline hydrolysis, Anal. Biochem., 49 (1972) 95-102.

7 Y. Tamada, A. Kishida, Y. Ikada, International Symposium on Polymer in Medicine, 1985, Capri, Italy.

8 H.K. Kleinman, R.J. Klebe, G.R. Martin, Role of Collagenous Materials in the Adhesion and Growth of Cells, J. Cell Biology, 88 (1981) 473-485.

Biomaterials and Clinical Applications,
edited by A. Pizzoferrato, P.G. Marchetti, A. Ravaglioli and A.J.C. Lee
Elsevier Science Publishers B.V., Amsterdam, 1987 — Printed in The Netherlands

THE DEGRADATION OF POLYHYDROXYBUTYRATE (PHB)

D. F. WILLIAMS[1] and N. D. MILLER[2]

[1]Institute of Medical and Dental Bioengineering, University of Liverpool, P. O. Box 147, Liverpool (England)

[2]Smith and Nephew Research Ltd., Gilston Park, Harlow, Essex (England)

SUMMARY

Polyhydroxybutyrate (PHB) has been proposed as a biodegradable implant material on the basis of its known degradation characteristics in certain biological environments. Monofilaments of PHB homopolymer and two PHB-PHV copolymers have been studied *in vivo* and *in vitro* and assessed for changes in mechanical properties and topography in order to determine susceptibility to degradation in the human physiological environment. The experiments have demonstrated that neither PHB, nor PHB-PHV copolymers in monofilament form, are biodegradable, although susceptibility to degradation may be increased by exposure to gamma irradiation.

INTRODUCTION

Poly-β-hydroxybutyrate, PHB, has long been known in microbiology as a natural storage material which is both synthesised and chemically degraded by a range of micro-organisms. It is a polymer of β-hydroxybutyric acid:

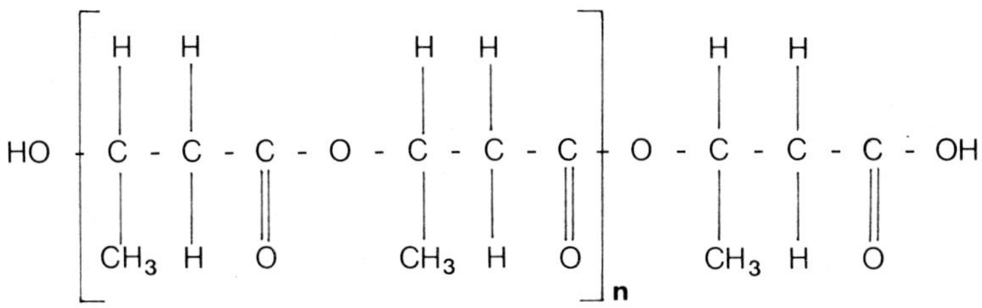

PHB may be isolated from micro-organisms quite readily and has been put to commercial use as a biodegradable material. Its degradability in certain biological environments has led to claims that it may be used as a degradable component of implantable materials and devices (refs. 1, 2). This is not an unreasonable expectation since extracellular degradation of PHB by soil bacteria (ref. 3) and enzyme-mediated degradation (ref. 4) have been demonstrated. However, claims of biodegradability within the human body seem premature and a study of this phenomenon, as part of a larger study on polymer degradation has been conducted in our laboratory. In addition to PHB, we have studied certain copolymers of PHB with PHV, the polyester of hydroxypentanoic acid:

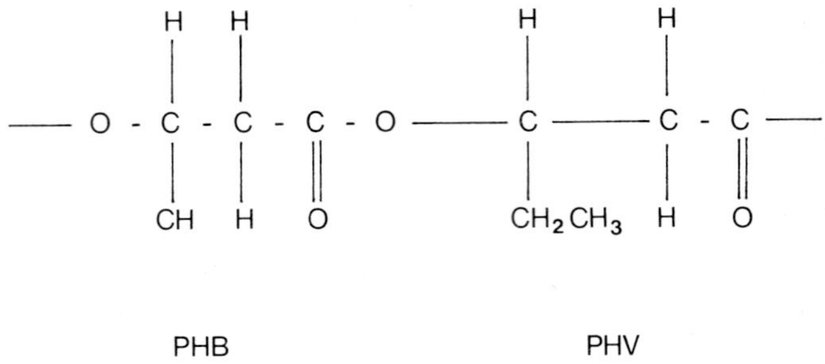

MATERIALS AND METHODS

PHB homopolymer and the copolymers 8% PHV-PHB and 17% PHV-PHB, all in monofilament fibre form were supplied by ICI PLC, Billingham, UK. The molecular weight of the homopolymer Mw was in the region of 200,000 Daltons. Both *in vivo* and *in vitro* experiments were carried out. In the former case, lengths of the polymer were weighed and implanted subcutaneously in black and white hooded rats of the Liverpool strain using standard aseptic techniques. Four specimens were separately implanted in each animal and two animals were used for each time period (2, 4, 7, 14, 21, 28, 56, 90 and 180 days).

At the end of each time period, the fibres were removed, cleaned of adherent tissue, washed in distilled, deionised water and vacuum dessicated. The fibres were separated into shorter lengths and tested in tension to failure on an Instron at a cross-head speed of 3cm/min and with a gauge length of 2.5cm. Each specimen was mounted on a guide card window to ease handling and alignment, as described in BS3411:1971.

A simultaneous *in vitro* experiment was performed in which lengths of fibre were maintained in sealed bottles of sterile phosphate buffered saline (PBS), pH 7.2 at 37°C. These were removed at selected times, washed, dessicated, weighed and tested in the manner described above.

Finally, in a separate series of experiments, PHB homopolymer was subjected to different levels of gamma irradiation in a Vickers Co-60 unit, up to a total of 10 Mrads, before *in vivo* or *in vitro* study.

In all experiments, the topography of the polymer fibres was examined by SEM on virgin material and after exposure. Implant holders in the form of 8mm o.d., 5mm i.d., 2.8mm thick acrylic rings with transverse notches were made to hold small lengths of the fibres such that they could be implanted, explanted, cleaned, coated and examined without touching the polymer itself.

RESULTS

Fig. 1 shows the variation in load at break of PHB homopolymer monofilament

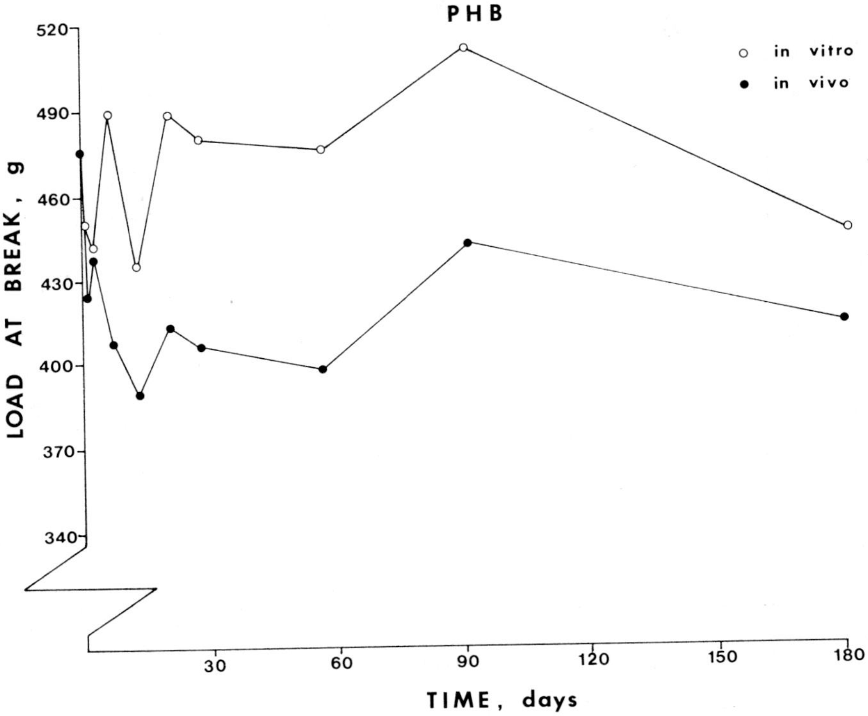

Fig. 1. Change in load at break for PHB homopolymer *in vitro* and *in vivo*.

as a function of time in subcutaneous sites in rats and in PBS, pH 7.2 at 37°C (in this series cross-sectional areas of specimens were not measured; tensile strength data is not, therefore, available). No weight changes were noted in any specimen and, topographically, no evidence of surface degradation was seen. Clearly on the basis of this evidence PHB homopolymer monofilament of the form described does not appear to degrade significantly, either *in vivo* or *in vitro*.

Fig. 2 illustrates the behaviour of the 8% PHV-PHB copolymer over the same time period. Again, no significant differences were observed between *in vivo* and *in vitro* conditions, and overall, although fluctuations in tensile strength are seen, there is no evidence of degradation. A similar conclusion was drawn from the 17% PHV-PHB copolymers.

Fig. 3 (a and b) illustrates the effect of prior gamma-irradiation on the degradability of PHB homopolymer. The 2.5 and 5 Mrad doses had no effect on the basic properties of the material, nor its degradability in the short term. 10 Mrad caused a significant change in mechanical properties but not in degradability *in vitro*. However, specimens receiving this 10 Mrad dose lost all strength by 7 days *in vivo*, indicating some influence of the tissue environment. Doses of 20 Mrad destroyed all mechanical integrity.

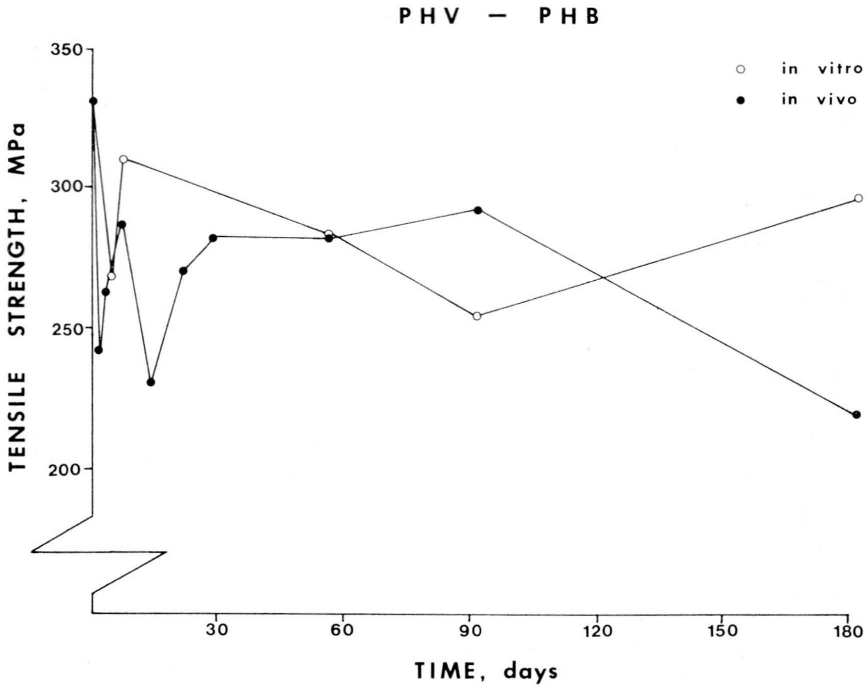

Fig. 2. Tensile strength of 8% PHV-PHB *in vitro* and *in vivo* over 180 period.

DISCUSSION

Within the limits of these studies, little degradation has been seen with PHB homopolymer monofilament, either *in vivo* or *in vitro*. Copolymer additions of PHV did not appear to alter the susceptibility to degradation under the conditions studied. The degradability of PHB is increased, however, by prior gamma irradiation at levels of 10 Mrad. All mechanical integrity was lost after 7 days *in vivo*, although tensile properties were altered very little after 14 days *in vitro*.

Two points are of interest. First, evidence of PHB in other environments had suggested that PHB was degradable in biological systems and claims had been made that the human body provided such a system. It is suggested here that this is not the case with high molecular weight PHB that, after microbial production, has been purified and processed. It is known that the intracellular degradation of native PHB by the micro-organisms in which it is produced cannot proceed until the polymer has been activated by what may be a proteolytic enzyme. The

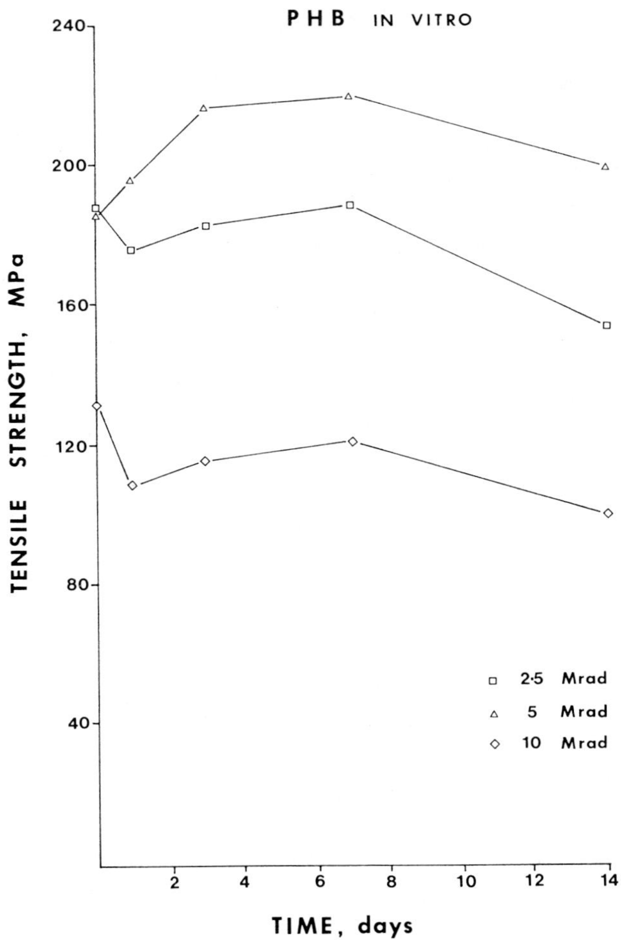

Fig. 3a. Effect of gamma irradiation on PHB homopolymer *in vitro* over 14 days.

degradation by a depolymerase requires such initiation and it is likely that the extracellular degradation of PHB (eg. by bacteria in soil) is enzymatically controlled (ref. 3). There is no reason to suppose that the human body presents the right enzymes for this attack.

It is possible, however, that changes to the structure of PHB by prior irradiation may increase the susceptibility to degradation. This is presumably accompanied by a reduction in molecular weight and the present evidence would suggest that 10 Mrad is sufficient to cause significant changes. After this irradiation a greater susceptibility to degradation is seen *in vivo* compared to *in vitro*, possibly associated with enzyme activity.

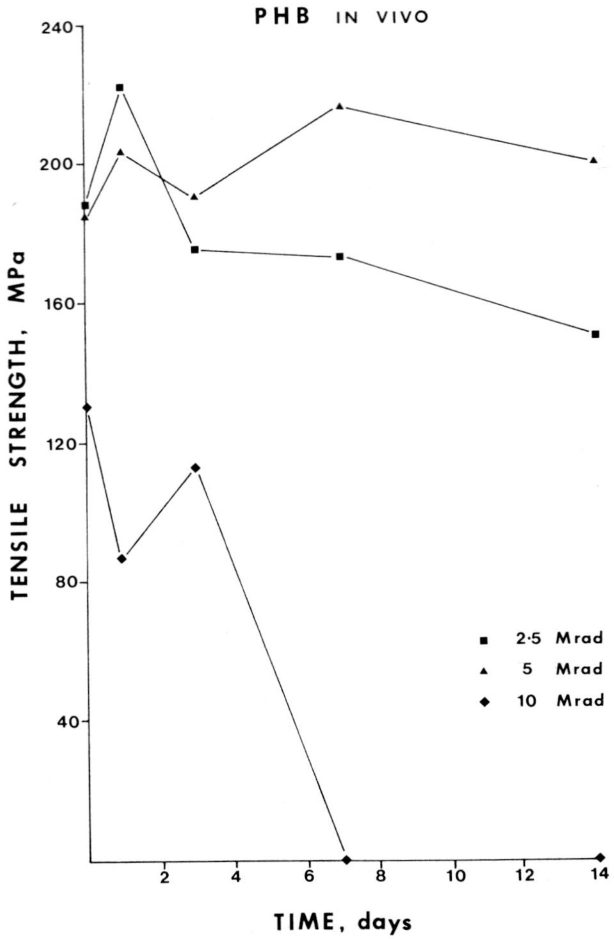

Fig. 3b. Effect of gamma irradiation on PHB homopolymer *in vivo* over 14 days.

REFERENCES

1. P. Holmes, Applications of PHB - a microbially produced biodegradable thermoplastic, Phys. Technol. 16 (1985) 32-36.
2. M. C. Bissery, F. Puisceux, S. Summerfield, T. Lenk and C. Thies, Biodegradable microspheres fabricated from β-hydroxybutyrate-hydroxyvalerate copolymers. First Biointeractions Conf., City University, London 1984.
3. A. Chowdury, Bacteria and exoenzymes capable of degrading poly-β-hydroxybutyric acid. Archiv. fur Mikrobiologie 47 (1963) 167-200.
4. R. Y. Slaner, M. Doudoroff and E. A. Adelberg, General Microbiology. 3rd ed., MacMillan, London, 1971.

Biomaterials and Clinical Applications,
edited by A. Pizzoferrato, P.G. Marchetti, A. Ravaglioli and A.J.C. Lee
Elsevier Science Publishers B.V., Amsterdam, 1987 — Printed in The Netherlands

PHYSICO-CHEMICAL CHARACTERISTICS OF CERAMICS FOR MEDICAL APPLICATIONS.

A.RAVAGLIOLI* and A.KRAJEWSKI
Institute for Technological Research on Ceramics of C.N.R. - Faenza (Italy)
*Invited lecturer

ABSTRACT

A review will be reported on biomaterials with particular reference to bioceramics involved in such field. Assessments on the properties of the used materials will be displayed with particular reference to those obtained through sintering. The applications and the technological methodologies for production will be further reported, putting attention also on their specific problems.

On the basis of the overall conclusions about the physico-chemical and physico-mechanical potentiality of such materials, new products for surgical applications with standardized characteristics may be made available. The use of ceramics either as bulk or coating materials will be taken into consideration.

GENERAL REMARKS ABOUT CERAMIC BIOMATERIALS

The term biomaterial includes a wide range of substances related to various qualities. Thus, biomaterials belong to that class of materials (ref.1) which includes metals, polymers and the inorganic non-metallic solids. Products manufactured from the metal and the polymer classes are normally prepared for casting into moulds from their melts, therefore the heating and casting processes precede those of moulding. When using inorganic non-metallic substances, only the glasses may employ a similar sequence of working. The remaining inorganic materials, primarily those with very high melting points, require a sintering process instead of a melting one and then the manufacture of a product from these substances requires a finishing stage prior to heating and partial casting. Unlike the metals, polymers and glasses, the moulding stage takes place before the maximum temperature to which the substance is subjected, is reached. The material of the tools and containers employed in the making of sintered objects are limited by a temperature of definable limits. Above this temperature, refractory substances capable of containing the sinter material as melt do not exist without the melt being seriously contaminated by the refractory, or a suitable refractory capable of reaching the desired temperature for the casting does not exist. Observing the range of casting temperatures for various substances, it is apparent that standard procedures include sintering for pure substances which melt above about 1700°C. Among these we find objects made of some special metals, such as Tantalum and Niobium, the manufacture of which requires a procedure typically corresponding to sintering.

Those bodies made of inorganic non-metallic substances obtained by sintering are called "ceramics". In the field of biomaterials pure substances are usually employed, rather than mixed systems or substances which originate from a complex closely mixed compound of various substances. The characteristic initially researched in manufactured ceramics for biomedical use was the great chemical inertness due mainly to the high binding energy found among the atomic components of the substance constituting the ceramics. Such inertness coincides with the characteristic called refractivity, since chemical stability reflects also stability at high temperatures, either in term of high melting point, or in terms of non-chemical reaction with hot gases with which the material defined as refractory comes into contact.

In a biological system the chemical stability looked for does not correspond precisely to the concept of refractivity, however, refractory materials are usually chemically stable in the human organism at standard temperatures.

Recently, attention has been given to ceramic substances which have a correspondence or closeness to those which constitute the mineral fraction of bone tissue, such as hydroxylapatite, β-whitlockite and bioglasses. They are not chemically inert but play an interaction role (which we shall

define as positive) with the surrounding tissue, developing biochemical interference allowing the ceramic part to be recognized and to become an integral part of the body.
These ceramic-like substances are then called "bioactive" ones. Such bioactive action of a substance may cease if some particular compounds (also at an impurity level in some cases), are present, such as Al_2O_3 for bioglasses.

Following is a brief view of the ceramic substances which, thus far, have been considered interesting for experimental application in the field of orthopedic, maxillary facial, dental and general surgery.

ZIRCONIUM OXIDE

In order to consider the behaviour of zirconium oxide, it is necessary to evaluate the transformations which it may undergo in relation to the cooling process once the preshaped object has been sintered. The ZrO_2 undergoes the phase transformations at the temperatures and with the properties shown in the table (Table 1).

The zirconium oxide is not suitable for use as the only material from which a body is manufactured because, in the transition from tetragonal to monoclinic during cooling, tensions are generated inside the ceramic body, by the different contraction relationships between the granules which can cause fractures. The transformation from the tetragonal to monoclyne phase is accompanied by an increase of volume of about 5% and by a change in shape, both factors generate a relevant tangential effort along particular cristallographic axes. This phenomenon, which has a destructive action, prevents the use of zirconium oxide as a massive material. Usually a stabilized ZrO_2 is used, with additions such as CaO, MgO and Y_2O_3, which promote the formation of the stable cubic phase. For proper additions and treatments, the zirconia may be partially stabilized. In this case, it may contain an appreciable quantity of tetragonal phase as a precipitate of the cubic phase, therefore avoiding fracture. Since objects made from partially stabilized ZrO_2 show high mechanical properties, it was supposed (ref. 2) that, in a similar way to steels, the good qualities would be the result of a martensitic transformation. Such transformation usually takes place without diffusion, without significant exotherm and implies a change of shape. This last aspect is considered as typical for such a transformation, and it is particularly important because, as for steels, it is the main reason for the toughening produced in ceramics. The reaction takes place during cooling at a temperature between 1000°C and 800°C, but particles of ZrO_2 scattered in another type of matrix, may be retained in the tetragonal form, also at a lower temperature. In this transformation an hysterisis process exists, in which the phase change temperature differs during the heating and cooling (Fig.1).

From the dilatometric point of view, the pattern of the transformation consequent to the existence of this hysterisis, which is a function both of the size of the ZrO_2 granules and of the different nature od the matrix surrounding each grain (this phenomenon will be examined later on), involves the possibility (ref.s 2-4) that particular particles may pass from the tetragonal to the monoclyne phase at variable temperatures during cooling. Under particular conditions such a transformation temperature may also be lower than the room temperature and the martensitic transformation temperature is related to the content of some stabilizers. Now, the cost of objects constituted of stabilized ZrO_2 is lower than in the past, primarily due to new knowledge, and in particular, to the new technologies of powder preparation according to orientative classification schemes which determine the destination of the various systems in zirconia, as recently proposed by Claussen (ref. 3). However, the cost level is not sufficiently low to guarantee this material in bulk for biomedical application.

Plasma spray coating with stabilized ZrO_2 is a much more difficult procedure than that of Al_2O_3. The heating process of the granules in the plasma flame may determine the partial evaporation or resolution of the stabilizing additives. In this

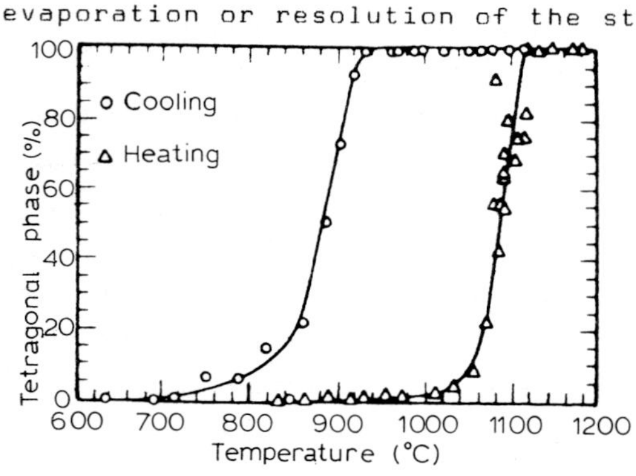

Fig. 1 - Tetragonal phase percent (by X-rays diffractometry) in the monoclinic:tetragonal transformation, during heating and cooling of ZrO_2. Note the well thermal hysteresis (ref. 3).

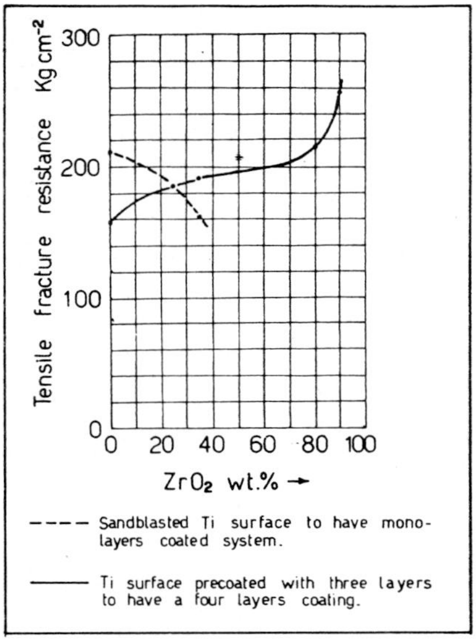

Fig. 2 - Effect of ZrO_2 content onto the cited bioglass admixture plasma-spayed on the metallic surface, treated as indicated.

way, the cubic phase becomes more critical and consequently the number of failures is significantly larger. This is probably the reason why ZrO_2 has not been widely used as a ceramic material for biomedical purposes, although some present tests would seem to show a proteic wedding incompatibility between cells and ZrO_2 surface. It is now certain that a stabilized ZrO_2 coating may prove very effective since the energy of the Zr-O bond is higher than that of the Al-O bond. Many believe that the higher stability of the bond strengthens the material against chemical erosion, partially shown by the allumina contained in spray plasma. It should, however, be emphasized that the technology of coating by spray plasma involves an extensive training period more than a great knowledge of the theory of its behaviour, especially for the satisfactory deposition of suitable surfaces for the substrate passage.

Tests of ZrO_2 coatings on 316L steel substrates and of titanium through spray plasma, have been explored in the past by the authors (ref. 5) in cooperation with Dr. G. Perugini of the Donegani Institute of Novara, in the presence and absence of percentages of bioglass 45S5F (flourized Hench's composition) (ref. 6).

The metallic samples to be coated with zirconia were previously treated by degreasing and heating, and were carefully coated with the sample maintained at a temperature around 600°C. Before the final coating, the samples underwent a preparatory coating with an intermediate layer according to the scheme reported in Table 2. The sprayed samples underwent post thermal treatment for about 1 hour at 1000°C in an air kiln to achieve oxidation conditions. For the spray a direct arco-plasma current, fed with fluid argon was used. The temperature level of the plasma flame was kept at around $10-13 \times 10^3$ °K. The primary gas used for the injection of the powders was nitrogen.

The mechanical strength of the ZrO_2 sprayed on the titanium is over 400 Kg/cm^2, while the pattern of Fig. 2 shows the decrease caused by the presence of the bioglass.

On the AISI 316L, coating with zirconia oxide was deleterious because of the maximum mechanical resistance for the coating with only glass, sprayed with plasma.

PHASE	Trasformation Temperature (C°)	unit cell constants (A°)	Space group	Kg m^{-3} density
Monoclinic		a=5.156 b=5.191 c=5.304 β=98.9°	$P2_1/c$	5560
	1000-2000			
Tetragonal		a=5,094 c=5.177	$P4_2/nmc$	6100 (calc) 5720 (exp)
	2000-2400			
Cubic		a=5.124	Fm3m	6090

TABLE 1 - Picture of the salient properties of Zirconium oxide.

Layer number	thickness (mm)	quality and composition	powders size (um; ±0.1%)
1	0.05	metal powder admixture of 50% wt Co; 50% wt Ti	75
2	0.05	metalceramic powder admixture of 60% wt Ti; 40% wt Al_2O_3	75
3	0.05	ceramic stabilized zirconia: 95% wt ZrO_2; 5% wt CaO	75

TABLE 2 - coating layers arranged techniques.

ALUMINA

The Al_2O_3 is the compound to which the greatest attention has been paid. This is due to the fact that it was a ceramic material widely used for porcelains, and therefore characterized more from an engineering point of view than any other known ceramic.

The various phases of the Al_2O_3, except for α, are meta stable phases which tend to undergo transformations, primarily during cooling, towards the more stable α phase. The phase transforamtion is encouraged by the grain size, by the disorder or degree of activity of the powders, by gases used in the kiln atmosphere, by humidity, or by impurities and additives which may promote or inhibit the crystalline increase. As an example, the presence of small percentages of Th^{4+} or Hf^{3+} or alkaline ions inhibit the transformation of both γ and δ phases into α by increasing the transition temperature. On the other hand the transition temperature from γ toward α- Al_2O_3 is reduced in the presence of metal oxides of the first transition series, as well as TiO_2 and SiO_2. The presence of MgO should promote the η and γ phases since the unit cell of the $MgAl_2O_4$ spinel is arranged as a cubic close stacking of 32 oxygen atoms in tetrahedral holes. The γ phase is universally considered to be formed at high temperatures by the hot flame of the plasma spray.

Experience has demonstrated how Al_2O_3 may undergo delayed fracturing in massive pieces (ref. 1). The main factors causing this effect are firing temperature, kiln atmosphere, grain shape (tabular alumina is worse than that with a roundish grain), and the sintering speed. Usually, modern industrial procedures for the production of Al_2O_3 balls require firing temperatures above 1700°C in an H_2 atmosphere to favour the formation of Al_2O_3 traces, which are extremely reactive and promote sintering, in the presence of SiO_2 and MgO traces to limit the size of the grains. In order to prevent the occurrrence of delayed fractures, the method of halting the tip of the crack by inseminating the ceramic body with partially stabilized tetragonal ZrO_2 can be used. Taking care not to add quantities above 15% of ZrO_2 to the ceramic powders with excessively larger grains than the medium ones obtained after the sintering of the Al_2O_3, the trapping condition may be reached for the tetragonal phase of ZrO_2 by physical constriction around the grains of the sintered Al_2O_3. In the case of development of cracks, its tip may be captured by a near metastable ZrO_2 grain, thus restricting the development of the crack and absorbing the energy of advancement. The sensitivity to the martensitic transformation of the ZrO_2 may be modified by properly adjusting its doping, as shown in Fig.2. Adding a 15 vol % of mixed crystals ZrO_2/HfO_2=1:1 to the Al_2O_3 matrix, an austenitic temperature shift (A_s) to 1460°C may be reached, indicating that compressive stresses would be retained up to this temperature. This energy may prove useful for the accomplishment of the martensitic transformation from the tetragonal phase into the monoclinic phase of the zirconia which, because it involves an increase of volume, occludes the volume of the final part of the crack (ref. 7). Insemination with ZrO_2 of an Al_2O_3 mass prevents the possibility of delayed fracture, and at the same time slows down the advancement of the microcracks, which are determined by induction from the overcoming of critical conditions in particular occasions.

A proposed suggestion (ref. 8) for practical application of this technique is that it may prolong average life of ceramic femoral-heads.

Another use of Al_2O_3 as a coating for metallic prostheses, was and still is, a known protective technique (ref 9). An arco plasma is used in order to reach temperatures above 2500°C, with Ar as carrier gas. When using this technique the metallic parts must be kept hot while carrying out multilayer adjusting procedures. An example of intermediate coating is that recently proposed (ref. 10), which illustrates the deposition of a layer of molybdenum on 316L steel (with powders ϕ=69±16μm, laid by spray plasma in air), on a carefully activated, cleaned and sandblasted surface. The coating was deposited on the stainless steel as an intermediate layer to reduce stresses caused by the different thermal expansion coefficients between the metallic supports and the ceramic band. All the plasma spray operations are carried out on rotating (in order to produce layers of homogeneous thickness) and heated specimens, to give a certain margin of elasticity, thus avoiding cracking during the exercise. Al_2O_3 powder size must range between 20 to 40 μm. In this case the crystalline phase of the coating is not the stable α type, but the γ one, which transforms with difficulty into the α phase. Even though the transformation takes place over a very long period of time, it can lead to a mechanical weakening of the layer.

It is therefore convenient to try to stabilize this γ phase with suitable doping procedures of the flux powders in the spray plasma (e.g. with MgO). In many cases these coatings show a diffused porosity (ref. 10) or pinholes (ref. 5), that may be conveyers for cationic release from the metal substrate.

TITANIA

Relative to TiO_2, nowadays prostheses in bulk were not experimented. TiO_2 shows polymorphic characteristics in its three modifications, where the thermally stable phase is the rutile.

This is the most interesting phase, crystallizing as a bipyramidal rhombic, which however originates formation geminating by reticular pseudomeriedria. The germinated is caused by specular growing on a plane derived from the representation of a pseudo-rhombical cell instead of a tetragonal one. While in the rutile the Ti^{4+} shows a octahedral regular field of coordination of the oxigens, in the two other forms such coordination field of the TiO_6 groups is less distorted in the anatase form which maintains the same symmetry while crystallizing in a different spatial group and more in the brookite, which symmetry is instead bipiramidal rhombic. Of course the chaining of the octahedrons is very different in the three phases. The anatase instead is formed also in particular conditions but at ordinary pressures, while the brookite is a high pressure phase, and therefore difficult to obtain during the ceramization procedures. As it happens for the Al_2O_3 the polymorphic phases are not interested in the constitution of massive bodies but in the particular coating procedures through plasma due to the high temperatures and to the uncommon conditions involved in the formation of the titania solid.

Coatings with TiO_2 have been tested for several years. Recently, also the one on AISI 316 L coated with molibdenum under the same conditions as the corresponding coating with Al_2O_3 have been tested. Molibdenum and titanium are known as efficient band coats for plasma spray and oxide layers[11]. The permeability to the ionic release seems to be lesser with this kind of coating than with the Al_2O_3 one, showing so its more compactness, and than its more efficiency as coating system.

SPECIAL NEW CERAMICS

Nowadays, famous surgeons have come to consider other ceramic materials at a very high chemical stability. In fact, much attention has been given to tests for coating metal prostheses with special refractory substances, in particular carbides and nitrides of titanium and tantalium (TiC, TaC, TiN, TaN). These materials, due to the high sintering temperatures, are not suitable for massive pieces, but may instead (ref. 11) be suitable for coating by means of particular technological procedures for ceramic formation on the surface of the substrata to be covered. The usual methods employ CVD techniques (chemical vapor deposition) achieving formation in the gas phase by chemical reaction of the activated carbide or nitride and their forced deposition under pressure and temperature conditions controlled through gas flux (Fig.3). In most cases the carbide and nitride coatings of refractory metals are obtained by reduction of the metallic halides working at temperatures ranging between 700 and 1100°C. At these temperatures and at deposition times which can go up to several hours, changes in structure and composition of the substrate bulk, the coating and the interface can occur, and will strongly influence the mechanical and corrosive behaviour of these composite materials. In other cases, ionic deposition or sputtering procedures (Fig.3) are used through PVD techniques (physical vapour

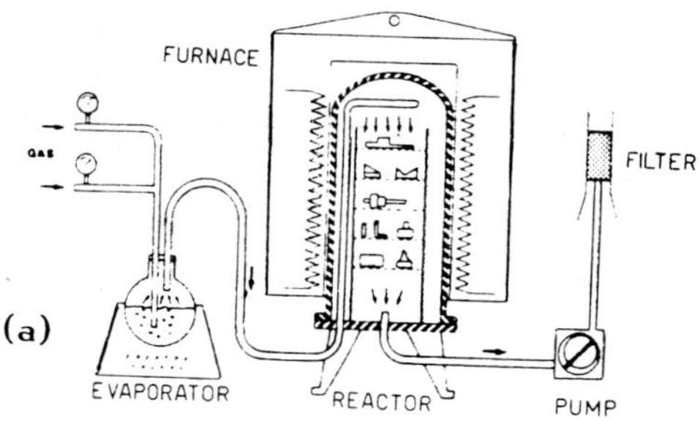

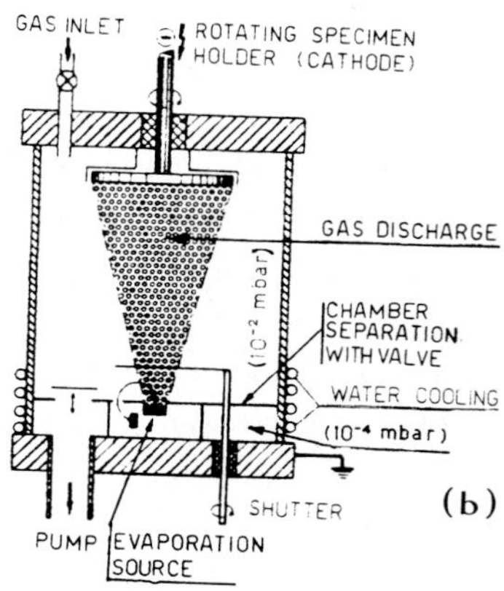

Fig. 3 - Schematic drawn of:
(a) CVD apparatus;
(b) ion plating unit;
(c) sputtering unit.

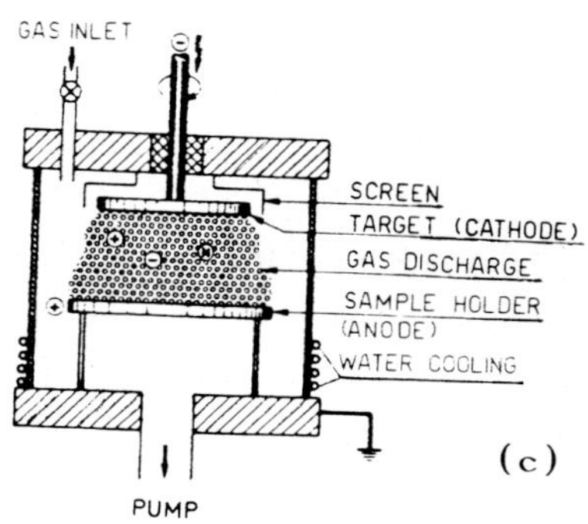

deposition). In the ionic deposition method a superficial film at deposition process of the substance to be used is employed in which the substrate surface and/or the deposition of film is subjected to a flux of high energy atomic or molecular particles. These cause changes in the interfacial region or in the film properties. Such changes may be reflected in the adhesion, morphology, stress, and density of the film or the coverage of the surface by the deposited film material. In this method, argon is admitted into a vacuum chamber at a pressure of about 1Pa, and a high voltage source is connected to the substrate holder. A gas discharge is set up with a positive charge. Because of the strong negative substrate potential, the ionized particles strike the substrate at high speed. In comparison with ordinary vacuum evaporation, this process gives both better adhesion and a more uniform coating for these substances, and for non-flat substrates. In the sputtering method the argon is emitted at the same conditions, where a rectified pulse radiofrequency current source at high voltage is connected to the target.

A gas discharge forms between the target and the surface of the substrate holder, previously enriched in carbon (ref. 12), which is electrically connected to the vacuum chamber, achieving a surfacial chemical reaction by admitting a reactive gas during the sputtering. It is used for the production of the layer on metal substrates.

PHOSPHATE CERAMICS

Phosphate materials are used in bioactive substances. Such materials may be easily ceramized and are obtained through hot pressing techniques in order to increase the final density. They provide the appropriate surface for cell bonds and connection to the mineral fraction is constituted through enzymatic action by the cells themselves. This action comes from the transfer of Ca^{2+} and phosphates groups. Some of the biochemical inertness of hydroxylapatite can be explained by the fact that it is already similar to the basic bone mineral phase and therefore the action of reconstructive readsorption, found for other substances, is probably made slower.

Massive ceramic objects do not show sufficient mechanical resistance properties (they range from 300 to 800 kg/cm^2).

The β-TCP is a material that undergoes a biochemical

rearrangement and induces an osteogenetic activity. Its manufacture is made easy by the presence of Mg^{2+} ions which prevents the formation of HA and helps that of β-TCP.

Phosphate ceramics are considered for dental roots and maxillofacial applications.

SUMMARY AND CONCLUSIONS

A description of the potential applications of ceramics in the field of biomaterials was reported considering various substances, their qualities and defects.

In relation to every substance the possible applications either as bulk or coatings of other materials (particularly metals) were put in evidence.

The substances coming from the ceramic field suitable for surgical applications are, particularly, zirconium oxide for bulk products and titanium oxide and TaN, TaC, TiN and TiC for coatings and the passivation of metallic prostheses.
The strengthening criterion of the alumina by loading with zirconium oxide grains is also proposed.

Some new and/or traditional ceramic moulding techniques were reported at disposal for the products suitable for the medical field too.

The authors with this paper wish to focus on standardization, considering that some ceramized substances lack a precise definition of their characteristics and application limits which should be recorded within specific normatives.

REFERENCES

1- A.Ravaglioli, A.Krajewski; "Bioceramica e Corpo Umano: aspetti scientifici, tecnologici ed applicativi" Ed. Faenza Editrice and C.E.L.I., 336 p., 162 f, 52 t, 976r, 1(1984).

2- R.C.Garvie, R.H.Hannink and R.T.Pascoe, Nature (London) 258 (1975) 703

3- E.C.Subbarao, "Zirconia - an overview" Science and Technology of Zirconia (Advance in Ceramics Vol.3) Edited by A.H.Heuer and L.W.Hobbs, by Amer.Ceram.Soc. (1981) 1

4- N.Claussen; "Microstructural design of zirconia-toughened ceramics (2TC)", reported in: "Science and Technology of Zirconia II", on vol. 12 of "Advances in Ceramics" series; Ed. by N.Claussen, M.Ruhle, A.H.Heuer on the sign of "The Amer. Ceram. Soc. (Columbus, Ohio, 1984) 325-351.

5- A.Krajewski, A.Ravaglioli, G.Perugini "Bioglass composition as coating for metal prostheses", Science of Ceramics vol. 11 (1981) 85-90

6- L.L.Hench, Ceramurgia 5 (1977) 253

7- G.De Portu, La Ceramica 1 (1985) 6-18

8- R.Davidge, Engineering performance prediction for ceramics" Courses lessons held at ISPRA, ASFM 1985/86 on "Fracture mechanics on non metallic materials".

9- M.Calderale, V.Vullo "Proceedings of 2nd CERP, Faenza Editrice (1979) Sez. "Special Ceramics".

10- F.Brossa et alii, Proceedings of 6th CIMTEC, 6 (1986) Milano.

11- S.Safa' and H.Herman; Int. Conf. on Advances in surface coating technology, London 13/15 February 1978

12- H.Boving and H.E.Hintermann, CVD and PVD ion friction/antiwear coatings", Science od Ceramics 13p. C1/111 Ed. P.Odier, F.Cabannes, B.Cales; printed on Journ. de Physique Supp. N°2, 1986).

Biomaterials and Clinical Applications, 491
edited by A. Pizzoferrato, P.G. Marchetti, A. Ravaglioli and A.J.C. Lee
Elsevier Science Publishers B.V., Amsterdam, 1987 — Printed in The Netherlands

COMPARISON OF TWO SYNTHETIC ROUTES TO SYNTHESIZE POLYSTYRENE-POLY(ETHYLENE OXIDE)-HEPARIN BLOCK COPOLYMERS

I. VULIĆ, T. OKANO*, S.W. KIM* and J. FEIJEN+

Department of Chemical Technology, Twente University of Technology, P.O. Box 217, 7500 AE Enschede (The Netherlands), and * Department of Pharmaceutics, College of Pharmacy, University of Utah, Salt Lake City, 84112, Utah (U.S.A.)
+ To whom all correspondences should be addressed.

SUMMARY

Anionically and radically prepared polystyrene with one terminal primary amino group was coupled to amino-telechelic poly(ethylene oxide) to afford amino-semitelechelic polystyrene-poly(ethylene oxide). These diblock copolymers were coupled to heparin using EDC or coupled to nitrous acid-degraded heparin using $NaBH_3CN$ to yield polystyrene-poly(ethylene oxide)-heparin block copolymers. Measurement of plasma recalcification times of plasma in contact with surfaces coated with the synthesized block copolymers demonstrated prolonged clotting times.

INTRODUCTION

In a previous paper we reported the synthesis and characterization of new polystyrene-poly(ethylene oxide)-heparin block copolymers (1). One possible route to prepare blood-compatible surfaces is to anchor the hydrophobic block into a hydrophobic substrate by swelling with a proper solvent. The coating process results in the exposure of heparin coupled via a hydrophilic spacer at the surface, see Fig. 1. As shown by Ebert et al.(2), who recently immobilized

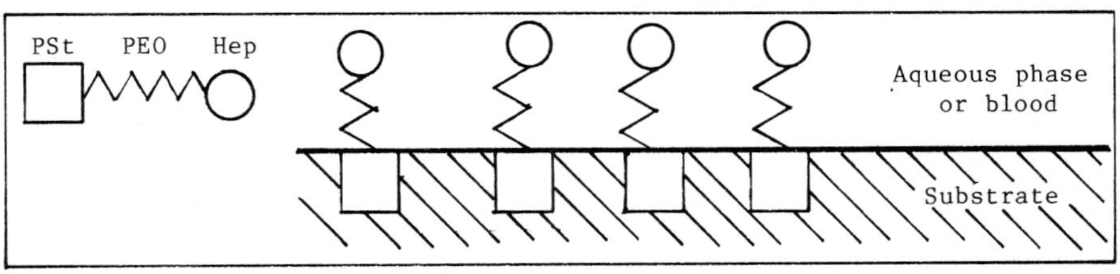

Figure 1. Schematic representation of coating block copolymers onto hydrophobic surfaces.

heparin via its carboxyl groups to diaminoalkane agarose gels, heparin directly affixed to the surface does not provide optimal, solution-like anticoagulant behavior. However anticoagulant activity does increase for 10-carbon unit spacer groups and longer.

Block copolymer surfaces that exhibit heterogeneous microphase separated surface structures of hydrophilic and hydrophobic microdomains have shown an ability to suppress platelet adhesion (3) and morphological changes of adhering platelets (4). Blood-compatible surfaces could be prepared by coating block copolymers onto materials so that a coating of heterogeneous microphase-separated microdomains would be exhibited, or by fabricating the block copolymer into the desired products (e.g. cardiovascular prostheses or catheters). This paper describes two different routes to synthesize polystyrene-poly(ethylene oxide)-heparin block copolymers. These polymers were further investigated as possible compounds for the improvement of the blood-compatibility of material surfaces.

METHODS

Materials

Amino-telechelic poly(ethylene oxide) with molecular weights 500 and 4000 (H_2N-PEO-NH_2) was a generous gift of Nippon Oil & Fats Company, Ltd., Tokyo, Japan. 2,2'-Azobisisobutyronitrile (AIBN, E. Merck, Darmstadt, Germany) was recristallized from EtOH. sec-Butyllithium (BuLi, Janssen Chimica, Beerse, Belgium) was used as a 1.3 M solution in cyclohexane. This BuLi-solution was freed of solids by filtration using a glass-sintered funnel under a N_2 atmosphere and was analyzed using the double titration procedure with 1,2-dibromoethane (5). 1,2-Dibromoethane (DBE, Fluka, Buchs Switzerland), N,N-dimethylformamide (DMF, Merck) after drying over anhydrous $MgSO_4$ (100 g/l), styrene (St, Merck) and toluene 2,4-diisocyanate (TDI, Fluka) were distilled under N_2 at reduced pressure. Dioxane (Merck) was first stirred with KOH-powder (10 g/l), refluxed and then distilled over CaH_2. Heparin, a sodium salt (Hep) from porcine mucosa had a specific activity of 165 U/mg, as indicated by the manufacturer (Diosynth B.V., Oss, Holland). N-(Benzylidene)trimethylsilyl-amide (BTMSA) with bp 101°C/18 mmHg was synthesized from sodium bis(trimethylsilyl)amide and benzaldehyde (Merck) in 34 % yield, following the method of Krueger et al.(6). Nitrous acid-degraded heparin (NADHep) was prepared by a slightly modified procedure as described by Hoffman et al.(7). All other chemicals were used as received.

Free-radical oligomerization of St

Polystyrene with a terminal primary amino function (PSt-NH_2) was synthesized by a free-radical oligomerization of St in DMF, using AIBN as initiator and 2-aminoethanethiol (AESH) as chain transfer agent, according to the procedure of Vulić et al.(1).

Anionic polymerization of St

Polymerizations were carried out under an inert N_2 atmosphere in a glove-box. Anionic polymerizations of St were initiated by BuLi in cyclohexane solution at 50°C. After 1 hr reaction time an excess (5 eq to initiator) of BTMSA was added dropwise to the solution of the living polymer at RT and the reaction mixture was allowed to stand for at least 3 hrs at RT. The polymer was then precipitated by slow addition to a 10-fold excess of MeOH. Subsequent deblocking of the N,N-bis(trimethylsilyl) terminal groups by hydrolysis in dilute HCl (pH 4) resulted in PSt-NH_2. This was performed according to the procedure of Schulz and Halasa (8).

Coupling of PSt-NH_2 and H_2N-PEO-NH_2

PSt-NH_2 was converted into PSt-N=C=O using TDI, Scheme 1 [1]. Subsequent coupling with H_2N-PEO-NH_2 afforded PSt-PEO-NH_2 diblock copolymers with a terminal primary amino group as previously reported (1), Scheme 1 [2].

Coupling of PSt-PEO-NH_2 and heparin

Coupling of Hep with PSt-PEO-NH_2 was performed in a DMF-H_2O (40:1, v/v) mixture, first by activating the Hep carboxyl groups with 1-ethyl-3-(3-dimethylaminopropyl)carbodiimide hydrochloride (EDC) at pH 5.1-5.2 and subsequently reacting the activated carboxyl groups with the amino groups of PSt-PEO-NH_2 at pH 7.5 as previously described (1), Scheme 1 [3].

Coupling of PSt-PEO-NH_2 and nitrous acid-degraded heparin

Coupling of NADHep and PSt-PEO-NH_2 was performed according to a modified procedure of Hoffman et al.(7). To a solution of NADHep in DMF-H_2O (40:1, v/v, c=2.0 g/l) were added a solution of PSt-PEO-NH_2 in DMF-H_2O (40:1, v/v, c=4.9 g/dl) and sodium cyanoborohydride ($NaBH_3CN$), and the reaction mixture was stirred for 24 hrs, Scheme 1 [4]. The pH was maintained at 7 by adding 1N HCl. The resulting PSt-PEO-Hep was precipitated in MeOH, collected by filtration, suspended in water to remove unreacted NADHep and $NaBH_3CN$ and after isolution suspended in tetrahydrofuran (THF) to remove unreacted PSt-PEO-NH_2. After filtration the PSt-PEO-Hep was dried at reduced pressure.

PSt-NH_2 + O=C=N-R-N=C=O ⟶ PSt-N=C=O [1]

PSt-N=C=O + H_2N-PEO-NH_2 ⟶ PSt-PEO-NH_2 [2]

a) Hep-COOH + H_2N-PEO-PSt $\xrightarrow{EDC}$ PSt-PEO-Hep [3]

b) Hep-CHO + H_2N-PEO-PSt $\xrightarrow{NaBH_3CN}$ PSt-PEO-Hep [4]

Scheme 1. Schematic representation of the synthesis of polystyrene-poly(ethylene oxide)-heparin block copolymers.

Characterization

(i) IR-spectra and NMR-spectra, (ii) molecular weights, (iii) amino end group concentrations and (iv) heparin contents of the synthesized polymers were determined according to the assays as previously described (1).

Plasma recalcification time (PRT)

PRTs of plasma in contact with uncoated and with polymer coated glass were determined. Glass tubes were cleaned by treatment with 5 % w/v Na_2CrO_4 in HNO_3. After washing 3 times with double distilled water and 2 times with MeOH the tubes were dried in an oven. The clean tubes were filled with a 2 % w/v solution of polymer in DMF-H_2O (40:1, v/v). After emptying the tubes, they were placed vertically in an oven at 37°C. After 10 min and 1 hr, any remaining solution was removed from the bottom using a pasteur pipette. After 6 hrs, the tubes were vacuum dried overnight. PRTs were measured as follows: Human CPD plasma (150 µl, Bloodbank Twente and Achterhoek, Enschede, The Netherlands) was pipetted into a tube. After an incubation time of 5 min at 37°C, $CaCl_2$ (50 µl, 50 mM in H_2O) was added and the clotting time was detected with a Lode LC-6 Coagulatometer (optical method).

RESULTS AND DISCUSSION

Table 1 shows the results of characterization of PSt-NH_2 and PSt-PEO-NH_2. PSt-NH_2 with a broad MWD was synthesized by a free-radical oligomerization of St, using AESH as a chain transfer agent and PSt-NH_2 with a narrow MWD was synthesized by an anionic polymerization of St, initiated by BuLi and terminated by BTMSA. PSt-NH_2 was then converted into PSt-N=C=O using TDI and subsequent coupling with H_2N-PEO-NH_2 afforded AB type block copolymers with terminal amino groups. Copolymer formation was indicated by disappearance of the -N=C=O IR band (2270 cm^{-1}) and appearance of the -NH-CO-NH- absorbance (1660 cm^{-1}). The deviation of the $\overline{M}_n{}^4/\overline{M}_n{}^3$-value from the theoretical value 1 may be explained by the formation of some ABA type block copolymers without reactive end groups as reported before (1) from NMR-analysis.

Table 2 shows the results of characterization of PSt-PEO-Hep. PSt-PEO-Hep was synthesized either by coupling of PSt-PEO-NH_2 with Hep using EDC as coupling agent in a DMF-H_2O (40:1, v/v) mixture (1) or by the new coupling reaction of PSt-PEO-NH_2 with NADHep using $NaBH_3CN$ as reducing agent in a DMF-H_2O (40:1, v/v) mixture. In the latter coupling reaction NADHep aldehyde groups react with the primary amine of PSt-PEO-NH_2 at pH 7 in the presence of $NaBH_3CN$ <u>via</u> reductive amination of the carbonyl group (9) to yield PSt-PEO-Hep triblock copolymers. With the EDC-method 16-29 % w/w Hep was coupled, while with the $NaBH_3CN$-method 28-49 % w/w Hep was incorporated. As shown before (1), using the EDC-method, on the average 2-5 PSt-PEO chains were coupled to 1 Hep molecule, depending on the molecular weight and composition of PSt-PEO-NH_2. With the new $NaBH_3CN$-method it can be calculated from the results of Table 2

TABLE 1

Preparation and analysis of $PSt-NH_2$ and $PSt-PEO-NH_2$

code	$PSt-NH_2$					PEO	$PSt-PEO-NH_2$				
	$\overline{M}_n{}^1$	$\overline{M}_w/\overline{M}_n$	$\overline{M}_n{}^2$	$\overline{M}_n{}^3$	$\overline{M}_n{}^1/\overline{M}_n{}^3$	$\overline{M}_n$	[St mol%] calcd.	found[5]	$\overline{M}_n{}^2$	$\overline{M}_n{}^3$	$\overline{M}_n{}^4/\overline{M}_n{}^3$
PE1	2800	1.46	3300	3500	0.80	500	74	87	7400	6600	0.58
PE2	9100	4.53	-	12700	0.72	4000	49	51	-	36400	0.36
PE3	9300	4.54	-	11300	0.82	4000	50	62	-	30200	0.44
PE4	11900	2.98	-	10300	1.16	4000	56	56	-	16300	0.98
PE5	15700	2.87	-	15900	0.99	4000	62	61	-	20900	0.94
PE6	8500	1.11	-	12500	0.68	4000	47	53	15000[6]	21500	0.58
PE7	23000	1.12	-	23700	0.97	4000	71	67	-	40400	0.67

PE1-PE5: free-radical oligomerization and PE6-PE7: anionic polymerization. 1) $\overline{M}_n$ and $\overline{M}_w$ determined by HPLC in THF, 2) $\overline{M}_n$ determined by VPO in toluene at 37°C, 3) $\overline{M}_n$ determined by end group analysis, 4) $\overline{M}_n=\overline{M}_n(PSt)+\overline{M}_n(PEO)$ calculated, 5) From NMR-spectroscopy, 6) $\overline{M}_n$ determined by VPO (Hallikainen 1361) in THF at 30°C.

TABLE 2

Preparation and analysis of PSt-PEO-Hep

code	$PSt-PEO-NH_2$	[g]	Hep [mg]	EDC [mg]	NADHep [mg]	$NaBH_3CN$ [mg]	Yield [g]	Hep in block [% w/w] (s.e.m.).
PEH1	PE1	2.53	737	264	-	-	1.37	29 (± 2)
PEH2	PE4	2.63	376	132	-	-	1.19	25 (± 4)
PEH3	PE5	2.03	180	66	-	-	0.62	-
PEH4	PE2	1.49	461	79	-	-	1.24	19 (± 6)
PEH5	PE7	1.50	820	14	-	-	0.99	16 (± 4)
PEH6	PE7	1.50	-	-	223	105	0.75	28 (± 7)
PEH7	PE6	1.49	-	-	204	100	0.40	49 (± 7)

TABLE 3

Plasma recalcification times (PRT) of control, $PSt-PEO-NH_2$ and PSt-PEO-Hep

		Block copolymer			
control	PRT [s]	$PSt-PEO-NH_2$	PRT [s]	PSt-PEO-Hep	PRT [s]
glass	130 ± 2 (s.e.m)	PE1	360 ± 13	PEH1	1700 ± 210
PSt	260 ± 14	PE4	580 ± 70	PEH2	1300 ± 310
		PE5	650 ± 70	PEH3	1500 ± 340
		PE2	290 ± 17		
		PE6	390 ± 14		
		PE7	380 ± 18		

(assuming $\overline{M}_n$ of NADHep is 6000 (10)) that only 1 PSt-PEO chain was coupled to 1 Hep molecule, affording PSt-PEO-Hep triblock copolymers.

Table 3 shows the plasma recalcification times (PRT) of uncoated glass and glass tubes coated with PSt, $PSt-PEO-NH_2$ and PSt-PEO-Hep. Modification of Hep carboxyl groups, e.g. in the coupling of $PSt-PEO-NH_2$ with Hep or NADHep, leads to a decreased anticoagulant activity (11). The bioactivity greatly increases as the immobilized heparin molecules are removed from the surface to a bulk-like plasma environment via spacer groups (2). From the results of Table 3 it can be concluded that glass coated with PSt-PEO-Hep block copolymer shows a prolonged recalcification time, possibly due to the exposure of the covalently coupled heparin into the plasma via the spacer PEO. The PSt-PEO-NH_2 diblock copolymers coated on glass also show prolonged clotting times, compared to glass and PSt coated on glass. Coatings of diblock copolymers could be composed of heterogeneous microphase-separated microdomains which have an effect on the adhesion of plasma proteins (12) and possibly on the adhesion of clotting factors, thereby retarding the clotting process.

The authors wish to thank Mr. G. van de Ridder for his help with HPLC and VPO, Mr. G.H.M. Engbers for his suggestions on preparing NADHep and Mr. D. Grainger for critically reviewing the manuscript. This work was supported by NIH Grant HL-17623-12.

REFERENCES

1 I. Vulić, T. Okano, S.W. Kim and J. Feijen, Synthesis and characterization of polystyrene-poly(ethylene oxide)-heparin block copolymers, J. Polym. Sci., (1986) submitted for publication.
2 C.D. Ebert, E.S. Lee, J. Deneris and S.W. Kim, The anticoagulant activity of derivatized and immobilized heparins, Biomaterials: Interfacial Phenomena and Applications in; Adv. Chem. Ser., 199 (1982) 161-176.
3 P.N. Sawyer, C. Burrowes, J. Oganiak, A.O. Smith and S.A. Wesolowski, Ionic architecture at the vascular wall interface, Trans. Amer. Soc. Artif. Int. Organs, 10 (1964) 316-319.
4 T. Okano, T. Aoyagi, K. Kataoka, K. Abe, Y. Sakurai, M. Shimada, and I. Shinohara, Hydrophilic-hydrophobic microdomain surfaces having an ability to suppress platelet aggregation and their in vitro antithrombogenicity, J. Biomed. Mater. Res., 20 (1986) 919-927.
5 H. Gilman and F.K. Cartledge, The analysis of organolithium compounds, J. Organomet. Chem., 2 (1964) 447-454.
6 C. Krueger, E.C. Rochow and U. Wannagat, Ueber die Einwirkung von Natrium-bis-trimethylsilyl-amid auf Benzophenon, Benzaldehyd und Benzochinon, Chem. Ber., 96 (1963) 2132-2137.
7 J. Hoffman, O. Larm and E. Scholander, A new method for covalent coupling of heparin and other glycosaminoglycans to substances containing primary amino groups, Carbohyd. Res., 117 (1983) 328-331.
8 D.N. Schulz and A.F. Halasa, Anionic polymerization initiators containing protected functional groups.II, J. Polym. Sci., Polymer Chem. Ed., 15 (1977) 2401-2410.
9 R.F. Borch, M.D. Bernstein and H.D. Durst, The cyanohydridoborate anion as a selective reducing agent, J. Amer. Chem. Soc., 93 (1971) 2897-2904.
10 A.J. Knipmeijer, Masters Thesis, Twenty University of Technology, Enschede, The Netherlands, (1985).
11 I. Danishefsky and F. Siskovic, Heparin derivatives prepared by modification of the uronic acid carboxyl groups, Throm. Res., 1 (1972) 173-182.
12 T. Okano, S. Nishiyama, I. Shinohara, T. Akaike, Y. Sakurai, K. Kataoka, and T. Tsuruta, Role of microphase separated structure on the interfacial interaction of polymer with blood, Polymer Preprints, 20 (1979) 571-574.

Biomaterials and Clinical Applications,
edited by A. Pizzoferrato, P.G. Marchetti, A. Ravaglioli and A.J.C. Lee
Elsevier Science Publishers B.V., Amsterdam, 1987 — Printed in The Netherlands

THE INFLUENCE OF SURFACE ROUGHNESS AND ELECTRICAL POTENTIAL UPON THE FRICTION AND WEAR OF POLYETHYLENE

M. ZAKI[1] and D. DOWSON[2]

[1]Department of Industrial Production, Mansoura University, Faculty of Engineering, Mansoura (Egypt)

[2]Department of Mechanical Engineering, Leeds University, Leeds LS2 9JT (England)

SUMMARY

The influence of counterface surface roughness and applied electrical potential upon the friction and wear of ultra-high molecular weight polyethylene (UHMWPE) sliding on surgical grade stainless steel has been studied on a pin-on-flat reciprocating testing machine. The tests were carried out under dry and lubricated conditions using distilled water.

The results have clarified that under dry sliding conditions, the wear rates and the coefficients of friction of UHMWPE displayed minimum values at specific steel counterface surface roughness in the range 0.08-0.12 μm Ra. Such optimum values were not found under lubricated sliding conditions as the friction and wear increased simultaneously with the increase in counterface surface roughness while tramendous increases were encountered under electrical potential.

The study has showed that the dominant effects upon friction and wear of UHMWPE against stainless steel are the topography of the counterface and the surface charges formed on the rubbing surfaces.

INTRODUCTION

One of the combination of materials favoured internationally for many years for total replacement load bearing joints in the human body has been UHMWPE in association with stainless steel. The useful life of endoprotheses is generally limited by the penetration of the metallic component into the opposite polymeric members, which results mainly from wear.

During the last ten years, since Buckley (ref. 1) has postulated his view that UHMWPE exhibited a minimum rate of dry wear against ground steel, having an initial roughness of 0.37 μm (r.m.s.), the subject has attracted detailed and sophisticated attention of many workers (refs. 2-4) due to its great technological and economic significance in both bio-engineering and normal engineering fields.

Up to now, there has been no consistent viewpoint with regards to the question of the role of surface electric charges in the human body upon the tribological characteristics of the joints. This results from different evaluations of the relative role of the forces of attraction and repulsion connected with the friction, wear and lubrication processes (refs. 5-7).

In the present paper, the friction and wear characteristics of UHMWPE against stainless steel, under dry and lubricated conditions, were described.

APPARATUS

To study the influence of counterface surface roughness and electrical potential upon friction and wear, experiments were performed on a pin-on-flat testing machine, shown diagrammatically in Fig. 1. The machine was driven by a variable speed motor which transmitted the mechanical power to a gear-box where the drive was changed by an off-set crank to allow reciprocating motion to the carriage supporting the steel counterface specimen. The electrically insulating UHMWPE pin was gripped in a pin-holder arm supporting by air bearing to enable precise evaluation of the friction and wear. The extreme end of the pin-holder arm was restrained by a load transducer which converted the output signal to a bridge. The output from the bridge was displayed on an X-Y pen recorder.

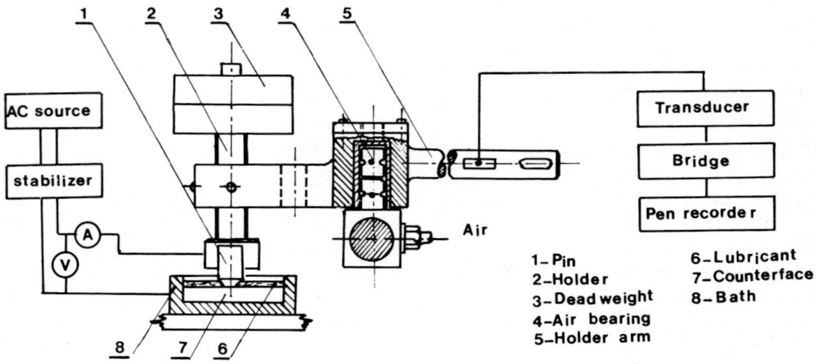

Fig. 1. Diagrammatic Layout of the Machine

MATERIAL AND EXPERIMENTAL PROCEDURE

The polymeric pins were all machined from a single block of Hoechst RCH 1000 Surgical Grade Polyethylene. One end of the pin was machined into a truncated conical form to cause the initial machining marks to be removed rapidly during rubbing, such that the subsequent wear would be representative of the bulk material.

The stainless steel plates were machined from (EN 58J) surgical grade stainless steel. All counterfaces were initially ground to a similar roughness and then lapped to the required Ra values. Table 1. summary some of the specimen properties.

The UHMWPE pins and the steel plates were ultrasonically cleaned during a rigid cleaning procedure which preceded each test. The volume of UHMWPE lost from the pin was measured and recorded periodically. The wear rate was calculated by dividing the slope of the graph relating the wear volume (V) in mm^3 to the sliding distance (L) in m, by the normal load (P) in Newtons:

$$\text{Wear Rate} = V/(P.L) \qquad mm^3/(N.m)$$

The experiments were carried out at low sliding speeds in the range 0.06-0.09 m/s, and at normal load of 10 N.

Table 1. Properties and Dimensions of Tested Specimen

PROPERTY	UHMWPE	STAINLESS STEEL
Specific gravity	0.94	7.96
Hardness (Vickers)	5.30	160
Modulus of elasticity (MPa)	500	210×10^3
Tensile strength (MPa)	30	540
Poisson's ratio	0.45	0.28
Shape and dimensions in mms.	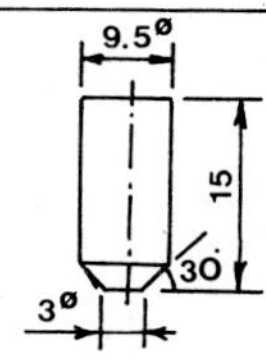	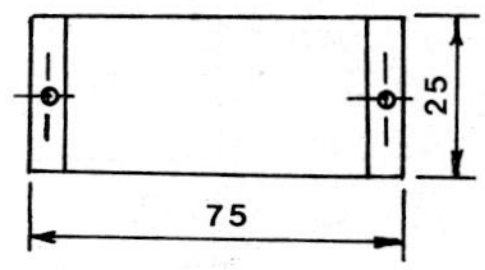

RESULTS

The values of the coefficient of friction and the wear rate have been plotted against the initial surface roughness of the stainless steel counterfaces for dry sliding conditions in Fig. 2., for distilled water lubricated studies in Fig. 3. and in the presence of an electrical potential of 1.5 volts in Fig. 4.

Under dry sliding conditions, Fig. 2. shows that there is a distinct rise in both the coefficient of friction and the wear rate as the counterface roughness was reduced to produce the finest possible finishes. In general, the results clarify the existence of an optimum surface roughness at which the wear rate was a minimum. Beyond the optimum roughness, the wear rates increased substantially with the increase in the initial counterface surface roughness, while the coefficients of friction were little affected, but still there is some features for a minimum coefficient of friction.

The results of the studies conducted using distilled water as a lubricant, showed a marked increase in coefficient of friction and wear rate as counterface roughness increased, as shown in Fig. 3.

The tests carried out under an electrical potential showed that higher wear rates occurred than under comparable dry or wet sliding conditions in the absence of an electrical potential. Based on friction measurements, the results have also clarified that a roughly linear relationship might exist between the coefficient of friction and the initial counterface surface roughness values. Although the wear rates exhibited a significant rise from 0.68×10^{-7} to 29.7×10^{-7} $mm^3/N.m$, with an increase in surface roughnesses from 0.009 to 0.2 μm Ra, the coefficient of friction showed slight variations from 0.09 to 0.10 which indicates that friction was little affected by surface roughness variations.

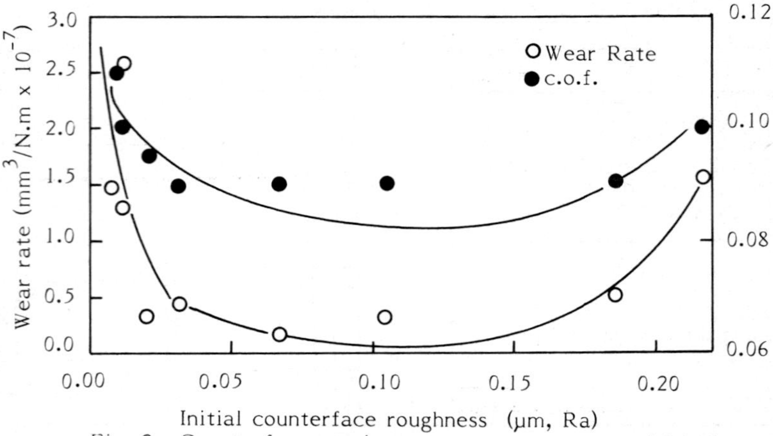

Fig. 2. Counterface roughness versus wear rate and friction in dry sliding conditions.

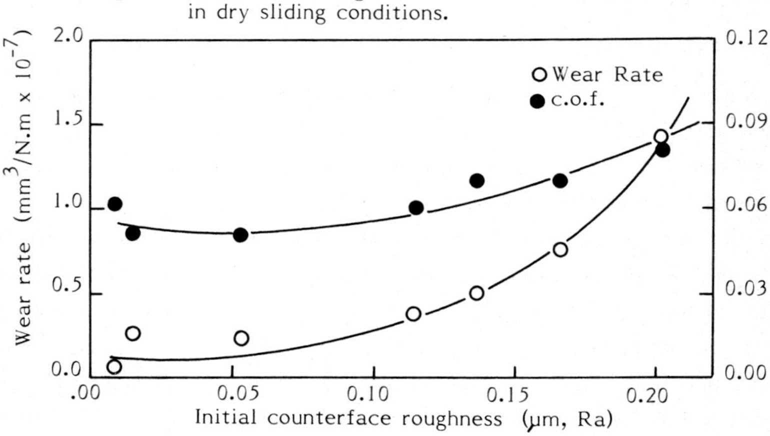

Fig. 3. Ra values against wear rate and coefficient of friction in wet sliding conditions.

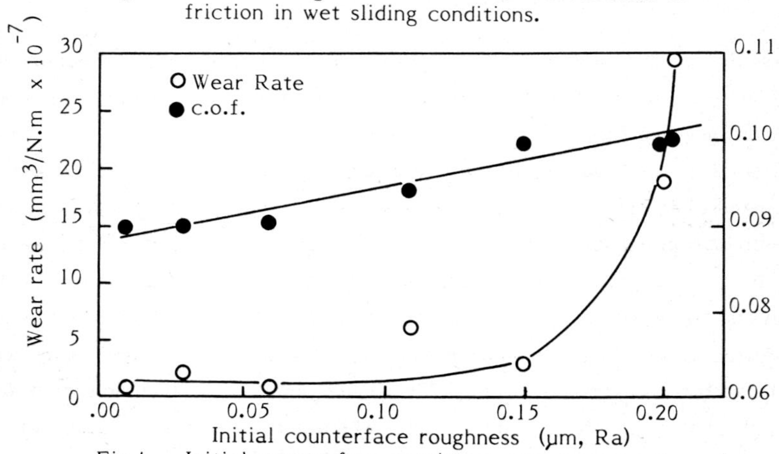

Fig.4. Initial counterface roughness versus wear rate and coefficient of friction for UHMWPE in wet sliding applying an electrical potential of 1.5 volts.

DISCUSSION OF RESULTS

Dry sliding of UHMWPE on stainless steel

Under dry sliding conditions, smooth counterfaces (Ra $<$0.08 μm) exhibited a gradual deposition of relatively thick and lumpy polymeric transfer which adheres to the steel surface. The results indicated that high wear rates and coefficients of friction were obtained on these surfaces due to the greater abrasive capability of new formed surfaces as they became rougher with the formation of lumpy transfer and due to adhesive wear which took place on the smooth areas between the lumps.

On rough surfaces (Ra$>$ 0.1 μm), little transfer was measured and thus the wear rates were dictated by the effectiveness of the abrasive mechanism which resulted in an increase in wear rates with increasing roughness.

At the optimum roughness (Ra=0.06-0.1 μm), the transfer due to adhesion and the ploughing effect due to abrasion were both low and this accounted for the (U) shape of the friction and wear graphs.

Wet sliding of UHMWPE on stainless steel using distilled water

The studies conducted under water lubricated conditions showed a marked increase in wear rates and coefficients of friction as counterface roughnesses increased. The contribution of abrasive and ploughing actions to the wear and friction processes against rough surfaces remained high due to the inhibiting effect of the water upon transfer film formation.

Sliding of UHMWPE on stainless steel under electric potential of 1.5 V

In the present set of experiments, there is clearly a very substantial increase in the wear rates of UHMWPE. The rough surfaces (Ra$>$0.15 μm), in particular, produced the most significant increases in wear which attained thirty time higher than that obtained during wet tests at identical roughness in the absence of potential.

The coefficient of friction values were also substantially higher by about 50% compared with the values obtained in the absence of potential.

A gradual increase in the amount of polymer which adhered to the stainless steel surface was evident during these tests. The results suggested that the adhesive and abrasive wear mechanisms were combined with a more severe form of wear characterised by surface disturbances and the generation of fine powdery debris. This mechanism appears to be a form of degradation related to surface fatigue and accelerated by the application of electrical potential. These actions would contribute to the more rapid wear rates against rougher counterfaces.

CONCLUSIONS

In the dry, reciprocating sliding of UHMWPE against stainless steel, the initial counterface surface roughness has profound effect upon the friction and wear through the transfer film formation and its topography, resulting in a minimum wear at surface roughnesses in the range 0.06-0.09 μm Ra.

The presence of distilled water restricts the transfer film formation and diminishes the adhesive action, therefore it facilitates a steady increase in the abrasive wear with an increase in surface roughness of the counterface.

Under an electrical potential of 1.5 V, the wear rates and the coefficients of friction increased significantly and substantially as the counterface roughness increased and they exceeded the values recorded under otherwise identical wet sliding conditions in the absence of electrical potential.

REFERENCES

1 D.H. Buckley, Introductory Remarks - Friction and Wear of Polymeric Composites, in: L-H. Lee (Ed.), Advances in Polymer Friction and Wear, 5B, Plenum Press, New York and London, 1974, pp. 601-603.
2 K. Holmes, A Study of the Effects of Contact Conditions and Surface Quality Upon the Wear of High Density Polyethylene, Ph.D. Thesis, Mechanical Engineering, The University of Leeds, U.K., 1975.
3 D. Dowson, J.M. Challen, K. Holmes and J.R. Atkinson, The Influence of Counterface Roughness on the Wear Rate of Polyethylene, in: D. Dowson, D. Godet and C.M. Taylor (Eds.), The Wear of Non-Metallic Materials, Proc. of the 3rd Leeds-Lyon Symposium on Tribology, Mech. Engrg. Publications, London, 1976, 99-102.
4 H. Czichos, Influence of Adhesive and Abrasive Mechanisms on the Tribological Behaviour of Thermoplastic Polymers, Wear, 88, 1983, pp. 27-43.
5 A.S. Akhmatov, Molecular Physics of Boundary Friction, Translated from Russian by N. Kaner, Israel Program for Scientific Translations, Jerusalem, 1966.
6 S.N. Postnikov, Electrophysical and Electrochemical Phenomena in Friction, Cutting and Lubrication, Translated from Russian by Ben Teague, Van Nostrand Reinhold Company, London, 1978.
7 A.R. Savkoor and T.J. Ruyter, Experimental Investigation of the Effect of Electrical Potential on Adhesive Friction of Elastomers, in: L.-H. Lee (Ed.), Advances in Polymer Friction and Wear, Plenum Press, New York,5A, 1974, pp. 333-351.

Biomaterials and Clinical Applications, 503
edited by A. Pizzoferrato, P.G. Marchetti, A. Ravaglioli and A.J.C. Lee
Elsevier Science Publishers B.V., Amsterdam, 1987 — Printed in The Netherlands

DESIGN AND SYNTHESIS OF BIODEGRADABLE POLY(ETHER-ESTERS)

D. COHN, G. MAROM, and H. YOUNES
Casali Institute of Applied Chemistry, The Hebrew University of Jerusalem, 91904 Jerusalem, Israel

INTRODUCTION

The synthesis and development of biodegradable polymers is one of the major research fields in Biomedical Polymer Science. They are used in such diverse applications as drug-releasing implants (1-3), bioabsorbable surgical sutures (4-6), and in more novel applications, as the absorbable component in selectively biodegradable vascular grafts (7,8). A biodegradable material is required to be biocompatible both when implanted as well as during the degradation process. Additional important attributes include the mechanical properties of the material and, for some applications, the matching of the polymer biodegradation kinetics to that of the healing process.

The paucity of polymers which meet these demainding requirements has prompted a continuous search for new, improved biodegradable polymers.

This study is part of a research project aimed at developing new biodegradable polymers, tailored to meet different requirements, as a function of the application and implantation site. Our objective was to develop a series of segmented block copolymers, in which polyester segments, especially glycolic (GA) and lactic (LA) based, create the hard, and generally crystalline blocks of the copolymer, while flexible polyether glycols (e.g., PEO, PPO, PTMO) were chosen to form the soft blocks of the segmented chains. The present paper will introduce these polymers, focusing especialy on copolymers based on PEO and PLA blocks.

EXPERIMENTAL

Materials

Lactic acid (L^+) was obtained from Merck (90%, extra pure). Glycolic acid, polyglycolic acid and polylactic acid were purchased from Polysciences Inc., U.S.A.. The different polyether glycols were purchased from Aldrich. The antimony III oxide catalyst was obtained from Fluka, and the phosphoric acid was supplied by Frutarom, Israel. Analytical grade solvents (99% purity) supplied by Frutarom, were used without further purification.

Apparatus and procedures

A Mettler TA3000 thermoanalyzer was used for the thermal analysis of polymers. An Analect fx-6260 Fourier Transform infrared spectrometer was used to obtain the specta of the different polymers. The stress/strain testing was performed on an Instron Universal Testing Machine (model 1114) with a 0.3 cm/min crosshead speed. The proton NMR spectra were recorded using a Bruker 300 High resolution H-NMR spectrometer.

The copolymers were synthesized through the polyesterification reaction of LA or GA, in the presence of polyether glycol chains, using an antimony oxide catalyst and phosphoric acid. The polymerization reaction was carried out in a 250 ml three-necked flask, fitted with a mechanical stirrer, under nitrogen flow.

RESULTS AND DISCUSSION

The "multicomponent" nature of the copolymeric systems affords the required versatility both in terms of mechanical and physical properties as well as specific biodegradation considerations. The existence of covalent, block copolymers, as opposed to physical blends was demonstrated by selective extraction and by I.R., D.S.C. and N.M.R. studies.

Figure 1 presents the DSC thermograms of a PEO/PGA (PEGA) copolymer and that of its basic components.

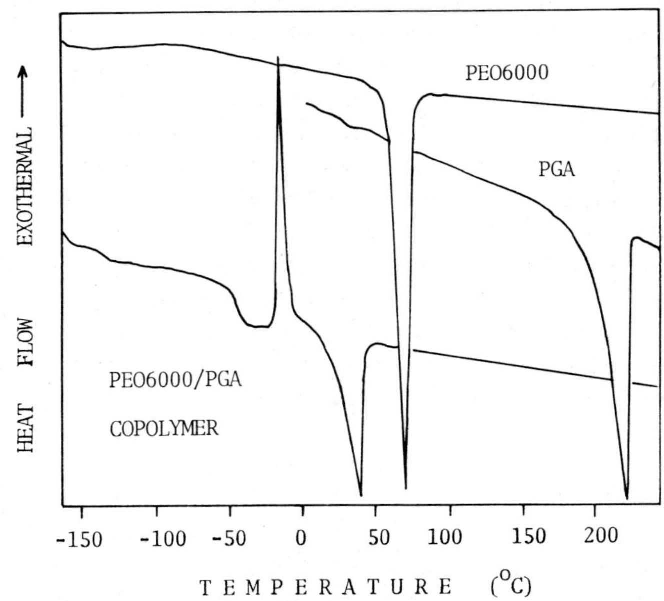

Fig. 1. DSC thermograms of PGA, PEO6000 and PEGA copolymer containing PEO6000 segments.

PGA homopolymer is a crystalline, rather hydophilic polymer melting at high temperature (222°C), with an almost undetectable Tg at about 30°C. The DSC trace of PEO6000 shows a sharp melting endotherm at 70°C and a glass transition at approximately -60°C. The copolymer exhibits a substantially different thermal behaviour, the most important features of it being the melting endotherm at 39°C, corresponding to the soft PEO segments. It is evident that the incorporation of the PEO oligomer into the copolymeric chain has caused a shift of the fusion peak to lower temperatures. It is also worth noting that there is no PGA related melting phenomena apparent in the thermogram. Both aforementioned phenomena seem to indicate a certain degree of phase blending. A glass transition due to the soft segments of the copolymeric chain is evident at -45°C. At temperatures higher than Tg, the additional thermal energy supplied to the segmented chains, and their enhanced degree of freedom allow further crystallizaiton to occur, as shown by the crystallization exotherm at -10°C. Since the most important characteristic of the basic components of PEGA copolymers, namely PEO and PGA, is their hydrophilicity, the copolymers absorbed large amounts of water; furthermore, their water contact angle couldn't be measured due to the instant spreading of the water drop and, sometimes, the local swelling and deformation of the polymeric surface.

Clearly contrasting with PEGA, PPLA matrices comprising PPO and PLA segments, exhibit an amorphous morphology, only a glass transition being evident at 26°C. This can be readily attributed to the limited molecular symmetry and cohesion caused by the pendant methyl groups present in the repeating unit of both components. Furthermore, the apolar methyl substituents rendered the molecule substantially hydrophobic, as expressed by both low equilibrium water absorption levels (below 10%) and relatively high contact angles (approximately 70°).

The remainder of this paper will focus on PELA matrices, where the copolymeric chain comprises PEO soft segments and PLA hard blocks. Figure 2 schematically illustrates the basic structure of the copolymeric system, where special attention is given to the end unit of each block, connecting the PEO and LA sequences.

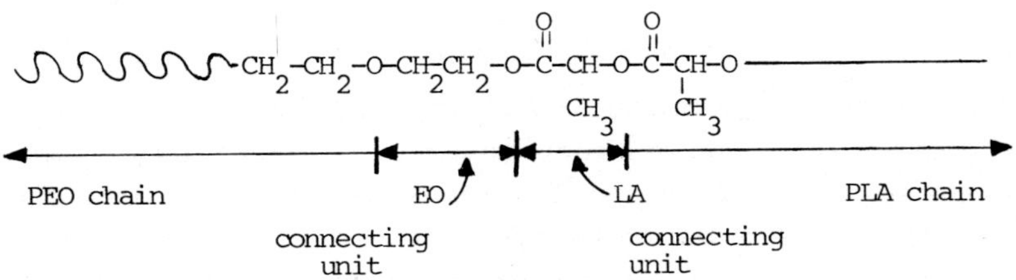

Fig. 2. Structure of PEO/PLA block copolymer

A series of PELA copolymers, covering a wide range of compositions was synthesized; the average segmental length of both components was also varied. The composition of the copolymers was calculated from ^{1}H-NMR spectra; more specifically, for PEO/PLA systems, the EO to LA molar ratio was calculated by comparing the EO methylene and the lactoyl methine integrations, centered at 3.65 and 5.15 ppm, respectively (see Fig. 3).

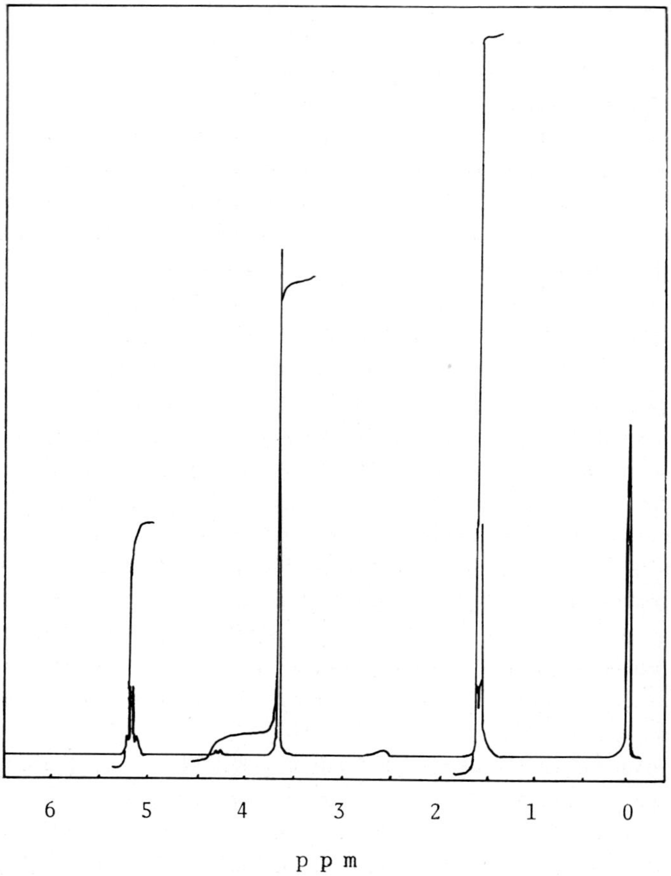

Fig. 3. NMR spectra of PEO3400/PLA copolymer dissolved in $CDCL_3$.

PELA is the generic name used to designate this family of PEO and LA based copoly (ether-esters). The molecular weight of the PEO oligomer comprising the soft segments, is given following the name, while the number after the slash refers to the average number of lactoyl units in the hard blocks.

Since the materials are designed to be implanted and degraded in the biological environment, and given the hydrophilic nature of PEO, the water absorption behaviour of these polymers is an important property. The incorporation of PEO segments enhanced substantially the hydrophilicity of PELA matrices, when compared to PLA, as expressed by the equilibrium water uptake as well as by the water contact angles. This issue can be illustated by comparing the 6% water content shown by PLA homopolymer, as compared with 31% for PELA 3400/164 and 55% for PELA 1500/45. The contact angles of PELA copolymers decreased markedly, when compared to PLA (76°), some matrices exhibiting angles as low as 27°.

Stress/strain curves are presented in Figure 4; the data plotted show a gradual transition from a strong but stiff and brittle PLA homopolymer, to materials exhibiting lower UTS values, but characterized by a more flexible and ductile overall mechanical response, with much larger elongation at failure values.

Figure 5 shows the DSC thermograms of three PELA copolymers, displaying unambigously different behaviours. The matrices shown, while being characterized by an almost identical overall composition (approximately 60 molarr percentage LA), differ in the length of the blocks along the chain. PELA600/16 is an essentially amorphous, waxy solid, displaying a glass transition temperature at 15°C and a very small, ill-defined melting endotherm around 115°C. The lack of any significant degree of crystallinity is attributed to the short segmental length of both components which prevents any crystallization. PELA3400/126 is a semi-crystalline polymer with a clear melting point at 125°C due to fusion of PLA blocks. The material containing the longer segments, PELA 6000/196 exhibits a different morphology, where a two phase matrix is evident, with both components being able to crystallize. The thermogram shows a clear endotherm at 40°C, corresponding to the melting of PEO6000 segments, whereas the triple endotherm, covering the 125-140°C range, corresponds to the fusion of the LA blocks. A microphase segregation phenomenon is demonstrated by the existence of two distinct, separate melting endotherms, corresponding to the two components of the copolymer. It should be stressed, however, that, even though phase separation is, undoubtedly, the determinant phenomenon taking place, some degree of phase blending has occurred, as revealed by the significant drop in the melting point of both components, as compared to that of the respective homopolymers.

The IR spectra of two PELA3400 copolymers containing different LA sequences are presented in Figure 6. Beyond the expected increase in the LA carbonyl band, at 1759 cm^{-1}, as compared, for example, to the EO related C-H stretching band centered at 2884 cm^{-1}, important information about the morphology of the matrices can be obtained by exploring in more detail the 1000-700 cm^{-1} spectral region. By comparing the 755 cm^{-1} and 869 cm^{-1} peaks, corresponding to the LA crystalline and amorphous bands (9,10) respectively, the crystallinity of the LA phase can be assessed.

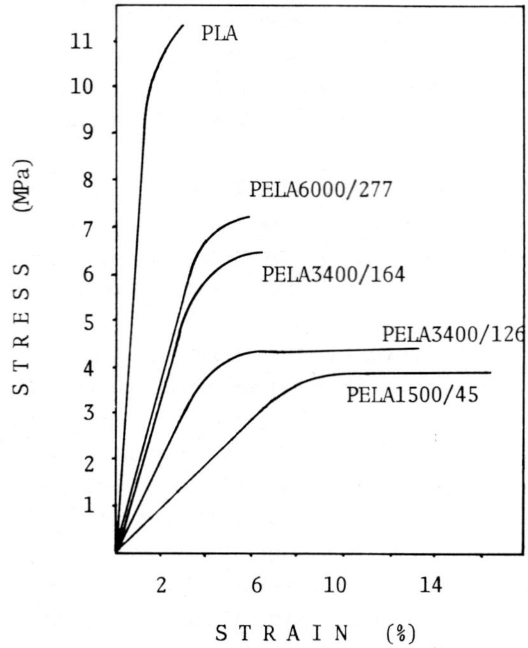

Fig. 4. Stress/strain curves for PLA and for PELA copolymers

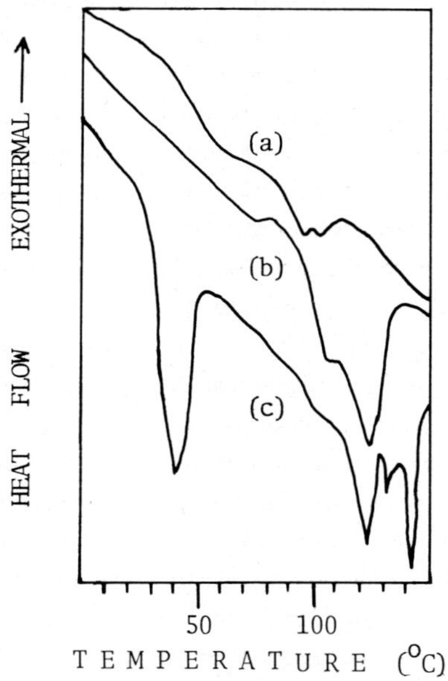

Fig. 5. DSC thermograms of three PELA copolymers: (a) PELA600/16; (b) PELA3400/126; (c) PELA6000/196.

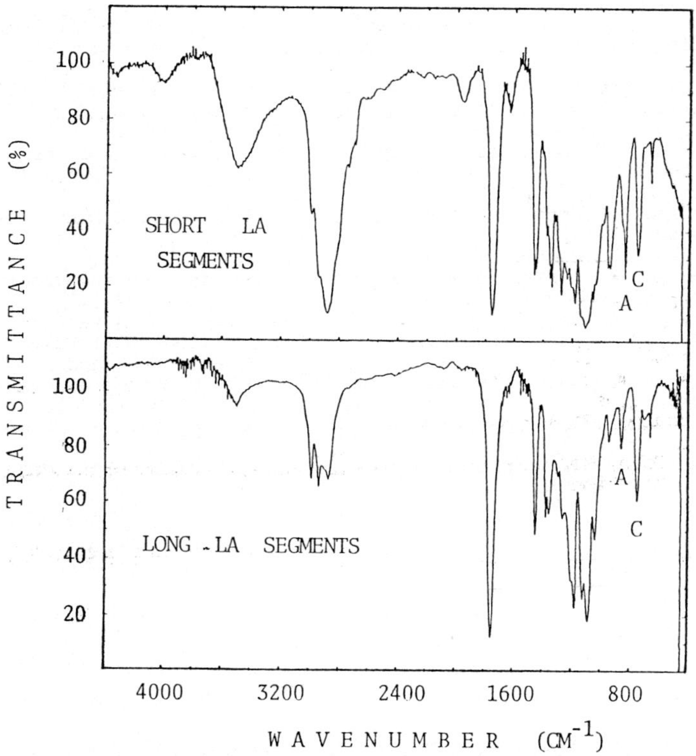

Fig. 6 IR spectra of two PEO3400-containing copolymers: (a) PELA3400/19; (b) PELA3400/209.

These bands are designated C (crystalline) and A (amorphous). The C/A ratio changes dramatically as a function of the lactoyl sequences, from 2.4 for the PELA containing the long LA blocks, down to 0.8 for the short LA sequences. These findings are consistent with the expectation that the crystallizability of the LA blocks will increase with segmental length, and are in full accordance with the DSC data presented.

This introductory paper has presented a family of biodegradable polymers, intended for use in a variety of biomedical applications. The hydrophilicity of the different segments (PGA versus PLA, or PEO veersus PPO), their degree of crystallinity (e.g. the length of the blocks), and their sensitivity to hydrolytic processes can be ccontrolled. By doing so, a variety of biodegradable polymers were produced, exhibiting a wide range of mechanical properties and biodegradation kinetics.

REFERENCES

1 T.M. Jakanicz, H.A. Nash, D.L. Wise and J.B. Gregory, Polylactic Acid as a Biodegradable Carrier for Contraceptive Steroids, Contraception, 8, 227 (1973).

2 L.R. Beck, D.R. Cowsar, D.H., Lewis, R.J. Coxgrove, C.T. Riddle, S.L. Lowry and T. Epperly, A New long-acting Injectable Microcapsule System for the Administration of Progesterone, Fert. Ster. 31, 545 (1979).

3 J. Heller, D.W.H. Penhale and R.F. Helwing, Preparation of Poly(ortho esters) by the Reaction of Diketene Acetals and Polyols, J. Polym. Sci., Polymer Lett. Ed., 18, 619-624 (1980).

4 E.J. Frazza and E.E. Schmitt, A New Absorbable Suture, J. Biomed. Mater. Res., 1, 43-58 (1971).

5 A.K. Schneider, (Du Pont), U.S. Patent 2,703,316.

6 D.K. Gilding and A.M. Reed, Biodegradable Polymers for Use in Surgery - PGA/PLA Homo and Copolymers: 1, Polymer, 20, 1459-1464 (1979).

7 R.J. Ruderman, A.F. Hegyeli, B.G. Hattler and F. Leonard, A Partially biodegradable Vascular Prosthesis, Trans, ASAIO, 28, 30-36 (1972).

8 E. Lommen, S. Gogolewski, A.J. Pennings, Ch. R.H. Wilderuur and P. Neiewenhuis, Development of a Neo-Artery Induced by a Biodegradable Polymeric Vascular Prosthesis, Trans, ASAIO, 29, 255-259 (1983).

9 D. Cohn and H. Younes, Biodegradable PEO/PLA Block Copolymers, Manuscript in preparation.

10 H. Younes and D. Cohn, Morphology of Biodegadable PEO/PLA Block Copolymers, Manuscript in preparation.

Biomaterials and Clinical Applications, 511
edited by A. Pizzoferrato, P.G. Marchetti, A. Ravaglioli and A.J.C. Lee
Elsevier Science Publishers B.V., Amsterdam, 1987 — Printed in The Netherlands

VIBRATIONAL (RAMAN-LASER AND INFRARED) STUDY ON $Ca(PO_3)_2$-Al_2O_3 GLASSES

A. BERTOLUZZA, C. FAGNANO, A. MARINANGELI, R. SIMONI, A. TINTI and M.A. MORELLI+

Istituto Chimico "G. Ciamician", Universita' di Bologna (Italy), via Selmi 2
+Istituto di Scienze Chimiche, Universita' di Bologna (Italy), via San Donato 9
Centro Studi Interfacolta' sulla Spettroscopia Raman, Istituto Chimico "G. Ciamician", Universita' di Bologna (Italy), via Selmi 2

SUMMARY

Calcium and aluminium oligophosphate glasses $CaO.yAl_2O_3.P_2O_5$ have been obtained by melting at 1300° C for one hour β-calcium metaphosphate ($Ca(PO_3)_2$) and Al_2O_3 (alumina).

Raman spectra are discussed in relation to the increase of Al_2O_3 molar ratio y and in relation to calcium and sodium and calcium oligophosphate glasses previously studied.

The increase of the ν_S POP frequency for aluminophosphate glasses suggests a breakdown of the indefinite linear structure of calcium metaphosphate glass and the formation of oligomers with a shorter chain. The anomalous behaviour of ν_S PO_2^- and ν_S PO_3^{2-} frequencies can be explained on the ground of a coordination of PO_3^{2-} terminal and PO_2^- inner chain groups with aluminium, by Al-O bonds with partial covalent character.

INTRODUCTION

The use of bioglasses with high biocompatibility, as orthopedic prosthesis or as coating for prosthetic materials with better mechanical properties, has received wide practical and scientific (in particular structural) interest in the literature over the last few years.

In this field glass biomaterials made of phosphate (in particular calcium phosphates) offer the advantage of having a composition similar to the inorganic components of bone, and they are therefore provided with characteristics that can help their biological tolerance.

Among phosphate materials, polyphosphates formed from linear chains with different average chain lengths, depending on their composition, show different properties due to the chain lengths, to the partial substitution of the oxygen atom with different groups (i.e. fluorine), to the cross-linking of the chains themselves.

Our research group has been working in this direction for some years. We have characterized the structure of some of these polyphosphates by means of vibrational Raman-laser spectroscopy measurements (ref.1,2,3,4) and we have related the structural properties to the mechanical characteristics (in particular modulus of elasticity), obtained from thermomechanical measurements (ref.5).

In this paper we give the results obtained for a new bioglass made from calcium metaphosphate and Al_2O_3, two of the main components used as biomaterials for orthopedic prostheses.

In this sense this biomaterial combines and improves the characteristics of their components, that is a high biocompatibility and good mechanical properties.

METHODS

Calcium metaphosphate glass, $Ca(PO_3)_2$ was prepared by melting the crystalline metaphosphate β-$Ca(PO_3)_2$ at 1300°C for one hour in a platinum crucible and then quickly cooling it between two copper plates. The β-$Ca(PO_3)_2$ was obtained by dehydration of monocalcium phosphate monohydrate, $Ca(H_2PO_4)_2.H_2O$, according to the literature (ref. 6). Alumina was a Erba RP product. $CaO.yAl_2O_3.P_2O_5$ glasses have been prepared using the same thermal process, starting from monocalcium phosphate monohydrate and alumina so as to obtain the expected y value.

Raman spectra were recorded using a Jasco R 300 spectrophotometer and 600 mw of 488.0 nm radiation from a Spectra-Physics argon ion laser.

Dynamic load thermomechanical measurements (TMA) were carried out by means of a Mettler TA 3000 system equipped with a TMA 40 accessory.

DISCUSSION

In previous studies (ref.1-4), we proved by vibrational Raman spectroscopy that sodium (Graham salt) and calcium metaphosphates have an indefinite polymeric linear structure characterized by the presence, in the Raman spectra, of two strong bands at about 1170 and 690 cm^{-1}.

These bands can be assigned to the symmetrical stretching vibrations of PO_2^- groups perpendicularly to the polymeric chain direction (the first) and to the symmetrical stretching vibrations of P-O-P bonds parallel to it (the second).

The symmetrical stretching band of PO_3^{2-} chain terminal groups does not appear in these spectra.

The addition of a basic oxide (alkaline, alkaline-earth or both) involves a demolition of the metaphosphate linear polymeric indefinite structure and the formation of oligomers with shorter average chain length. The average chain length is related to the molar ratio x between basic and acidic oxide by this relation:

$$x = \frac{\bar{n}+2}{\bar{n}}$$

In fact, as molar ratio x increases, the ν_S PO_3^{2-} stretching vibration at about 1020-1040 cm^{-1} increases; at the same time the intensities of the ν_S PO_2^- at 1170 and of ν_S POP at 690 cm^{-1} grow weaker, and new bands, at lower and higher wave numbers respectively, appear.

We have confirmed this behaviour by oligophosphate glass spectra with molar ratio x=1.65 which are analogous to the tri- and tetraphosphate fused salts. In fact the average chain length for the oligophosphate glass for which x=1.65 is 3.3, that is between the tri- and tetrametaphosphate values.

Raman spectra of the new glass material formed from calcium metaphosphate and aluminium oxide are shown in Fig. 1.

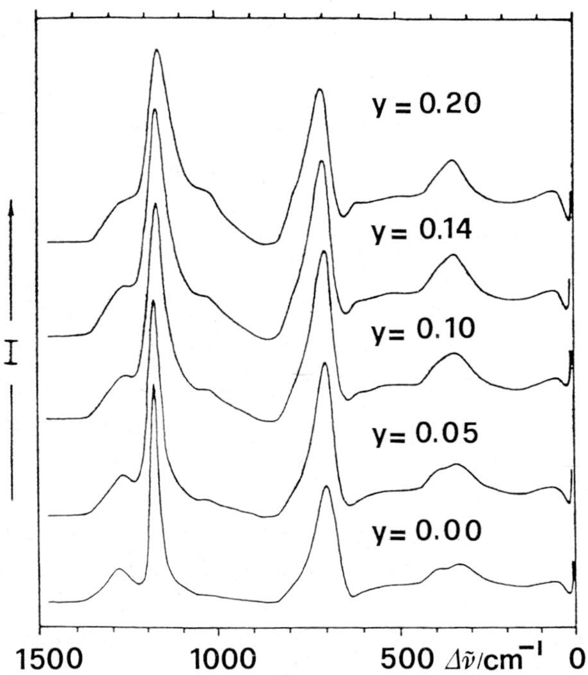

Fig. 1 Raman spectra of calcium metaphosphate (y=0) and calcium aluminophosphate glasses for wich y⩽0.2.

The calcium metaphosphate spectrum (for which y=0) is given at the bottom; the other spectra refer to oligophosphate glasses for which $0<y\leqslant 0.2$. The highest value allowed to y for the glass state goes to 0.2, which corresponds in this case to a molar ratio P/Al=5.

Considering that the aluminium oxidation number is +3, the limit value for the basic/acidic oxide molar ratio corresponding to the glass state is of the same order (1.6) of that peculiar to the glass state for the alkaline or alkaline earth oligophosphate glasses.

The spectral behaviour of oligophosphate glasses when y increases is not exactly coincident with that of alkaline or alkaline earth oligophosphate glasses. We observe a similar increase in the frequency of the ν_S P-O-P Raman band at about 690 cm^{-1}. This band rises from an average value $\Delta\nu$= 17 cm^{-1} going to the oligophosphate glass for which y=0.2.

On the contrary, the frequency decrease in the ν_S PO_2^- band at 1170 cm^{-1} is less marked. For calcium oligophosphate glasses $\Delta\nu$=35 cm^{-1}, while for the examined calcium and aluminium $\Delta\nu$=11 cm^{-1}, only. A band (practically absent in the spectrum of calcium metaphosphate and appearing only in the spectra of calcium oligophosphate glasses at ~1040 cm^{-1}), appears in the spectrum of calcium and aluminium oligophosphate glass with the limit molar ratio y=0.2, but it is much less intense and localized at lower wavenumbers, that is at 1025 cm^{-1}.

The spectroscopical trend of calcium and aluminium oligophosphate glasses can be interpreted by considering that the addition of aluminium oxide to the glass causes a lowering of the indefinite polymeric chain of the calcium metaphosphate.

Shorter chains, with an average length related to the ratio between basic and acidic oxide, can thus be formed.
We can oberve that, for y=0.2, the lowering of ν_S POP is of the same order as that observed for alkaline and alkaline earth oligophosphates with the same molar ratio between basic and acidic oxide.

This means that oligophosphates with a corresponding average chain length are formed, and that the presence in the chains of aluminium oxide breaks the vibrational chain coupling.

On the contrary, the behaviour of the symmetrical stretching band of the terminal PO_3^{2-} group, and that of the lateral PO_2^- group, suggests a partial covalent interaction Al-O as regards the prevailingly ionic one of alkaline and alkaline earth ions. Probably, the Al-O bands are masked in the spectra by strongher bands of calcium oligophosphate.

This conclusion on the structure of $CaO.yAl_2O_3.P_2O_5$ obtained from Raman spectra agrees with the model proposed for $NaPO_3.Al_2O_3$ oligophosphate glasses (ref. 6).

Fig. 2 shows that TMA measurements, performed on some glass samples of $Ca(PO_3)_2$-Al_2O_3 system, reveal some differences of dynamic elastic modulus as a function of the composition and of the chain length of the glass. The Young modulus calculated with TMA measurements corrected for blank is of the order of GPa.

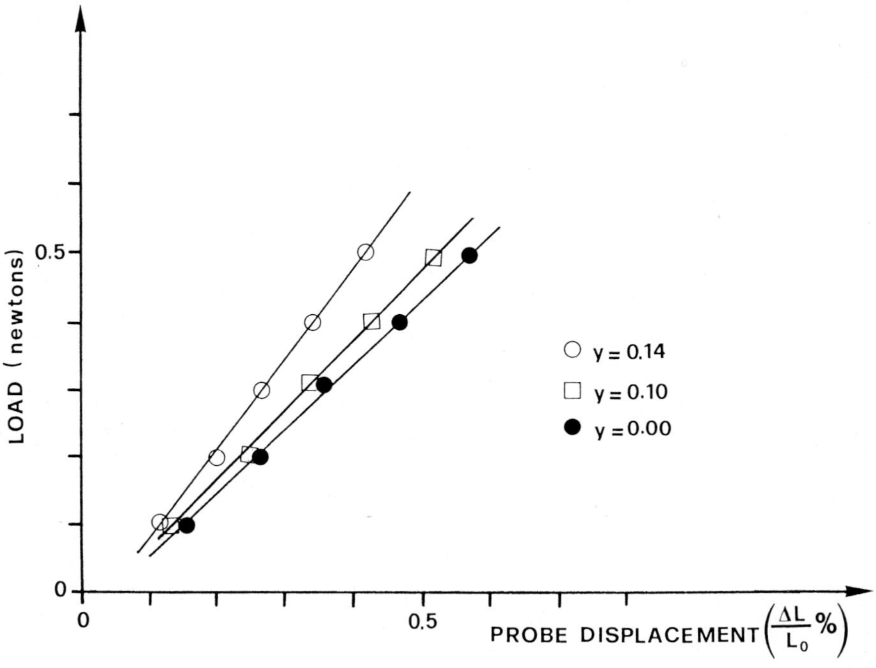

Fig. 2 Dynamic load thermomechanical analysis of calcium metaphosphate (y=0) and two calcium aluminophosphate glasses.

REFERENCES

1 a) A. Bertoluzza, M.A. Morelli and C. Fagnano, Indagine vibrazionale Raman e Ultrarossa di vetri polifosfati sodici: sale di Graham e vetri oligofosfati, Rend. Accad. Naz. Lincei, 54(6) (1973) 138-150.
b) A. Bertoluzza, M.A. Morelli, C. Fagnano and M.A. Battaglia, Indagine vibrazionale Raman e Ultrarossa di vetri oligofosfati sodici di composizione $xNa_2O \cdot P_2O_5$, con x compreso fra 1 e 1,625, Rend. Accad. Naz. Lincei, 56(3-4) (1976) 269-273.

2 A. Bertoluzza, C. Fagnano, V. Fawcett, D.A. Long and L.H. Taylor, Vibrational spectroscopic studies of a new class of oligophosphate glasses of biological interest, J. Raman Spectr., 11(1) (1981) 10-13.

3 A. Bertoluzza, M.A. Battaglia, R. Simoni and D.A. Long, Vibrational spectroscopic studies of a new class of oligophosphate glasses of biological interest. Part 2, J. Raman Spectr., 14(3) (1983) 178-183.

4 A. Bertoluzza, A.M. Marinangeli, P. Monti and R. Simoni, A Raman study on the structure of glasses of the $NaPO_3$-NaF system, Can. J. Spectr. 27(6) (1982) 171-177.
5 Results not yet published.
6 E.P. Egan, Jr., and Z.T. Wakefield, Thermodynamic properties of calcium metaphosphate, 10 to 1400° K, J. Am. Chem. Soc., 78 (1956) 4245-4249.
7 M. Watanabe, S. Sato and H. Saito, Thermal products in the system of $NaPO_3$ glass - Al_2O_3, Bull. Chem. Soc. Jpn. 48(3) (1975) 893-895.

Biomaterials and Clinical Applications,
edited by A. Pizzoferrato, P.G. Marchetti, A. Ravaglioli and A.J.C. Lee
Elsevier Science Publishers B.V., Amsterdam, 1987 — Printed in The Netherlands

MICROSTRUCTURE AND MECHANICAL PROPERTIES OF POLYMETHYLMETHACRYLATE COMPOSITE CEMENTS

A. CASTALDINI, A. CAVALLINI and D. CAVALCOLI

Department of Physics,University of Bologna, Unità GNSM-CISM
Bologna (Italy)

SUMMARY

Previous analyses on the mechanical behavior of PMMA bone cement with added hydroxyapatite (HA) showed that the porosity patterns strongly affect the load-bearing ability of these composites for orthopaedic implants.

This paper concerns the results of an extended investigation on porosity, assumed as microstructural control factor. Since the porosity by itself is not sufficient to describe the cement mechanical properties, Simplex P bone cement was mixed with a varying amount of HA to understand the correlation between resin morphology and mechanical behavior: since the fillers act as porosity condensation centers, changes in their concentration modulate the porosity patterns. Optical microscopy of thin layers brought into evidence the existence of a relative maximum of the void density and a correspondent diameter minimum at X_o=3%. These results are in agreement with previous investigation data, which showed sharp improvement in the cement performances right at this HA percentage.

INTRODUCTION

The long-term survival of cemented joint prostheses depends to a great extent on the polymethylmethacrylate (PMMA) bone cement strength.

In recent years, many solutions have been suggested to improve the mechanical behavior of PMMA.

These may be brought back to the following two fundamental conceptions:

1) the use of a low viscosity cement (ref.1), whose practical handling, however, causes some difficulties (ref.2),

2) the reduction of the PMMA porosity, that affects the mechanical properties to a great extent (ref.3).

For such reduction, dough centrifugation after mixing (ref.4-5) and vacuum mixing (ref.5) were proposed.

The solution presented as follows for the improvement of the mechanical properties of the cement pertains to this second conception.It consists in the introduction of hydroxyapatite (HA)crystals in the cement composition: the presence of HA inclusions acts, as this study will demonstrate, as a controlling factor on the cement porosity morphology.

However, this idea differs from those mentioned above: in fact the previous methods suggest modifying the porosity by means "external" to the cement itself, whereas the procedure suggested here acts directly on its void coalescence.

EXPERIMENTAL

The bone cement employed in this analysis was Simplex P plain (Howmedica, Rutherford, New Jersey). To investigate the effects induced on its microstructure by introducing inert dispersions in the continuous acrylic matrix, a weight fraction Xo of the polymer powder from commercial batches was substituted with an equal weight of crystalline hydroxyapatite (grain size 2μm) synthetically sinterized. The fraction Xo ranged up to 25 %.

After mixing the polymer with the HA fillers, the dough was prepared in the standard way suggested by the manufacturer.

For each hydroxyapatite weight percent tested, two series of specimens were made: the former was prepared according to the ASTM F451-76 specifications (ref.7), the latter by applying a pressure equal to 5 MPa to the dough during polymerization, so as to eliminate the voids trapped (hereafter these specimens will be indicated with the label HP (high pressure)).

The sample density ρ was measured with the hydrostatic scales method, and the porosity P was calculated by the expression:

$$P=(1-(\rho_{porous}/\rho_{HP})) \quad (1)$$

where ρ_{porous} and ρ_{HP} are the density of porous and HP samples, respectively.

Porosity morphology was analyzed by optical microscopy: void counting measurements and diameter determinations were made upon random plane surfaces produced through the specimens. Also scanning electron microscopy observations were carried out after coating the surfaces with a thin layer of gold.

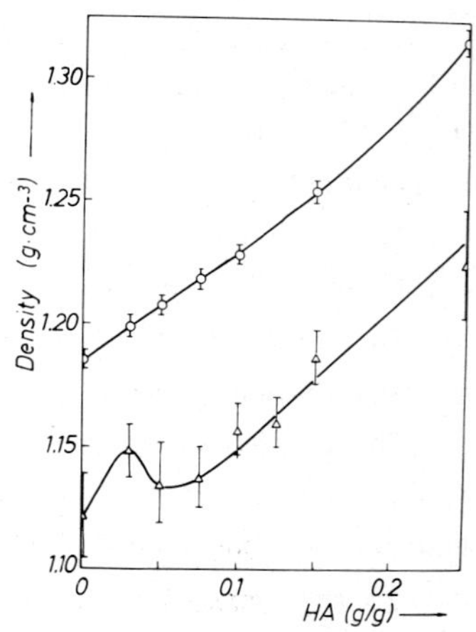

Fig.1 Density vs. HA percentage —o— HP samples, —△— standard preparation samples.

RESULTS

Density data are reported in Fig.1 for both the porous and HP specimen series. As can be seen, while the diagram referred to the HP samples shows a strictly monotonic increase, the porous set presents a significant ($p<0.05$) maximum at 3 wt % HA.

This phenomenon,not justifiable by the calculation of mixture (bone cement+ hydroxyapatite) density, can be interpreted by the porosity behavior,

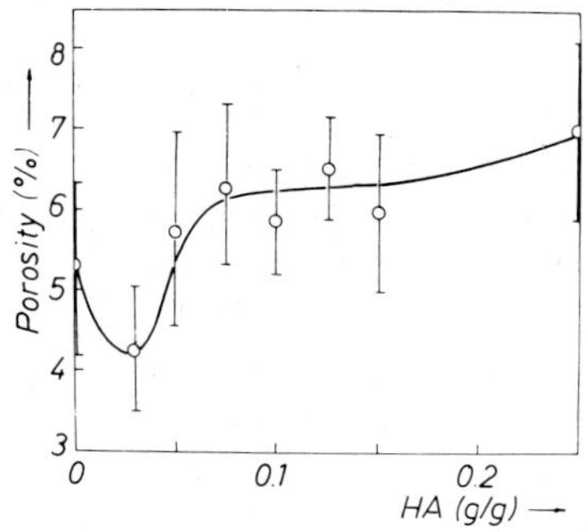

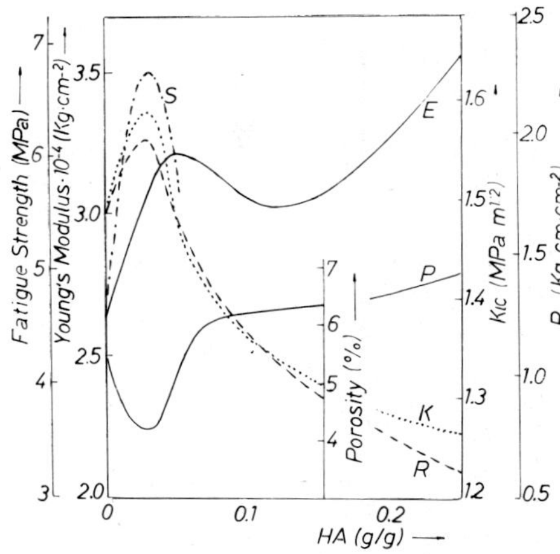

Fig.2. Porosity vs. HA percentage
Fig.3. Comparison of mechanical properties with the porosity P trend vs.HA percentage:S=fatigue strength, E=Young's modulus, K=toughness, R=impact strength, determined by both the expression (1) and weight-to-volume ratios (Fig.2).

The above diagram can be compared to the behavior of some mechanical properties, reported in previous works. On that subject, Figure 3 shows the trends of fatigue strength S (ref.8), Young's modulus E (ref.9), impact strength R (ref.10),and critical stress intensity factor K_{Ic} (ref.10) versus HA percentage in the cement.

The material performances present a sharp maximum in correspondence of the porosity minimum, as, on the other hand, could have been foreseen. However, the mechanical property changes are not quite justifiable with the porosity profile: also in the HA content range (7.5%,25.0%) where the pore volume fraction P remains nearly constant, the cement behavior shows dramatic changes.

The cause can be found in the relevant variations induced by HA fillers on the continuous polymeric matrix morphology (Fig.4): the pore surface density, N, increases with increasing hydroxyapatite percentage, and it presents a clear maximum at 3 wt% HA. In correspondence, the pore diameter Ø has a minimum, and also in the remaining part of the curve the void size keeps substantially below the starting value. Table I gives the Student t-test values about the above data, where DF refers to the freedom degrees.

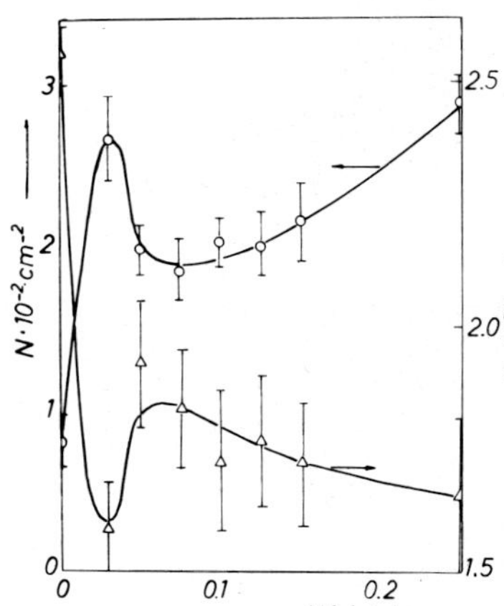

Fig.4. Surface void density N (—o—) and diameter Ø (—Δ—) vs. HA percentage.

TABLE I

T-test difference in means

HA %	0-3	3-5	5-7.5	7.5-10	10-12.5	12.5-15	15-25
N	-33.68	11.18	-1.64	-0.18	0.95	-1.68	-9.49
DF	33	28	16	16	16	10	16
Ø	30.02	-7.37	1.33	1.46	-0.39	0.43	0.78
DF	33	27	16	16	16	10	12
ρ	-5.80	2.46	-0.30	-4.06	-0.56	-4.59	-4.23
DF	42	39	25	20	19	10	15
P	3.40	-4.63	-0.96	1.40	-2.46	1.23	-2.09
DF	46	40	22	19	20	13	19

It is to be noticed, too, that these estimates must be made on a very large sample population to obtain sufficiently unbiased results: the microscopy measurements resulted widely spread, even if in different extent for different HA percentages. The frequency pore size distribution of the standard cement, for example, exhibits a larger scatter than the 3 wt % one (Fig.5).

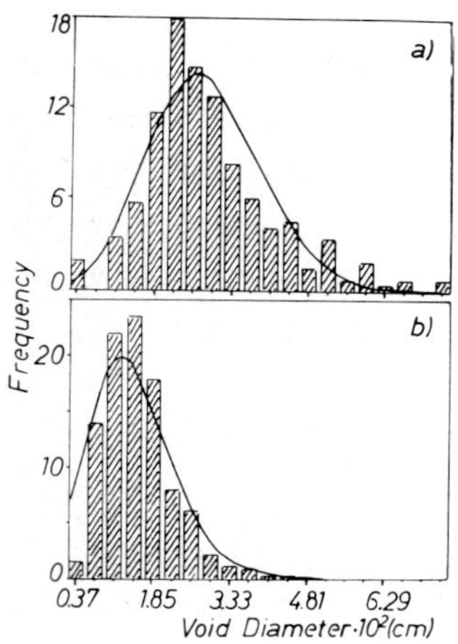

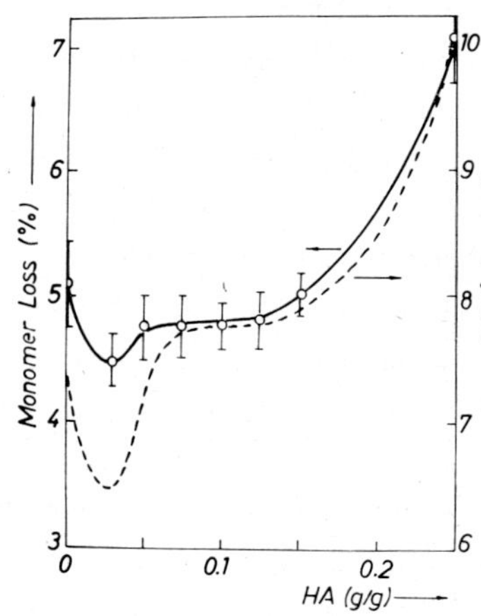

Fig.5. Distribution graphs of the diameter frequencies: (a) without HA, (b) with 3 wt% HA. The correspondent Poisson probability density function is represented by the continuous curve.

Fig.6. Weight loss percent (—o—) and rate B (dashed line) vs. HA percentage.

For performance comparison, the continuous curve in each graph represents the Poisson function corresponding to the calculated mean μ:

$$P_p(x,\mu)=\mu^x e^{-\mu}/\ \Gamma(x) \quad (2)$$

where Γ is the gamma function

$$\int_0^\infty y^{x-1}\, e^{-y}\, dy \tag{3}$$

Interpretation of the previous results led to measuring the cement weight loss during the polymerization (Fig.6). Both weight loss percent and weight loss rate B present a minimum at the 3 wt % HA.

DISCUSSION AND CONCLUSIONS

As noted so far, the cement behaviour with regard to all the physical properties examined is strongly affected by the presence of the HA dispersions.

In particular all the trends, tested or calculated, exhibit a relative extreme in correspondence of the 3 wt% of hydroxyapatite.

Considerations regarding the pore features and monomer loss characteristics offered independent checks on the action carried out by the HA fillers to control the polymeric cement microstructure and, consequently, its mechanical performances.

During the dough polymerization, the HA inclusions affect the monomer leakage rate: in fact they act as condensation nuclei as regards the gas present.Because the fillers are homogenously distributed in the polymeric resin,in this way they exert a shattering action on the gas bubbles (Fig.7a,b).

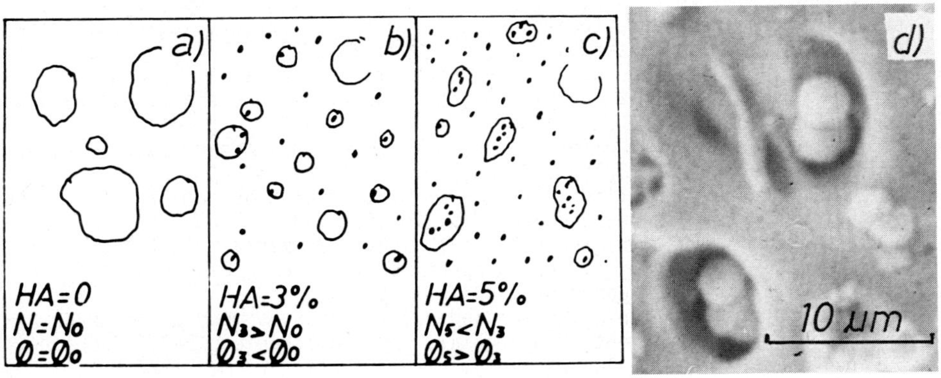

Fig.7:(a),(b),(c) sketches of the effect induced by the HA fillers on the porosity patterns.N and Ø indicate the void number and diameter, respectively; the index refers to the HA percentage. (d) scanning electron micrograph of a 5 wt% HA sample.

Therefore, the microstructure resulting after the hardening has void distribution more homogeneous than the standard cement one, and with smaller and more numerous pores. By increasing the HA filler concentration, the number of non disjointed particles increases (Fig.7 c, d); this fact produces, as an ultimate effect, larger size pores. Besides, another element could take part in the process: large HA weight fractions change substantially the polymer-monomer ratio involved in the polymerization reaction, with consequent further monomer release. In any case the voids, which can be regarded as a second phase in the brittle matrix, are elastic discontinuities, whose patterns condition the material behavior: the fracture strength So, computed by:

$$So = \{(6\gamma EP)/|\pi\emptyset(1-P)|\}^{\frac{1}{2}} \qquad (4)$$

(where the specific fracture surface energy γ is given by $K_{Ic}^2/(2E)$), results equal to 21.2 and 26.3 MPa for the standard and the 3 wt % HA cements, respectively.

By examining as a whole the mechanical performances of the composite cement versus the dispersion percentage, it is possible, in the last analysis, to assert that there exists an optimum HA content (3 wt %) that clearly improves the cement behavior.

REFERENCES

1 J.Miller, D.L.Burke, W.Krause, A.Ahmed, L.Kelebay and G.Tremblay, Improve fixation of knee arthroplasty components by the injection of acrylic cement into cancellous bone surfaces, J. Bone Joint Surg. Vol.61-B,(1979) 515-520.
2 R.S.M.Ling, Prevention of loosening of total hip components, The Hip Proc. Eighth Open Scientific Meeting of the Hip Society, Vol. 14 (1980) 292-307.
3 S.Pal and S.Saha, Stress relaxation and creep behaviour of normal and carbon fibre reinforced acrylic bone cement, Biomaterials,Vol.3,(1982) 93-96.
4 A.J.C.Lee,R.S.M.Ling and J.D.Wrighton, Some properties of polymethylmethacrylate with reference to its use in orthopaedic surgery, Clinical Orthopaedics and Related Research, Vol.95, (1973) 281-287.
5 D.W.Burke, E.I.Gates and W.H.Harris, Centrifugation as a method of improving tensile and fatigue properties of acrylic bone cement, J.Bone and Joint Surg. Vol.66-A, (1984) 1256-1273.
6 L.Lidgren,H.Drar and J.Moller, Strength of polymethylmethacrylate increased by vacuum mixing, Acta Orthop. Scand. Vol.55, (1984) 536-541.
7 A.Castaldini and A.Cavallini, Setting properties of bone cement with added synthetic hydroxyapatite, Biomaterials, Vol.6, (1985) 55-60.
8 A.Castaldini, A.Cavallini and F.Pirini, Fatigue behavior of composite bone cement. Presented at the European Conference on Biomechanics, in Berlin/West, Germany, September 8-10 th 1986.
9 A.Castaldini, A.Cavallini,A.Moroni and R.Olmi, Young's modulus of hydroxyapatite mixed bone cement, Biomaterials and Biomechanics 1983,P.Ducheyne, G.Van der Perre and A.E.Aubert (eds), Elsevier, Amsterdam, (1984), pp.427-432.
10 A.Castaldini and A.Cavallini, Fracture of acrylic composite bone cement, Biomechanics, Current Interdisciplinary Research, S.M.Perren and E.Schneider (eds), Nijhoff, Dordrecht, Boston, Lancaster,(1985) 147-152.

Biomaterials and Clinical Applications,
edited by A. Pizzoferrato, P.G. Marchetti, A. Ravaglioli and A.J.C. Lee
Elsevier Science Publishers B.V., Amsterdam, 1987 — Printed in The Netherlands

DIFFERENT NETWORK SYSTEMS FOR DIFFERENT GLASSMAKING OPERATIONS ON A BIOGLAZE.

C.B.Azzoni*, A.Krajewski**, A.Ravaglioli** and A.Piancastelli
*Dipartimento di Fisica "A.Volta", Unità GNSM-CISM, Università di Pavia (Italy);
**Istituto di Ricerche Tecnologiche per la Ceramica del CNR, Faenza (Italy)

SUMMARY

A previous study (Ref.1) emphasized the effect of changing some physical parameters on a bioglass system towards the addition of some doping oxides. In this study, however, an investigation was conducted on how the same parameters would change in connection with different possible glassmaking processes. This was carried out using systems at constant composition. Since paramagnetic spectroscopy looks at some ionic species, we decided to observe the change of the coordination field of Fe^{3+}. Therefore we prepared systems which all contained 8% wt. of Fe_2O_3. These systems were brought to a fixed temperature of 1300°C in all cases. The different glassmaking procedures were taken from actual ones used in the production of bioglazes. On each obtained glassy system obtained, thermal expansion and EPR (Electron Paramagnetic Resonance) data were collected.

Substantial differences were observed that confirm previous correlations between the thermal expansion coefficient values and the population abundance of specific coordination field arrangements around Fe^{3+} ions (indicating network rearrangement). Further, it was apparent that relevant differences in the properties of the glassy systems are due to the different glassmaking technologies. These are very important for the quality of the systems.

INTRODUCTION

It is known (Ref.2) that a close biochemical link between a biological tissue and a vitreous system characterizes the optimal condition of coupling to the bone of bioactive ceramics.

The vitreous system studied in this work must guarantee good adhesion to the metallic alloy (316 L steel). Such adhesion is favoured by suitable doping oxides: among them the iron oxide plays a fundamental role.

Consequently the influence of iron oxide on a suitable vitreous system has been studied, either with different quantities added or different operative techniques employed. On the basis of the tests, we tried to establish a correlation between the phenomenological (thermal expansion) and structural characteristics of the samples through Electron Paramagnetic Resonance (EPR) measurements.

METHODS

In a previous work (Ref 1) we proposed a model to interpret the trend of the linear thermal expansion coefficient $\beta=(1/L_0)(dL/dT)p/3$ in connection with the amount of the Fe_2O_3 added to a vitreous system based on SiO_2(45% wt.), CaO (24.5% wt.), Na_2O (24.5% wt.), P_2O_5 (6% wt.).

With EPR tests on Fe^{3+} ion it was possible to obtain a quantitative correlation between the percentage of Fe^{3+} ions inserted in cubic symmetry sites with a strong rombic distorsion and the linear thermal expansion coefficient β. In this work we will try to ascertain, using the same techniques, the influence of the modalities of the preparation of samples and particularly the modalities of insertion of Fe_2O_3 in the vitreous base system, on the dilatometric characteristics and on EPR signals. To that end we prepared three chemically identical systems, inserting into the base composition the same quantity (8% wt.) of Fe_2O_3 according to the following methodology:

a) we mixed all the oxides of base composition with Fe_2O_3, successively firing in a Pt crucible at a temperature of 1350°C. A part of the melt was poured into a graphite mould preheated to 600°C to create a small bar for dilatometric and EPR tests, thus obtaining the sample A.

b) the remaining part of the melt was quenched in water to obtain a frit that, having been finely ground in a alumina ball mill and carefully dried, was remelted at 1350°C in a Pt crucible. After the melting, it was poured into a graphite mould preheated to 600°C, and we thus obtained another bar, called sample B.

c) the third sample, named C, was prepared with the same methodology cited in literature (Ref.1). We mixed only the oxides of the base composition and later fired them at 1350°C in a Pt crucible. The melt was quenched in water, then dried and ground. At the frit stage, 8% wt. of Fe_2O_3 was added and the system so obtained was melted at 1350°C in a Pt crucible and then poured into a graphite mould preheated to 600°C to obtain a small bar. The dilatometric tests on the samples, 5 cm long, were carried out with Netzch dilatometer with dT/dt=0.8°C sec^{-1} in a temperature range 20 to 500°C. and the EPR measurements were performed with a Bruker spectometer at x-band (9,008 GHz) and at room temperature. In the table (besides the β values) the values of $y= x_r/x_c$ are reported representing the ratio between the x_r number of Fe^{3+} ions in octaedral coordination sites rombically distorted (C_{2v}, C_{3v}) and the number x_c of Fe^{3+} ions in regular octahedral coordination sites (Oh). The y values were obtained making the ratio of the areas calculated with numerical methods of EPR signals and with g_{eff}=4.27 and g 2.00 corresponding respectively to Fe^{3+} ions in C_{2v}, C_{3v} symmetry sites and to Fe^{3+} ions in Oh ones. The table also shows the values relative to the sample with 8% wt. of Fe_2O_3 coming from the previous study (sample D) (Ref. 1).

samples	$\beta \cdot 10^5$ (0°C^{-1})	$y_{20°C}$	addition (wt%)
A	1.25 ± .02	.35 ± .05	8
B	1.36 ± .02	.45 ± .05	8
C	1.36 ± .02	.67 ± .06	8
D	1.39 ± .02	.70 ± .06	8

The samples C and D, obtained with the same technology, have the same β and y values, taking into consideration the experimental error range.

The sample B has the same dilatometric characteristics of the sample C even if with a different y value. The values relative to the sample A differ considerably from those relative to B and C samples; it also differs substantially also for the preparation modalities since, unlike the B and C samples, it was subjected to a different treatment.

DISCUSSION AND CONCLUSIONS

Applying to B and C samples the same interpretative model used for D sample (Ref.1), we mantain that the lesser value of y of the sample B indicate that, in a matrix derived from a frit already containing Fe_2O_3, the availability of sites C_{2v} and C_{3v} at disposal are less than in sample C: this follows from the hypotheses already formulated according to which the low symmetry sites were occupied progressively by Fe^{3+} ions until they were completely filled up, while the further Fe^{3+} ions added settled into regular cubic symmetry sites with a continuous network rearrangement.

For sample C, the maximum number of Fe^{3+} ions which could be inserted in C_{2v} and C_{3v} sites is about 40.10^{-5} mol.g-3, while for sample B, (always at room temperature), it should be about 30.10^{-5}mol.g^{-1}.

Since in sample C the low symmetry sites are already all occupied (it contains 8% wt of Fe_2O_3 i.e. 100.10^{-5}mol/g), it can be assumed that the same results will be seen in sample B with a lesser value of β; furthermore having attributed to the Fe^{3+} ions in higher symmmetry sites the role of driving modifiers of the network rearrangement, we can infer that the sample prepared in a similar way to B may exhibit an anomalous behaviour of β in function of the Fe_2O_3 additions in the range of 0-2,5% wt, while the sample prepared similarly to C exhibited a such anomalous behaviour for Fe_2O_3 included in the range 0-3,2% wt.; with this last value the complete filling of low symmetry sites was reached by Fe^{3+} ions.

We can deduce that, with suitable Fe_2O_3 additions and with suitable methodological preparation, it is possible to obtain samples (as the sample B) for which β anomalous behaviour appears less evident and in a range more restricted in quantity of Fe_2O_3 added, in respect to the previously studied samples C and D.

It is important to ascertain - and we are continuing these kinds of studies - if there exists a correlation between the ascertained β anomalies and the stability of the system, from the chemical point of view (for example through the attack of the vitreous mass by a physiological solution simulating the biological environment in which the prostheses are inserted). Some tests already carried out on different compositions and prepared "ad hoc" (Ref.3) with the same methodologies of preparation of the system, are put as evidence that added quantities of Fe_2O_3 equal to 6%, will permit the possibility of obtaining systems of high chemical stability.

For sample A, the experimental value is decisively anomalous. In fact, according to the traditional equation attributed to Winkelmann and Schott (Ref. 4)

$$\beta teor.=\Sigma_i\beta_iC_i + \beta_{Fe_2O_3}C_{Fe_2O_3}$$

where C_i=%wt. of i oxide component and β_i, the relative Meyer-Havas coefficient, we obtain, for the Σ only of the components of the vitreous system, the value $\Sigma_i\beta_iC_i=1,29\times10^{-5}{}^\circ C^{-1}$ (beyond the experimental error) than the value of the sample. The sample, therefore, has no affinity, considering the dilatometric behaviour, with the other examined samples. This was foreseeable since the effect of the alteration of the amount of any oxide is not linear except to a limited degree; consequently, the best results my be expected only from comparison of similar systems prepared under like conditions (Ref.4).

REFERENCES

1 C.B. Azzoni, G.L. Del Nero, A. Krajewski and A. Ravaglioli, Thermal Expansion of silico-phosphate glasses with small additions of Fe_2O_3: EPR and dilatometric studies, J. Mater. Sci., 19, (1984) 3620-3625.

2 L. Hench, La fabbricazione sui bioceramici, Ceramurgia, 5 (1977) 253-

3 A. Ravaglioli, A. Krajewski, Q. Zini and R. Venturi, Short and long range silicate release from doped bioglass into 199 medium, Biomaterials, 1 (1986) 76-78.

4 C.V. Parmelee, Ceramic Glazes, Chaners Books, Boston, 1973, pp. 240-251.

Biomaterials and Clinical Applications,
edited by A. Pizzoferrato, P.G. Marchetti, A. Ravaglioli and A.J.C. Lee
Elsevier Science Publishers B.V., Amsterdam, 1987 — Printed in The Netherlands

CHEMICO-PHYSICAL CHARACTERIZATION OF BIOMATERIAL STRUCTURES IN RELATION TO THEIR UTILIZATION.

A. BERTOLUZZA[1], P. MONTI[1], R. SIMONI[1],
L. PRATELLI[2], A. PIZZOFERRATO[2]

[1]Istituto Chimico "G. Ciamician", Centro Studio Interfacolta' sulla Spettroscopia Raman, Universita' di Bologna (Italy)

[2]Centro di Ricerca per la Biocompatibilita' dei Materiali da Impianto, Istituto Rizzoli, Bologna (Italy)

SUMMARY.

The structure of an alumina-titania material (60% Al_2O_3, 40% TiO_2), which can be used in coating orthopaedic prostheses has been characterized by vibrational (i.r. and Raman-laser) spectroscopy.

The spectra have shown that this alumina-titania does not consist of a binary oxide, but of a mixture of Al_2O_3 (corundum) and TiO_2 (anatase). This result was also confirmed by X-ray diffraction measurements.

TG and DSC analyses have shown the thermal stability of the material and the presence of adsorbed water on its surface.

INTRODUCTION.

The study of the biocompatibility of a material needs a preliminary structural characterization in order to correlate the possible variations of the chemico-physical parameters with the effects of the biological environments.

For this purpose different instrumental techniques such as Raman and i.r. spectroscopy, thermogravimetric (TG), differential scanning calorimetric (DSC) and thermomechanical (TMA) analyses are utilized in our Center of Research.

In particular Raman spectroscopy, which provides a non-destructive and non-invasive vibrational probe, is a suitable method for directly investigating the structure of a material without affecting the sample.

In this work we present a chemico-physical characterization of an alumina-titania material that can be used in coating orthopaedic prostheses.

METHODS.

The material (e.g. Alumina 131 METCO) was composed of Al_2O_3 (60% w/w) and TiO_2 (40% w/w).

The infrared spectrum of the powdered sample was obtained from a nujol mull on CsJ disk and was recorded with a Jasco DS701G spectrophotometer.

The Raman spectrum was recorded using a Jasco R-300 spectrophotometer with a Lexel Ar^+ 4880 Å laser source.

X-ray diffraction pattern was obtained using a Philips diffractometer (CuKα).

TG and DSC measurements were performed in a Mettler TA 3000 system with TG 50 and DSC 20 equipments.

DISCUSSION.

Al_2O_3 exists in α and γ forms. α-Al_2O_3 possesses the same crystalline structure as mineral corundum while, under the name of γ form, a variety of phases are collected, which possess a defect spinel structure (ref. 1).

The three main polimorphs of TiO_2 are anatase, rutile and brookite, which are characterized by octahedral coordination groups with different Ti-O lengths (ref. 1).

X-ray diffraction patterns of both Al_2O_3 and TiO_2 forms are reported in the literature (ref. 2).

Al_2O_3-TiO_2 complex oxides, with different Al/Ti atomic ratios, are also known, which are not simply mechanical mixtures of Al_2O_3 and TiO_2, but consist of new complex oxides as shown by X-ray diffraction measurements (ref. 3). The infrared spectra of Al_2O_3-TiO_2 binary oxides have never been reported in the literature.

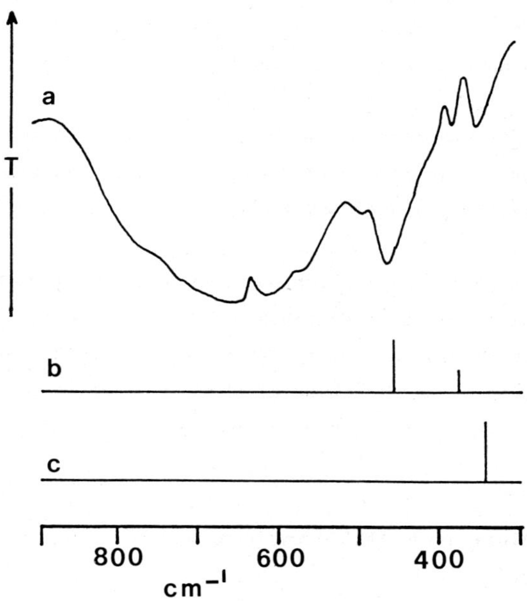

Fig. 1. Infrared spectra of: a) Alumina 131; b) α-Al_2O_3; c) anatase.

The i.r. spectra of the different forms of Al_2O_3 show strong and broad absorption bands between 900 and 500 cm^{-1} (ref. 4). Nevertheless the i.r. spectrum of α-Al_2O_3 is characterized by a strong band at 450 cm^{-1} and by a weaker one at $\sim$380 cm^{-1}.

Among the main forms of TiO_2, anatase and rutile are spectroscopically much more widely studied than brookite. The i.r. spectra of anatase and rutile are quite different especially in the low frequency range. In particular the i.r. spectrum of anatase shows a characteristic band at 347 cm^{-1}, which is absent in the spectrum of rutile (ref. 5).

In Fig.1a we report the i.r. spectrum of Alumina 131. It shows besides a broad absorption band centered at $\sim$650 cm^{-1} bands at 455, 375 and 345 cm^{-1}. These bands coincide with the most characteristic ones of the i.r. spectra of α-Al_2O_3 and TiO_2 (anatase) which are reported in Fig.1b and 1c respectively, thus verifying that Alumina 131 is a mechanical mixture of the two oxides and does not consist of a new complex oxide.

This conclusion is also supported by the trend of the Raman spectrum of Alumina 131 which is reported in Fig.2a. As can be seen it coincides with the Raman spectrum of TiO_2 (anatase) (ref. 6) which is shown in Fig.2c.

The absence of α-Al_2O_3 Raman bands (Fig.2b) (ref. 7) can be explained by considering that the intrinsic spectrum of anatase is much more intense than α-Al_2O_3 one and masks it.

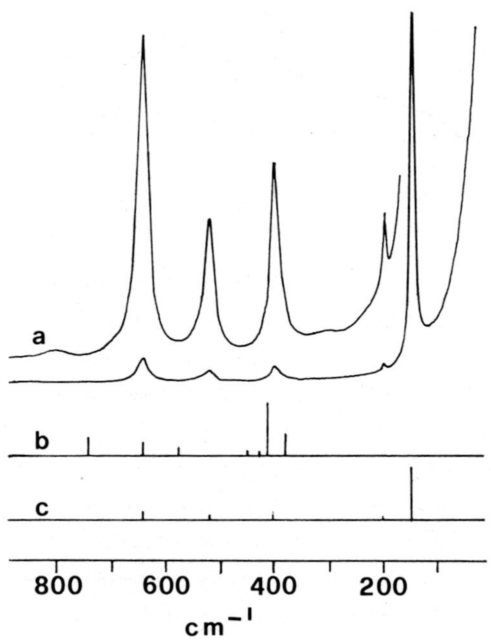

Fig. 2. Raman spectra of:
a) Alumina 131
b) α-Al_2O_3
c) anatase

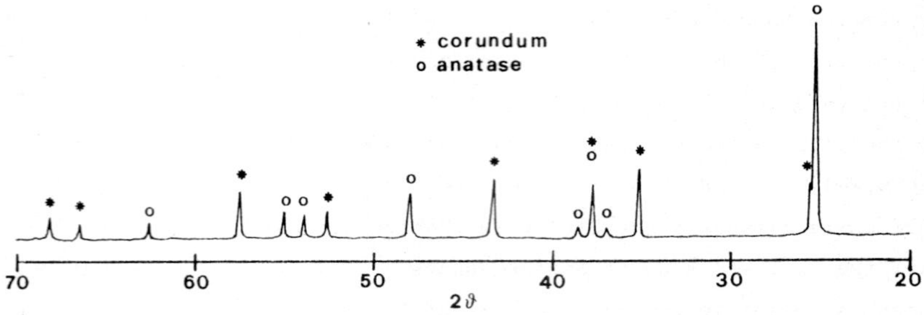

Fig. 3. X-ray diffraction pattern of Alumina 131.

The spectroscopic results are also confirmed by Alumina 131 X-ray diffraction pattern (Fig.3) which contains anatase and corundum peaks.

The thermogravimetric and differential scanning calorimetric curves of Alumina 131 are reported in Fig.4 and 5 respectively.

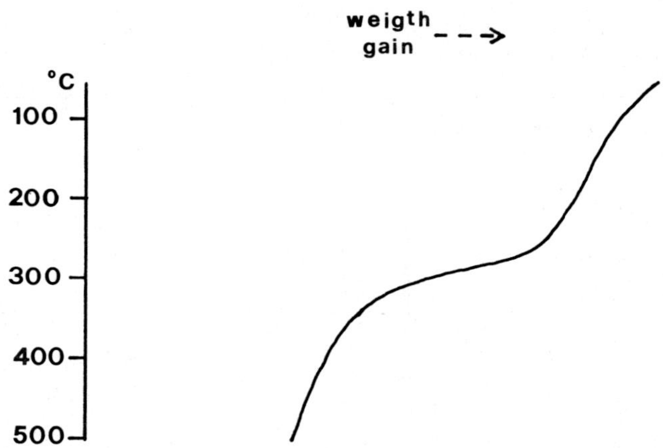

Fig. 4. TG curve of Alumina 131.

TG analysis show a 4% weight loss between 30 and 450°C. DSC analysis reveals endothermic peaks in the same temperature range.

It is well known that metal oxides as Al_2O_3 and TiO_2 retain water molecules adsorbed on their surfaces. Previous i.r. studies (ref. 8) showed that such water molecules are completely removed after heating at relatively high temperature in vacuum. On this basis we can reasonably conclude that the weight loss and the endothermic processes are probably related to the removal of adsorbed water rather than to a thermal degradation of the material.

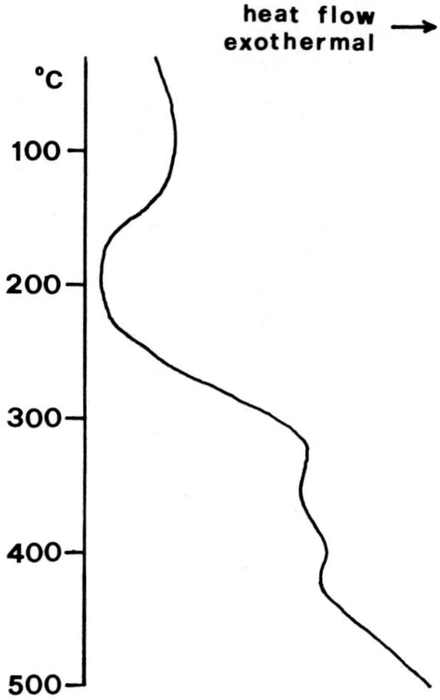

Fig. 5. DSC curve of Alumina 131.

Preliminary studies on the characterization of the material after interactions with biological systems have shown that there are no structural changes in Alumina 131 structure after being phagocyted by peritoneal macrophages (ref. 9).

The authors are indebted to prof. F. Lucchini for X-ray diffraction measurements.

REFERENCES.

1 A.F. Wells, Structural Inorganic Chemistry, 4th edn., Clarendon Press, Oxford, 1975.
2 X-ray powder data file, American Society for Testing Materials (ASTM), Phyladelphia.
3 E. Rodenas, T. Yamaguchi, H. Hattori and K. Tanabe, Surface and catalytic properties of TiO_2-Al_2O_3, J. Catal., 69 (1981) 434-444 and literature cited therein.
4 M.C. Stegmann, D. Vivien and C. Mazieres, Etude du spectra infrarouge des alumines de transition et du corindon, J. Chim. Phys., 71 (1974) 761-764.
5 N.T. Mc Devitt and W.L. Baun, Infrared absorption study of metal oxides in the low frequency region (700-240 cm^{-1}), Spectrochim. Acta, 20 (1964) 799.

6 I.P. Alekseeva, N.M. Belyaevskaya, Y.S. Bobovich, M.Y. Tsenter and T.I. Chuvaeva, Generation, interpretation, and some examples of the use of Raman spectra of titanium-dioxide activated devetrified glasses, Opt. Spectrosc., 45 (1978) 927-936.
7 S.P.S. Porto and R.S. Krishnan, Raman effect of corundum, J. Chem. Phys., 47 (1967) 1009-1012.
8 L.H. Little, Infrared spectra of adsorbed species, Academic Press, London, (1966) and literature cited therein.
9 A. Pizzoferrato, S. Stea, G. Ciapetti, C. Tarabusi, A. Ruggeri, S. Guizzardi, M. Morocutti, A. Bertoluzza, P. Monti and A. Tinti, Phagocytosis, ultrastructural evaluation and vibrational spectroscopy (Raman-laser and i.r.) of alumina titania, this issue.

This study has been funded by a grant from Ministero della Sanità, Progetto Finalizzato "Definizione di modelli di studio di biocompatibilità e di nuove protesi".

Biomaterials and Clinical Applications,
edited by A. Pizzoferrato, P.G. Marchetti, A. Ravaglioli and A.J.C. Lee
Elsevier Science Publishers B.V., Amsterdam, 1987 — Printed in The Netherlands

SURFACE ENERGY MEASUREMENTS ON PROTEIN LAYERS ADSORBED ONTO SYNTHETIC SUBSTRATA

Clay, C.S.[1] Lydon, M.J.[1,3] and Tighe, B.J.[2]

[1]Unilever Research, Colworth House, Sharnbrook, Bedford, U.K.

[2]Speciality Polymer Group, Aston University, Aston Triangle, Birmingham, U.K.

[3]Current Address: Convatec Biological Research Lab., c/o Squibb International Developmental Lab., Moreton, Wirral, U.K.

SUMMARY

Biological response to polymeric implants or cell culture substrata is influenced by the physicochemical properties of the polymer. We have carried out surface energy measurements on deposited layers on synthetic surfaces. These layers do not completely mask the underlying surface energy, however, it appears to be of no interest or relevence to the cells in deciding whether they will attach or spread on that surface.

INTRODUCTION

Biological response to polymeric implants or cell culture substrata is influenced by the physicochemical properties of the polymer. In investigations of the relevance of surface properties to biological response we have found cell culture models to be invaluable (refs. 1,2). However, these studies in themselves are of limited value in investigations of the mechanisms of cell/substratum interactions. Cellular response ultimately depends upon the deposition of biological molecules onto culture substrata or implanted materials (refs. 1, 3, 4, 5, 6). We have, therefore, set out to study the role of these "interface conversion" events (ref. 3) in our model systems.

Physicochemical properties of the synthetic substrata are an important consideration in interface conversion, at least in the initial stages (ref. 1). Previous work by our group and others has led to an overview of the relationships between chemical group expression (refs. 2, 7, 8, 9, 10), surface free energy (fractional polarity) (refs. 1, 2, 6) and cell adhesion. The surface energy of the substratum is clearly important in triggering interface conversion (refs. 1, 6) but is not the sole criterion as the expression of chemical groups at the surface does have a part to play (ref. 2).

As part of this programme, we have carried out surface energy measurements (by the sessile drop contact angle method) on deposited layers on synthetic surfaces, which either support or do not support cell adhesion in the presence of a foetal calf serum supplement (ref. 1). Serum is of particular importance as it is a required supplement for the culture of anchorage-dependent cell lines (refs. 1, 6, 11). It is, however, a complex substance with numerous constituents, some of which have been isolated and shown to promote cell adhesion to surfaces; these include fibronectin (refs. 5, 12) and vitronectin (refs. 5, 11). Other constituents of serum can also be used in cell adhesion studies, e.g. albumin can be used as a non-adhesion-promoting control (ref. 13).

MATERIALS AND METHOD

The polymers tested were:

- polyhydroxyethylmethacrylate (pHEMA)
- polyethylmethacrylate (pEMA)
- 50/50 pEMA/pHEMA
- Tissue culture plastic (surface treated polystyrene)
- Bacteriological grade plastic (native polystyrene)

The cleaned surfaces were then incubated with each of the following solutions for 2 hours at 37°C before measuring the contact angles:

- 10% foetal calf serum (FCS) in Dulbecco's Modified Eagles Medium (DMEM)
- 1% bovine serum albumin (BSA) in phosphate buffered saline (PBS)
- 5 µg/ml partially purified vitronectin in PBS
- 5 µg/ml pure fibronectin in PBS.

The vitronectin was prepared by glass bead column separation as described in Lydon and Foulger (ref. 4).

The surfaces were blotted dry with tissues ready for the contact angle measurements. Contact angles for distilled water and methyl iodide were measured, with the left and right contact angles being paired. Surface energies were calculated according to the method of Owens and Wendt (ref. 14).

Cell adhesion was tested using Baby Hamster Kidney (BHK) fibroblasts as previously described by Lydon et al (ref. 1), incubated at 37°C for 6 hours in both serum-free and serum-supplemented medium.

RESULTS

Table 1 shows the surface energies of the bare polymer surfaces and demonstrates that the hydrophillicity/hydrophobicity of the surface is best represented by the polar component, γp. The addition of serum or protein layers shifts the fractional polarity but the underlying surface energy is still expressed to an extent (Fig. 1). The cell adhesion properties of these surfaces with deposited layers is shown in table 2.

Table 1

Surface Energies of Bare Surfaces

Polymer Surfaces	Surface Energies (dynes cm-1) γp	γd	γt
pHEMA	23.7	32.1	55.8
pEMA	10.8	38.3	49.1
50/50 pEMA/pHEMA	19.8	31.8	51.5
Tissue culture p/s	15.2	36.9	52.1
Bacteriological p/s	1.5	45.5	47.0

Figure 1

Polar components of adsorbed layers on polymer surfaces.

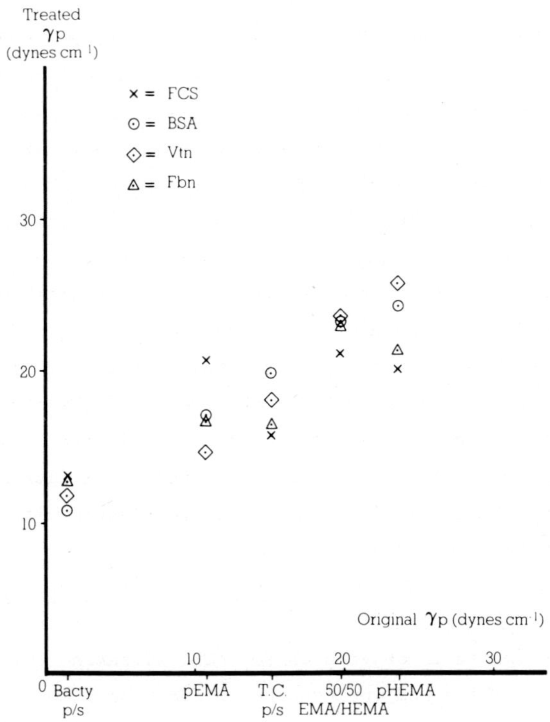

Table 2

Cell Response

Polymer Surfaces	Serum in Medium	Cell Adhesion on Deposited Layers +FCS	+BSA	+Fbn
pHEMA	+Serum	-	-	++
"	Serum Free	-	-	+
pEMA	+Serum	+	-	++
"	Serum Free	+	-	+
EMA/HEMA	+Serum	+	-	+
"	Serum Free	+	-	+
T.C. Plastic	+Serum	+++	+++	+++
"	Serum Free	++	-	+
Bacty Plast.+Serum	-	-		++
"	Serum Free	-	-	+

DISCUSSION

Cell adhesion has been demonstrated to be related to the polar component of the surface free energy (refs. 1,6). The results presented here show that the underlying surface energy (particularly the polar fraction) is still expressed to an extent even when deposited serum or protein layers are present (fig.1). However, the fractional polarities of surfaces coated with adhesive and non-adhesive proteins are very similar to one another. The resulting values do not bear any obvious relationship to one another or to the cell response to the surface. For example, tissue culture plastic is adhesive to cells in serum-free medium in the presence of FCS but pEMA in the presence of BSA is not adhesive and yet the fractional polarity values are very similar. The situation being reversed for pEMA with FCS (adhesive) and tissue culture plastic with BSA (non-adhesive) where the fractional polarities are also very similar. Also, tissue culture plastic coated with vitronectin or fibronectin have very similar fractional polarities to tissue culture plastic with BSA (non-adhesive) and are adhesive to cells.

When serum is present in the medium the cell response to a surface is enhanced compared to serum-free medium. In the case of tissue culture plastic coated with BSA the cell response is as good as for FCS indicating that the FCS in the medium can compete with and replace the preadsorbed BSA.

Similarly the other surfaces and the deposited layers show little correlation in their fractional polarities and cell adhesion capabilities. This suggests that the energy of the surface once coated with a deposited layer of protein is of no interest or relevance to the cells in deciding whether they will attach and spread on that surface.

"Interface conversion" is a complex event, therefore, as non-adhesive proteins like albumin can render a surface which is normally adhesive in the presence of FCS non-adhesive to cells. The converse of this also operates with the adhesion promoting proteins vitronectin and fibronectin rendering a surface (eg. bacteriological grade plastic) which is non-adhesive in the presence of FCS, adhesive to cells. This indicates that cell adhesion is a protein-specific event but that "interface conversion" depends on the composition, organisation, conformation and orientation of proteins in the deposited layers (refs. 15,16) and this is influenced by the surface properties of the underlying substrata.

It is our working hypothesis that in a non-adhesive surface energy zone "interface conversion" does not proceed in an appropriate manner thus preventing cell interaction with the synthetic surface. However, in a non-physiological situation as with deposited single protein layers cell adhesion may occur. In these cases the system cannot be a true test for biocompatability as it does not predict the behaviour of the material in a physiological environment as represented by mixed protein components such as serum.

REFERENCES

1. M.J. Lydon, T.W. Minett, B.J. Tighe; Biomaterials 6 (1985) 396.
2. K.D. Thomas, B.J. Tighe, M.J. Lydon; in P. Christel, A. Meunier, A.J.C. Lee, Advances in Biomaterials Vol 6 Biological and Biomechanical Performance of Biomaterials, Elsevier, Amsterdam, 1985. 379.
3. R.E. Baier; J. Biomech. Eng. 104 (1982) 257.
4. M.J. Lydon, and C.A. Foulger; (1986) This Symposium.
5. R. Neumeier and W. Reutter; Exp. Cell Res. 160 (1985) 287.
6. P. van der Valk, A.W.J. van Pelt, H.J. Busscher, H.P. de Jong, C.R.H. Wildervuir, J. Arends; J. Biomed. Mat. Res. 17 (1983) 807.
7. A.S.G. Curtis, J.V. Forrester, C. McInnes, F. Lawrie; J. Cell Biol. 97 (1983) 1500.
8. H.W. Gibson, and F.C. Bailey;Macromol. 13 (1980) 34.
9. H.G. Klemperer, and P. Knox; Lab. Pract. 26 (1977) 179.

10. N.G. Maroudas; J. Cell. Physiol. 90 (1976) 511.
11. R. Holmes; J. Cell Biol. 32 (1967) 297.
12. R.O. Hynes, and K.M. Yamada; J. Cell Biol. 95 (1982) 369.
13. B.R. Young, L.K. Lambrecht, S.L. Cooper, D.F. Mosher, in S.L. Cooper and N.A. Peppas, Biomaterials: Interfacial Phenomena and Applications, American Chemical Society, 1982, 351.
14. D.K. Owens, and R.C. Wendt; J. Applied Polym. Sci. 13 (1969) 1741.
15. F. Grinnell, and M.K. Feld; J. Biol. Chem. 257 (1982) 4888.
16. G.K. Iwamoto, L.C. Winterton, R.S. Stocker, R.A. van Wagenen, J.D. Andrade, D.F. Mosher, J. Colloid Interface Sci. 106 (1985) 459.

Biomaterials and Clinical Applications,
edited by A. Pizzoferrato, P.G. Marchetti, A. Ravaglioli and A.J.C. Lee
Elsevier Science Publishers B.V., Amsterdam, 1987 — Printed in The Netherlands

IN VITRO AND IN VIVO REACTIONS OF VARIOUS AMORPHOUS METALS

H. OONISHI M.D.[1], E. TSUJI Ph.D.[2], T. NABESHIMA M.D.[1], S. KUSHITANI M.D.[1], K. TSUYAMA M.D.[1], Y. UKON M.D.[1] and N. MURATA M.D.[1]

[1]Department of Orthopaedic Surgery, Artificial Joint Section and Biomaterial Research Laboratory, Osaka-Minami National Hospital, 677-6, Kido-Cho, Kawachinagano-Shi, Osaka 586, JAPAN
[2]Osaka Prefectural Industrial Research Institute

ABSTRACT

In order to pursue the possibility of application of thin twisted wire of amorphous metal of (1) the Fe-Cr-Si-B group as well as (2) Co-Fe-Si-B, Co-Fe-Nb-Si-B and Co-Si-B in the Co group to orthopaedic surgery, they were compared of biocompatibilities and reactions in vivo and in vitro. They had excellent corrosion resistance in vitro. Its wire was about 4 times stronger than the SUS 316 wire. However, they showed in vivo reaction quite different from those in vitro. Deposition of metallic elements in the living tissues as well as very marked corrosion in particular cases started early. It seems that they were unique reactions of non-crystaloid amorphous metal which was different from the usual crystalloid metal.

INTRODUCTION

The SUS 316 wire is often broken relatively early after clinical use as its diameter is not large enough. The surface of the SUS 316 has relatively a lot of pit corrosion. Thus the SUS 316 is more frequently broken in vivo due to stress corrosion breakage or fatigue breakage attributable to scars on the wire surface. In order to pursue the possibility of application of thin twisted wire of amorphous metal of the Fe-Cr-Si-B group or Co group to orthopaedic surgery, they were compared of biocompatibilities and reactions in vivo and in vitro.

Generally, amorphous metal attracts interest in various fields as a unique, new material having irregular atomic arrays. Since it has such properties as high tensile strength, long fracture elongation, high Vickers hardness, near roundness in cross section with radial isotropy and good flexibility, processing including twisting, weaving, knitting and combining is easy. In addition it has very good corrosion resistance.

EXPERIMENTAL METHODS AND RESULTS

The following experiment was made using (1) (A) and (B) in the Fe-Cr-Si-B group as well as (2) (A) Co-Fe-Si-B, (B) Co-Fe-Nb-Si-B and (C) Co-Si-B in the

Co group.

A) Corrosion resistance

(a) Methods

The corrosion resistance test was made using (1) the high-frequency corrosion resistance method, (2) the immersion test with pure water and 4% salt water and (3) the weight loss method (A sample of about 0.1g was cut into pieces of 3cm in length. They were dissolved at 34°C in an acid solution of 50ml by shaking for each time period, and their residual weight was measured).

(b) Results

(1) Corrosion resistance method : The corrosion resistance of the Fe-Cr-Si-B group against HCl was lower than the SUS 304. On the other hand, the wire materials of the Co group were high in corrosion resistance and this property did not change so substantially as HCl concentration increased. All the piano wires were broken due to partial corrosion during measurement in HCl of 0.1 to 1N. Thus, they could not be measured.

(2) Immersion test with pure water and 4% salt water : After immersion for 10 days, the (B) of the Fe-Cr-Si-B group and the Co group metal did not show any change on their surfaces.

(3) Weight loss method with acid solution : The Fe-Cr-Si-B group showed larger weight loss in HCl and H_2SO_4 of 0.5N. On the other hand, the corrosion resistance of the Co group was higher in HCl, but slightly lower in H_2SO_4 than the SUS 304 as corrosion gradually occurred in the Co group.

B) Strength test for twisted wires

(a) Methods

We prepared twisted wires (1.2 to 1.3mm in outer diameter) with 3 core cables made by twisting 7 element wires of 90μm in diameter and 9 side cables made by twisting 7 element wires of 100μm in diameter. Then, the following experiments were carried out:

(1) Since the tested wires could not be jointed like the currently used SUS 316 wire in the twisting method, the clamping method had to be employed with a metal pipe and a clamping tool was experimentally made. The jointing strength between the two was compared using the SUS 316.

(2) Using the SUS 316 wires, Ti wires, Ti twisted wires and amorphous wires (Fe-Cr-Si-B), the tensile strength test was made under the conditions of 5mm/min in cross head speed and 10cm/min in chart speed.

(b) Results

(1) The Ti wires were stronger in stress corrosion breakage, but weaker in fatigue breakage than the SUS 316 ones. When comparisons were made on the twisted wires and element wires of the same outer diameter, it was found that the twisted wires were lower by about 20% in strength than the element wires. However, the tensile strength of the amorphous wires was much stronger than

that of the Ti and SUS 316 wires, namely, about 6 times stronger and about 4 times stronger, respectively.

C) Biological reactions

(a) Methods

Amorphous metal ribbon pieces of the Fe-Cr-Si-B group and the Co group were implanted in the femoral condyles and muscles of mature rabbits. After 6 weeks, 3 months and 6 months, they were sacrificed and observed by using a light microscope and a SEM. Observations were also made on the state of element disposition to surrounding tissues by using X-ray microanalyzer. Furthermore, changes on the metal surfaces in vivo were observed with SEM.

The samples implanted in the bones were embedded with resin and hard preparations were made. In addition, after amorphous metal was removed from the bones, decalcified samples were prepared.

(b) Results

In the process of making the amorphous metal ribbons, one side became wavy and the other side smooth.

When the metal ribbons of the Fe-Cr-Si-B group was implanted in soft tissues including muscles and tendons, this connective tissue membrane was formed around the metal ribbons with no pathological reaction (Fig. 1). Similarly,

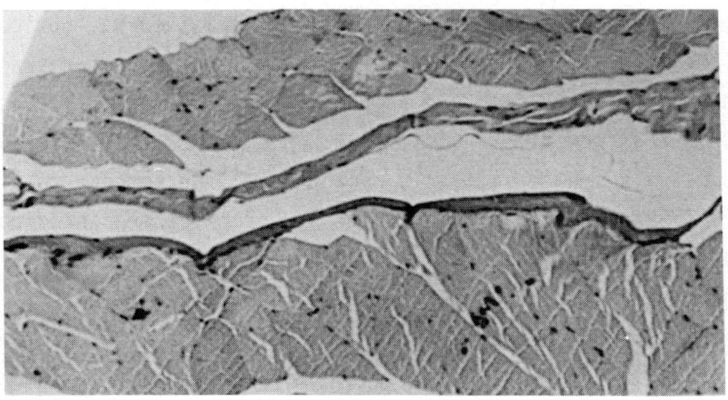

Fig. 1. Fe-Cr-Si-B group was implanted in the muscle of the rabbit for 12 weeks. There was no pathological inflammations.

in the case in which they were implanted in the bones, there was no pathological inflammation in peripheral tissues. New bone formation was observed around the metal ribbons and there existed only very thin connective tissue membrane on the surface contacting with the metal ribbons. After the metal ribbons were removed, soft tissues and bone tissues adhered to the metal surfaces. No corrosion was found, but after 12 weeks, deposition of Fe, Cr and Si elements to a medium degree was observed in tissues surrounding the metal (Fig. 2).

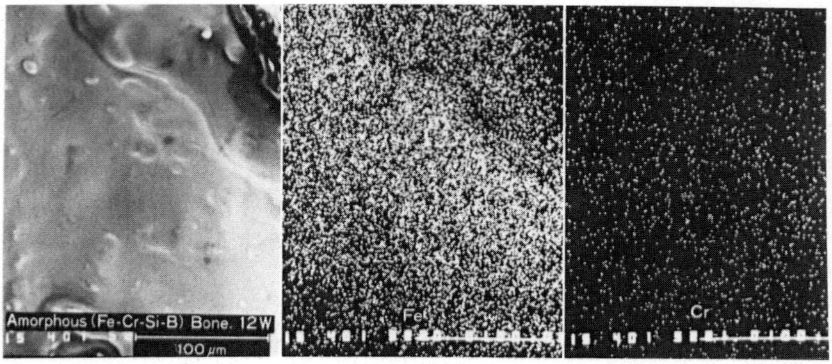

Fig. 2. Fe-Cr-Si-B group was implanted in the bone of the rabbit for 12 weeks. Deposition of Fe, Cr and Si elements was observed in tissues surrounding the metal.

When the metal ribbons of the Co-Fe-Si-B group were implanted in soft tissues, 6 weeks later a marked pathological inflammation was noticed around the metal ribbons, together with considerable cell infiltration and formation of thick connective tissue membrane as well as with necrotic tissues in some portions. When they were implanted in the bones, a very marked pathological inflammation was also quite similarly recognized. The removed metal ribbons completely lost their original shape. The SEM pictures presented conspicuous corrosion and changes into porous or sponge-like surfaces (Fig. 3). In addition, a large number of cracks were found on the surfaces. In soft tissues and bone tissues around the metal ribbons, especially in the part contacting with the bones, a large amount of deposition of Co, Fe and Si elements was found (Fig. 4). The metal of the Co-Fe-Nb-Si-B group showed almost the same reactions as that of the Co-Fe-Si-B group.

When the metal ribbons of the Co-Si-B group were implanted in soft tissues and bone tissues, as in those of the Fe-Cr-Si-B group, no pathological, inflammation was noticed in surrounding tissues. The reactions in the bones were also quite the same. Furthermore, the state of the deposition into the surrounding tissues was the same, namely, Fe and Cr deposited to a medium degree.

D) Long-term reaction in physiological saline solution

(a) Method

Ribbons of (A) Co-Fe-Si-B, (B) Co-Fe-Nb-Si-B and (C) Co-Si-B in the Co

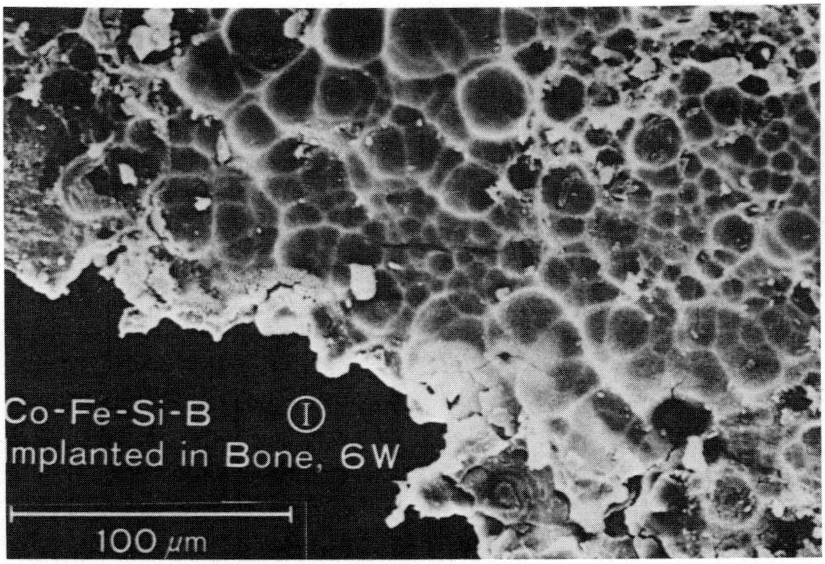

Fig. 3. Co-Fe-Si-B group was implanted in the bone of the rabbit for 6 weeks. The implanted metals completely lost their original shape. (SEM).

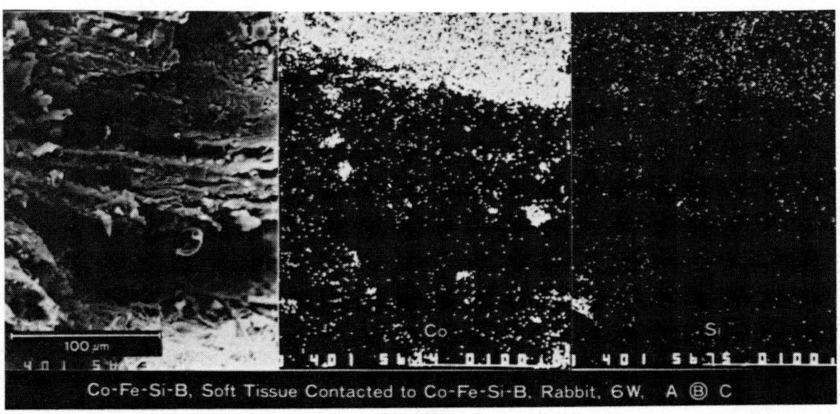

Fig. 4. Co-Fe-Si-B group was implanted in the soft tissues and the bone of the rabbit for 6 weeks. Deposition of Co, Fe and Si elements was found in tissues surrounding the metal.

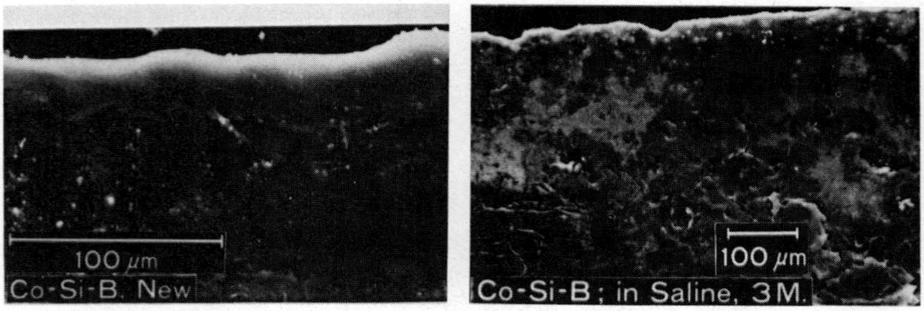

(a) (b)

Fig. 5. Co-Si-B in the Co group was allowed to stand in a physiological saline solution for 3 months. (a) is before the test and (b) is after the test. (SEM)

group were allowed to stand in a physiological saline solution at room temperature for 3 months and then their surfaces were observed by SEM.

(b) Results

Foreign matter was found to adhere to the Co-Si-B surface (Fig. 5 (a)(b)), but neither corrosion nor change in shape was noticed. On the surface of Co-Fe-Si-B and Co-Fe-Nb-Si-B, membrane was formed and the cracks and exfoliation of the membrane were found when the samples were prepared, but no corrosion was observed.

DISCUSSION

Amorphous metal has very good corrosion resistance in vitro. Its wire is about 4 times stronger than the SUS 316 wire, having very excellent wire properties in vitro. However, the amorphous metal we used showed in vivo reactions quite different from those in vitro. Deposition of metallic elements as well as very marked corrosion in particular cases started early.

We found that they were unique reactions of non-crystaloid amorphous metal which was different from the usual crystalloid metal.

REFERENCES

1 Oonishi, H. et al: Application of amorphous metallic wire as biomaterials to orthopaedic surgery —— the 1st report ——, the 58th Congress of Japanese Orthopaedic Surgery, 1985.
2 Oonishi, H. et al: Application of amorphous metallic wire as biomaterials to orthopaedic surgery —— the 2nd report ——, the 7th Congress of Japanese Society for Biomaterials, 1985.

Biomaterials and Clinical Applications,
edited by A. Pizzoferrato, P.G. Marchetti, A. Ravaglioli and A.J.C. Lee
Elsevier Science Publishers B.V., Amsterdam, 1987 — Printed in The Netherlands

TISSUE OR CELL CULTURE VERSUS IN VIVO TESTING OF SURFACE-REACTIVE BIOMATERIALS

U.GROSS, H.-J. SCHMITZ, R.KINNE, F.R.FENDLER, V.STRUNZ*

Institute of Pathology and Department of Maxillo-Facial and Plastic Surgery*, Klinikum Steglitz, Freie Universität Berlin, Hindenburgdamm 30, D 1000 Berlin 45, FRG

ABSTRACT

Tissue and cell culture test methods were assessed and compared with in vivo testing of two surface-reactive biomaterials: bone-bonding glass-ceramic KG Cera and non-bonding glass KG y 213. For tissue and cell culture tests, primary and first passage fetal rat calvaria osteoblasts were applied. Blocks of bone-bonding and non-bonding materials were implanted into the femur of adult male Sprague-Dawley rats and evaluated histologically and immuno- histologically.

The in vitro growth and multiplication pattern of osteoblasts revealed better results for the non-bonding material KG y 213 than for the bone-bonding material KG Cera. In vivo results showed well-known bone-bonding of KG Cera and non-bonding of KG y 213. Exclusive testing in vitro would have banned the bone-bonding material KG Cera and favored the non-bonding material KG y 213. Therefore exclusive in vitro testing of surface-reactive biomaterials for bone or tooth replacement must be avoided, and animal studies are indispensable.

INTRODUCTION

Cell culture test methods are widely used in assessment of medical devices by manufacturers. There exist different methods applicable for short-term evaluation of medical devices, e.g. direct-contact cell-culture method (ref.1, 2), agar diffusion method (ref.3), flask dilution method (ref.3). Some standardization of these methods was achieved (ref.4,5). The results obtained with these methods were rated in score systems or otherwise quantified (ref.1,2,3,6). Their reliability was compared with in vivo tests (ref.7.8) in which the material being tested in vitro was implanted into soft tissue and histologically evaluated. In vitro tests were found to be quickly performable, as reliable as in vivo tests and much cheaper. All these methods were established to assess cytotoxicity or biocompatibility of the materials. Therefore any material displaying cytopathogenic effects in vitro was banned from use in patients.

The principal question of this study is: can tissue or cell-culture test methods replace in vivo testing procedures if surface-reactive biomaterials are considered which are intended for replacement of bone or teeth? The problem evolved when Hench showed that some composition of glasses or glass-ceramics are bonded to bone (ref. 9,10), which was contrary to the accepted view in general pathology that every foreign body elicits a reaction resulting in demarcation and/or sequestration from the living system of an individual.

The use of cell lines derived from fibroblasts, lung cells, tumor cells or epithelia was proposed for cell culture test methods (ref.11). But since these cell lines were not considered to be closely enough related to the problem, osteoblasts were used in this study. Some support for this decision was given by studies in which, among other cell lines, osteoblasts were also used successfully in in-vitro tests of different substrates (ref.12). The materials used in this study were known to belong to the bone-bonding and non-bonding categories (ref.13).

MATERIALS AND METHODS

The bone-bonding material was glass-ceramic KG Cera (composition in wt%: SiO_2 46.2, $Ca(PO_3)_2$ 25.5, Na_2O 4.8, K_2O 0.4, MgO 2.9, CaO 20.2). The non-bonding material was KG y 213 (composition in wt%: SiO_2 38, $Ca(PO_3)_2$ 13.5, Na_2O 4, CaO 31, Al_2O_3 7, Ta_2O_5 5.5, TiO_2 1). Rectangular discs (10 x 10 x 0.5 mm) were used for tissue culture and rectangular blocks (1.1 x 1.1 x 4 mm) with a surface roughness below 10 /um for implantation. Sterilization was done by dry heat.

TISSUE AND CELL CULTURES

Osteoblasts were prepared from the calvaria of 15 - 18-day-old fetal rats (ref. 14). Culture medium was minimum essential medium (MEM) Eagle, L-glutamine (5 ml/500 ml medium), 10 % fetal bovine serum, 100 units of penicillin and 50 /ug/ml of streptomycin. In additional experiments, a medium favorable for calcification was used with 20 % fetal bovine serum, 50 /ug/ml fresh ascorbic acid and 10 mM ß-glycerol phosphate (ref. 15).

For primary cultures the carefully minced bone chips from rat calvaria were transferred to plastic culture dishes (diameter 35 mm, depth 10 mm) (Falcon) on glass or glass-ceramic discs mounted on inert thermanox plates.

For first-passage cultures, the osteoblasts were collected from tissue culture flasks with 0.25 % calcium-free trypsin in phosphate buffer solution (PBS) after 30 minutes at 37° C; the suspension was centrifuged with 600 g at 4° C for 16 minutes and the sediment resuspended in 10 ml of the culture medium with 10 % fetal bovine serum, counted and diluted to 10^5 cells/ml. Then 4 ml of the cell suspension were seeded in 35 mm culture dishes on the substratum and the discs mounted on thermanox plates. The control's substratum was thermanox. Incubation was at 37° C and 4.8 % CO_2 with over 90 % relative humidity.

In a first and second experiment, the incubation time was 24, 48, 72 hours and 7, 14, 21 days respectively. For each time period, 10 culture dishes were prepared. After incubation, the dishes were rinsed three times with Eagle's medium, the cells fixed in Carnoy's solution and stained with hemalum and eosin for light-microscopic evaluation. Cell counting was done with an ocular net at sites with a maximum density of cells on the substrate's thermanox (control), on KG Cera and KG y 213 and the thermanox in the surroundings of the substrates. In a parallel experiment, osteoblasts were removed from the KG Cera discs, the KG y 213 discs and the thermanox plates by incubation at 37° C for 30 minutes in 5 ml PBS solution containing 0.25 % trypsin . After this incubation, the substrates were free of adherent cells. The cell suspension was measured in a Coulter Counter for particles larger than 10 /um in diameter. Two cultures of each time interval were prepared for scanning electron microscopy (SEM), rinsed with MEM, fixed for 30 minutes in 3 % glutaraldehyde in 0.02 M TES buffer solution (N-tris (hydroxymethyl) methyl-2-aminoethanesulfonic acid), pH 7.4, dried with the critical point method and sputtered with gold-platinum for SEM with a Philips SEM 505.

IN VIVO STUDIES

Rectangular blocks of KG Cera and KG y 213 were implanted bilaterally into the femur of adult male Sprague-Dawley rats, collected after 7, 14, 21 and 28 days postoperatively and processed for light-microscopic evaluation as described (ref.16). Some specimens were perfused with Zamboni solution for fixation, embedded in Spurr's resin, cut in semithin sections, deplastified with sodium methylate and analysed immunohistochemically with the APAAP-method (ref.17). The rabbit antibodies were against fibronectin, procollagen I, collagen I, collagen II, procollagen III, proteoglycan, bone sialoprotein and bovine osteonectin.

RESULTS AND DISCUSSION

In two independent experiments, first-passage osteoblasts were determined quantitatively 1, 2, 3, 7, 14 and 21 days after seeding, and the results were similar. Osteoblasts multiplied best on the inert substratum. Thermanox was used as a control (Table 1). Their multiplication was more inhibited on the surface-reactive substrate KG Cera than on the less surface-reactive and less soluble substrate KG y 213. Osteoblasts were found in fewer numbers on the inert substrate thermanox in the surroundings of the surface-reactive materials KG Cera and KG y 213 than on the thermanox used as a control (numbers not given). In the medium, the highest cell counts were observed in culture dishes with KG Cera; the lowest cell counts were in the thermanox-containing dishes, and the cell counts in dishes with KG y 213 were intermediate (numbers not given). These findings indicate that some unknown factors were released from the two materials inhibiting cell multiplication on the substrates and in the adjacent area.

The morphology of osteoblasts in culture was described (ref. 18) and found to be dependent on density of the cell layer and on time. They lacked preferential arrangement on smooth surfaces (controls) but were aligned with grooves parallel on structured surfaces (Fig. 1,2). This behavior was found on the substrates KG Cera and KG y 213. Osteoblasts displayed long cell processes which were in contact (Fig. 1,5). The processes were flattened on surfaces where they adhered (Fig. 3-6). Fibronectin was demonstrated at the surface of the cell processes with different methods. There were small microvilli-like projections on the osteoblast surface (Fig. 1,4), as shown by others (ref.19). Expression of alkaline phosphatase, fibronectin, collagen type I and matrix vesicles was demonstrated in osteoblast cultures (ref. 18). Osteoblasts cultured on KG y 213 showed a tendency to develop slim cell processes (Fig. 2,4) whereas those on KG Cera were more flat or rounded (Fig. 3,5). In old cultures on KG Cera, osteoblasts were more oval and rounded than elongated and rather flat (Fig. 3). They rarely showed the above-mentioned small microvilli-like projections at the surface. In some of the first-passage osteoblast cultures and more often in the primary cultures, osteoblasts formed multilayers in small humps (Fig. 7), and staining with von Kossa suggested spots of mineralization in the humps. This phenomenon was more often observed on KG Cera as substrate than on KG y 213. Similar humps have been described and demonstrated (ref. 12).

These data from cell culture tests could be interpreted in the sense that the bone-bonding glass ceramic KG Cera was not as effective and biocompatible as the less soluble and less surface-reactive glass KG y 213. In vivo implantation of the two materials, however, repeatedly yielded strong evidence histomorphologically and morphometrically that KG Cera was bonded to bone, whereas KG y 213 was not (ref.13). Besides, biomechanical tests for tensile strength of the interface between bone and glass-ceramic KG Cera yielded up to 2.4 N/mm^2, 56 days after implantation into the femur of rabbits (ref.20). Therefore there are abundant data in favor of the bone-bonding material KG Cera and data indicating that materials like KG y 213 are not applicable for bone-bonding implants.

The reason for bone bonding is not yet fully clear. Comparison of the expression of fibronectin, procollagen I, collagen I, procollagen III, bone proteoglycan and bone sialoprotein at the interface of the bone-bonding material KG Cera and the non-bonding material KG y 213 did not reveal convincing differences in in-vivo studies 7, 14, 21 and 28 days postoperatively. There was, however, at the interface of KG y 213 a seam of non-mineralized tissue, osteoid or chondroid, indicating that the mineralization was inhibited. One reason for inhibited mineralization at the interface of glass KG y 213 could be the release of aluminum ions from the surface. Three days after osteoblast culture on KG y 213 discs, the culture medium contained 3.1 /uM/l aluminum, which is above the normal serum level of aluminum in humans, whereas the culture medium of KG Cera discs 3 days in culture showed only 0.8 /uM/l aluminum, as determined by atom-absorption spectroscopy. Aluminum ions were made responsible for considerable reduction of the crystallite size of apatite (ref. 21). It can be assumed that this effect of aluminum leaching from the surface of KG y 213 implants was also operative in the in vivo condition.

The conventional staining of cultures on the bone bonding material KG Cera revealed some necrotic cells among living cells with intact stainability of nuclei. The areas in which dead cells were situated displayed different degrees of substrate stainability, indicating some remnants of cells or cellular products. Considering the results of prior electron-microscopic studies of the interface, in which a more electron-dense seam was demonstrated at the interface (ref. 16), it can be speculated that the deposition of cellular material at the interface of bone-bonding glass or glass-ceramic favors the adhesion and function of osteoblasts and the bonding mechanism. There was some experimental support for this view: the precoating of bioglass with fibronectin favored the speading of cells and their attachment in-vitro (ref. 22).

What were the causes of the different results after in-vitro and in-vivo testing of surface-reactive materials? Up to now, it seemed that the tissue and cell culture conditions were more or less static with regard to both the cellular and the material response. The in vivo conditions, on the other hand, were more dynamic: there was a sequence of events in which the surgical trauma was followed by blood clotting and exudation, the development of organization tissue and tissue regeneration, the interaction of various cell lines capable of proliferation, differentiation and adaption to the implant function. The material response in in-vivo conditions cannot be static, there must be fluid turnover and transport phenomena from ions released from the surface being resorbed and excreted or deposited in the surroundings of the implant or in distant sites, in remote organs. Besides, the biomechanical situation must be different in-vitro and in-vivo. In-vitro, no biomechanical effects can be assumed. In-vivo static or dynamic load conditions can be expected to exert their influence on cell and tissue behavior.

Therefore in-vitro testing of surface reactive biomaterials cannot adequately reflect all aspects operative in-vivo. Thus in-vitro testing of surface reactive biomaterials is not a reliable method, and not the method of choice. Animal studies are indispensable for testing of surface-reactive biomaterials intended for bone or tooth replacement.

TABLE 1

Number of first-passage osteoblasts x 1000 ± SEM / cm^2 of substrates counted in a Coulter Counter.

days	KG Cera	KG y 213	Control
1	5.6 ± 0.4	4.8 ± 0.3	11.3 ± 0.3
2	7.8 ± 0.6	13.2 ± 0.5	12.7 ± 0.2
3	8.9 ± 0.7	8.9 ± 0.4	18.3 ± 1.1
7	64.2 ± 5.6	88.7 ± 8.6	73.0 ± 4.8
14	74.3 ± 7.5	79.9 ± 6.1	85.0 ± 4.6
21	44.1 ± 3.6	47.2 ± 6.6	57.2 ± 13.2

Fig.1. Osteoblasts 1 day after seeding on KG Cera. Alignment of the osteoblasts parallel with the grooves of the substrate. SEM. Bar 10 /um.

Fig.2. Osteoblasts 1 day in culture on KG y 213. Irregular surface structure and no preferential orientation of cells. SEM. Bar 50 /um.

Fig.3. Osteoblasts rounded and without pronounced surface structure 7 days in culture on KG Cera. SEM. Bar 5 /um.

Fig.4. Osteoblasts with microvilli-like surface projections and slim cell processes 7 days in culture on KG y 213. SEM. Bar 5 /um.

Fig.5. Elongated and rounded osteoblasts 14 days in culture on KG Cera. SEM. Bar 5 /um.

Fig.6. Flattened osteoblasts 14 days in culture on KG y 213. SEM. Bar 5 /um.

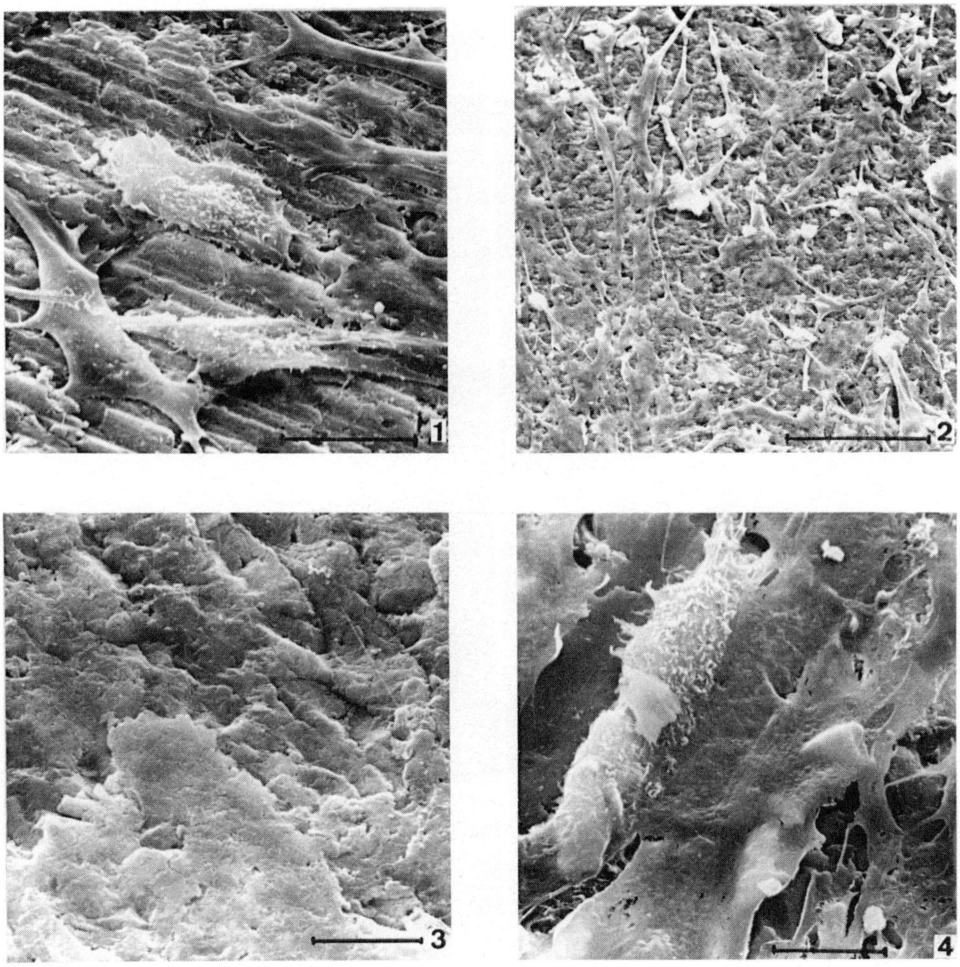
1
2
3
4
5
6

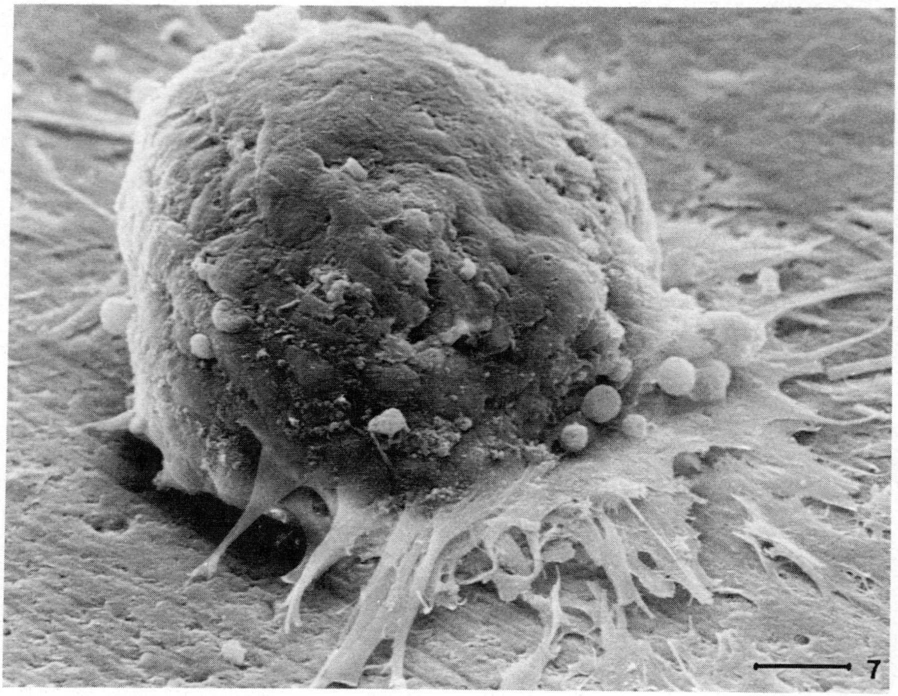

Fig.7. Hump of osteoblasts in a primary culture 14 days after seeding on KG Cera. SEM. Bar 16 /um.

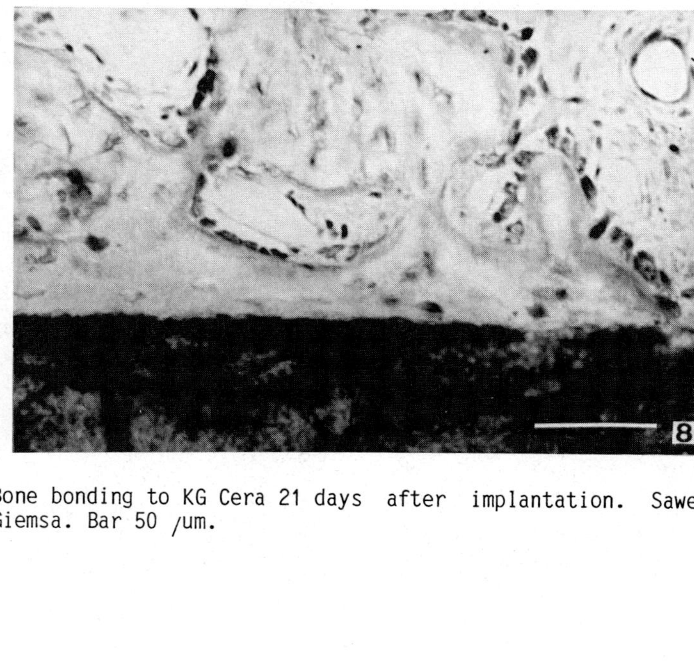

Fig.8. Bone bonding to KG Cera 21 days after implantation. Sawed section. Giemsa. Bar 50 /um.

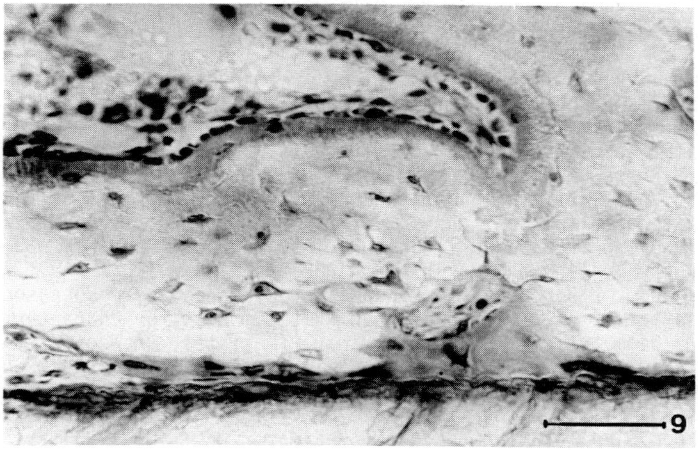

Fig.9. Seam of non-mineralized tissue at the interface of KG y 213 21 days after implantation. Sawed section. Giemsa. Bar 50 /um.

ACKNOWLEDGEMENTS

This study was supported by grant 01 ZQ 110 of the Ministry for Research and Technology, Bonn, FRG. Materials were supplied by E.Leitz Wetzlar, 6330 Wetzlar, FRG.

REFERENCES

1 L.M.Smith, Direct-contact cell-culture method, in: S.A.Brown (Ed.), Cell -Culture Test Methods, ASTM STP 810, American Society for Testing and Materials, Piladelphia, 1983, pp. 5 - 11.

2 L.M.Ettore, K.Phillips, Test method for human cell-culture elution to evaluate medical materials and devices for cytotoxicity, in: S.A.Brown (Ed.), Cell-Culture Test Methods, ASTM STP 810, American Society for Testing and Materials, Philadelphia, 1983, pp. 12 - 18.

3 H.J.Johnson, S.J.Northup, Tissue-culture biocompatibility testing program, in: S.A.Brown (Ed.), Cell-Culture Test Methods, ASTM STP 810, American Society for Testing and Materials, Philadelphia, 1983, pp. 25 - 34.

4 Designation: F 813-83, Standard practice for direct contact cell-culture evaluation of materials for medical devices, American Society for Testing and Materials, Philadelphia, 1983.

5 Fédêration dentaire international, J.W.Stanford, Int.Dent.J.30 (1980) 140 - 188.

6 C.R.Horres, H.G.Mears, R.E.Wilsnack, G.E.Moore, Evaluation of materials used for the fabrication of medical devices: cytotoxicity testing, in: S.A.Brown (Ed.), Cell Culture Test Methods, ASTM STP 810, American Society for Testing and Materials, Philadelphia, 1983, pp. 35 - 50.

7 E.O.Dillingham, Primary acute toxicity screen for biomaterials: rationale, in vitro / in vivo relationship and interlaboratory performance, in: S.A.Brown (Ed.), ASTM STP 810, American Society for Testing and Materials, Philadelphia, 1983, pp. 51 - 70.

8 T.F.Genova, S.Bodnar, M.Vaccarella, C.Stafford, K.M.Schady, Cytotoxicity Testing: Prediction of in vivo toxicity from in vitro tests, in: S.A.Brown (Ed.), Cell Culture Test Methods, ASTM STP 810, American Society for Testing and Materials, Philadelphia, 1983, pp. 71 - 76.

9 L.L.Hench, R.J.Splinter, W.C.Allen, T.K.Greenlee, Bonding mechanisms at the interface of ceramic prosthetic materials, J.Biomed.Mater.Res. Symp. 2 (1971) 117 - 141.

10 L.L.Hench, E.C.Ethridge, Biomaterials, an Interfacial Approach, Academic Press, New York-London 1982.

11 R.J.Hay, Availability and standardization of cell lines at the american type culture collection: current status and prospects for the future, in: S.A.Brown (Ed.), Cell Culture Test Methods, ASTM STP 810, American Society for Testing and Materials, 1983, pp. 114 - 126.

12 M.F.Harmand, L.Bordenave, R.Duphil, R.Jeandot, D.Ducassou, Human differentiated cell cultures: in vitro models for characterization of cell / biomaterial interface, in: P.Christel, A.Meunier, A.J.C.Lee (Eds.) Biological and Biomechanical Performance of Biomaterials, Elsevier, Amsterdam, 1986, pp. 361 - 366

13 U.Gross, V.Strunz, The interface of various glasses and glass ceramics with a bony implantation bed, J.Biomed.Mater.Res. 19 (1985) 251 - 271.

14 I.Bindermann, D.Duksin, A.Harell, E.Katzir, L.Sachs, Formation of bone tissue from isolated bone cells, J.Cell Biol.61 (1974) 427 - 439.

15 P.G.Robey, J.D.Termine, Human bone cells in vitro, Calcif.Tissue internat. 37 (1985) 453- 460.

16 U.Gross, J.Brandes, V.Strunz, I.Bab, J.Sela, The ultrastructure of the interface between a glass ceramic and bone, J.Biomed.Mater.Res. 15 (1981) 291 - 305.

17 J.L.Cordell, B.Falini, W.N.Erber, A.K.Gosh, Z.Abdulaziz, S.MacDonalds, K.A.F.Pulford, H.Stein, D.Y.Mason, Immunoenzymatic labelling of monoclonal antialkaline phosphatase, J.Histochem.Cytochem. 32 (1984) 219 - 229.

18 W.Roggendorf, V.Strunz, U.Gross, Osteoblasten-Zellkulturen, ein Modell zur Testung von Biomaterialien, Zschr.zahnärztl.Implantol. (1986) in press.

19 A.Boyde, S.J.Jones, Bone modelling in the implantation bed, J.Biomed.Mater.Res. 19 (1985) 199 - 224.

20 U.Gross, W.Roggendorf, H.-J.Schmitz, V.Strunz, Biomechanical and morphometric testing methods for porous and surface-reactive biomaterials, ASTM Special publication, American Society for Testing and Materials, Phildelphia, 1986, in press.

21 R.Z.LeGeros, M.H.Taheri, G.B.Quirolgico, J.P.LeGeros, in: Proc. 2nd International Congress on Phosphorus Compounds, Boston, April 21 - 25 1980, pp. 89 - 103.

22 T.L.Seitz, K.D.Noonan, L.L.Hench, N.E.Noonan, Effect of fibronectin on the adhesion of an established cell line to a surface reactive biomaterial, J.Biomed.Mater.Res. 16 (1982) 195 - 207.

Biomaterials and Clinical Applications,
edited by A. Pizzoferrato, P.G. Marchetti, A. Ravaglioli and A.J.C. Lee
Elsevier Science Publishers B.V., Amsterdam, 1987 — Printed in The Netherlands

DEVELOPMENT OF AN IN VITRO METHOD FOR ASSESSMENT OF BLOOD COMPATIBILITY OF BIOMATERIALS BASED ON QUANTITATIVE MEASUREMENTS OF THE ADHESIVENESS OF Cr-51-LABELLED HUMAN PLATELETS

R. KARWATH[1], M. SCHÜRER[2] and H. WOLF[1]
Humboldt University, School of Medicine (Charité),
[1]Biomaterials Research Unit and
[2]Clinic of Nuclear Medicine,
Schumannstr. 20/21, Berlin 1040, G.D.R.

SUMMARY

In this study an in vitro method for assessment of blood compatibility of biomaterial candidates was developed based on radiotracer technique suited for comparative quantitative measurements of platelet adhesiveness on artificial surfaces using human platelets and Cr-51 as nuclid. It was possible to obtain sufficient labelled human platelet suspensions, if 9.25 MBq Cr-51-sodium chromate were used for labelling of 1 ml platelet suspension containing more than 10^9 cells. The necessary well-defined conditions to perform the contact between platelets and test surfaces were achieved by means of coaxial rotation of test tubes at 0.2 rpm and 37 °C for 1 h. The "relative index of platelet adhesion" (RIPA) which relates the number of adherent platelets per unit area of a test material to the same one of a reference material (glass) was shown to be suited for quantification and comparison of test results. The sensitivity and reproducibility of method developed was demonstrated by investigation of different types of poly(vinyl chloride) and siliconized glass. The values of RIPA were found to differ significantly ($p < 0.05$) and to be in qualitative agreement with adhesion data measured by means of an independent in vitro method.

INTRODUCTION

The adhesion of blood platelets to surfaces is one of the first steps in thrombosis and hemostasis. Therefore platelet adhesiveness onto artificial surfaces is regarded to be an essential parameter for characterization of blood compatibility of biomaterials. Several in vitro methods were developed for material screening based on measurements of platelet adhesiveness. The number of adherent platelets was measured by means of optical methods, particle counting or radiotracer technique (refs. 1-5). The advantages of radiotracer technique consist in its independence of test material shape and transparency, good reproducibility of test results and relative easy performance provided that sufficient labelled platelet suspensions can be prepared without essential reduction of functional integrity of platelets. This was achieved so far for bovine and rabbit platelets using Cr-51 as radiotracer (refs. 4-5). Because there are essential differences in platelet function between animal and human platelets (ref. 6) the application of human platelets should be prefered for biomaterial assessment.

It was the aim of this study to develop an in vitro test procedure based on radiotracer technique for comparative quantitative measurements of platelet adhesiveness on artificial surfaces using human platelets and Cr-51 as nuclid.

MATERIALS AND METHODS

Blood was collected from healthy donors. Sodium citrate (3.8 %) and ACD-solution (Acid. citric, 6.6 g, Natr. citric. 18.5 g, Glucos. dep. 20.0 g, Aqua ad inj. ad 1000 ml) were used as anticoagulants. Cr-51 sodium chromate (3400 GBq/ g Cr, Isocommerz, G.D.R.) was used for labelling of platelets. Gamma-radiation was measured by means of a gamma sample handler (type GAMMASZINT BF 5300, Berthold, F.R.G.). The number of platelets in platelet rich plasma (PRP) was counted using a particle counter (type LABORSCALE, Medicor, Hungary).

Tubes of 5 mm inner diameter and 20 mm length of siliconized glass and two types (KWR or FA) of poly(vinyl chloride) (PVC) were used as test surfaces. Bare glass tubes (type ILMGLASS) served as reference surfaces.

RESULTS AND DISCUSSION

Labelling procedure

Starting from the question, wether Cr-51 is a suitable radiotracer to bind a sufficient activity on a sufficient high number of human platelets, at first the conditions for platelet preparation and labelling were investigated. Labelling and platelet yield were measured under different conditions of cell preparation and labelling. We found that citrated blood (1:10) has to be used for the preparation of platelets. PRP was obtained from 20 ml citrated blood by centrifugation at 200 g for 10 min. The pH of PRP was adjusted with ACD-solution to 6.5. After centrifugation at 2000 g for 12 min platelets were resuspended

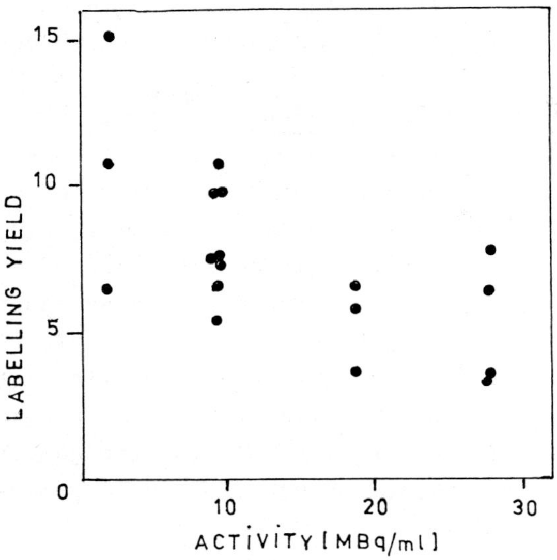

Fig. 1. Labelling yield in dependence on used activity of Cr-51-sodium chromate for labelling of platelet concentrates.

in platelet poor plasma (PPP) with physiological pH. After that the concentrated platelet suspension was incubated with Cr-51-sodium chromate for 30 min at 37 °C. After incubation ascorbic acid (2 mg/ml) was added to stop the labelling and then ACD-solution was added to adjust the pH to 6.5. After centrifugation at 2000 g for 12 min the platelets were resuspended in PPP.

In Fig. 1 the found dependence of labelling yield on used activities is shown. From the results in Fig. 1 it was concluded that sufficient labelling results can be obtained, if approx. 9.25 MBq Cr-51-sodium chromate in 1 ml platelet suspension containing more than 10^9 platelets are used. The mean ratio between platelet bound activity and platelet count was found to be 360 Bq/10^6 pt.

The functional integrity of Cr-51-labelled platelets was checked by means of measurements of ADP-induced aggregation with 5 μM ADP in the platelet suspension. In comparison with non-labelled platelet suspension only a slight decrease of aggregability was found which was in agreement with corresponding data in literature (ref. 7). From these results it was concluded that the Cr-51-labelled platelets are in such a functional state that their application in adhesion studies should be possible.

In vitro method for assessment of platelet adhesion

Before contact with test surfaces the number of Cr-51-labelled platelets in the suspensions was measured by means of a particle counter. After that the Cr-51-labelled platelet suspensions were filled into the test tubes avoiding formation of air bubbles and closed with siliconized glass stoppers. The necessary well-defined conditions to perform the contact between platelets and test surfaces were achieved by means of slow coaxial rotation of test tubes at 0.2 rpm and 37 °C for 1 h. After rinsing the test tubes with physiological saline solution the number of adherent platelets was determined by means of their gamma-radiation.

Quantification of test results

In Fig. 2 the results are given for the number of adherent platelets on different surfaces. The highest platelet adhesiveness was measured for bare glass, the lowest one for PVC, type FA. Additionally it was found that the platelet adhesiveness at one and the same material depends on both, platelet concentration in PRP and donor of blood. Therefore it was necessary to introduce a normalized parameter, which allows the quantitative comparsion of several tests. As such a parameter the "relative index of platelet adhesion" (RIPA) was shown to be suited (ref. 4), which relates the number of adherent platelets per unit area of a test surface to the same one of a reference surface (eqn 1). In our experiments bare glass was chosen as reference surface.

$$\text{RIPA} = \frac{\text{counts at test surface}}{\text{counts at reference surface}} \qquad (1)$$

Fig. 3 represents the values of RIPA for the materials used in this study. The values are found to differ significantly ($p < 0.05$) and to be in qualitative agreement with adhesion data obtained by us for the same materials applying an independent in vitro method (ref. 8). As the results in Fig. 3 demonstrate

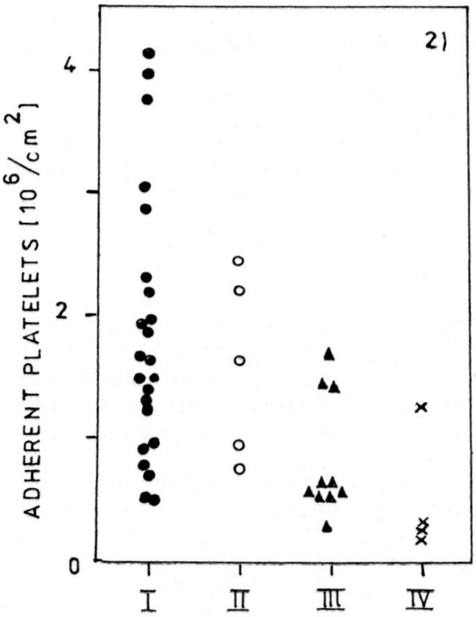

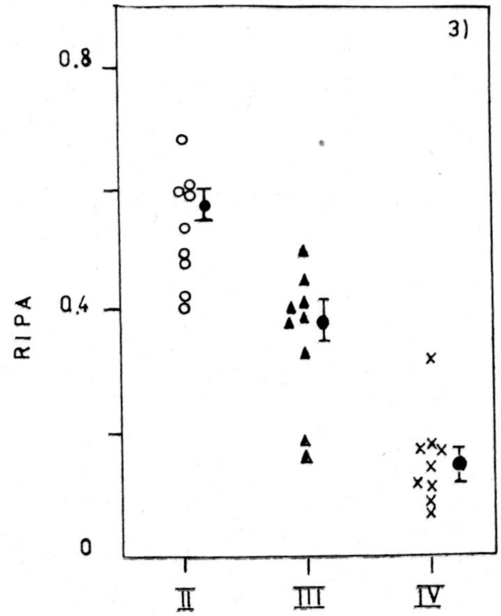

Fig. 2. Number of adherent platelets onto different surfaces: I - glass; II - siliconized glass; III - poly(vinyl chloride), type KWR; IV - poly(vinyl chloride), type FA.

Fig. 3. Individual values and means ± S.E.M. of "relative indices of platelet adhesion" (RIPA) of test surfaces calculated from data in Fig. 2 (reference surface: glass).

the method developed allows also to discriminate between different types of one polymer, i.e., the sensitivity and the precision of method are high enough to be applied as screening method for material selection.

CONCLUSIONS

This study has demonstrated that the problem of radioactive labelling of suspensions of human platelets to obtain a sufficient high number of sufficient labelled cells can be solved by use of Cr-51 as nuclid. These Cr-51-labelled platelet suspensions were shown to be suited for an easy and sensitive test procedure developed for comparative assessment of blood compatibility of biomaterial candidates based on quantitative measurements of platelet adhesiveness.

ACKNOWLEDGEMENTS

We are grateful to Mrs. Dr. S. Ziemer (Institute of Pathological and Clinical Biochemistry) for support in measuring the ADP-induced platelet aggregation and for helpful discussions.

This work was supported by HFR "Artificial Organs and Biomaterials" of Ministry of Health of G.D.R.

REFERENCES

1 O.S. Hum, D.N. Ghista and J.L. Brash, Thrombogenetic studies of bioprosthetic heart valve surfaces. I. In vitro platelet adhesion in a static system, Thromb. Res., 38 (1985) 163-172.
2 D.J. Magilligan, C. Oyama, S. Klein, J.M. Riddle and D. Smith, Platelet adherence to bioprosthetic cardiac valves, Am. J. Cardiol., 53 (1984) 945-949.
3 K. Dolowy and L.W. Cunningham, Adhesion of human platelets to collagen: Evidence for two states of platelet activation, Collagen Rel. Res., 4 (1984) 111-118.
4 V.I. Sevastianov, Z.M. Belomestnaia and N.K. Zimin, In vitro assessment of the hemocompatible properties of polymers, Artif. Organs, 7 (1983) 126-133.
5 R. Thiele, Ch. Grosse-Siestrup, V. Unger, W. Lemm, P. Bensch and E.S. Bücherl, Platelet adhesion from platelet rich blood to polyurethane and silicone surfaces before and after protein coating, Proc. Eur. Soc. Artif. Org., 7 (1980) 80.
6 W. Zingg and B.S. Leibel, Modification of platelet adhesion by antiplatelet drugs helps prevent cardiovascular complications of diabetes mellitus, Med. Hypotheses, 18 (1985) 119-127
7 W.A.L. Heaton, Indium-111 (^{111}In) and Chromium-51 (^{51}Cr) labeling of platelets. Are they comparable?, Transfusion, 26 (1986) 16-19.
8 R. Karwath and H. Wolf, A modification of an in vitro method for assessment of blood compatibility, Adv. in Biomaterials, Vol. 6, Elsevier, Amsterdam, in press.

Biomaterials and Clinical Applications,
edited by A. Pizzoferrato, P.G. Marchetti, A. Ravaglioli and A.J.C. Lee
Elsevier Science Publishers B.V., Amsterdam, 1987 — Printed in The Netherlands

BIOCOMPATIBILITY OF DIFFERENT BIOACTIVE GLASSES FOR COATING METALLIC PROSTHESES IN RELATION TO CELL ADHESION MECHANISMS

M. CANNAS[1], M.R. AMEDEO[1], A. KRAJEWSKI[2] and A. RAVAGLIOLI[2]

[1]Dept. Human Anatomy and Physiology, University of Torino, C.so M. D'Azeglio 52, 10126 Torino

[2]Research Institute for Ceramics Technology of CNR, Via Granarolo n.64, 48018 Faenza

SUMMARY

Some bioactive glasses that have proved to be useful in coating 316L steel, with a special kind of doping agent, have been developed. The interface compatibility of such glasses in cell culture was tested. Fibronectin adsorption values of the three materials were also determined.

INTRODUCTION

From the initial studies, bioactive glasses are proposed as suitable materials for implants, thanks to their good biocompatibility, although their mechanical properties are rather poor. Scanning and trasmission electron microscope studies of ceramic bone interface demonstrated intimate bonding between glass-ceramics and bone, as well as a seam of partially ossified osteoid, interpreted as enhanced ossification of unmineralized tissue at the interface (ref. 1). A combination of ceramics and metal results in a good compromise for some applications; this is the case of bioactive glass coating a metallic prosthesis. For this combination we developed some bioactive glass materials that proved usuful to coat 316L steel, with special kind of doping (ref. 2). The addition used to modify the bonding properties of the bioactive glass to the metal of particular interest is the Fe_2O_3, in different concentrations. The coating procedure involves ionic diffusion and redox processes in which nickel and iron are in competition with each other for oxidation. This process may be decisive in the biological phase of adhesion, involving cells and proteins, as the doping agents consist in the addition of particular oxides, known in the glasses industry as favouring the linking the metallic support and the glass.

As the knowledge of the behaviour of cells at the tissue-material interface is essential to establish the tissue biocompatibility of materials, we have tested a "base" bioactive glass (from Hench 45S, 1, cit.) and one of the vitreous compositions for prosthetic metallic alloys, called AKRA 15, showing a good adhesion to the metal. The hystological behaviour of this composition was tested and previously published (ref. 3).

A second experimental phase regards the fibronectin (FN) binding test, a radioimmunological method able to quantify the ability of materials to act as substrate for FN. FN is a glycoprotein of cell surfaces and blood involved in cell-to-substratum interaction (ref. 4); on its capacity to link a surface depends the cellular behaviour on the same surface.

MATERIALS AND METHODS

In this study we have used Baby Hamster Kidney (BHK) cells, subcultured in Dulbecco's Modified Eagle medium (DMEM). Metabolic labeling of cells was carried out by incubating sub-confluent cells as described in Cannas et al. (ref. 5). Adherent cells were quantified by measuring the amount of biomaterial-bound radioactivity.

Fibronectin (FN) was purified from human plasma by affinity chromatography on denatured collagen. The final protein was 95% pure, as judged by SDS acrylamide gel electrophoresis. For coating with FN the biomaterials were incubated in sodium phosphate buffer pH 7.4 (PBS) containing 50 mcl/ml of the purified FN. Samples were then incubated with a dilution (1/500) of anti-FN in PBS. The amount of antigen-antibody complex was determined with 125-I-Labeled Staphylococcus protein A, and the radioactivity was expressed as c.p.m./mm squared of surface.

RESULTS

The results on BHK adhesion are shown in Fig. 1. The data is the result of counting particle emission for ten minutes and as units of counts per minute (c.p.m.). Bars represent standard error (S.E.). Controls were done with carbon fibres (Howmedica Corp.), a material that domonstrated a very good cell adhesion in all our preliminary experiments. Two experiments were done with samples in quadruplicate. As it is possible to observe, AKRA appears to have a highest number of adherent cells in respect to the "base" glass, with a

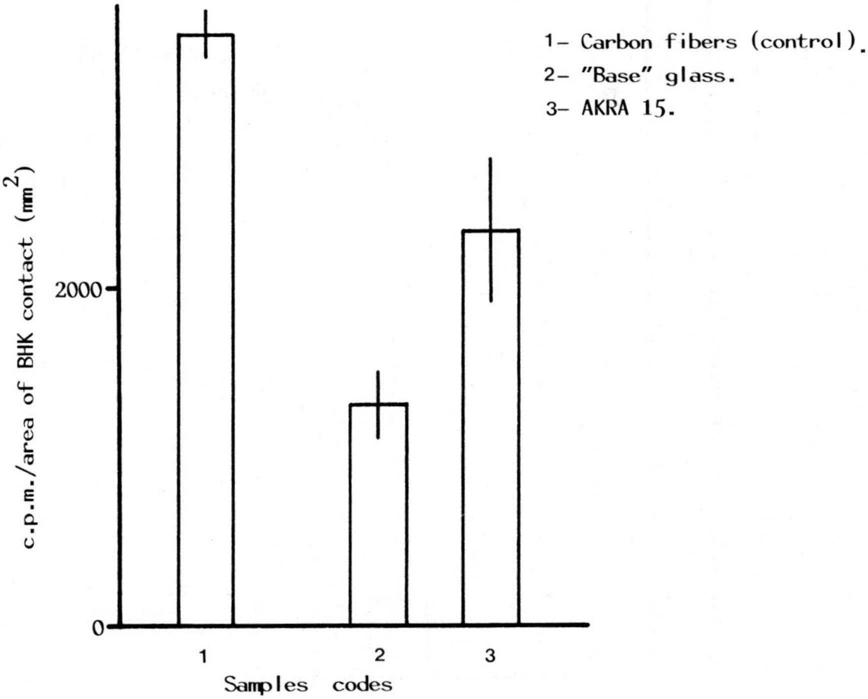

Fig. 1. Adhesion of BHK cells to Biomaterials. See test for explanation.

significant difference.

The result on Fibronectin adsorption is presented in Fig. 2. Data ara expressed as c.p.m. of 125-I/area of fibronectin adsorption. The "Base" glass shows a highest capacity to link fibronectin respect to AKRA, but the difference is not significant. Controls are the same as in the previous experiment.

DISCUSSION

Mechanisms for biocompatibility are different and tests in vitro are not able to predict the complete response to materials in human. In every case they permit us to define some characteristics of a new material.

During preliminary experiments involving three types of AKRA bioactive glass and a biological glass, doped with different agents in order to improve its adherence to the metal surface of steel prostheses, it was evident that silicon release ends and reaches a steady concentration after about 270 days (ref. 6). This was observed after the immersion in a biological simulating solution.

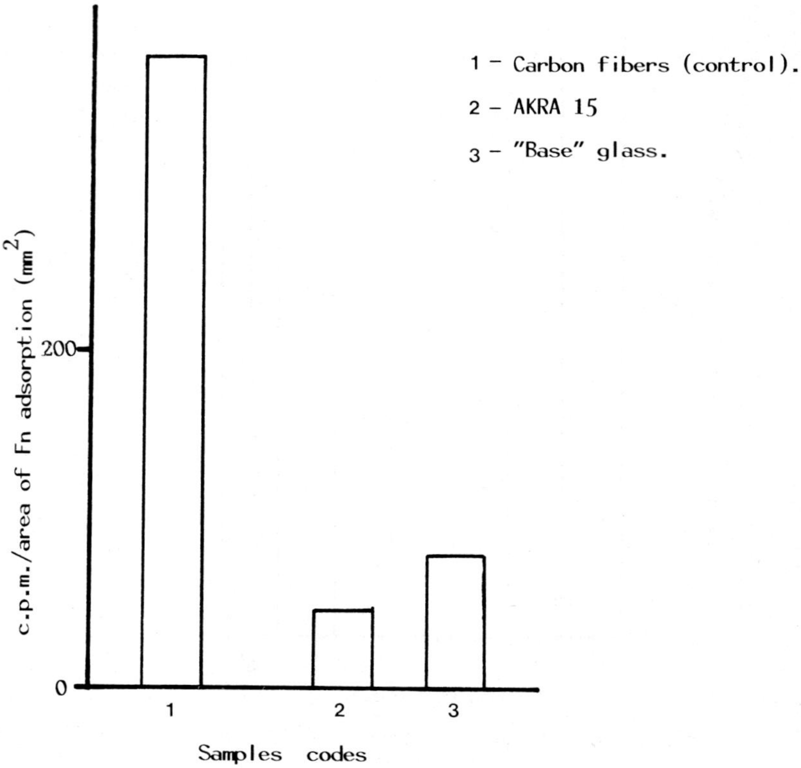

Fig. 2. Adsorption of fibronectin on Biomaterials. See test for explanation.

The surface of AKRA resulted more stable than the others, and this data has importance in the evaluation of our observation on FN adsorption. In fact the initial stage of interaction between blood and tissues with foreign surfaces is the adsorption of plasma proteins, as FN. Its importance in biocompatibility may be summarized by three points: i) it has been localized during bone formation (ref. 7), ii) it contributes to the inflammatory processes (ref. 8) and iii) there is a relationship between adherence of pathogen bacteria on biomaterials and the quantity of FN deposited on the surface of the same biomaterials (ref. 9). Here we have seen the possibility for FN to link the AKRA surface, but in a quantity similar to the other glass surface. The cell adhesion on our tested materials showed differences, with a good adhesion on AKRA. This data confirms the optimum joint point at the vitreous implanted samples with the cortical bone in vivo; particularly the bone tissue ingrowth gave rise to both cortical or cancellous bone as it was needed (ref. 3).

The importance of surface free energy on fibroblast spreading (ref.10) must also be considered in the discussion of the results. The increase of the iron quantity, that involves a decrease of the release rate of the analyzed ions (Calcium, Sodium, Iron, etc.) results in a different capacity of cell adhesion (data not published). As we can use different types and quantities of doping agents, we have the possibility to control partially the release rate and consequently to obtain the best biological adaptability.

The results obtained from these two tests provide a good basis for further studies directed towards improving the acceptability by part of cells of the glass surface, which in every case is in the present acceptable.

REFERENCES

1 L. L. Hench et Al., J. Biomed. Mater. Res., 2-117, 1971.
2 A. Krajewski et Al., J. Mater. Sci., 21-1625, 1986.
3 S. Contoli et Al., Ceramics in Surgery, P. Vincenzini edt., Elsevier Sci. Publ. Comp., Amsterdam, 187, 1983.
4 M.W. Mosesson et Al., Bioch. Biophys. Acta, 386-50, 1975.1.
5 M. Cannas et Al., Biomechanics: Current Interdisciplinary Research, S.M.Perren e E. Schneider edts., M. Nijhoff Publ., 2-117, 1985.
6 A. Ravaglioli et Al., Biomaterials, 7-76, 1986.
7 R.E. Weiss and H. Reddi, J. Cell Biol., 88-630, 1981.
8 B.J. Mc. Creedy, abst ASBC, 1984.
9 P.E. Vaudaux et Al., Infect. Immun. 45-768, 1984.
10 P. Van der Valk et Al., J. Biomed. Mater. Res., 17-807, 1983.

Biomaterials and Clinical Applications,
edited by A. Pizzoferrato, P.G. Marchetti, A. Ravaglioli and A.J.C. Lee
Elsevier Science Publishers B.V., Amsterdam, 1987 — Printed in The Netherlands

PHAGOCYTOSIS, ULTRASTRUCTURAL EVALUATION AND VIBRATIONAL SPECTROSCOPY OF ALUMINA-TITANIA.

A.PIZZOFERRATO[1], S.STEA[1], G. CIAPETTI[1], C. TARABUSI[1], A. RUGGERI[2], S.GUIZZARDI[2], M. MOROCUTTI[2], A. BERTOLUZZA[3], P. MONTI[3] and A. TINTI[3]

1 Centro di Ricerca per la Biocompatibilità dei Materiali da Impianto, Istituto Rizzoli, 40136 Bologna (Italy)

2 Istituto di Anatomia Umana Normale, Università di Bologna, 40126 (Italy)

3 Istituto di Chimica 'G. Ciamician', Università di Bologna, 40126 (Italy)

SUMMARY

The Authors tested the biocompatibility and the biostability of an Alumina-Titania material. They injected a suspension of the powdered material into mice peritoneal cavity. After seven days the cell population was collected,counted and maintained in vitro for 24 hours. Morphological observations were carried out by means of both optical and electron microscope.The chemico-physical structure of Alumina - Titania was characterized before and after phagocytosis by vibrational spectroscopy.

INTRODUCTION

Alumina and Titania can be used in coating orthopedic prostheses since they are characterized by high biocompatibility and biostability. To evaluate the biocompatibility of an Alumina-Titania material (Alumina 131, Metco Inc. NY, USA), a cell culture method, performed "in vivo" and "in vitro" was developed to evaluate numerical and morphological modifications of mouse macrophages after contact with alloplastic materials (ref.1).

Moreover a chemico-physical characterisation of the Alumina - Titania, before and after phagocytosis was carried out to evaluate its biostability.

MATERIALS AND METHODS

The material structure was characterized by infrared spectroscopy and X-ray diffraction techniques.

The infrared spectra were recorded with a JASCO DS 701G spectrophotometer. The spectra of powdered samples were obtained from nujol mulls on KRS5 disks, while those of the powder phagocytosed by macrophages were obtained from thin layers of cells deposited on a KRS5 disk.

The phagocytosis test was carried out by intraperitoneally injecting 10 mice with 0.5 ml of the Alumina-Titania powder suspension in saline (1 mg/ml). Intraperitoneal injection of saline was used as a control.

After seven days the exudate with macrophages was collected by peritoneal lavage and cells were counted in order to ascertain their number in each peritoneum. A sample of this suspension was then cytocentrifuged and the smear was Giemsa stained to determine the phagocytosis index and the percentage of different types of cells. The remaining suspension was 'in vitro' maintained for 24 hours and morphological observations were then carried out on the monolayer.

Beside these researches an ultrastructural investigation on the samples of cell suspension was carried out: the specimens were dehydrated in acetone and epon embedded. 800 Å thick slices were stained with uranil acetate and lead citrate.

RESULTS

The infrared spectrum of Alumina 131 showed that the material did not consist of a binary oxide but was a mixture of Al_2O_3 and TiO_2 and evidenced that the oxides are present as corundum and anatase forms respectively (ref.2).

This result was also confirmed by X-ray diffraction means. In Fig.1 the infrared spectrum of the material between 900 and 300 cm^{-1} is reported (b).

The spectrum shows, besides a broad absorption centered at 650 cm^{-1}, bands which are characteristic of Al_2O_3 (corundum) (d) and TiO_2 (anatase) (e). In the same figure the i.r. spectra of macrophages before (a) and after (c) phagocytosis are also shown.

The infrared spectrum of phagocytic macrophages (c) shows bands at 455,375 and 345 cm^{-1} which appear in the infrared spectrum of alumina-titania material and coincide with the most characteristic absorptions of Al_2O_3 (corundum) and TiO_2 (anatase). The infrared spectrum of macrophages (a) lacks these bands.

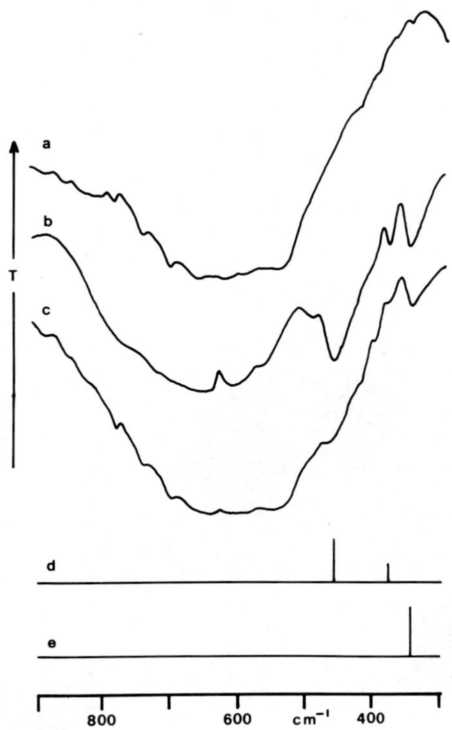

Fig.1. Infrared spectra of: a) control macrophages, b) alumina - titania material, c) phagocytic macrophages, d) Al_2O_3 as corundum, e) TiO_2 as anatase.

The phagocytosis test results are illustrated in Tab.1

	MØ phag.	MØ non phag.	Lymph.	Polym.	Other cells
Control	/	77.6±15.9	10.9±8.2	1.6±0.8	9.9±2.4
Alumina 131	34.1±2.4	58.3± 1.0	0.3±0.5	1.2±1.2	6.1±5.2

TABLE 1. % differential cell count on mouse peritoneal lavage collected 7 days after injection.

In our hands peritoneal cell population, as collected 7 days after Alumina-Titania injection was mainly composed by macrophages (MØ 92.4%) and the phagocytosis index was quite high (37%). Negligible was the percentage of other cells (lymphocytes,poly-morphs, mast cells, multinucleated cells). Macrophages appeared to be viable and non suffering despite the high number of vacuoles containing the powdered material (Fig.2)

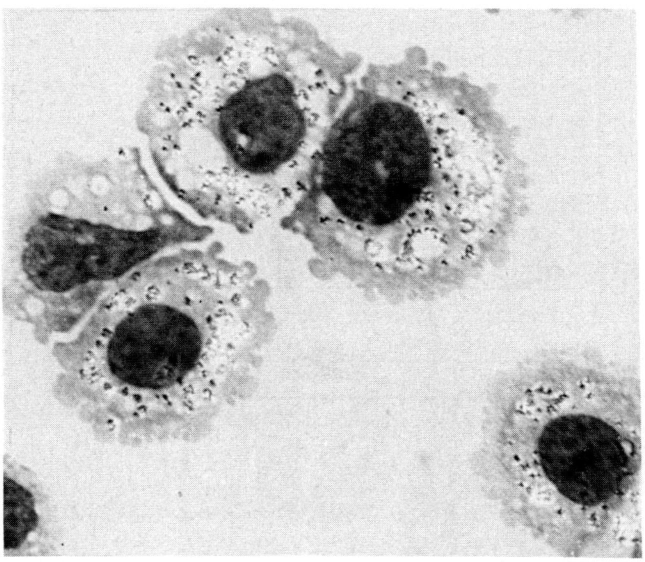

Fig.2 Cells collected 7 days after intra peritoneal inoculum of Alumina-Titania; the phagocytosis of the particles is particularly evident in polarized light (Giemsa, 100x pol.)

After 24 hours 'in vitro' maintenance the percentage of suffering cells in the samples obtained after Alumina 131 injection is high, as illustrated in Table 2.

TABLE 2

	Non ingesting	Particle phagocytosing	Suffering and non viable
Control	69.9±13.2	/	30.4±13.3
Alumina 131	5.0±4.5	20.8±7.4	74.2±32.0

At ultrastructural examination the cell membrane appeared to be ruffled with an increase of the number and the lenght of surface processes and of the number of invaginations. The nucleus did not present differences if compared to the control macrophages while in the cytoplasm an increase of the intracytoplasmatic organelles was evident. The rough endoplasmic reticulum appeared to be well developed with a particular localization near the nucleus; it was also evident an amount of free ribosomes, mitocondria and smooth endoplasmic reticulum.

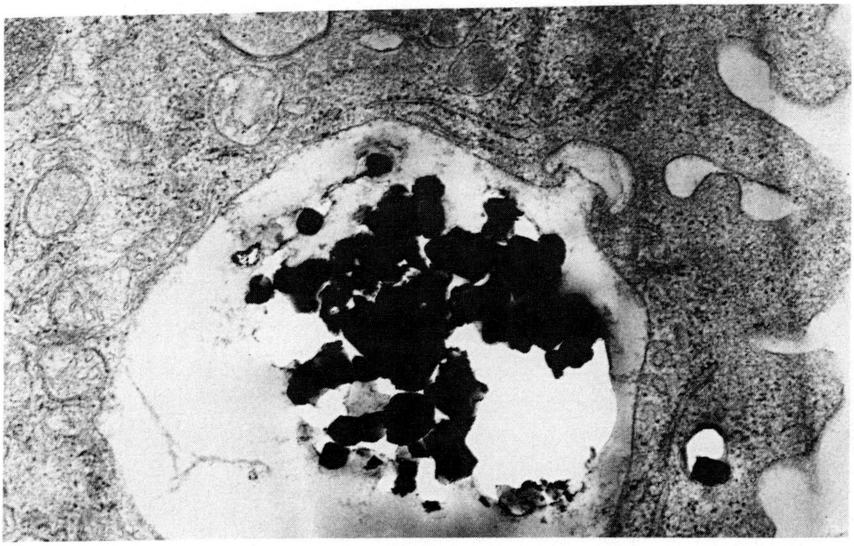

Fig.3 Vacuole of a macrophage containing polygonal electrondense granules (Alumina 131).

Many vacuoles were detectable in the cytoplasm, both free and containing electrondense structures or cytoplasmic bodies surrounded by a membrane. Some vacuoles, as shown in Fig. 3 contained polygonal electrondense granules which are also present in the extracellular spaces.

CONCLUSIONS

The spectroscopic results confirm that the Alumina-Titania is present in phagocytic macrophages and evidence that both oxides did not change their structures after being phagocyted. The possibility of directly monitoring the material inside phagocytic cells is an exciting result since the method can give a response at molecular level.

Moreover the morphological observations, both optical and ultrastructural, confirm the good cytocompatibility of the Alumina-Titania tested that however is widely used in clinical practice.

REFERENCES

1 A. Pizzoferrato, A. Vespucci, G. Ciapetti and S. Stea, Biocompatibility testing of prosthetic implant materials by cells cultures, Biomaterials, 6, (1985), 346-351.

2 A. Bertoluzza, P. Monti, R. Simoni and A. Pizzoferrato, Chemico-physical characterization of biomaterial structures in relation to their utilization, This issue.

Biomaterials and Clinical Applications,
edited by A. Pizzoferrato, P.G. Marchetti, A. Ravaglioli and A.J.C. Lee
Elsevier Science Publishers B.V., Amsterdam, 1987 — Printed in The Netherlands

EVALUATION OF BIOLOGICAL PROPERTIES OF THE POLYHEMA-COLLAGEN COMPOSITES IN A POPLITEAL REGION OF RATS

M. ŠTOL[1], I. CÍFKOVÁ[2], R. HOLUŠA[3] and M. ADAM[1]

[1]Research Institute for Rheumatic Diseases, Prague (Č.S.S.R.)
[2]State Institute for Drug Control, Prague (Č.S.S.R.)
[3]Institute of Hygiene and Epidemiology, Prague (Č.S.S.R.)

SUMMARY
This paper only summarizes the results obtained with implantation of the polyHEMA-collagen composites into a popliteal region of rats. Alterations of the implanted material and its surroundings were followed by usual histological techniques and electronmicroscopically. Moreover, calcification of the implants was examined by using radioindicator.

Since 1980, we have studied new composite materials based on biopolymer collagen and synthetic poly(2-hydroxyethyl methacrylate); the latter being well known as polyHEMA and widely used in the form of contact lenses[1-3].

Main principle of the composite material preparation consists in utilization of a lyotropic agent, usually the cosolvent mixture of suitable organic solvent and water. It enables good mutual mixing of the two polymers in any desired ratio. The solid polymer matrix arises from the starting liquid mixture following solvent evaporation[4].

In our previous study, we have shown that the composites are able to support attachment, growth and differentiation of primary chicken embryo muscle cells in culture[5].

In order to investigate changes taking place *in vivo*, these materials were implanted into experimental animals. Solid discs, 1 mm thick and 10 mm in diameter, made of the composite materials with different collagen or polyHEMA contents were implanted into the popliteal region of Wistar rats. Alterations of the implants were examined histologically and electronmicroscopically 3, 6 and 12 months after the surgery. A special care was devoted to calcification processes in the implanted materials and their surroundings with use of ^{99m}Tc as radioindicator[6].

The following results were obtained:

(1) It has been confirmed again that pure polyHEMA is fairly stable and is not substantially biodegraded within the "aggressive" environment of living tissues. The host organism responds by formation of a rather thick and nonadherent fibrous capsule.

(2) Presence of the fibrillar collagen within the synthetic hydrogel matrix has a dramatic effect on its biological behaviour.

The composites containing 10-20 wt.-% fibrillar collagen remained compact for the whole implantation period, while cellular penetration into the superficial layers of the implant was already well-pronounced. The implants were surrounded by a thin closely attached fibrous capsule.

The composites with 30-50 wt.-% fibrillar collagen were invaded to an increasing depth by fibrous tissue containing capillaries. The polyHEMA matrix became exposed as globular particles of different size. The central part of the implant was edematous and deformed. A fibrous capsule was quite thin, often missing (see Figs. 1 and 2).

The implants containing 60-90 wt.-% fibrillar collagen were totally disintegrated within 12 months following the implantation. Very thin capsules were found only in connection with implants containing 60-70 wt.-% fibrillar collagen. However, no capsules and even no rests of the implants containing originally 80-90 % of the collagen were found in the site of implantation.

Accordingly, the samples of pure collagen were fully absorbed within the first 3 months after their implantation.

(3) The mass of implants containing less than 50 wt.-% fibrillar collagen did not differ considerably from the control samples of pure polyHEMA. However, the mass decreased steeply in implants containing more collagen and in correspondence with an increasing implantation time.

(4) Calcification of the implants was dependent on the collagen content and the implantation time. The degree of calcification was more pronounced in correlation with an increasing collagen content, up to 60-70 wt.-%. However, for the highest collagen content, it was again much lower. Surprisingly, the highest degrees of calcification were observed three months after the implantation. In the course of the highest degrees of calcification, following long-term implantation, the implants were markedly decalcified. The control samples of pure polyHEMA maintained their relatively low degree of calcification practically constant during the whole time period.

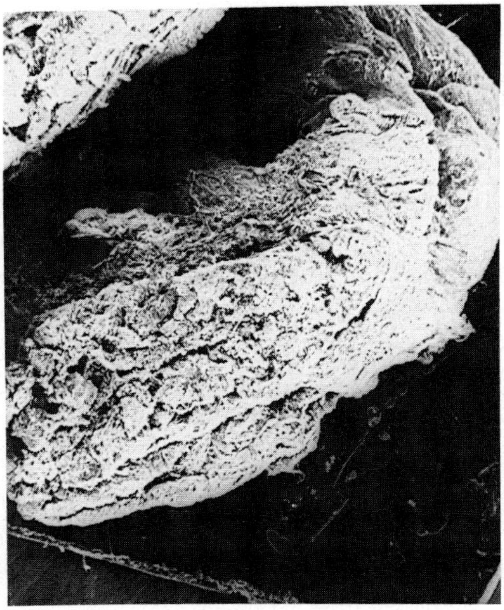

Fig. 1. Scanning-electron-micrograph of cross-section of the solid disc following 3 months of implantation into the popliteal region of Wistar rat. The composite implant consists of 50 wt.-% fibrillar collagen and 50 wt.-% polyHEMA. Magnification x20.

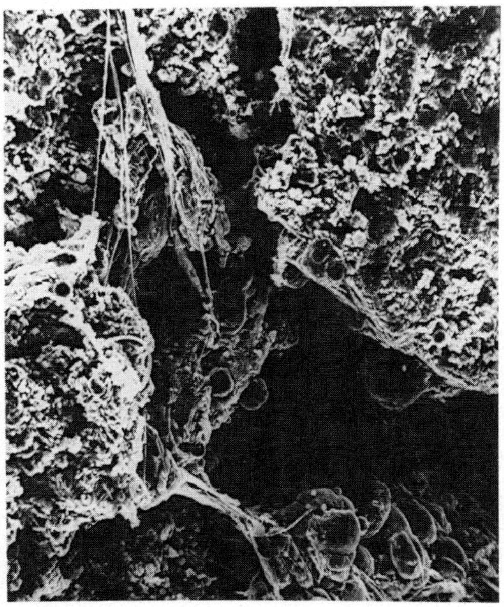

Fig. 2. The same implant as shown above, viewed with S.E.M. at higher magnification. Penetration and disintegration of the implant by cells is quite apparent. Notice the infiltration of fibrous connective tissue containing capillaries into the deep layers of the implant. Magnification x1000.

If the implant cannot be penetrated and degraded by cells (low collagen content), the organism´s response consists in formation of the fibrous connective tissue capsule eliminating the "foreign body".

It was here demonstrated that high collagen content induced cellular infiltration and degradation of the implant as a whole. The more was the implant degraded by the host organism, the more pronounced cellular "cleaning" reaction and the lower fibrous encapsulation of the implant occurred. Biodegradation processes proceded to such an extent that after the long-term implantation only small rests of implants were found or were completely absent in the site of implantation.

We can conclude that the composites containing maximally 20 % of fibrillar collagen are well suited for long-term implantation. In this case, the recipient´s fibrous tissue invades only surface layers of the implant, while its core remains unchanged.

ACNOWLEDGEMENTS

We wish to express our gratitude to Professor M. La Placa, chairman, and all members of the Organizing Committee of the European Congress on Biomaterials, Istituto Rizzoli, Bologna, September 14-17, 1986, for kind invitation of one of us (M.Š.) and generous hospitality during all the days of that exceptional meeting.

REFERENCES

1 O. Wichterle and D. Lím, Hydrophilic gels for biological use, Nature, 185 (1960) 117-118.
2 J.D. Andrade (Ed.), Hydrogels for medical and related applications, ACS Symp. Ser. No. 31, ACS, Washington, 1976.
3 D.G. Pedley, P.J. Skelly and B.J. Tighe, Hydrogels in biomedical applications, Brit. Polym. J., 12 (1980) 99-110.
4 Czechoslovak Patent Application No. PV 5125-80, 1980.
5 M. Štol, M. Tolar and M. Adam, Poly(2-hydroxyethyl methacrylate)-collagen composites which promote muscle cell differentiation in vitro, Biomaterials, 6 (1985) 193-197.
6 I. Cífková, M. Štol, R. Holuša and M. Adam, Calcification of the poly(2-hydroxyethyl methacrylate)-collagen composites implanted into a popliteal region of rats, Biomaterials (in press).

Biomaterials and Clinical Applications,
edited by A. Pizzoferrato, P.G. Marchetti, A. Ravaglioli and A.J.C. Lee
Elsevier Science Publishers B.V., Amsterdam, 1987 — Printed in The Netherlands

INTERACTION BETWEEN PRIMARY BONE CELL CULTURES AND BIOMATERIALS PART 1: METHOD; THE IN VITRO AND IN VIVO STAGES

J.E. DAVIES, S.F. TARRANT and *T. MATSUDA.
Department of Anatomy, University of Birmingham Medical School,
Birmingham B15 2TJ, England.

SUMMARY

This paper describes a combined in vitro/in vivo technique which permits examination of the interface created by primary bone cell cultures and bone-substitute biomaterials. The technique described is not only applicable to the use of other cell types but also the introduction of biomaterials testing using primary human cell populations. Other papers in this Congress discuss preliminary results using these techniques.

INTRODUCTION

The examination and understanding of the interface created between the biological environment and an artificial material are of central and fundamental importance to the field of biomaterials research. Inevitably, such an interface will initially comprise an interaction between the material surface and the components of tissue fluid. Of the latter, ion exchange at the solid/liquid interface, the adsorption of proteins and possibly lipids could be essential pre-requisites to either the establishment or prevention of a cell/substrate interface.

In the case of many biomaterials, particularly those used as replacements for various connective tissues, the colonization of the biomaterial by host connective tissue cells which retain their phenotype and thus an ability to synthesize a particular extracellular matrix, is essential to their long-term clinical success. Although morphologically close or chemically intimate relationships have been demonstrated at the interface between many biomaterials (e.g. metals and bioactive ceramics respectively) and host bone, from a fundamental point-of-view little is known about either the behaviour of osteoblasts, osteoprogenitor cells or the surface physico-chemical characteristics of a biomaterial which will "allow" cellular expression of the osteoblast phenotype. Indeed, in vivo experiments, by their very nature, do not allow the examination of the reaction of single cell types to the substrate since, on implantation, the latter will be bathed in blood, tissue fluid and an heterogeneous cell population.

* Visiting Research Fellow (Permanent Address: Dept. of Orthodontics, Kagoshima University Dental School, Kagoshima, Japan.

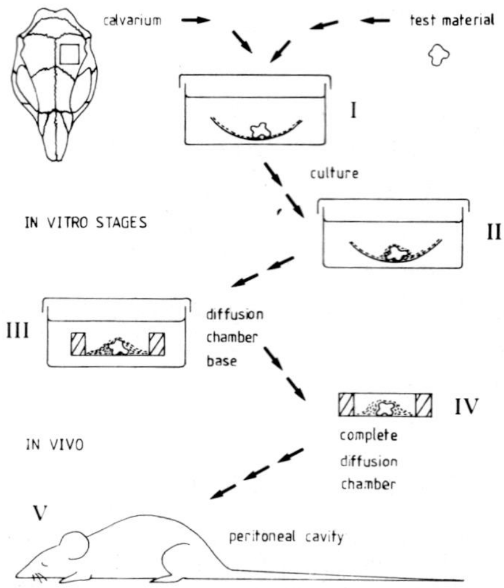

Fig. 1.: Diagrammatic representation of the five principle preparatory stages for the examination of the interactions between primary bone cell cultures and test biomaterials:- I: Introduction of test material as an overlay in a periosteally-stripped bone organ culture. II: Colonization of the test substrate by bone cells. III: Removal of the colonized substrate to diffusion chamber base. IV: Completion of diffusion chamber. V: Implantation in peritoneal cavity of littermate of donor animal.

To circumvent these problems we describe the development of new techniques which, while not clinically analogous, do allow the examination of the interface created between bone cells and biomaterial surfaces. The techniques described not only avoid the problems associated with long term in vitro maintenance of primary bone cell populations, but also are applicable, in the future, to the establishment of biological assays of biomaterials using human bone cell cultures (ref. 1). This paper describes these techniques and their rationale while preliminary results are reported in three further papers at this Congress (refs 2,3,4).

METHOD

Neonate Albino Wistar rat litters (1-4 days old) were divided into two groups of equal numbers. The first group was left with the dam, the second group was isolated. Each of the animals in group 2 was killed and the calvaria removed aseptically. The subsequent preparatory stages are summarized, diagrammatically, in Fig. 1.

In vitro stages I and II

The calvaria are stripped of endocranial and exocranial periostea, to expose, on the host bone, a tesselated arrangement of osteoblasts interupted

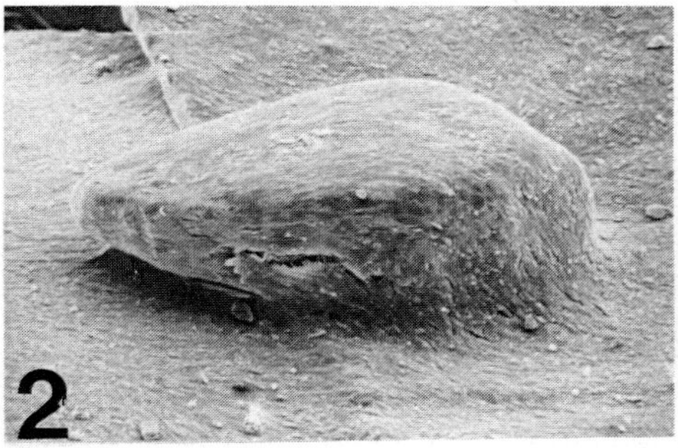

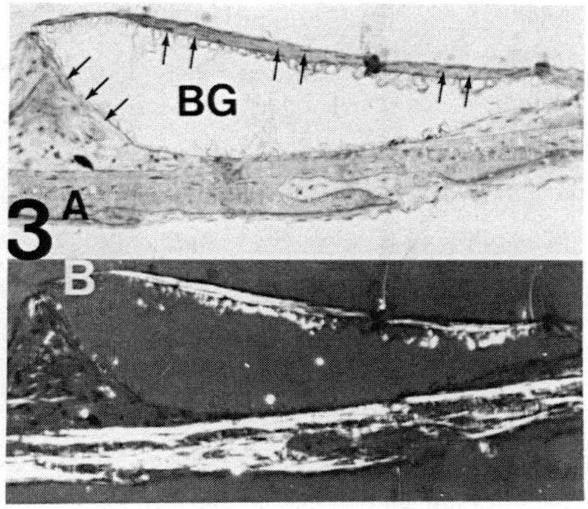

Fig. 2: SEM photomicrograph of a single calcium phosphate particle maintained in culture for 11 days on two pieces of overlapping periosteally stripped endocranial bone. Note that the cell morphology is almost identical on both substrata. Field Width = 1.55mm.
Fig. 3: Light micrographs of a section through a fragment of bioactive glass (BG), maintained in culture for 4 weeks. [A] Bright field. Note the firm anchoring of the glass to the host bone by cells and tissue (arrows). [B] Same field viewed with crossed polars to demonstrate the birefringent (collagenous) extracellular matrix produced by migrated osteoblasts.

occasionally by osteoclasts. The calvaria are then trimmed with fine dissecting scissors to remove the sutural areas and produce small (2-3mm^2) squares of frontal or parietal bone fragments. These provide a source of primary bone cells and are maintained as an organ culture (Bigger's culture medium [Fitton Jackson modification - Flow Laboratories] containing 10% foetal calf serum, glutamine 20µl/ml, Penicillin/Streptomycin 10µl/ml and Hepes 25 µl/ml - [sFJm]) for a period of 11 days with the test biomaterial lying on the endocranial osteoblastic surface. During this time the bone cells migrate to colonize the test material (Fig. 2). This method has been used to observe the migration of osteoblasts over a variety of substrata (ref. 5) and compare the morphologies of osteoblasts on commercially available calcium phosphate bioceramics (ref. 6). Both osteoblasts and, under certain conditions, osteoclasts will migrate onto the test material during this preliminary *in vitro* stage and we have developed a combined incident light and SEM technique to demonstrate the presence of such cells (ref. 7). This organ culture system can yield important information concerning the migratory morphology (ref. 8) and synthetic activity (ref. 4) of osteoblasts. The production, by osteoblasts, of a collagen-containing extracellular matrix precedes mineralisation and Fig. 3 shows the collagenous extracellular cellular matrix produced by migrated osteoblasts over a fragment of bioactive glass (Nippon

Kogaku K.K., Tokyo) maintained in vitro for 4 weeks. No such organised fibrous matrix was found, on light microscopical examination, on quartz glass in identical culture conditons.

Although it is feasible to create in vitro conditions wherein migrated osteoblasts will produce a mineralized extracellular matrix (ref. 9,), such techniques are not easily applied to the establishment of an interface with a three-dimensionally complex sample of bone-substitute biomaterial. We have therefore extended our in vitro stages, in the following way, in preparation for transfer of the samples to the in vivo environment.

In vitro stages III and IV

On the 12th day the fragments of test material were removed from the host bone tissue and transferred to rafts floating in culture fluid contained within a petri dish. Each raft, effectively a "Millipore" diffusion chamber (DC) base, comprised a 10mm internal diameter plexiglass ring to which a single filter had been glued. Several particles of cell colonized test material were transferred to each floating raft and maintained in culture (in sFJm) for a further 12 days (cell particles in each raft were initially cultured on bone fragments from the same donor).

During this time cells confined to the raft but maintained by a large volume of culture medium, continued to divide and migrate. Some cells left the test material to migrate over the surface of the filter (see Figs. 5 & 6 in ref. 3) and during this phase cell processes of re-migrated osteoblasts were seen to penetrate the pores of the filter while being in continuity with the confluent cell layer over the test material. This culture stage allowed the cells to anchor the test material onto the new substrate i.e. the diffusion chamber filter. After 12 days, the second (top) filter was glued down onto the perspex ring of each diffusion chamber to complete the chamber structure.

In vivo stage V

These chambers containing up to 10-cell colonized test fragments were implanted in the peritoneal cavities of litter mates of the original donor animal. The DC filter (pore size 0.45 microns) was chosen to allow exchange of nutrients but prevent cell contact with the host.

The use of diffusion chambers (DC's) for the long term culture of cells of osteogenic capacity is not new (refs 10,11). However, our method differs from all previously reported DC experiments in the following ways:- (i) Cell colonized biomaterial particles were used as an inoculum rather than cell suspensions, (ii) the initial seeding density was relatively low (approx. 10^4 cells per 150 l chamber) due to the nature of the initial in vitro stage and (iii) the bone cell population was primary and was obtained from calvaria by a non-enzymatic isolation procedure.

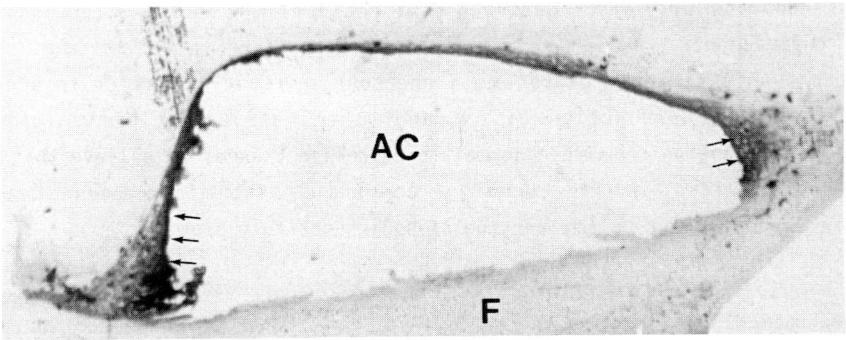

Fig. 4: Photomicrograph of a section through an apatite ceramic particle [AC] (decalcified during preparation) anchored to a diffusion chamber filter [F] by tissue elaborated by the colonizing cells. Note calcified matrix apposed to the ceramic surface [arrows].

The cells in our system were considered to be osteoblasts for two reasons. First, the cells had migrated in the initial in vitro stage from the host bone surface. Second, DC experiments favour the survival of osteoblasts (OB's) rather than cells derived from the haemopoietic system, such as osteoclasts (OC's). Such evidence was provided by Friedenstein et al (ref. 12) and Bab et al (ref. 13) who reported that bone marrow stromal (i.e. fibroblastic) cell populations proliferated whilst haemopoietic cells degenerated in DC's. The in vitro stage in our system would further inhibit OC proliferation according to Chambers (ref. 14) who observed that in a culture consisting of OC's, macrophages and fibroblast-like cells , both the OC and macrophage populations were overgrown by the fibroblast-like cells and very few OC's remained after 7 days in culture.

The low seeding density in our initial experiments produced a degree of osteoblast modulation which resulted in production of a mesenchymal-type extracellular matrix. The temporal re-organization of the latter may be analogous to stages in hard tissue wound repair and these phenomena are described in more detail in ref 2. As the number of cells transferred to each DC is limited by the degree of colonization during the in vitro stages, we have increased the relative seeding density in subsequent experiments by reducing the DC volume. A reduction from 150 l to 50 l using the same number of cell-colonized particles has resulted in the production of a mineralized extracellular matrix by OB's directly on the surface of a calcium phosphate ceramic biomaterial within a 6 week implantation period (see Fig. 4 and ref. 3). We are currently inoculating prototype 3 l volume DC's with particles of colonized bone-substitute biomaterials to further increase the relative initial cell seeding density and reduce the time required by the cells to condition their environment.

With such a range of DC volumes, the concommitant variation in seeding density and the production of extracellular matrix, by the colonizing osteoblasts, ranging from mesenchymal to calcified tissue, we believe that this combined in vitro/in vivo technique can be used to mimic wound healing phenomena which occur on implanation of bone-susbtitute biomaterials.

ACKNOWLEDGEMENTS

We are grateful to Yvonne Bovell and Lyndsey Davies for technical assistance and manuscript preparation respectively. This work is financially supported by the Science and Engineering Research Council, U.K. (Grant No. GR/D/53913) and The West Midlands Regional Health Authority.

REFERENCES

1 J.E. Davies, Human bone marrow cell synthesize collagen, in diffusion chambers implanted into the normal rat, in press.

2 S.F. Tarrant and J.E. Davies, Interaction between primary bone cell cultures and biomaterials, Part 2: Osteoblast behaviour, in: European Congress on Biomaterials, Sept. 14th-17th, Bologna, Italy, 1986.

3 P.G.J. Rout, S.F. Tarrant, J.W. Frame, J.E. Davies, Interaction between primary bone cell cultures and biomaterials, Part 3: A comparison of dense and macroporous hydroxyapatite, ibid.

4 R.M. Shelton, I.M. Whyte, J.E. Davies, Interaction between primary bone cell cultures and biomaterials, Part 4: Colonization of charged polymer surfaces, ibid.

5 S.J. Jones and A. Boyde, Colonization of various natural substrates by osteoblasts in vitro, Scannin Electron Microscopy (1979/) 529-538.

6 J.E. Davies, R.P. Hurst, N.T. Spooner, Surface emission and biological probes for inorganic interfaces. To be published in "Interactions of Cells with Natural and Foreign Surfces" [Eds: N. Crawford, D.E.M. Taylor] Plenum Press, New York.

7 Y. Bovell, J.E. Davies and S. Tarrant, Incident light and SEM observations of bone cell colonized bioceramics, Histochem. J. (1986), in press.

8 J.E. Davies, B. Causton, Y. Bovell, K. Davy and C.S. Sturt, The migration o osteoblasts over substrata of discrete surface charge, Biomaterials, 7, (1986) 231-234.

9 B. Ecarot-Charnier, F.H. Glorieux, M. Van der Rest and G. Pereita, Osteoblasts isolated from mouse calvaria initiate matrix mineralization in culture. J. Cell Biol. 96, (1983) 639-643.

10 A.J. Friedenstein, Precursor cells of mechanocytes, Int. Rev. Cytol., 47, (1976) 327-355.

11 B.A. Ashton, T.D. Allen, C.R. Howlett, C.C. Eaglesom, A. Hattori and M. Owen, Formation of bone and cartilage by marrow stromal cells in diffusion chambers in vivo. Clinical Orthopaedics and Related Research, 151, (1980) 294-307.

12 A.J. Friedenstein, I.I. Piatetzky-Shapiro and K.V. Petrakova, Osteogenesis in transplants of bone marrow cells, J. Embryol. Exp. Morph. 16(3) (1966) 381-390.

13 I. Bab, B.A. Ashton, D. Gazit, G. Marx, M.C. Williamson and M. Owen, Kinetics and differentiation of marrow stromal cells in diffusion chambers in vivo, J. Cell Sci., 84 (1986) 139-151.

14 T.J. Chambers, Phagocytosis and Trypsi-resistant glass adhesion by osteoclasts in culture, J. Pathol. 127 (1979) 55-60.

Biomaterials and Clinical Applications,
edited by A. Pizzoferrato, P.G. Marchetti, A. Ravaglioli and A.J.C. Lee
Elsevier Science Publishers B.V., Amsterdam, 1987 — Printed in The Netherlands

INTERACTIONS BETWEEN PRIMARY BONE CELL CULTURES AND BIOMATERIALS PART 2 : OSTEOBLAST BEHAVIOUR

S.F.TARRANT and J.E.DAVIES*
Department of Anatomy, University of Birmingham Medical School,
Birmingham B15 2TJ England.

SUMMARY

The behaviour of primary bone cell populations cultured on biomaterials within diffusion chambers is reported. Low initial cell seeding density resulted in non-uniform colonization of the chamber. Extracellular matrix production occurred directly onto the surface of the biomaterial and included an unorganized matrix containing a complex collagen fibre network. Limited mineralization of the matrix was observed. Initial seeding density and cell modulation within the chamber are discussed.

INTRODUCTION

The culture conditions for osteoblasts, conducive to normal behaviour (i.e. synthesis of a calcified extracellular matrix) are complex and critical (ref. 1) and as a result, a reliable method for investigating long term osteoblast behaviour _in vitro_ is not available. The Diffusion Chamber (DC) method discussed in Part I of this series of papers (ref. 2), enables maintenance of cells in physiological conditions by diffusion of metabolites across filters which prevent direct cell contact with the host. This method has an advantage over _in vivo_ experiments in that the contents of the DC are isolated from the heterogeneous host cell population and can be removed, intact, for examination. Similar systems have been used previously to assess the osteogenic potential of rabbit bone marrow and murine calvarial cells (refs. 3,4).

In this paper we present the results of an investigation of the behaviour of primary bone cells seeded on the surface of artificial bone-substitute ceramics maintained in-vivo, in DC's.

MATERIALS AND METHODS

DC's containing rat bone cells and bioceramics particles were implanted in rats as described in ref. 2. Following implantation times of up to 19 weeks, the host animal was killed and the DC retrieved from the peritoneal cavity, fixed immediately in Paraformaldehyde and dehydrated in a graded ethanol series. Samples were then embedded in L.R. White (hard grade) acrylic resin,

* To whom correspondence should be addressed

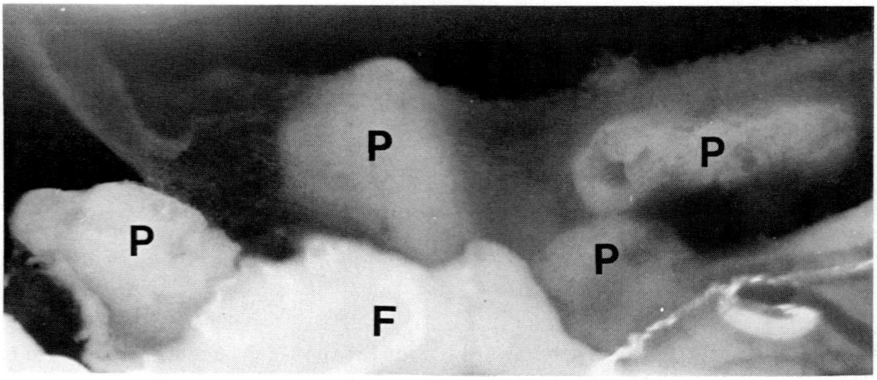

Fig. 1: Photomicrograph of "Calcitite"TM calcium hydroxyapatite ceramic particles (P) surrounded by a Fibrin clot after 8 weeks implantation. Part of the DC filter (F) can be seen in the lower part of the photograph.

sectioned using a Tungsten Carbide knife in a Reichert-Jung 1140/Autocut and stained with either Toluidine Blue or by the Von Kossa method. Samples for examination by transmission electron microscopy (TEM) were embedded in resin as above, trimmed to the surface of a biomaterial particle, decalcified using 10% EDTA in 0.1M Tris/HCl and re-embedded in resin. Sections were cut on a Reichert Jung OMU2 Ultramicrotome using glass knives, mounted on 400 mesh uncoated grids, stained with Uranyl Acetate and Lead Citrate and viewed using a Jeol 100 CX II TEM.

RESULTS AND DISCUSSION

Primary bone cells colonizing artificial bone-substitute materials, transplanted _in vivo_ in DC's, survived for periods of up to 19 weeks. Following introduction into the DC, the cells proliferated and migrated in an attempt to populate the inner surface of the chamber. On visual examination of the chambers following retrieval from the peritoneal cavity a jelly-like substance, identified as fibrin (using Masson's Trichrome stain) surrounded the biomaterial particles and occupied a variable volume of the chamber (Fig. 1).

As the diffusion chamber filter pore size allows exchange of tissue fluid and macromolecular species, blank chambers used as controls were also seen to accumulate a fibin/fibronectin clot. Such an organisation, visible both at light and electron microscopic levels (vide infra) was inevitably included in any extracellular matrix (ECM) produced by the cells colonizing the biomaterial sample.

It is a fibrin/fibronectin clot which provides a three dimensional scaffold

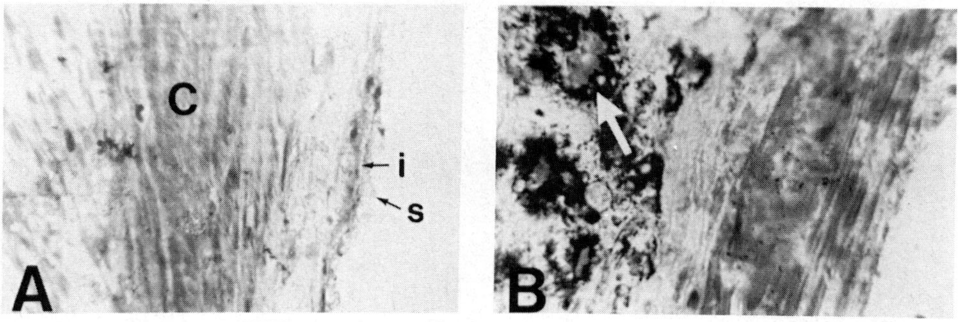

Fig. 2A: Viewed with crossed polars at the extinction position for the vertically aligned collagen fibre bundles, this photomicrograph of a resin embedded section shows the complex collagen fibre network (C) near to but not directly against the biomaterial surface. The bulk of the biomaterial has shattered and been lost during sectioning to leave only fragments of the substrate (s) at the biomaterial/tissue interface (i) (6 week implant). Field width = 170μm
Fig. 2B: Viewed with crossed polars, this photomicrograph illustrates mineralizing foci in a 19 week implant. The black precipitate (arrow) indicates a positive Von Kossa reaction for calcium. Note also the ordered cellular arrangement to the right which is similar to that seen in both figures 2A and 3A. Field width = 170μm

through which cells may migrate and into which matrix components are secreted during wound healing. Indeed, a fibrin clot produced at fracture sites is invaded by fibroblasts which secrete collagen to form a fibrous callus (ref. 5). The fibrous tissue then undergoes osteogenesis and is replaced by newly formed bone. It is known that fracture repair recapitulates embryonic bone development and Ashton et al (ref. 6) reported that the development of osteogenic tissue in DC's was reminiscent of the formation of long bone anlagen. As both endochondral and intramembraneous ossification have been observed in single diffusion chambers (ref. 6) this would suggest that bone formation in DC's reflects fracture repair.

In the present experiments, cells produced ECM directly onto the surface of the biomaterial. In some areas the ECM had an unorganized appearance and contained very few cells. During these low seeding density experiments the osteoblasts underwent extensive proliferation, migration and modulation as exhibited by their changing synthetic function. Modulation of cell activity between chondroblasts and fibroblasts involving changes in synthetic activity and morphology, are known to occur. Deshmukh (ref. 7) for example, reported modulation of synthetic activity of bovine articular chondrocytes in culture involving a change in collagen type from $[\alpha 1(II)]_3$ Type II collagen, to a fibroblastic $[\alpha 1(I)]_2\alpha 2$ Type I collagen. Osteoblast migration has been shown to

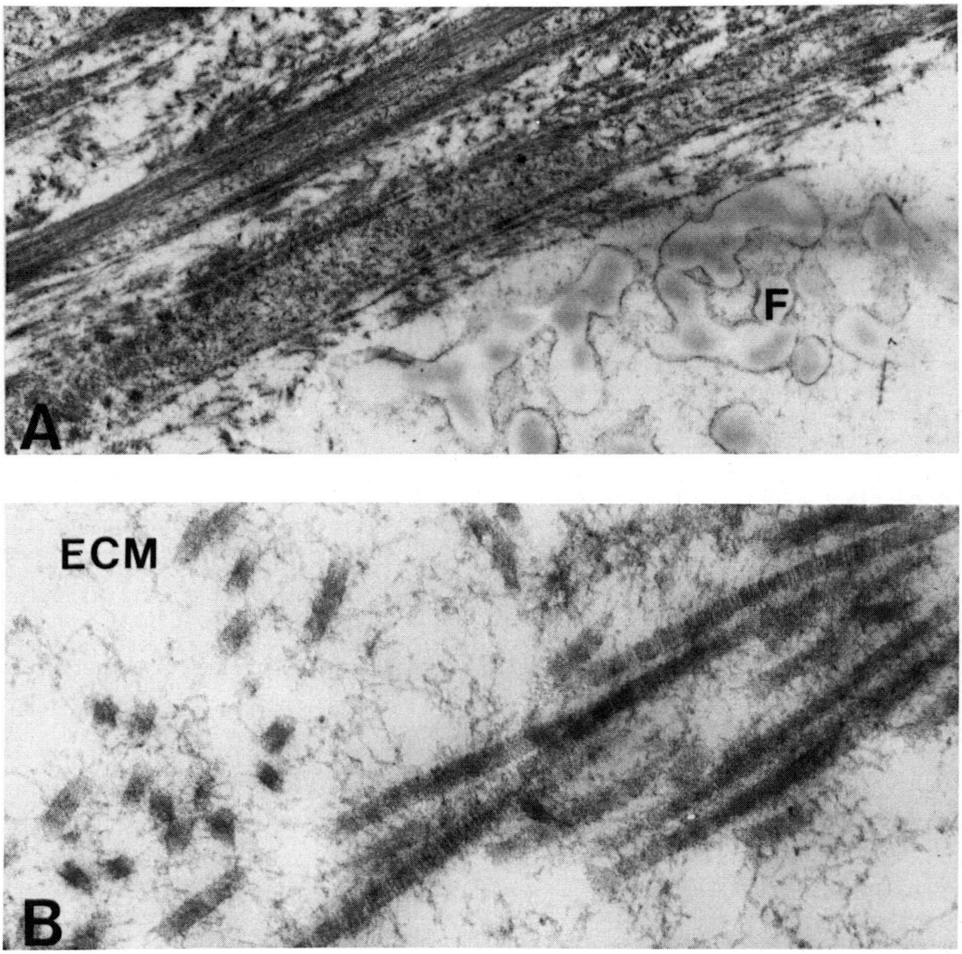

Fig. 3A: TEM photomicrograph showing filter septa (F) surrounded by a condensed material assumed to be fibrin and supporting a complex collagen fibre network comprising collagen fibres sectioned along both transverse and longitudinal planes (6 week implant). Field width = 8.5 microns
Fig. 3B: Higher power TEM of the above sample showing the diffuse reticular appearance of the material surrounding the collagen fibres which exhibit characteristic (64nm) banding. Field width = 1.7 microns

result in a change in cell shape, from a typical tesselated osteoblast to a fibroblast-like form (ref. 8) Furthermore, the morphology of OB's has been shown to be influenced by the nature of the substrate over which they migrate (ref. 9) Such migratory morphology is considered to reflect, or affect, cellular metabolic activity (ref. 10). It is therefore likely that the unorganized ECM is an embryonic type mesenchymal tissue which at electron microscopic levels is similar in appearance to Wharton's Jelly (ref. 11) and whose production is associated with a modulation of osteoblast synthetic activity.

Fig. 2A illustrates the complex, collagen fibre network near to, but not directly against the biomaterial surface. This arrangement, of alternatively orientated sheets of tissue is also seen in Fig. 3A, where the collagen is apposed to the filter surface. Surrounding the filter septa (F) and condensed onto its surface, a reticular substance, assumed to be fibrin, can be seen. Fig. 3B shows the characteristic banding of the collagen and the fibrin clot into which it has been secreted. The tissue seen in these figures is indicative of organized cellular behaviour. Similar alternate arrangements of collagen fibre bundles was attributed (ref. 12) to the secretion of collagen in "pulses", the thickness of the layer being determined by the duration of the pulse and amount of collagen secreted, all collagen secreted during one pulse being orientated in the same direction. It is therefore possible that the cells in our experiments are secreting collagen and other ECM products in this manner, however, we are unable at the present time to specify the duration of the secretory pulse.

It was also noted that the most organized ECM (i.e. collagen containing) was distanced from the biomaterial surface by a less organized ECM (Fig. 2A). The in-vivo implantation studies of Yamamuro et al (ref. 13) for bioglass and Kurokawa et al (ref. 14) for calcium phosphate ceramic particles showed similar directional organization of tissue with respect to an implant surface. Their results demonstrated that mineralized tissue was formed from the traumatized bone towards the biomaterial surface, and not primarily on the implant surface. Bab et al (ref. 15) reported that osteogenesis within DC's containing marrow stromal cells was preceded by production of fibrous tissue and it is assumed that the primary osteoblasts in this system will progressively mineralize the fibrous tissue they have produced towards the implant surface.

Little calcification of the ECM was observed in our experiments (Fig. 2B), but osteogenesis in DC's is known to be dependent upon the initial cell-seeding density (ref. 16) where 210 bone marrow cells/0.05mm^2 were required for bone formation in DC's. In the work reported in this paper, the initial seeding density provided approximately 2 primary bone cells/0.05mm^2. However, the colonization of the chamber surface by these differentiated cells was not uniform and resulted in a higher cell density in localized areas with correspondingly more complex ECM. In order to increase the relative cell density in this system chambers with smaller volumes, which we have already shown to promote mineralization of fibrous tissue directly against the biomaterial surface (ref.2), are currently under investigation.

CONCLUSIONS

This preliminary work has demonstrated that primary bone cell populations, colonizing artificial bone-substitute materials, can produce an extracellular matrix on the surface of the latter. The composition of the elaborated extracellular matrix is dependant upon the initial cell population density. Areas of high cell density will result in calcified tissue formation.

ACKNOWLEDGEMENTS

We are grateful to Alan Murdoch and Yvonne Bovell for technical assistance and Lyndsey Davies for preparation of the manuscript. This work was financially supported by both the Science and Engineering Research Council, U.K. (grant number GR/D/53913) and the West Midlands Regional Health Authority.

REFERENCES

1 H.C. Tenenbaum and J.N.M. Heersche, Differentiation of osteoid-producing cells in vitro: Possible evidence for the requirement of a microenvironment, Calcif. Tiss. Int., 38 (1986) 262-267.
2 J.E. Davies, S.F. Tarrant, T. Matsuda, Interaction between primary bone cell cultures and biomaterials. Part 1: Method; the in vitro and in vivo stages, Proc. Europ. Congr. on Biomaterials. Sept. 14-17, Bologna, Italy 1986.
3 D.J. Simmons, G.N. Kent, R.L. Jilka, D.M. Scott, M. Fallon and D.V. Cohn, Formation of bone by isolated, cultured osteoblasts in Millipore diffusion chambers, Calcif. Tiss. Int. 34 (1982) 291-294.
4 I. Bab, B.A. Ashton, G.T. Syftestad, M.E. Owen, Assessment of an in vivo diffusion chamber method as a quantitative assay for osteogenesis, Calcif. Tissue Int. 36 (1984) 77-82.
5 J. Lindner, Bone healing, Clin. Plast. Surg., 4(3) (1977) 425-437.
6 B.A. Ashton, T.D. Allen, C.R. Howlett, C.C. Eaglesom, A. Hattori and M. Owen, Formation of bone and cartilage by marrow stromal cells in diffusion chambers in vivo, Clin. Orth. Rel. Res. 151 (1980) 294-307.
7 K. Deshmukh, Synthesis of tissue nonspecific collagen by bovine articular cartilage as a result of aging in vitro, Proc. Soc. Exp. Biol. Med. 147 (1974) 726-729.
8 S.J. Jones & A. Boyde, The migration of osteoblasts, Cell Tiss. Res. 184 (1977) 179-193.
9 J.E. Davies, R.P. Hurst, N.T. Spooner, Surface emission and biological probes for inorganic interfaces, in: "Interactions of cells with natural and foreign surfaces", Plenum Press, New York, in press.
10 Y. Bovell, J.E. Davies, S.F. Tarrant, Incident light and SEM observations of bone cell colonized bioceramics, Histochem. J., 1986, in press.
11 E.W. Parry, Some electron microscope observations on the mesenchymal structures of full-term umbilical cord, J. Anat. 107 (1970) 505-518.
12 J. Gross, Collagen, Sci. Am. 204 (1961) 120-130.
13 T. Yamamuro, T. Nakamura, S. Higashi, R. Kasai, Y. Kakutani, T. Kitsugi, T. Kokubo, Artificial bone for use as a bone prosthesis, Prog. Artif. Orgs. 1983, 810-813.
14 H. Kurokawa, M. Kajiyama, N. Nomura, K. Rin, T. Kodama, I. Akama, M. Sako, I. Suenaga, A fundamental study on the application of calcium phosphate ceramics in bone defects. J. Kyushu Dent. Soc. 40(3) (1986) 686-693.
15 T. Bab, B.A. Ashton, D. Gazit, G. Marx, M.C. Williamson and M. Owen, Kinetics and differentiation of marrow stromal cells in diffusion chambers in vivo, J. Cell Sci., 84 (1986) 139-151.
16 A.J. Friedenstein, I.I. Piatetzky-Shapiro and K.V. Petrakova, Osteogenesis in transplants of bone marrow cells, J. Embryol. Exp. Morph. 16(3) (1966) 381-390.

Biomaterials and Clinical Applications,
edited by A. Pizzoferrato, P.G. Marchetti, A. Ravaglioli and A.J.C. Lee
Elsevier Science Publishers B.V., Amsterdam, 1987 — Printed in The Netherlands

INTERACTION BETWEEN PRIMARY BONE CELL CULTURES AND BIOMATERIALS PART 3: A COMPARISON OF DENSE AND MACROPOROUS HYDROXYAPATITE

P.G.J. ROUT[1], S.F. TARRANT[2], J.W. FRAME[1] and *J.E. DAVIES[2]
[1]Department of Oral Surgery and [2]Department of Anatomy,
University of Birmingham Medical School,
Birmingham, B15 2TJ, England.

SUMMARY

The interaction between primary bone cell cultures and dense and macroporous hydroxyapatite ceramics was examined in a controlled environment using an *in vitro/in vivo* technique. Using light and electron microscopy, the colonization of the biomaterials by bone cells, the production of extracellular matrix and appearance of mineralising foci was observed. In particular, the infiltration of pores by migrating osteoblasts was found to be dependent on pore size.

INTRODUCTION

Hydroxyapatite (HAp) is becoming widely used for augmentation and implantation in the maxillofacial region (ref. 1). It is particularly valuable in the management of patients with atrophy of the jaws following loss of the natural dentition (ref. 2). Such patients often have difficulty wearing dentures and have problems with mastication due to of lack of bony support. Particulate HAp is placed between the mucoperiosteum and the alveolar bone to produce a stable augmentation of the jaw (ref. 3). To examine the suitability of differing implant materials for this type of surgical procedure we are currently evaluating two forms of commercially available particulate hydroxyapatite. First, "Calcitite"™, a solid dense non-resorbable form (Calcitec Inc., San Diego, California): the preparation and properties of this dense hydroxyapatite have been reported (ref. 4). Second, "Interpore 200"™, a macroporous form derived by hydrothermal exchange from the aragonite skeleton of a common scleractinian reef-building coral, genus: porities (Interpore International, Irvine, California); the technique of preparation has been described in ref. 5.

Experience in patients and in clinically-analogous animal models confirms that both materials are biocompatible and rapidly consolidate to produce relatively stable augmentation of the host bone (refs. 3 and 6). However, the surgical and functional parameters involved in clinical and *in vivo* procedures do not allow the examination of the reaction of osteoblasts and osteoclasts to

*To whom correspondence should be addressed

the artificial material in a controlled environment. The aim of this study was to compare the interaction of bone cells to these two bioceramics, with the intention of bridging the gap between laboratory investigation and clinical practice.

METHODS

The technique involved two stages. First an in vitro procedure involving the organ culture of the calvaria of Albino Wistar rats upon which the test material had been placed. Second, an implantation of the test material within a diffusion chamber into the peritoneal cavity of a littermate rat. These procedures have been described in detail, in a previous paper (ref. 7). The bone fragments and test material were maintained in organ culture for periods of up to 11 days. At this stage some samples were examined microscopically and the migration of osteoblasts and osteoclasts onto the hydroxyapatite was studied using a modified azo-dye acid phosphatase technique and scanning electron microscopy (SEM) (ref. 8).

The other bone-cell colonised particles of hydroxyapatite were transferred to the in vivo environment for long term culture in Millipore-type diffusion chambers for periods of between 6 and 12 weeks. After retrieval from the animal each complete diffusion chamber (DC) was embedded in L.R. White (hard) acrylic resin prior to sectioning.

RESULTS AND DISCUSSION

In vitro stage

(i) Scanning Electron Microscopy (SEM) Examination. On SEM examination, bone cells were seen to have migrated on to both the "Calcitite"™ and the "Interpore 200"™ granules (Figs. 1 and 2). The morphology of the migrating cells on both types of ceramic particle were similar. This finding was expected because of the similar chemical composition and rugosity of the solid surfaces. The colonising cells were polygonal, tesselated and exhibited many pseudopodial and filopodial extensions both anchoring the cells to the substrata and forming inter-cellular communications. In areas of close packing, the appearance was identical to that of the cells remaining on the host natural bone tissue although cells actively migrating from the host bone onto the bioceramic particles assumed a more elongated, fibroblast-like, morphology. The maintainence of a normal morphology, by the cells which had migrated onto these two materials, is significant since it has been reported (ref. 9) that other calcium phosphate ceramic preparations will affect osteoblast morphology.

Cells colonizing "Interpore 200"™ particles were seen, at 3 days, to

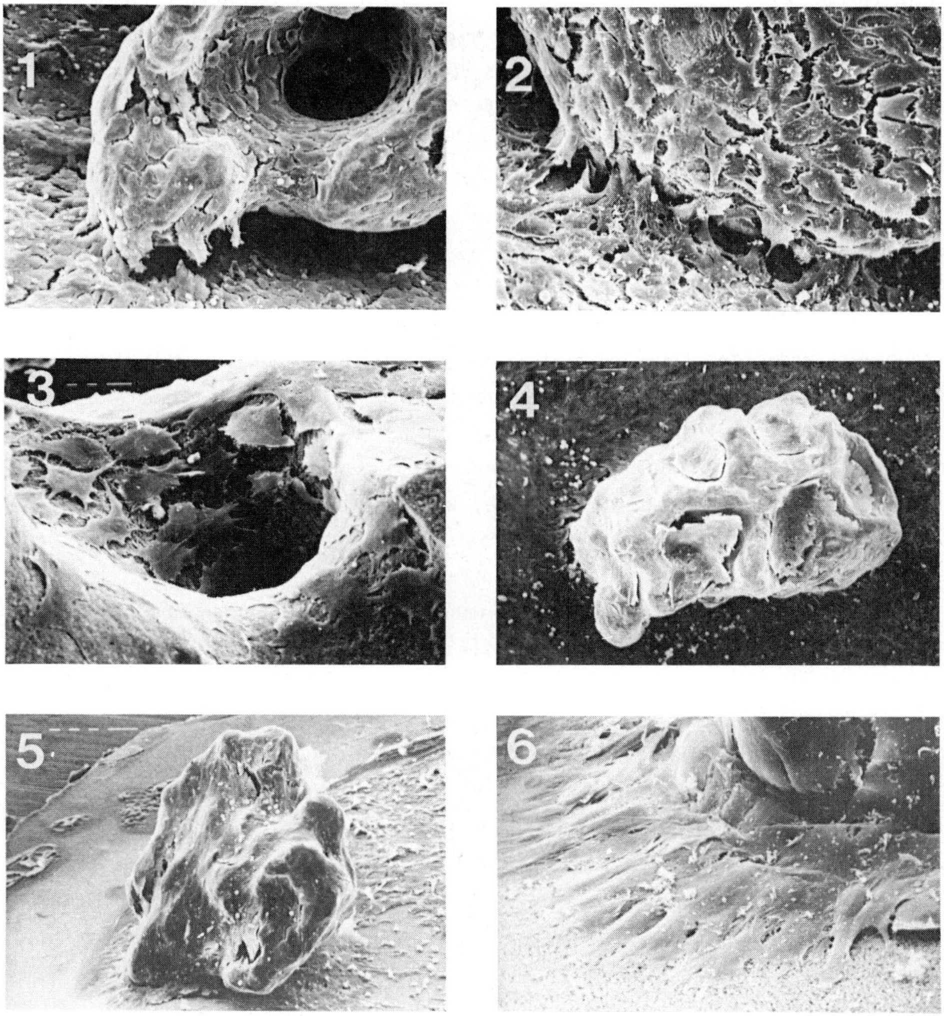

Figs. 1 and 2: SEM photomicrographs of primary bone-cell populations migrating onto "Interpore" and "Calcitite" calcium phosphate bioceramic particles respectively. Note that the morphology of the migrated cells is similar on both ceramic materials and the host bone surface. Field Widths = 513 and 290microns.
Fig. 3: Following a 3day culture period, cells can be seen migrating into the pore structure of this macroporous material. Note also the filopodial extensions which maintain both cell/substrate and cell/cell contact. Field Width = 186microns.
Fig. 4: Following 10days in culture, the colonizing cells have formed sheets of tissue covering the pore openings (only visible here due to peripheral shrinking during critical point drying). Such cellular enveloping will retard further ingrowth into the pore structure. Field Width = 1.52mm.
Figs. 5 and 6: A bioceramic particle after 10days culture on a diffusion chamber filter. The cells which have previously colonized the particle have now proliferated and migrated to anchor the former to the filter surface. Field Widths = 1.52mm and 300microns.

migrate from the outer surface into the pores of this material (Fig. 3). This would concur with reports of tissue ingrowth into this macroporous ceramic *in vivo* (ref. 10). However, by 10 days, migrating cells had formed continuous sheets over the orifices of the pores (Fig. 4) with smaller diameter pores being covered over preferentially. This finding suggested that while cells do migrate into the pores, covering over the pores by sheets of cells will limit tissue ingrowth within the pore structure.

(ii) Acid Phosphatase Staining and Light Microscopy Examination. It has been noted (ref. 11) that sterilization by high energy irradiation (^{60}Co-gamma) will cause an increase in the cell population colonizing some calcium phosphate ceramics. Using acid phosphatase histochemistry we have observed both osteoblasts and osteoclasts on "Calcitite"™ which had been irradiated prior to use *in vitro* (ref. 8). However, in short term culture, no osteoclasts were identified, in the present study, on the surface of "Interpore 200"™ either by incident light microscopy or SEM. Nevertheless, on sectioning a single DC which had become invaded by host tissue, we observed multinucleate giant cells within the pore structure of this material.

In vivo stage

After periods of 6-12 weeks the chambers were retrieved and macroscopic examination indicated that the particles had become firmly attached to the diffusion chamber filters. In the in vitro stage, attachment of the particles took place to one filter by cellular migration (Figs. 5 and 6), but on removal after implantation a small number (2 or less/chamber) of particles had re-attached to the opposite filter. Loss of attachment of these particles was due to insufficient numbers of cells anchoring the particles to the filter, which would indicate that cell migration during the first *in vitro* stage was variable.

The amount of tissue which formed in the diffusion chambers increased with the duration of implantation of both "Calcitite"™ and "Interpore 200"™. The outer surfaces of both materials were always covered with a confluent multi-cell layer of varying thickness containing organised collagen fibre bundles. This layer was continuous with that on the filter resulting in a smooth flowing, bow-shaped layer providing mechanically efficient anchorage within the DC volume. Of the two materials examined, the potential clinical advantage of "Interpore 200"™ is the ingrowth of tissue into the pore structure. While some cells did migrate into pores initially, as noted in the *in vitro* stage (vide supra), with increasing culture time developing fibrous tissue enveloped the surface of the particle reducing the likelihood of cell migration into the pores. This was evident when sections were examined (Fig. 7). However, studies of "Interpore 200"™ particles in a clinically-analogous animal model showed

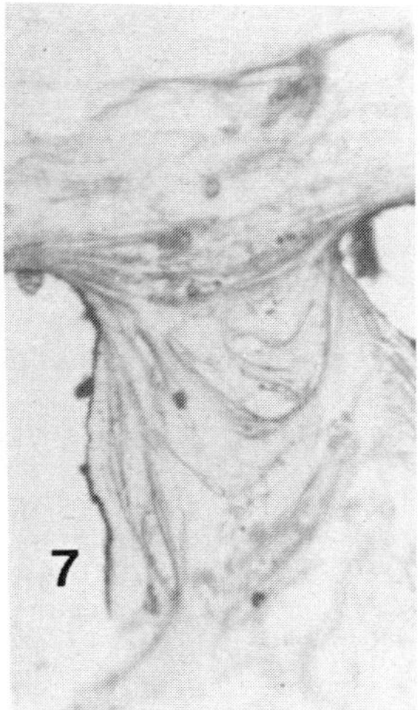

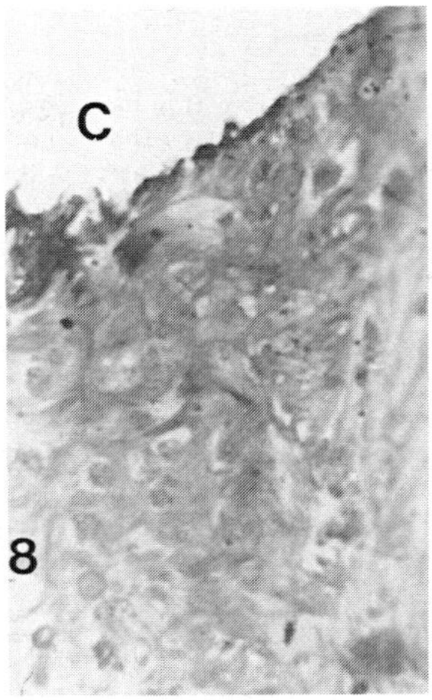

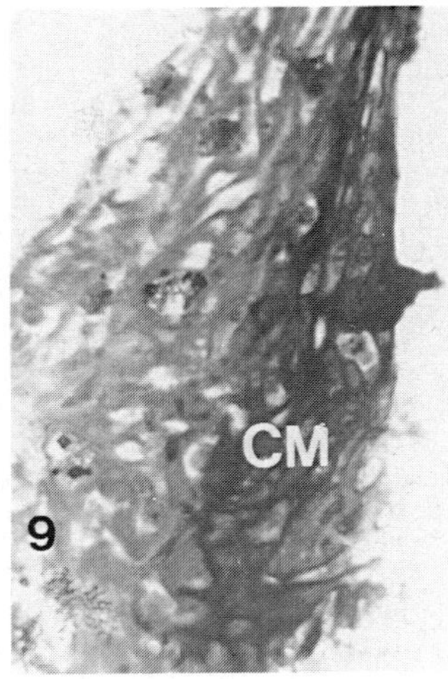

Fig. 7: Area of low tissue density at the opening of a pore. Note that while tissue is developing within the pore structure, sheets of cellular material are now bridging the pore opening. Compare with figs. 3, 4 and 5.
Fig. 8: Area of higher cell density apposed to the ceramic surface above (C). Note the dense, matted, collagen fibre network enclosing rounded cells.
Fig. 9: Similar area to that seen in fig. 8. Here, on the surface of the ceramic particle, the extracellular matrix has started to calcify. The cells trapped within this matrix (CM) may now be identified as osteocytes.
All specimens stained with Toluidene Blue. Field Width = 160microns.

that after 6 months the porous particles had become completely infiltrated with fibrous tissue and bone (ref. 6).

The dynamics of the in vitro/in vivo model employed, in this initial study, were such that the effective seeding density of cells within the diffusion chamber was low, and thus osteogenic tissue formation was low. The reasons for this have been discussed in detail by Tarrant and Davies (ref. 12). However, it has been possible to increase the relative seeding density by reducing the size of the diffusion chamber. This has resulted in the production of a mineralized extracellular matrix by migrated osteoblasts directly on the surface of the ceramic biomaterial (see Figs. 8, 9 and also Fig. 4 in ref. 7). While the initial matrix produced was of an un-organized type (ref. 12), this was followed by the laying down of linear sheets of collagenous extracellular matrix. This linear arrangement, itself, is re-organized into an inter-woven mat appearance wherein the synthesizing cells change in shape from an elongated fibroblastic form to a more rounded morphology (fig. 8). This tissue is reminiscent of the formation of osteoid and is followed by mineralization of the extracellular matrix to create woven bone. This work is now continuing, with the use of 3μl volume DC's, within the aim of quantifying the rate of mineralized ECM production in the presence of these two bioceramics.

ACKNOWLEDGEMENTS

Our thanks to Yvonne Bovell and Mark Dallas for technical assistance and Lyndsey Davies for manuscript preparation. This work is financially supported by the West Midlands Regional Health Authority and the S.E.R.C. (Grant. No. GR/D/53913).

REFERENCES

1 J.W. Frame & C.L. Brady, The versatility of hydroxyapatite blocks in bone augmentation, B.J. Oral Max. Surg., in press.
2 J.W. Frame, Hydroxyapatite as a biomaterial for alveolar ridge augmentation, Int. J. Oral Max. Surg., in press.
3 J.N. Kent, I.M. Finger, J.H. Quinn and L.R. Guerra, Hydroxyapatite alveolar ridge reconstruction: Clinical experiences, complications and technical modifications, J. Oral Maxillofac. Surg., 44 (1986) 37-49.
4 M. Jarcho, C.H. Bolen, M.B. Thomas, J. Bobick, J.F. Kay and R.H. Doremus, Hydroxyapatite synthesis and characterization in dense polycrystalline form, J. Mater. Sci., 11 (1976) 2027-2035.
5 D.M. Roy, S.K. Linnehan, Hydroxyapatite formed from coral skeletal carbonate by hydrothermal exchange, Nature, 247 (1974) 220-222.
6 J.W. Frame, P.G.J. Rout, R.M. Browne, A comparison of solid and porous particulate hydroxyapatite for alveolar ridge augmentation, submitted for publication.
7 J.E. Davies, S.F. Tarrant and T. Matsuda, Interaction between primary bone cell cultures and biomaterials, Part 1: Method; The in vitro and in vivo stages, Proc. European Congress on Biomaterials, Bologna, Sept. 14-17, 1986.
8 Y. Bovell, J.E. Davies, and S.F. Tarrant, Incident light and SEM observation of bone-cell colonized bioceramics, Histochem. J. (1986), in press.
9 J.E. Davies, R.P. Hurst, N.T. Spooner, Surface emission and biological probes for inorganic interfaces, to be published in "Interactions of Cells with Natural and Foreign Surfaces", [Eds. N. Crawford, D.E.M. Taylor] Plenum Press New York.
10 J.F. Piecuch, R.G. Topazian and S. Skoly, Experimental ridge augmentation with porous hydroxyapatite implants. J. Dent. Res. (1983) 62, 148-154.
11 J.E. Davies, Exoemssion for Biomaterials Research, Japan J. Appl. Phys., 24 S-4 (1985) 43-47.
12 S.F. Tarrant and J.E. Davies, Interaction between primary bone cell cultures and biomaterials, Part 2: Osteoblast behaviour, European Congress on Biomaterials, Bologna, Sept. 14-17, 1986.

Biomaterials and Clinical Applications, 597
edited by A. Pizzoferrato, P.G. Marchetti, A. Ravaglioli and A.J.C. Lee
Elsevier Science Publishers B.V., Amsterdam, 1987 — Printed in The Netherlands

INTERACTION BETWEEN PRIMARY BONE CELL CULTURES AND BIOMATERIALS PART 4: COLONIZATION OF CHARGED POLYMER SURFACES

R.M. SHELTON, I.M. WHYTE and J.E. DAVIES*
Department of Anatomy, University of Birmingham Medical School, Birmingham, B15 2TJ, England.

SUMMARY

Osteoblasts migrating in vitro over polymers exhibited a flattened morphology and a "stand off" relationship on positively and negatively charged surfaces respectively. Synthesis of extracellular matrix was only seen when the cells were colonizing polymers displaying negative surface charge.

INTRODUCTION

A knowledge of the interaction between osteoblasts (OB's) and polymer surfaces is of considerable importance in the development of both bone substitute and ligament replacement biomaterials. The early migration of OB's onto bone substitute materials may be analogous to the colonization of tissue culture polystyrene. The cellular covering of differently treated polystyrene can be related to surface charge (refs. 1-3). Surface treatments also influence serum protein adsorption (refs. 4, 5), which in turn affects the rate of cell spreading (ref. 6). This in-vitro study is an extension of previous work (ref. 7) which demonstrated that OB's migrating over positively charged ion exchange resin beads were flattened and closely adapted to the substrate, with little dorsal cell surface membrane activity (the dorsal surface being exposed to medium in culture, the ventral surface overlying the bead). OB's on negatively charged substrata adopted a "stand off" morphology with considerably more dorsal surface activity in the form of blebs and ruffles. In the present work we have examined the interface between charged polymer substrata and OB's using transmission electron microscopy (TEM).

METHODS

Four types of "Amberlite" (Rohm & Haas Co., Philadelphia) polystyrene ion exchange resin beads were used in the study, selected according to their surface morphology (smooth gel or rough macroporous) and charge sign (see Table 1). The ion exchange resin beads were cut in half under distilled water to create a flat base, which was later placed on a periosteally stripped rat parietal bone fragment. The bone fragments were transferred to individual wells

* To whom correspondance should be addressed.

TABLE 1. Ion Exchange Resin Beads

Bead No.	Type	Bead Surface Group	Surface Morphology	Exchange ion
200	strong acid cation exchanger	HSO_3^-	rough	Na^+
IRC 84	weak acid cation exchanger	$R\text{-}COO^-$	smooth	H^+
IRC 50	weak acid cation exchanger	$R\text{-}COO^-$	rough	H^+
IRA 900	strong base anion exchanger	$R\text{-}CH_2N^+$	rough	Cl^-
IRA 400	strong base anion exchanger	$R\text{-}CH_2N^+$	smooth	Cl^-

in a Linbro tissue culture multiwell plate in 2mls of Fitton-Jackson modified Biggers medium. Two halves of resin beads were placed flat surface down on the endocranial surface of the parietal fragment and maintained _in vitro_ for up to 7 days in a 5% CO_2 atmosphere at 37°C. Specimens for electron microscopic examination were fixed in 2.5% glutaraldehyde in 0.1M cacodylate buffer pH 7.2 at 4°C for 24hrs, washed using 0.25M sucrose in 0.1M cacodylate buffer pH 7.2 several times and post fixed in 1% osmium tetroxide in 0.1M cacodylate buffer for 1hr at room temperature. Samples were dehydrated through a graded series of ethanols, critical point dried from CO_2 and gold coated to a thickness of 200A for scanning electron microscopical examination (SEM), using an ISI 100A microscope. Some samples were prepared directly for TEM observation, using the same fixation procedure and embedded in "Epon". Sections of 750-800 A were cut using glass knives, stained with uranyl acetate and lead citrate and viewed using a Jeol CX11 electron microscope.

RESULTS

Scanning Electron Microscopy

Over the culture period, OB's migrated over approximately 60% of the beads surface area, although occasionally beads cultured under identical conditions would be sparsely covered. The least consistent and poorest coverage was noted on IRC 84. The observations of Davies et al (ref.7) were confirmed; OB's adapted very closely to strongly positively charged beads and showed little dorsal surface activity (Fig.1A and B). Contact was maintained with adjacent cells by filopodia around the entire margin of the cells. OB's on the weakly negatively charged beads did not adapt closely to their substrate, but maintained a more "stand off" (Fig. IC and D) position as previously observed. These cells had a greater dorsi-ventral depth, made more numerous contacts via microextensions with the bead surface and demonstrated considerably more dorsal surface activity, in the form of blebs and ruffles, than their counterparts on

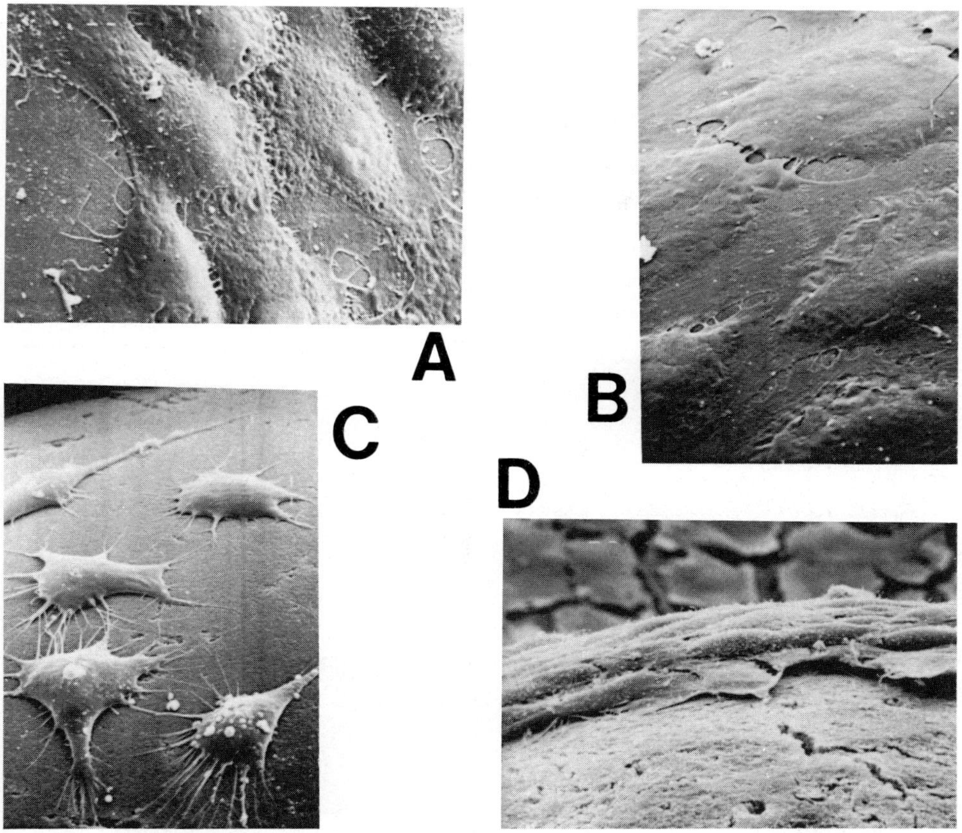

Figure 1. Scanning electron micrographs of OB's on ion exchange beads. [A] IRA 900 and [B] IRA 400 showing flattened OB's with little dorsal surface activity. [C] IRC 84 and [D] IRC 50 showing plump cells with dorsal blebs and ruffling. Field widths; 57μm, 40μm, 40μm and 71μm respectively.

positive substrata.

Transmission Electron Microscopy

Obtaining thin sections of the OB's adhering to the beads was difficult due to incomplete infiltration of the embedding resin into the bead. Sectioning at gold or silver thickness resulted in fragmenting of the bead such that the cell/substrate interface could not be seen. A compromise of decreased resolution at an increased section thickness of 750-800Å was accepted. Despite this, examination of cells on both rough and smooth surfaced positive beads revealed common characteristics. The OB's demonstrated a flattened morphology (as seen at SEM) very closely apposed to the bead surface, so that the ventral cell membrane could not be seen, minimal dorsal membrane surface activity and a flat elongated nucleus. There was little cytoplasm dorsally or ventrally

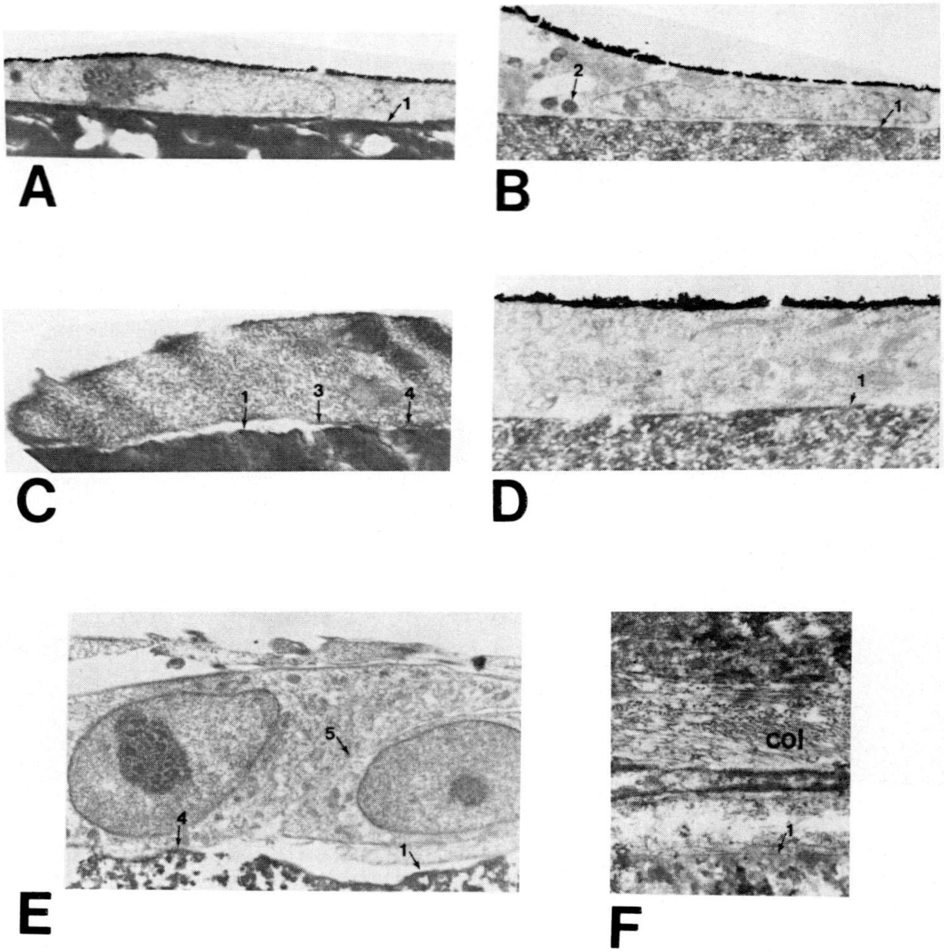

Fig. 2. TEM photomicrographs. [A] and [B], flattened cells on IRA 400 and IRA 900 respectively with ventral cell membrane not visible; [C] and [E], plump cells on IRC 84 and IRC 50 showing adhesions only in discrete areas; [D], higher magnification of cell on IRA 900, cell membrane still not visible; [F], demonstration of collagen above surface of 200 bead. Field widths; 15μm, 12μm, 5μm, 7μm, 13μm and 2.5μm respectively. 1= bead surface 2 = secretory vesicle 3 = cell surface 4 = electron dense cytoplasm over adhesion area 5 = close cell-cell contact.

between the cell margin and the nuclear envelope. The dark staining line on the dorsal surface of the cells (Fig. 2A and B) was from the gold sputter coating used during preparation for SEM. At higher magnification the bead surface was delineated by a near continuous electron dense line, yet it was not possible to visualize the ventral cell membrane of the cell (Fig. 2D).

The macroporous bead IRC 50 revealed a discontinuous surface (probably as a result of fragmentation during sectioning) but a continuous one on the smooth gel IRC 84. The OB's showed similarities on both negative beads, having a plump morphology, rounded nuclei and adhering closely to the substrate only in discrete areas. The ventral cell membrane was visualized even at low power (Fig 2C and E). Preliminary examination of a strongly negatively charged macroporous bead, 200, indicated a similar "stand off" morphology of the osteoblasts with respect to the bead surface and also the synthesis of extracellular collagen. Collagen appeared to be laid down along two axes approximately perpendicular to one another (Fig. 2F).

DISCUSSION

The "stand off" and flattened cell morphology seen previously (ref. 7) were confirmed in this TEM examination on negatively and positively charged substrata respectively. These results strongly indicate that substrate charge sign plays an important role in determining the nature of adhesion to the substrate and the migratory morphology of osteoblasts. There are two theoretical models of cell adhesion. The DLVO model of colloid stability suggests a balance between electrostatic forces of repulsion (from the negatively charged cell surface) and electromagnetic attraction due to fluctuating dipole moments in the substrate and cell surface, in addition to any interposed medium. The contact hypothesis involves not only dipole and electrostatic forces, but also hydrogen and hydrophobic bonding. Since all vertebrate cell surfaces may be assumed to have a net negative charge (ref. 8) the "stand off" relationship of OB's on negatively charged beads can be accounted for by the mutual repulsion of like charges. Similarly the close adaptation of osteoblasts on positive beads would be expected between surfaces of opposite charge sign. The discrete regions of cellular attachment seen on negative beads were characterized by an electron dense area of cytoplasm immediately deep to the cell membrane. The appearance of the cellular attachments was similar to "adhesion plaques" (ref. 9). Although little is known about these plaques it is possible they may be areas of decreased negativity, sufficient for that area of the cell to overcome electrostatic forces of repulsion. The cell membrane is the first contact a cell has with its surrounding environment and as such must play an important role in determining cellular activity and function. Pilla (ref. 10) proposes that charge fields may produce local structural modifications in the cell membrane and thereby transfer information which modifies cell regulation. Fibroblasts exposed in culture to both continuous and pulsed electrostatic fields, have demonstrated an increase in the number of mitochondria, free ribosomes and secretory vesicles (ref. 11). Whilst the latter is not analagous to the model presented, the implication is that charge influences cellular behaviour. The very close approximation of OB's on positively charged beads could inhibit their synthesis of extracellular matrix, either due to the close relationship with the substrate or to a modification in cell membrane function. Interestingly, the only synthetic activity we have observed on these charged surfaces is on the strongly negatively charged 200 bead, where collagen has been laid down above the bead surface (Fig. 2F).

We believe that it is of central importance in understanding these interfacial phenomena that the morphological and metabolic effects brought about by surface charge are distinguished. Our work is currently concerned with the surface charge effects on protein adsorption and the synthesis of extracellular matrix by the migrated osteoblasts.

ACKNOWLEDGEMENTS

We are grateful to A. Murdoch and J. Wallington for technical assistance and L. Davies for preparing the manuscript. Part of this work contributed to a B.Sc. degree in Anatomical Studies (I.M.W.). R.M.S. is grateful for financial support from The Wellcome Trust.

REFERENCES

1 N.G. Maroudas, Adhesion and spreading of cells on charged surfaces, J. Theor. Biol., 49 (1975) 417-424.
2 A.S.G. Curtis, J.V. Forrester, C. McInnes and F. Lawrie, Adhesion of cells to polystyrene surfaces, J. Cell Biol., 97 (1983) 1500-1506.
3 M.J. Lydon and C.S. Clay, Substratum topography and cell traction on sulphuric acid treated bacteriological-grade plastic, Cell Biol. Int. Rep. 9(10) (1985) 911-921.
4 K.L. Bentley and R.J. Klebe, Fibronectin binding properties of bacteriologic petri plates and tissue culture dishes, J. Biomed. Mater. Res. 19 (1985) 757-769.
5 A.S.G. Curtis and J.V. Forrester, The competitive effects of serum proteins on cell adhesion, J. Cell Sci., 71 (1984) 17-35.
6 P. Knox, Kinetics of cell spreading in the presence of different concentrations of serum or fibronectin depleted serum, J. Cell Sci., 71 (1984) 51-59.
7 J.E. Davies, B. Causton, Y. Bovell, K. Davy and C.S. Sturt, The migration of osteoblasts over substrata of discrete surface charge, Biomaterials 7 (1986) 231-233.
8 L. Weiss, A Biophysical Consideration of Cell Contact Phenomena, in: R.S. Manly (Ed.) Adhesion in Biological Systems, Academic Press, New York, 1970,
9 M. Abercrombie, J.E.M. Heaysman and S.M. Pegrum, The locomotion of fibroblasts in culture, IV, Electron microscopy of the leading lamella, Exp. Cell Res., 67 (1971) 359-367.
10 A.A. Pilla, Electrochemical Information Transfer and its Possible Role in the Control of Cell Function, in: C.T. Brighton, J. Black and S.R. Pollack (Eds.) Electrical Properties of Bone and Cartilage. Grune and Stratton, New York, 1979, pp455-489.
11 C.A.L. Bassett, Biophysical Principles Affecting Bone Structure, in: G.H. Bourne (Ed.) The Biochemistry and Physiology of Bone, 2nd Edition Vol III, Academic Press, New York and London, 1971, pp1-76.

Biomaterials and Clinical Applications,
edited by A. Pizzoferrato, P.G. Marchetti, A. Ravaglioli and A.J.C. Lee
Elsevier Science Publishers B.V., Amsterdam, 1987 — Printed in The Netherlands

MORPHOLOGICAL STUDIES OF NEW BONE FORMATION FAVOURED BY ß-TCMP IMPLANTS.

A.Ruggeri[1], M.Franchi[1], A.Evangelisti[1], V.De Pasquale[1], A.Bigi[2], A.Ripamonti[2], N.Roveri[2].

1 Institute of Human Anatomy, University of Bologna.

2 Chemistry Department - G. Ciamician, University of Bologna.

SUMMARY

Magnesium substituted ß-tricalcium phosphate (ß-TCMP) has been used as a new alloplastic biodegradable material aimed to fill bone cavities and to restore bone defects in dentistry. The material, which was partly sintered before use, was implanted in tibia and maxillary bone cavities of monkeys and studied by radiographic follow-ups and light and transmission electron microscopy observations.

The results suggest two different mechanisms of resorption: a) a cell-mediated dissolution of unsintered ß-TCMP grains accompanied by an accelerated extracellular calcification and b) a passive dissolution of sintered ß-TCMP grains accompanied by a rapid new bone formation around these grains. The influnce on the process of new bone formation is discussed.

INTRODUCTION

Among the calcium phosphates which are present in calcified tissues, ß-$Ca_3(PO_4)_2$ (ß-TCP) is second only to hydroxyapatite in its stability under most physiological conditions(1). Furthermore, it represents the inorganic phase present in several pathological calcifications (2,3) and is the product of thermal conversion of biological apatites (4). The different solubilty of ß-TCP and hydroxyapatite (1) suggests that, when used as bone implant materials, ß-TCP materials should be more resorbable than hydroxyapatite materials. It is known that magnesium plays an important role in the selective precipitation of a hydroxyapatite and ß-TCP in aqueous medium (4,5). On the other hand an appreciable amount of magnesium ion is present in human bone (6).

On this basis we have prepared ß-TCMP with a substitution of magnesium for calcium such that the relative amounts of these two ions were equivalent to those found in human bone (6) and utilized it to fill bone cavities. The new bone implant material, part of which was sintered, was tested in monkeys. The biocompatibility, the rate and the modality of resorption and the osteostimula tion of the material was investigated by radiographic follow-ups and light and transmission electron microscopy observations.

METHODS

ß-TCMP with a substitution of magnesium for calcium of 2.5 atom % was prepared by solid state reaction at 1000° C of ß-$Ca_3(PO_4)_2$ and $Mg_3(PO_4)_2$. Part of the ß-TCMP powder was compressed in a stainless steel up to an applied pressure of 3.5 tons/cm^2. Sintering temperature of 1000° C was reached at a rate of 100° C/h and held for 5h. Thereafter the temperature decreased at a rate of 100° C/h. Sintered material was ground to a grain size of 200-300 um . Specimens containing 50 % unsintered and 50 % sintered powder mixed with fibrin clot (Tissucol-Immuno) were implanted in tibia and maxillary bone cavities of monkeys. Several bone cavities were left empty for control evaluations . Postsurgery periodic oral hygienic treatments and radiographs were carried out starting 1 wk after implantation. 2, 4 and 8 wks after surgery, biopsies were taken for light and transmission electron microscopy. The samples were fixed in Millonig buffered glutaraldehyde solution (2 %). Specimens for light microscopy were decalcified, dehydrated and embedded in paraffin. Sections of 5 um were prepared and stained with Haematoxylin-Eosin, Azan Mallory, Sirius Red and Masson's Tricromic. Specimens for electron microscopy were either decalcified with EDTA or directly post fixed in 1 % buffered (Millonig) OsO4. After the dehydration in graded alcohols, the specimens were embedded in Araldite. Thin sections were stained with Uranil Acetate and Lead Citrate. Semi-thin sections were stained with Toluidine Blu.

OBSERVATIONS

In the radiographs carried out immediately after surgery and 1 and 2 wks later, the implant material was distinguishable from the surrounding bone while it was no longer appreciable 4 wks after surgery.

Histological sections carried out 2 wks after surgery showed dense connective tissue filling the spaces within the ß-TCMP grains. Scarse inflammatory cells were detectable. According to their dimensions, unsintered grains were histologically distinguishable from the sintered ones. The formers were usually grouped in clusters. Around and within these clusters, fibroblasts, few macrophages and giant cells could be detected (fig.1). On thin sections these last cells contained single grains . Furthermore areas of precipitated calcium crystal needles on a background of collagen fibrils were observable close to these cells(fig.2).

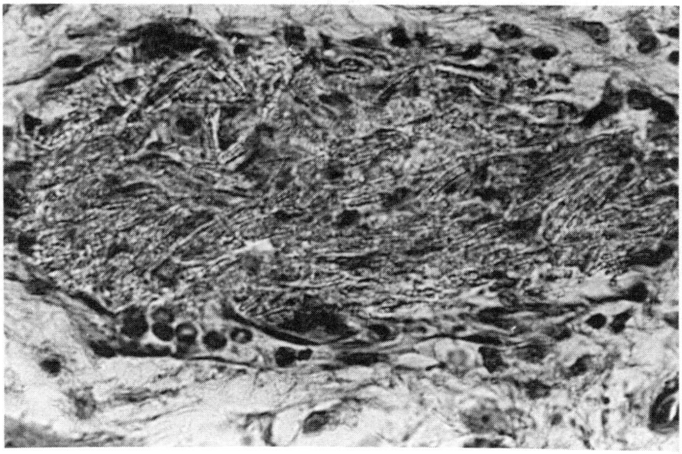

Fig. 1

Among clusters of unsintered grains, sintered ß-TCMP grains were detectable.On paraffin sections they appeared to be permeated by stainable material and surrounded by fibroblasts and osteoblasts-like globous cells. On thin sections,these cells, close to the grains, showed a high secretory activity. Moreover most part of the material penetrating the grain micropores was represented by thin cells foldings and collagen fibrils containing extracellular matrix (fig.3).

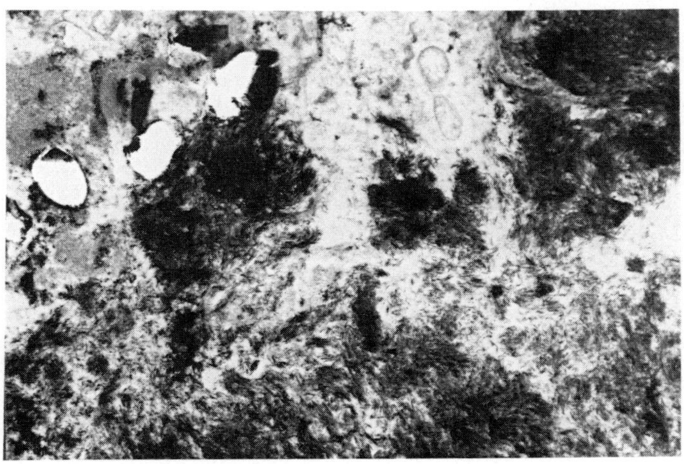

Fig. 2

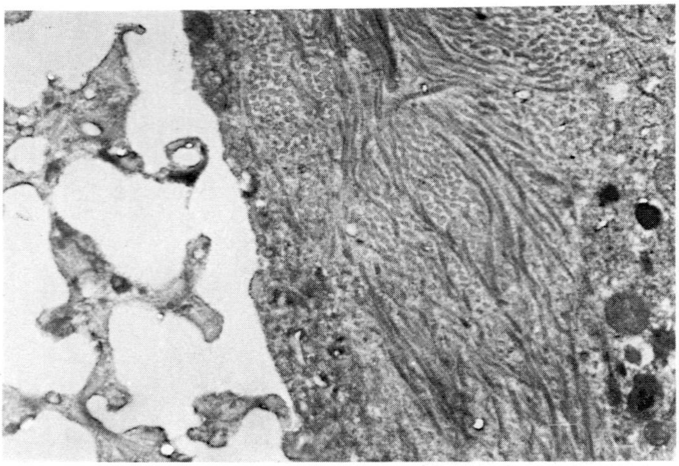

Fig. 3

4 wks after surgery very few unsintered grains were still detectable both in paraffin and thin sections. It is noteworthy that new bone spicules, remnants of unsintered grains and scattered in the cavity were observable. On the other hand the majority of the sintered grains was close to or surrounded by large areas of bone-like tissue(fig. 4).

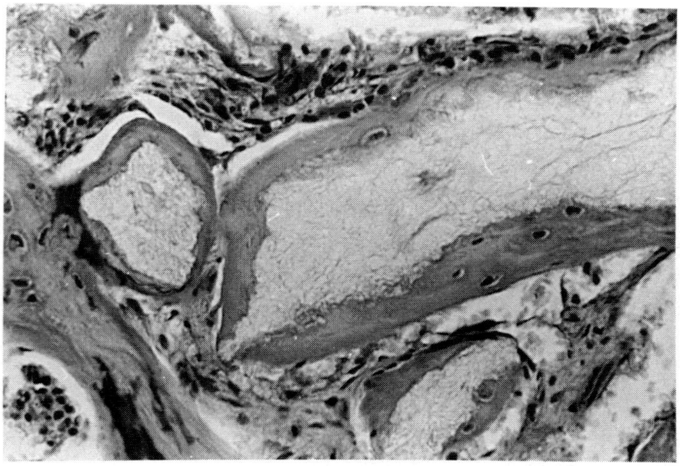

Fig. 4

On thin sections, tightly close to the grains a bone-like extracellular matrix was observed; osteoid-like tissue with highly secreting cells was externally surrounding this matrix (fig.5).

8 wks after surgery very few sintered grains were still detectable. Each

grain was surrounded by both primary and lamellar bone. Moreover other thick lamellar bone spiculae were also observed in the central part (fig.6).

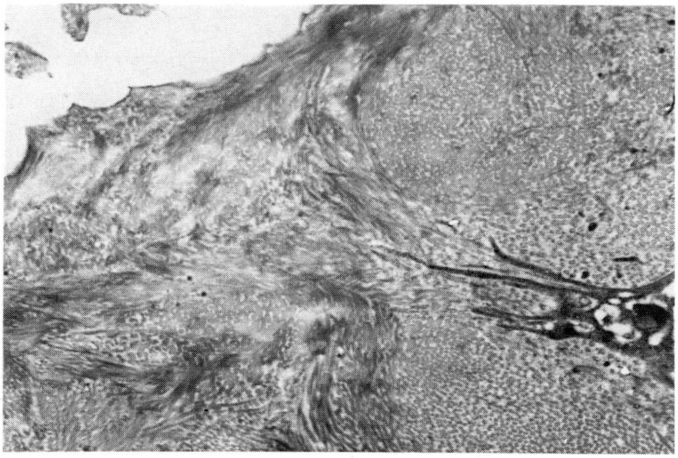

Fig. 5

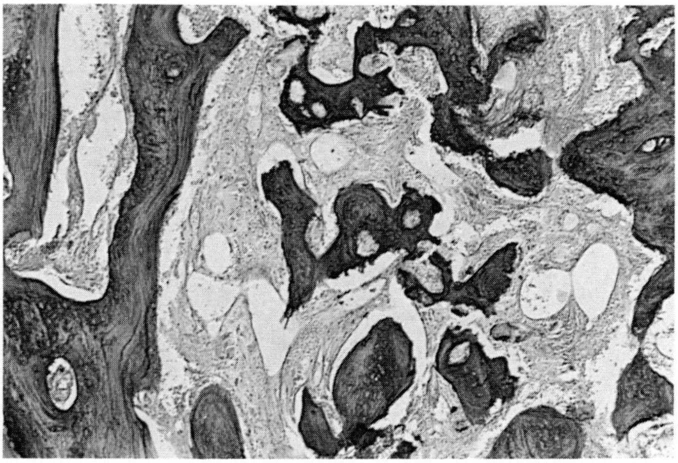

Fig. 6

Histological sections of 8 wks control samples showed new formed bone trabeculae mainly at the periphery of the cavities, while a dense connective tissue was still present in the central part.

DISCUSSION

According to our observations, clusters of unsintered ß-TCMP grains are quickly surrounded by fibroblasts and giant cells. The latters always contain grains. Close to these grain clusters, calcified areas are shown on an extracellular matrix of dense connective tissue. It is suggested that a cell-mediated dissolution of unsintered ß-TCMP grains is accompanied by an accelerated extracellular calcification.

The ß-TCMP sintered grains appear to be surrounded and penetrated by fibroblasts and osteoblasts-like cells and connective tissue matrix. Around the grains giant cells or macrophages are not detectable. At the electron microscopy this matrix shows to undergo a gradual process of calcification which begins from the areas tightly close to the grains. It is suggested that a passive dissolution of sintered ß-TCMP grains and an early new bone formation around these grains take place.

In conclusion, the early presence of newly calcified areas tightly close to both unsintered and sintered grains suggests that the bone implant material containing a mixture of unsintered and sintered (1:1)magnesium substituted ß-TCP accelerate the process of new bone formation.

REFERENCES

1 G.H.Nancollas, Biological Mineralization and Demineralization, Springer-Verlag, New York,1981.

2 R.Z.Le Geros,S.R.Contiguglia and A.C.Alfrey, Pathological Calcifications Associated with Uremia, Calcif.Tissue Res.,13 (1973) 173-185

3 A.Bigi,E.Foresti,A.Incerti,A.Ripamonti and N.Roveri,Strctural and Chemical Characterization of Inorganic Deposits in Calcified Human Aortic Wall,Chim. Acta,55 (1980) 81-85

4 S.Baravelli,A.Bigi,A.Ripamonti,N,Roveri and E.Foresti, Thermal Behavior of bone and Synthetic Hydroxyapatites Submitted to Magnesium Interaction in Aqueous Medium, J.Inorg.Biochem. 20 (1984) 1-12

5 R.Z.Le Geros,M.H.Taheri,G.B.Quirologico and J.P.Le Geros, Formation and Stability of Apatites: Effects of some Cationic Substituents, Proc.2nd International Congress of Pjosphorous Compounds, Boston (1980)89-103

6 J.E.Eastoe in Biochemestry Handbook (G.C.Long ed.)London, (1961) 715

Biomaterials and Clinical Applications,
edited by A. Pizzoferrato, P.G. Marchetti, A. Ravaglioli and A.J.C. Lee
Elsevier Science Publishers B.V., Amsterdam, 1987 — Printed in The Netherlands

TISSUE REACTION AND BIODEGRADATION BEHAVIOR OF VARIOUS CALCIUM PHOSPHATE MATERIALS

W. WAGNER*, U.W. WAHLMANN* and D. HEIDEMANN**

* Clinic for maxillo-facial surgery, Augustusplatz 2, D-6500 Mainz, FRG

** Dept.Cons.Dent.&Periodont., Dental School, Augustusplatz 2, D-6500 Mainz, FRG

SUMMARY

Various types of calcium phosphate ceramics have attracted major attention during the last decades because they are biocompatible with bone and soft tissue. In this study we compared tricalcium phosphate (TCP) ceramics and hydroxyapatite (HA) ceramics either as almost dense materials or specimen with microporosity and macroporosity.

All calcium phosphate materials were biocompatible with bone and soft tissue. Histologic investigations showed no significant difference with very good tissue reaction. New bone without any interlayer of connective tissue was found in direct contact with the surface of HA (96% of surface), TCP (97% of surface) and glass ceramic (92% of surface) pins after 3 month.

A biological degradation took place in all types of ceramics. The biodegradability of the ceramics depended on the porosities and size of the particles. Results for dense tricalcium phosphate and hydroxyapatite showed that tricalcium phosphate ceramics are only slightly more biodegradable than hydroxyapatite. We believe that the porosity and the crystallographic structure of the ceramics are much more important than the Ca/P ratio of the ceramics. However both factors are a cause for the difference in biodegradation behavior. The different advantages and disadvantages of the various ceramics imply a selection of the best ceramics for the particular indication.

INTRODUCTION

Calcium phosphate ceramics are biocompatible with bone and soft tissue. New bone of a lamellar or woven structure proliferatesonto the surface, in the macroporous types and between the granulates without an interlayer of connective tissue (ref. 1-5). Recently there have been several papers published on chemistry, preparation and biocompatibility of calcium phosphate ceramics, for both solid and porous forms. Biodegradable tricalcium phosphate (ref. 6-8), nondegradable hydroxyapatite (ref. 9-10) and CaP containing glass ceramics (ref. 11-12) are the common groups of CaP-materials. Dense and porous forms of all ceramics are available. A lot of different types of ceramics have been developed (see Tab 1.) without a comparable experimental or clinical study. The aim of this study is to compare the tissue reaction and biodegradation behavior of various commercially available calcium phosphateceramics.

MATERIALS:

Commercially available calcium phosphate granulates with microporosity and/or macroporosity (6 HA/ 2 TCP) and dense ceramics (4 HA/ 1TCP) were compared. Furthermore the tissue reaction of a porous tricalcium phosphate ceramic impregnated with fixed gentamycin-salt was investigeted. Gentamycin is used to decrease the inflamation rate of the porous types.

CaP-MATERIALS	investigated specimen
I. natural primary materials	
a) marine corals	INTERPORE
b) bovine bone	PYROST
II. synthetic materials	
a) dense ceramics (>5% pores)	CALCITITE, ALVEOGRAF
	HA-FUA, HA-FRIEDRICHSFELD
	HA-PHILIPS, ALLOTROPAT
b) porous ceramics (50-60% pores)	OSPROVIT (50%), CEROS 80 (60%)
III. glass ceramics	CERAVITAL

TABLE 1
Investigated HA-granulates

Dense cylindrical pins of three different materials (HA/TCP/glass ceramic) with a diameter of 2 mm were implanted into bone to compare the osseous layer on the surface of the implants. Cross sections of these pins were used for morphometric analysis.

METHODS:

To compare the osseous reaction and biodegradation, specimens of each type of ceramic were implanted into the left and right femur and abdominal muscles of rats. The animals were anesthetized with sodium Ketamin (Ketanest, 50mg/ml, Parke-Davis) 125mg/kg by intraperitoneal injection. The granulates were implanted through a window made in the distal cortical bone of the femur. The cylindrical pins were implanted into a drill-hole of 2mm in diameter. The animals were sacrificed at 1,2,3 and 6 months after implantation. The specimens were embedded in methyl methacrylate and cut into microslices. The sections were examined after Giemsa staining. Morphometric analysis of the sections of the dense cylindrical pins (ref. 12) were done using the M.O.P. equipment (manufactured by Kontron Co).

RESULTS:

Clinically an uneventful wound healing was observed in all rats. None of the implants were mobile. The radiographic examinations revealed no difference between the numerous materials and showed good bony healing arround the ceramics. Radiographically was there no sign of degradation.

The histological appearances of the healing processes of all ceramics were similar. The ceramics were well accepted and rapidly incorporated into the host bone. The new bone had been deposited directly on the surface after 14 days or grew onto the surface during the following weeks. In porous specimens the tissue ingrowth was completed after 4 weeks. Synthetically porous granulates occasionally demonstrated empty pores while larger blocks only showed an ingrowth of bone or soft tissue into an outer layer of 2 to 4 mm thickness. There was similar bone formation in the group containing gentamycin.

Great differences exist in the degradation behavior of the different ceramics. Afer 14 days a great degradation of porous tricalcium phosphate took place and macrophagus cells carried off particles of the ceramics. The same behavior exists although less pronounced in porous hydroxylapatite The degradation increases in the soft tissue of the muscle, with increase of the porosity and with decrease of particle size. The natural materials -Pyrost and Interpore- varied in degradation in different areas of the same specimen, perhaps due to different contents of calciumcarbonate or tricalcium phosphate.

In dense hydroxyapatite there was no evidence of resorption. In high magnification there appears a disintegration of the supperficial ceramic-layer. This disintegration was more pronounced in the dense TCP and glass ceramic specimens. In all dense ceramics superficial degradation occured in areas with soft tissue contact after 6 month. The greatest degradation of the dense pins was seen in Ceravital followed by TCP and less pronounced in hydroxyapatite.

Morphometric results

After 3 months bone contact averaged 96% (range: 92-100%) of the surface of hydroxyapatite, 97% (range: 87-100%) of tricalcium phosphate surface, and 92% (range: 86-98%) of the surface of the glass ceramic (see Fig. 1). There was no signifficant difference between the 3 ceramics. The contact between bone and these CaP-materials increased very quickly during the first 12 weeks with a negligible gain thereafter up to 6 months (see Fig. 2).

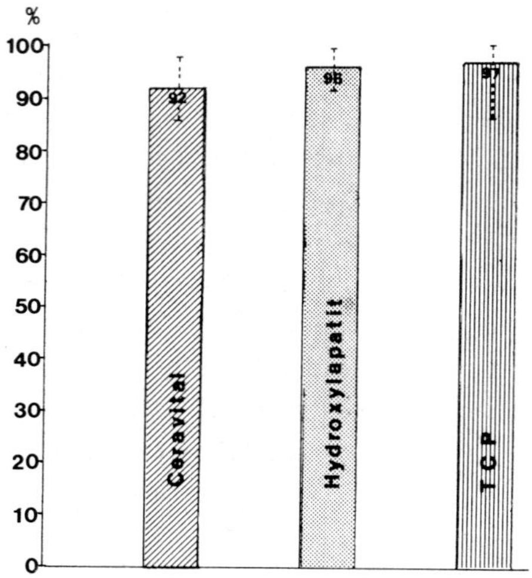

Fig. 1. Morphometric results: percentage of bone contact 3 months after implantation of Ceravital, HA and TCP in the femora of rats. (n=12 for each material)

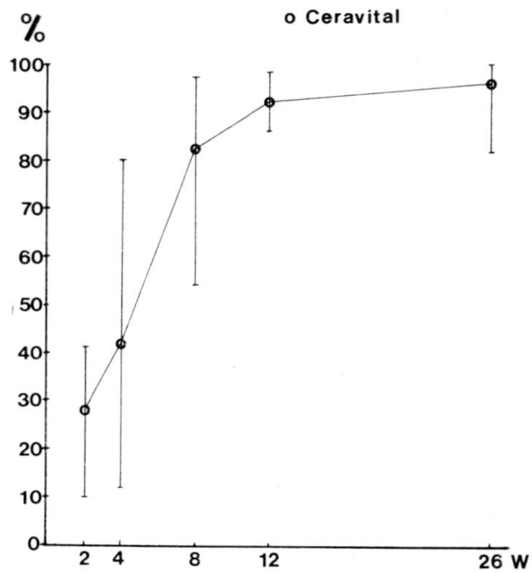

Fig. 2. Morphometric results: increasing percentage of bone contact for Ceravital after implantation from 2 to 26 weeks. (n=12 for each time measured)

DISCUSSION

All calcium phosphate materials were biocompatible with bone and soft tissue (ref. 1-10). New bone of a lamellar or woven structure proliferated onto the surface, in the macroporous types and between the granulates without an interlayer of connective tissue. Histologic investigations showed no significant difference in the tissue reaction. Porous ceramics allowed ingrowth of soft tissue and bone which enhances retention and produces a very satisfactory interface layer. Synthesized porous specimens however contained empty pores. The controlled interconnected porosity of natural porous materials has not been copied synthetically (ref. 3). Therfore ceramics from natural porous materials with an uniform pore size and complete interconnection of pores are preferred to block materials.

The biological degradation took place in all types of ceramics (ref. 13). The biodegradability of porous tricalcium phosphate was greater than hydroxyapatite particles. Results from dense and porous hydroxyapatite showed that this material is also biodegradable. Results from dense tricalcium phosphate and hydroxyapatite showed that the tricalcium phosphate ceramic is only slightly more biodegradable than hydroxyapatite. We believe that the porosity of the ceramics is much more important than the Ca/P ratio or crystallographic structure of the ceramics, as also mentioned by Klein and coworkers (ref.14). However both factors are a cause for the difference in biodegradation behavior. The biodegradation rate was much higher in soft tissue than in bone. The porosity can lead to degradation of the implant especially in soft tissue. Thus when the implant has to be permanent and withstand functional forces, a more dense, solid form of hydroxyapatite is indicated. On the other hand in unstressed areas (ref.15) of bone porous types of TCP and HA are prefered, which allow an ingrowth of bone and only slow substitution of the implant material. Different specimens of CaP-ceramics have different advantages and disadvantages and these offer a selection of the best ceramics for the particular surgical indication.

REFERENCES

1 J.F. Osborn, Implantatwerkstoff Hydroxylapatitkeramik, Quintessenz, Berlin Chicago London Rio de Janeiro Tokio, 1985

2 H.P. Drobeck, S.S. Rothstein, G.I. Kenneth, A.D. Sherer and R.G. Slighter, Histologic observation of soft tissue responses to implanted, multifaceted particles and discs of hydroxylapatite, J. oral Maxfac. Surg., 42 (1984) 143-149.

3 R. Holmes, V. Mooney, R. Bucholz and A. Tencer, A coralline hydroxyapatite bone graft substitute, Clinical Orthop. Tel. Res. 188 (1984) 252-262.

4 K. DeGroot, Bioceramics consisting calciumphosphate salts, Biomaterials 1 (1980) 47-50

5 H. Denissen, C. Mangano and G. Venini, Hydroxylapatite implants, Piccin, Padua, 1985.

6 S.N. Bhaskar, J.N. Brady, L. Getter, M.F. Growner and Th. Driskell, Biodegradable ceramic implants in bone. Electron and light microscopic analysis, Oral Surg., 32 (1971) 336-346.

7 K. Köster, H. Erhard, J. Kubicek und H. Heide, Experimentelle Anwendungen von Kalziumphosphatgranulat zur Substitution von konventionellen Knochentransplantaten. Z. Orthop. u. Grenz. 118 (1979) 398-403

8 W. Wagner und U.W. Wahlmann, Vergleichende tierexperimentelle Untersuchungen nach der Implantation verschiedener Kalziumphosphat-Keramiken, Dtsch. Zahnärztl. Z. 40 (1985) 664-667.

9 M. Jarcho, Calcium phosphate ceramics as hard tissue prosthetics, Clin. Orthop. 157 (1981) 259-278.

10 P.J. Boyne, S.S. Rothstein, K.I. Gumaer and H.P. Drobeck, Long-term study of hydroxylapatite implants in canine alveolar bone, J. oral Maxfac. Surg., 42 (1984) 589-594.

11 L.L. Hench, R.J. Splinter, W.C. Allen and T.K. Greenlee, Bonding mechanisms at the interface of ceramic prosthetic materials, J. Biomed. Mater. Res. 2 (1971) 117-121.

12 V. Strunz, Enossale Implantationsmaterialien in der Mund- und Kieferchirurgie, Hanser, München Wien, 1985
13 K. Donath, F. Sitzmann and G. Bauer, Experimentelle Untersuchungen über das Einwachsverhalten verschiedener Kalziumphosphat-Keramiken -Morphologische Ergebnisse, Dtsch. Z. Zahnärztl. Implantol. in press
14 C.P.A.T. Klein, A.A. Driessen, K. De Groot and A. van den Hooff, Biodegradation behavior of various calcium phosphate materials in bone tissue, J. Biomed. Mater. Res. 17 (1983) 769-784.
15 B.D. Katthagen, Knochenregeneration mit Knochenersatzmaterialien, Springer, Berlin, Heidelberg New York Tokyo, 1986

Biomaterials and Clinical Applications,
edited by A. Pizzoferrato, P.G. Marchetti, A. Ravaglioli and A.J.C. Lee
Elsevier Science Publishers B.V., Amsterdam, 1987 — Printed in The Netherlands

QUANTITATIVE STUDIES ON THE EARLY INFLAMMATORY CELL RESPONSE TO IMPLANTS IN THE ABDOMINAL WALL OF THE RAT

P. THOMSEN, A.S. ERIKSSON, R. OLSSON, L.M. BJURSTEN and L.E. ERICSON

Department of Anatomy, University of Göteborg, P.O. Box 33031, S-400 33 Gothenburg (Sweden)

SUMMARY

The tissue reaction to implants of titanium and Teflon was studied using a new experimental model. The cellular composition of the tissue was evaluated 8 h, 1, 3, 7 days and 9 weeks after insertion.

Around titanium implants a transient inflammatory response, similar to that in wound healing, was observed during the first week. After 9 weeks a thin layer of collagenous tissue devoid of inflammatory cells surrounded the implants.

Teflon implants induced a pronounced inflammation. At 8 h the concentration of inflammatory cells was twice that seen close to titanium implants. The number of inflammatory cells, predominantly monocytes-macrophages, remained high during the first week. After 9 weeks multi-nucleated giant cells and active macrophages formed a zone at the surface of the Teflon implants and outside this a thick, reactive fibrous capsule was present.

Our observations indicate that the initial interaction between the implant and the inflammatory cells determines the development of the tissue response and the late composition of the interfacial tissue.

INTRODUCTION

Implant materials induce different types of tissue reactions (ref. 1). Conceivably the tissue reaction is of decisive importance for the healing-in and function of an implant. It is quite possible that it is the primary, very early interaction at the implant-tissue interface that determines the further changes in the tissue surrounding the implant (refs. 2, 3). However, at present very little biological evidence supporting this view is available and virtually nothing is known about the nature of the interaction between implants and tissue.

The aim of the present study was to study the early interaction between implants and tissue. From a previous study (ref. 4) we know that the tissue reactions to titanium and Teflon are quite different after 9 weeks. Knowing these late results we have therefore used such implants as models for quantitative studies of changes in the tissue during the first week after implant insertion.

MATERIALS AND METHODS

Details of the implantation procedure are described elsewhere (ref. 3). Sprague-Dawley rats, weighing 250-300 g, were used. Plugs of non-alloyed

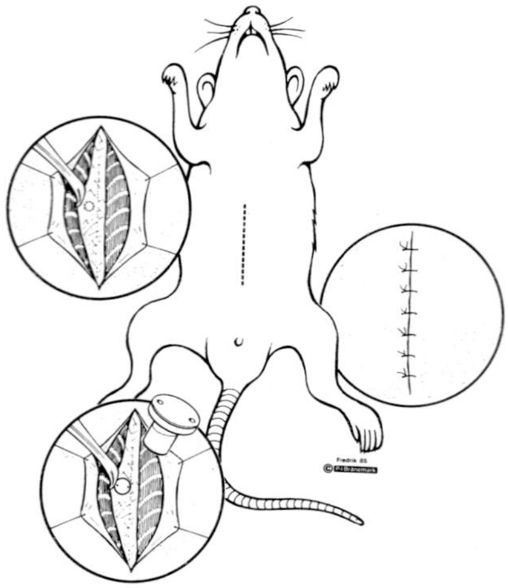

1

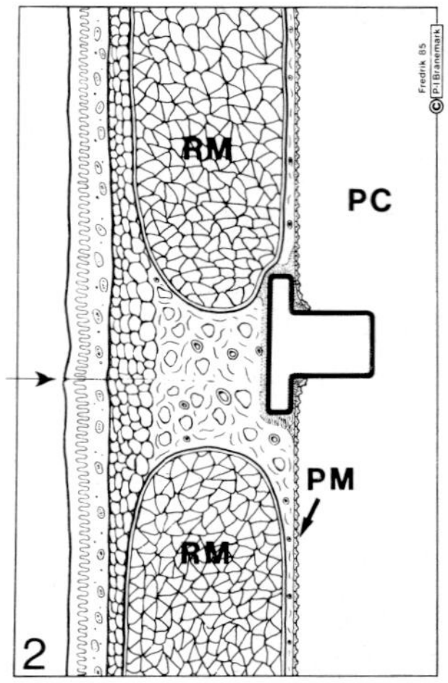

2

Fig. 1. The surgical procedure. The rectus muscle is moved laterally (upper left), the plug is inserted through the peritoneal membrane (bottom left) and the rectus sheath, fascia and skin are sutured (right).

Fig. 2. Position of the implant. PC = peritoneal cavity. PM = peritoneal membrane. RM = rectus muscle.

titanium and Teflon (surgical grade) consisting of a cylindrical rod (length 3 mm; diam. 2 mm) and a circular plate (thickness 0.5 mm; diam. 4 mm) were used (Fig. 1). The plugs were cleaned ultrasonically and sterilized before insertion.

As shown in Fig. 1, the rectus sheath was opened, the rectus muscle moved laterally, and the rod part of the implant inserted through a hole in the peritoneal membrane. The circular plate remained outside the peritoneum covered by the rectus muscle (Fig. 2).

The implants were removed 8 hours, 1, 3, 7 days and 9 weeks after insertion. For each time interval and each type of implant 4 or 5 rats were examined.

The abdominal wall was fixed by perfusion via the left heart ventricle with 2.5% glutaraldehyde in 0.05% sodium cacodylate. The implant and surrounding tissue were then excised en bloc. In general the tissue was removed before post-fixation in 2% osmium tetroxide which was followed by dehydration and embedding in epoxy resin.

One µm thick sections for light microscopy, cut on an ultramicrotome, were stained with 0.5% Azur II and 0.5% methylene blue in 1% disodium tetraborate.

The composition of the interfacial tissue was analyzed by counting the number of different cells within a square given by a grid in the microscope eye piece with an area of 2×10^4 μm^2. For each implant the average cell content in 5 squares was evaluated. The quantification was performed on the tissue located adjacent to the surface of the circular plate facing the peritoneum (Fig. 2). One side of the test-square coincided with the implant-tissue border.

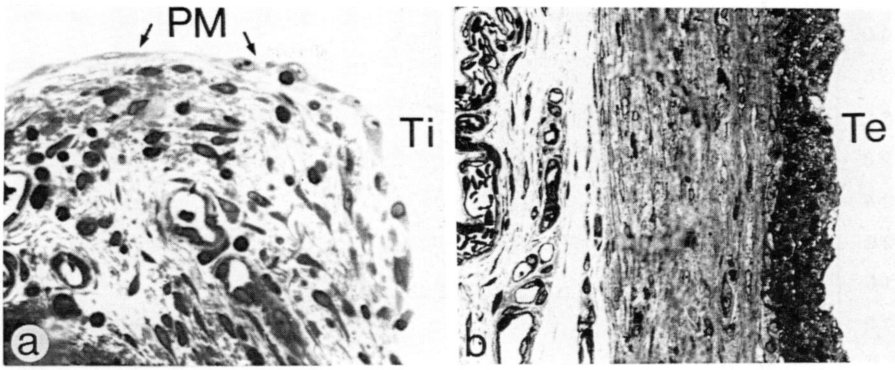

Fig. 3 a. Tissue close to the rod portion of a (removed) titanium (Ti) implant after 9 weeks. PM = peritoneal membrane. Fig. 3 b. Tissue surrounding the rod portion of a Teflon (Te) implant after 9 weeks. Note inner zone of inflammatory cells and outer fibrous capsule.

RESULTS

Tissue composition 9 weeks after implantation

The two types of implant materials, titanium and Teflon, used in the present study of the early tissue response around implants were chosen because they have previously been found to cause quite different late responses (ref. 4). To provide a background for the description and discussion of the early changes we will first describe the tissue morphology 9 weeks after implantation.

The circular plate of the titanium implants was surrounded by orderly arranged collagenous connective tissue closely adhering to the implant surface (Fig. 3 a). The thin layer of connective tissue was composed of elongated fibroblasts and collagen bundles following the contours of the implants. Inflammatory cells were not present (Fig. 3 a). The cylindrical rod projecting into the peritoneal cavity was covered by an incomplete monolayer of non-activated peritoneal macrophages attached to surface of the implant.

The composition of tissue around Teflon plugs after 9 weeks was quite different (Fig. 3 b). The rod portion was encapsulated. The inner zone of this capsule consisted of macrophages and multi-nucleated giant cells and the outer zone of a reactive fibrous capsule. The tissue adjacent to the circular plate had a similar composition with an inner zone of inflammatory cells and an outer zone of fibrous tissue.

Tissue composition during the first week after implantation

The amount of polymorphonuclear granulocytes (PMNGs), monocytes/macrophages, mast cells and fibroblasts in the tissue adjacent to titanium and Teflon implants

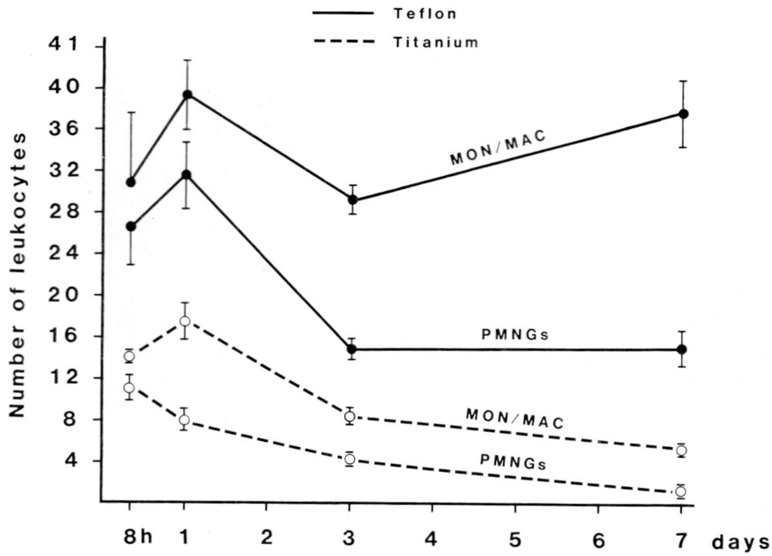

Fig. 4. The number of leukocytes per 2 x 10^4 μm^2 is given. Mean ±SE of 5 rats. MON/MAC = monocytes/macrophages; PMNGs = polymorphonuclear granulocytes.

was evaluated. Considerable differences in the inflammatory response were already apparent within 8 h (Fig. 4).

In the tissue surrounding titanium implants PMNGs and monocytes/macrophages predominated 8 h and 1 day after insertion of the implant. These cells decreased progressively at 3 and 7 days. The number of fibroblasts increased markedly between 1 and 3 days and was the predominant cell type (Fig. 5). At this time the fibroblasts were orderly arranged along collagen bundles arranged in parallel to the implant surface.

A similar transient inflammatory response and gradual increase in the amount of fibroblasts was seen in rat abdominal walls in which the surgical procedure was imitated by insertion and immediate removal of an implant. Thus, the tissue reaction around a titanium implant resembled qualitatively and quantitatively a normal wound healing process.

The composition of the tissue surrounding Teflon implants was quite different. At 8 h and 1 day the amount of inflammatory cells, both PMNGs and monocytes/macrophages, was about twice that present close to titanium implants (Fig. 4). Monocytes/macrophages became the predominant cell type at 3 and 7 days while PMNGs decreased. However, the number of PMNGs was at all time intervals higher than found at any time around titanium implants. Compared to titanium implants many fewer fibroblasts were present close to Teflon implants (Fig. 5).

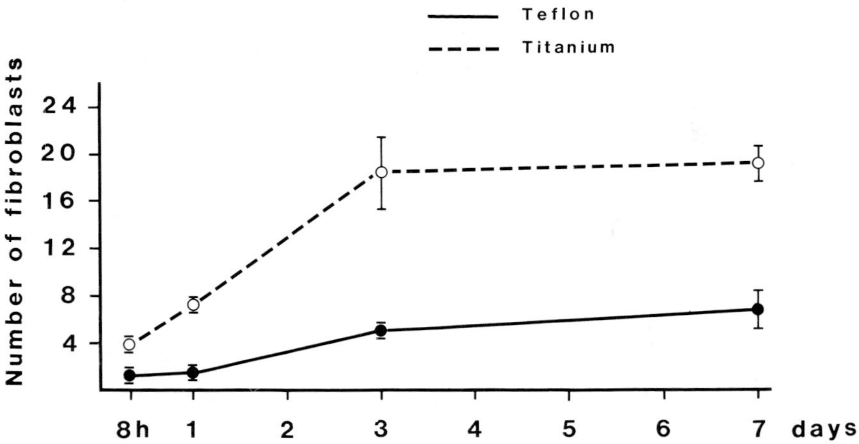

Fig. 5. Number of fibroblasts per 2 x 10^4 μm^2. Mean ±SE of 5 rats.

DISCUSSION

In the present study we found that 9 weeks after insertion titanium implants had healed into the abdominal wall without any remaining inflammation whereas Teflon implants were surrounded by a zone of macrophages and multinucleated giant cells and peripherally to this zone, by a thick, reactive fibrous capsule. The knowledge of these different late response led us to study the early reaction to the two implant materials. A corresponding difference in the early tissue changes was found. Insertion of titanium implants evoked an acute inflammation which was transient and qualitatively and quantitatively similar to a wound healing response after the surgical trauma caused by the implant insertion. Thus, it appears that the presence of a titanium implant per se had little influence on the tissue response. On the other hand, insertion of Teflon implants induced a pronounced acute inflammatory response, evident within 8 h, and a large number of leukocytes remained close to the implant throughout the first week. Thus, Teflon implants rapidly induced an inflammation that persisted.

Together our observations suggest that the early interaction between the implant and the tissue determines the development of the tissue response and the late result of the healing-in process. At present very little is known about the nature of this interaction. Our observations of an early and persistent increase of PMNGs and monocytes around Teflon implants point to the importance of the inflammatory cells. Such cells will always be present close to a newly inserted implant as a consequence of the inevitable surgical trauma. The further development of the tissue response might then depend on whether or not, and to what extent, these inflammatory cells are influenced by the implant. For instance, an activation of the leukocytes, as might occur at Teflon implants, could lead to a reinforcement and perpetuation of the inflammatory reaction ultimately leading to secondary effects as formation of reactive fibrous tissue. Absence of an activation of leukocytes, as might be the situation at titanium implants, might lead to a normal healing and integration of the implant with the tissue without any persistent inflammatory reaction.

At present very little is known about possible mechanism for the interaction between an implant and leukocytes leading to their activation and to a perpetuation of the inflammatory response. One possibility is that the cells interact directly with the implant surface. In vitro studies indicate that this surface is covered by adsorbed proteins (refs. 5, 6) and it is therefore possible that it is the protein adsorption pattern that determines the reactivity of the implant surface towards inflammatory cells. Implant materials differ considerably in their protein binding properties (ref. 5) and might therefore differ in their putative capacity to influence leukocytes. Another possibility is that protein molecules are structurally and functionally modified by interaction with the implant surface which might lead to secondary events such as attraction and activation of inflammatory cells. It is known that artificial surfaces can activate the complement system (ref. 6). Apart from surface properties also other properties of the implant, as for instance leakage of substances into the surrounding tissue, might be of great importance for the interfacial cellular response.

In conclusion, our morphological observations on the tissue response to two types of implant materials, titanium and Teflon, strongly suggest an important role of the inflammatory cells for the development of the early tissue response and for the late healing-in result.

REFERENCES

1 D.F. Williams (Ed.), Biocompatibility of Clinical Implant Materials, Vols. I-II, CRC Press, Boca Raton, (1982).
2 L.M. Bjursten, L.E. Ericson, J. Hed, B. Kasemo, J. Lausmaa and P. Thomsen, Interfacial mechanisms in tissue integrated prostheses, in: P.-O. Glantz, S.A. Leach, T. Ericsson (Eds.), Oral Interfacial Reactions of Bone, Soft Tissue and Saliva, IRL Press, Oxford, (1985).
3 B. Kasemo and J. Lausmaa, Surface science aspects on inorganic biomaterials, CRC Crit. Rev. Biocomp., 2(4) (1986).
4 P. Thomsen, L.M. Bjursten and L.E. Ericson, Implants in the abdominal wall of the rat, Scand. J. Plast. Reconstr. Surg. In press. (1986).
5 B. Ivarsson and I. Lundström, Physical characterization of protein adsorption on metal and metaloxide surfaces, CRC Crit. Rev. Biocomp., 2(1) (1986).
6 J. Hed, M. Johansson and M. Lindroth, Complement activation according to the alternate pathway by glass and plastic surfaces and its role in neutrophil adhesion, Immunology Letters, 8 (1984) 295-299.

This study was supported by grants from Swedish National Association against Rheumatism; Gothenburg Medical Society; King Gustav V 80-years Fund; Medical Faculty, University of Göteborg.

Biomaterials and Clinical Applications,
edited by A. Pizzoferrato, P.G. Marchetti, A. Ravaglioli and A.J.C. Lee
Elsevier Science Publishers B.V., Amsterdam, 1987 — Printed in The Netherlands

THERMOPLASTIC POLYURETHANES. HYDROPHILIC-HYDROPHOBIC BALANCE.

Richard J. Zdrahala, Donald D. Solomon, David J. Lentz* and Charles W. McGary, Jr.

Deseret Polymer Research, Dayton, OH, USA
*Deseret Medical Inc., Sandy, UT, USA

ABSTRACT

A series of thermoplastic polyurethanes (TPU) based on 4,4'-diphenylmethane diisocyanate/1,4-butanediol (MDI/BDO) hard segment and polytetramethylene ether glycol (PTMEG) and/or polyethylene ether glycol (PEG) soft segment was synthesized and evaluated as biomaterials. The hard segment content (MDI + BDO) was 55 weight percent. The soft segment molecular weights varied between 1000 and 3000 and the weight content of PEG in the polymers was 0, 15, 30 and 45 percent. The variations in soft segment composition were designed to achieve different hydrophilic-hydrophobic balance at the polymer surface.

Hemocompatibility was evaluated via fibrinopeptide A (FPA) generation and complement activation (C3a, C5a) assays and in an ex vivo canine A/V shunt. Although FPA and complement activation did not show any significant trends, the platelet deposition in the canine model varied significantly with the polymer composition. An increase of hydrophilic PEG content resulted in a higher number of platelets deposited when the molecular weights of PTMEG and PEG in the soft segment blends were similar (1000/1000 and 2900/3350). Utilization of different molecular weight PTMEG/PEG soft segment blends (1000/3350 and 2900/1000) rendered materials with very low affinity for the platelets, presumably by the formation of differently sized hydrophilic and hydrophobic microdomains on the polymer surface.

INTRODUCTION

Development of a biomaterial, resembling normal vascular endothelium for ultimate hemocompatibility, represents a major effort in current biomaterials research. Sawyer et al. (ref. 1) postulated in the early sixties that vascular endothelium is composed of hydrophilic and hydrophobic microdomains. Feasibility of this concept for synthesis of biopolymers, in order to improve their hemocompatibility, was investigated by Sasaki, Ratner and Hoffmann (ref. 2), Okano et al. (ref. 3), and Gnanou, Hild and Rempp (ref. 4), to name a few.

Thermoplastic polyurethanes (TPU) are microphase-separated $(AB)_n$ block copolymers. Hard, relatively hydrophilic hard segment microdomains are joined by soft segment microdomains. If polyether glycols are used as soft segments, their hydrophilicity can be varied by the carbon to oxygen ratio of their alkylene oxide moieties. Overall surface and bulk microdomain morphology depends on the hard/soft segment ratio, soft segment composition and molecular weight and, to a lesser extent, on the method of sample preparation.

In our work, a series of twelve, melt processable TPUs was synthesized. Hydrophilic PEG was copolymerized with a relatively hydrophobic PTMEG as co-soft-segment at 55 weight percent of MDI/BDO hard segment content. Molecular weights of PTMEG and PEG were 1000 and 2900 and 1000 and 3350, respectively. The PEG content in the polymers was 0, 15, 30 and 45 weight percent. Hemocompatibility was evaluated as a function of the soft segment composition.

EXPERIMENTAL

All polymers were synthesized at 100% solids by a one-shot hand casting technique (ref. 5). No leachable catalysts were used for attainment of highest purity. Upon synthesis, the polymers were extruded into ribbons and tubings for subsequent testing.

Tensile properties were determined on ribbons after two days equilibration at 23°C and 55% RH. Water absorption and simulated softening in the body were determined in 37°C n-saline. An 48 hour exposure was needed to achieve equilibrium. Static water contact angles (sessile drop) and dynamic (Wilhelmy plate) advancing and receding water contact angles were measured on non-hydrated and fully hydrated ribbon samples (48 hours, 23°C distilled water).

Hemocompatibility was evaluated on extruded, fully hydrated tubing samples. FPA generation and complement activation assays, and an *ex vivo* canine A/V shunt were the tests used. Detailed description of these tests was published previously (ref. 6).

RESULTS AND DISCUSSION

To achieve variation in surface hydrophilic-hydrophobic balance, similar and different molecular weight PTMEG and PEG were blended. As can be seen from Table 1, the maximum content of PEG in the polymer was 45 weight percent.

Tensile Properties

Tensile modulus (at 100%), tensile strength and ultimate elongation of studied polymers are summarized in Table 1. As the PEG content in the polymer increases the tensile modulus and strength decrease and ultimate elongation increases. In summary, all the polymers had excellent tensile properties which can satisfy the highest performance requirements.

Bulk/Surface Hydrophilicity

Hydrophilicity of a material can be determined, by water absorption and water contact angles. As summarized in Table 2, the polymers absorbed 1.5-32 wt.% of water at 37°C. The increase in water absorption depends on the weight fraction and molecular weight of PEG. Upon exposure to 37°C n-saline, significant, but reversible softening of the materials was observed. In general, the softening decreases with an increase in the PEG content and its molecular weight.

TABLE 1

Tensile Properties as a Function of Soft Segment Composition.

Material Code	Soft Segment			Tensile Properties		
	PTMEG MW	PEG MW	PEG Wt. Fract.	100% Tens. Modulus (psi)	Tensile Strength (psi)	Ultimate Elongat. (%)
H/H-1	1000	--	0	2400	10700	400
H/H-7	1000	1000	1/3	2000	9300	370
H/H-8	1000	1000	2/3	1500	7900	460
H/H-4	--	1000	1	1000	5800	570
H/H-3	2900	--	0	3100	8200	310
H/H-17	2900	3350	1/3	2900	8300	340
H/H-18	2900	3350	2/3	1700	7300	430
H/H-6	--	3350	1	1100	5100	520
H/H-15	2900	1000	1/3	2800	7000	330
H/H-11	1000	3350	1/3	1900	10000	410
H/H-16	2900	1000	2/3	1800	7500	490
H/H-12	1000	3350	2/3	1300	7500	510

TABLE 2

Water Absorption and Softening in 37°C n-Saline.

Material Code	Soft Segment			% Water Absorbed at 37°C	% Softening in 37°C N-Saline as Change of:	
	PTMEG MW	PEG MW	PEG Wt. Fract.		5% Tens. Modulus	100% Tens. Modulus
H/H-1	1000	--	0	1.7	-58	-54
H/H-7	1000	1000	1/3	1.5	-40	-40
H/H-8	1000	1000	2/3	10.5	-34	-27
H/H-4	--	1000	1	17.8	-27	+ 4
H/H-3	2900	--	0	1.6	-28	-16
H/H-17	2900	3350	1/3	4.3	-27	-24
H/H-18	2900	3350	2/3	14.7	-20	-12
H/H-6	--	3350	1	31.5	+13	+36
H/H-15	2900	1000	1/3	2.2	-72	-25
H/H-11	1000	3350	1/3	5.7	-43	-26
H/H-16	2900	1000	2/3	10.6	-40	-33
H/H-12	1000	3350	2/3	19.6	-16	0

Water contact angles provide additional information about surface hydrophilicity. Both static and dynamic contact angles were determined on non-hydrated and fully hydrated samples and results are summarized in Table 3. Clearly, an increase in surface hydrophilicity can be observed with an increase in PEG content and molecular weight.

TABLE 3

Static and Dynamic Water Contact Angles.

Material Code	MW/Wt.% of PEG in Polymer	Static Contact Angles with water		Dynamic Contact Angles in Water			
		Non-Hydrated	Hydrated	Non-Hydrated		Fully Hydrated	
				Advanc.	Reced.	Advanc.	Reced.
H/H-1	0/0	80.8	80.1	89.0	55.0	90.4	57.4
H/H-7	1000/15	72.3	71.7	86.3	45.1	76.7	32.0
H/H-8	1000/30	65.5	69.0	84.0	39.4	76.2	39.7
H/H-4	1000/45	51.5	57.2	64.3	37.0	70.2	42.8
H/H-3	0/0	80.7	83.7	93.3	58.0	91.3	59.5
H/H-17	3350/15	78.5	81.5	92.2	51.5	86.6	49.3
H/H-18	3350/30	74.3	75.5	77.5	41.4	75.8	43.1
H/H-6	3350/45	29.2	33.6	50.8	34.4	52.0	35.4
H/H-15	1000/15	79.7	78.8	92.6	49.3	84.7	44.7
H/H-11	3350/15	66.1	65.9	81.2	40.4	77.5	39.4
H/H-16	1000/30	74.1	75.7	81.4	42.6	77.3	45.6
H/H-12	3350/30	60.3	56.5	64.8	35.4	54.6	31.7

Hemocompatibility

No clear trend was indicated by FPA generation assay. Most polymers generated 200-450 ng of FPA per ml of blood. However, H/H-4 (45 wt.% PEG-1000) and H/H-6 (45 wt.% of PEG-3350) generated over 600 ng of FPA, indicating potentially poor hemocompatibility. All materials were non-activating to the complement system (C3a and C5a).

Platelet deposition, which is to a certain extent indicative of hemocompatibility, was studied in an ex vivo canine model and the results are summarized in Table 4. In this procedure, a femoral A/V shunt is constructed from selected materials and deposition of In-III labeled platelets is followed as a function of time by gamma counting.

Two trends are clearly visible: (1) the number of deposited platelets increases significantly with increasing PEG content when the molecular weight of PTMEG and PEG is 1000. Additionally, but to a lesser extent, this trend prevails for materials containing higher, but similar molecular weight PTMEG and PEG components; and (2) very low platelet deposition was detected for materials utilizing blends of dissimilar molecular weight co-soft segments (1000/3350 and 2900/1000, respectively).

TABLE 4

Hemocompatibility Determined via Ex Vivo Canine A/V Shunt Model.

Material Code	Soft Segment: PTMEG MW	Soft Segment: PEG MW	Soft Segment: PEG Wt. Fract.	Platelet Deposition per 1000 μm^2 (Ex Vivo Canine A/V Shunt; Minutes): 1	5	15	30	60
H/H-1	1000	--	0	63	129	258	199	481
H/H-7	1000	1000	1/3	67	140	273	299	819
H/H-8	1000	1000	2/3	64	151	260	263	926
H/H-4	--	1000	1	59	156	172	418	1516
H/H-3	2900	--	0	23	78	115	155	279
H/H-17	2900	3350	1/3	47	92	139	169	747
H/H-18	2900	3350	2/3	41	104	156	263	1015
H/H-6	--	3350	1	40	104	134	437	1082
H/H-15	2900	1000	1/3	32	97	65	88	65
H/H-11	1000	3350	1/3	23	89	60	87	54
H/H-16	2900	1000	2/3	31	103	81	158	319
H/H-12	1000	3350	2/3	22	91	58	101	107

Since the extent of microphase separation of the TPUs depends on molecular weight of co-segments, it is plausible to speculate that higher molecular weight polyether glycols render more complete phase separation and better surface organization, which in turn affects positively the hemocompatiblity. Furthermore, potential heterogenicity of surface domain sizes generated by dissimilar molecular weight PTMEG and PEG co-segments could have a very significant positive effect.

Unexpectedly high platelet deposition was detected for H/H-1 and H/H-3 materials which, according to previous testing, have had very low affinity for platelets. It was concluded that the relatively high thrombogenicity of all PEG-soft-segment materials (H/H-4 and H/H-6) triggered higher overall platelet sensitivity to foreign surfaces. This hypersensitivity resulted in higher platelet deposition for all materials in the shunt at longer circulation intervals. The effect was not isolated to the arterial or venous portion of the shunt. No significant difference in platelet adhesion was noted between randomly placed identical material segments, i.e. no correlation was made with position in the shunt.

To test this conclusion, a shunt composed of H/H-1, 3, 11 and 15 polymers was re-tested at 60 minutes and 60, 46, 65, and 50 platelets per 1000 μm^2 were counted. By the merits of this model, the results indicate excellent hemocompatibility. Furthermore, the results show an eight-fold decrease in platelet deposition for the H/H-1 material in the absence of H/H-4. These data are supported by previous work (ref. 6) which show H/H-1 to be a relatively benign material.

CONCLUSIONS

Increased hydrophilicity of MDI/BDO/PTMEG based TPUs caused by incorporation of PEG co-soft segments significantly affects the TPU's performance. Specifically: (1) water absorption and surface hydrophilicity is increased; (2) platelet deposition (*ex vivo* canine shunt) increased significantly when PEG content increased and molecular weight of both PTMEG and PEG was 1000. A similar, but weaker trend was observed when molecular weight of PTMEG was 2900 and PEG 3350; and (3) very low platelet deposition was observed when PTMEG/PEG soft segment blends were based on 1000/3350 and 2900/1000 respectively.

These trends can be rationalized in terms of microphase separation of the TPUs. Higher molecular weight of segments promotes microphase separation and domain formation. Variation in co-soft-segment molecular weight can produce differently sized, heterogeneous surface domains. These phenomena do affect hemocompatibility of the TPUs. Further investigation of these principles is in progress.

REFERENCES

1 P.N. Sawyer, C. Burrowes, J. Oganiak, A.O. Smith and S.A. Wesolowski, Ionic Architecture at the Vascular Wall Interface, Trans. Am. Soc. Artif . Intern. Organs, 10, (1964), pp. 316-319.

2 T. Sasaki, B.D. Ratner and A.S. Hoffman, Radiation-Induced Co-Graft Polymerization of 2-Hydroxyethyl Methacrylate and Ethyl Methacrylate onto Silicone Rubber Films, in: J.D. Andrade (Ed.), ACS Symposium Series, Hydrogels for Medical and Related Applications, Am. Chem. Soc., 71, (1976) pp. 283-294.

3 T. Okano, S. Nishiyama, I. Shinohara, T. Akaike and Y. Sakurai, Interaction between Plasma Protein and Microphase Separated Structure of Copolymers, Polym. J., 10 (1978) pp. 223-228.

4 Y. Gnanou, G. Hild and P. Rempp, Hydrophilic Polyurethane Networks based on poly(ethylene oxide). Synthesis, characterization and properties, Macromolecules, 17, No. 4 (1984) pp. 945-952.

5 R.J. Zdrahala, R.M. Gerkin, S.L. Hager and F.E. Critchfield, Polyether-based thermoplastic polyurethanes. Effect of the hard segment content., J. Appl. Polym. Sci., 24 (1975) pp. 2041-2050.

6 R.J. Zdrahala, D.D. Solomon, D.J. Lentz and C.W. McGary, Jr., Thermoplastic polyurethanes. Materials for vascular catheters, presented at 2nd International Conference on Polyurethanes in Bioengineering, Stuttgart, FRG, June 1986.

Biomaterials and Clinical Applications,
edited by A. Pizzoferrato, P.G. Marchetti, A. Ravaglioli and A.J.C. Lee
Elsevier Science Publishers B.V., Amsterdam, 1987 — Printed in The Netherlands

COMPARISON OF CALCIUMHYDROXYLAPATITE CEROS 80^R AND β-TRICALCIUMPHOSPHATE CEROS 82^R IN VIVO WITH STABLE SOFT TISSUE INTERFACE

V. GERET[1], W. MUELLER[2], M. TEPIC[1], B.A. RAHN[1], S.M. PERREN[1]

[1]Laboratory for Experimental Surgery, Obere Str. 22, CH-7270 Davos, Switzerland
[2]R. Mathys & Co., Surgical Instruments, CH-2544 Bettlach, Switzerland

SUMMARY

Calciumhydroxylapatite and β-Tricalciumphosphate as technical bone graft materials have received frequent use in reconstructive surgery. Both materials are available in different porosity and in compact shape. There is a difference in their resorption behavior. In order to test the tissue reaction, the in vivo screening test using grooved cylinders and a special histological technique revealed the biological tolerance as compared to the controls, steel and titanium.

INTRODUCTION

Bone replacement in reconstructive surgery requires materials of comparably high mechanical strength. This problem for a new implant material led us to test the in vivo biocompatibility of the compact version of Ceros 80^R and Ceros 82^R. Both materials, in different porous conditions, are degradable implants, therefore their tissue tolerance reaction will have to be tested in the future.

MATERIAL

The tested materials: Ceros 80^R (Calciumhydroxylapatite) and Ceros 82^R (β-Tricalciumphosphate) were compared with the conventional implant materials, stainless steel ISO 5832/I and pure titanium ISO 5832/II to which tissue tolerance is well established.

Ceros 80^R consists of polycrystallic hydroxylapatite which is essentially identical with natural bone mineral substance. Depending on the porosity Ceros 80^R can be designated as a non-degradable or an extremely slowly degradable material (refs. 1, 2).

Ceros 82^R is made of β-Tricalciumphosphate and depending on the porosity is a degradable material. The granulate, when implanted in bone, degrades in about 6 to 12 months. The compression resistance of Ceros 82^R is smaller than Ceros 80^R, therefore it is mainly used as granulate in closed defects for bone induction.

METHOD

Standard cylindrical implants with grooves to prevent tissue interface motion (ref. 3) were placed subcutaneously under sterile conditions in mice and observed for periods ranging up to 36 weeks. The implanted material, surrounded completely by soft tissue, was fixed and embedded in methylmetacrylate. The blocks containing tissue and implant were sectioned in 6 µm slices using the Zeiss-cut-all microtome. The special histological technique permits one to obtain the direct-contact-area of the tissue even if it consists of fluid phases. After dissolving the methylmetacrylate in benzol the slides were stained in Giemsa.

The histological samples were then evaluated using a digitizer tablet (refs. 4, 5). The number of giant cell nuclei is reported per mm length of the contact surface. The number of round cells is reported per area evaluated. The average is then evaluated and represented in median, upper and lower quartiles.

RESULTS

Table 1 Sample of raw data: Ceros 80[R], 36 weeks

Histo Number	Top/ Bottom	Length in mm	Number Nuclei Foreign Body Giant Cells	n/mm	Surface in mm^2	Number Round Cells	n/mm^2
9442 a	t	2.66	18	6.8	0.60	4	6.6
	b	2.65	29	10.9	0.66	5	7.6
9442 b	t	2.68	150	56.1	0.25	7	28.1
	b	2.63	63	24.0	1.21	28	23.1
9442 c	t	2.63	138	52.4	0.65	43	66.2
	b	2.64	83	31.4	0.67	47	69.8
9442 d	t	----	---	----	----	--	---- *
	b	2.61	43	16.5	0.68	2	3.0
9442 e	t	2.63	81	30.8	0.25	10	39.8
	b	2.63	49	18.6	0.19	8	41.9
9442 f	t	2.46	93	37.7	0.80	31	38.7
	b	2.53	92	36.3	0.64	42	65.6
9442	t	2.77	7	2.5	0.26	14	54.3
	b	2.29	34	14.8	0.20	36	180.9

*) missing within the preparation

Table 2 Statistical data of Ceros 80^R and Ceros 82^R

a) Nuclei foreign body giant cell/mm

		n	Upper Quartile	Median	Lower Quartile
Ceros 80^R	1 w	7	40.4	34.6	30.5
	3 w	10	38.0	32.6	23.4
	9 w	10	29.9	22.9	14.8
	18 w	10	40.7	28.5	24.4
	36 w	7	38.5	24.7	12.7
Ceros 82^R	1 w	9	50.1	43.8	37.1
	3 w	8	59.3	48.2	42.8
	9 w	10	42.0	34.8	19.0
	18 w	9	38.4	32.9	19.9
	36 w	7	32.7	28.3	27.2

b) Round cells/mm^2

		n	Upper Quartile	Median	Lower Quartile
Ceros 80^R	1 w	7	17.7	10.7	7.1
	3 w	10	23.8	14.4	12.2
	9 w	10	15.9	13.2	10.3
	18 w	10	21.8	13.7	10.3
	36 ..	7	60.1	40.9	16.4
Ceros 82^R	1 w	9	16.8	7.0	5.8
	3 w	8	10.8	8.9	7.3
	9 w	10	7.8	5.2	4.6
	18 w	9	22.9	17.4	13.9
	36 w	7	25.9	19.7	13.1

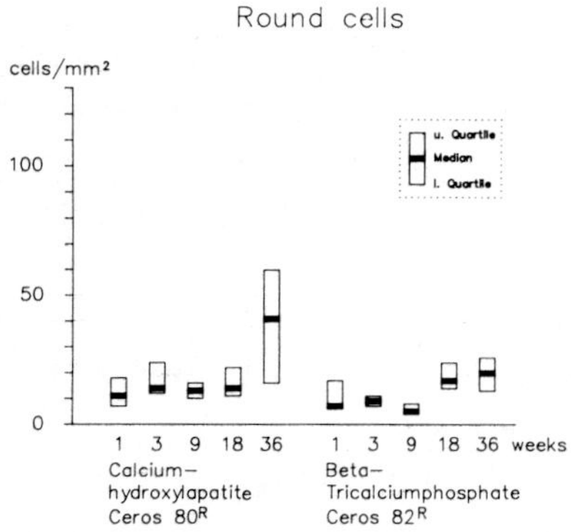

Fig. 1
The count of round cells was evaluated per area

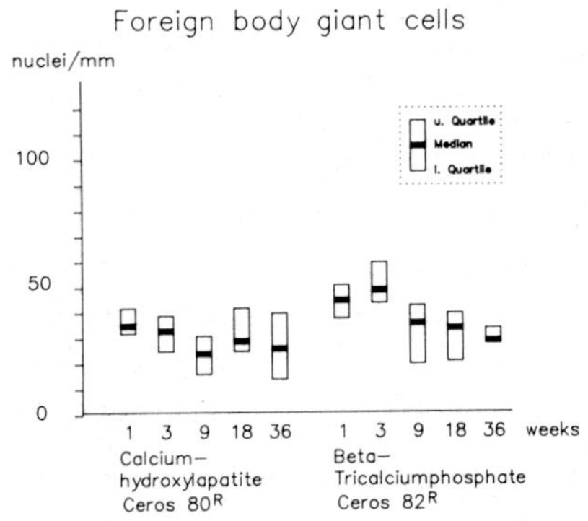

Fig. 2
The count of nuclei of foreign body giant cells was evaluated per mm length of the contact area

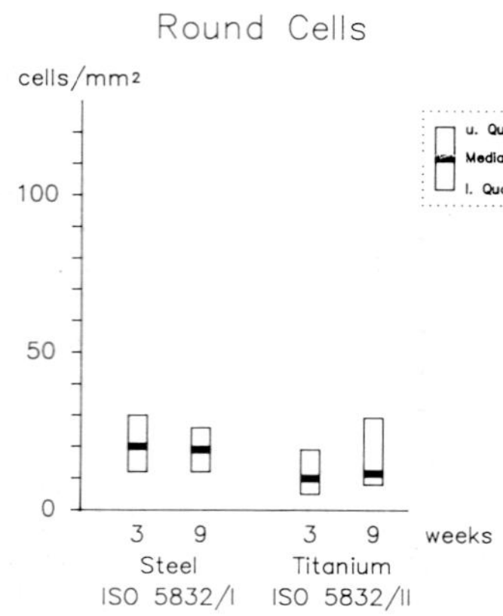

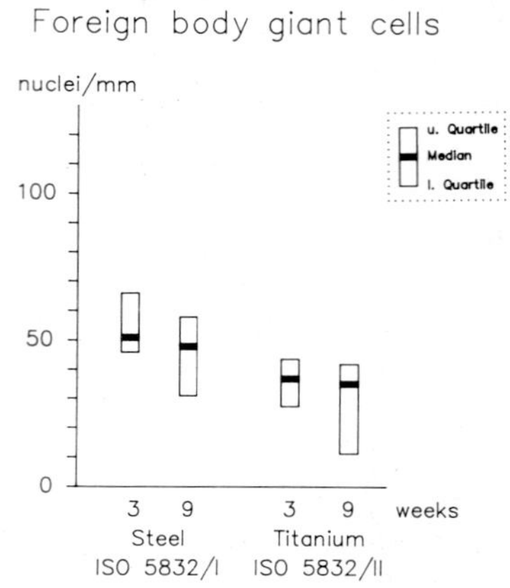

Fig. 3 and 4
These non porous "non degradable" materials are tested only up to 9 weeks. The count of round cells and nuclei of foreign body giant cells was identically evaluated as figure 1 and 2.

Ceros 80^R and Ceros 82^R show a number of round cells and foreign body giant cell nuclei comparable to the controls, steel and titanium. We observed within the implantation period of up to 36 weeks a number of round cells below $50/mm^2$. Ceros 82^R started with a low round cell reaction but increased toward 18 and 36 weeks. Ceros 82^R started with more marked foreign body giant cell reaction at 1 and 3 weeks. The data should show a baseline for further comparison of biodegradable materials. Visible Ceros 82^R degradation is reported to start at 6 months.

DISCUSSION

The standard method using cylindrical implants with grooves exhibit a low variance of the tissue reaction. The shallow grooves of the test implants prevent motion of the interface. The special histological technique, stabilizing the implant and tissue layer in methacrylate, prevent the trauma of the cell layer (ref. 6).

To evaluate the tissue reaction, comparing Ceros 80^R and Ceros 82^R in situation needing comparably high mechanical strength, it was felt appropriate to test the two materials in the compact quality first.

Both materials show similar tissue reaction. The histology slides and the tissue reaction evaluation do not reveal visible degradation of either material up to 18 weeks of observation. At 36 weeks Ceros 82^R demonstrates the start of degradation.

Future test series of Ceros 80^R and Ceros 82^R with different porosity will be performed and compared with degradable materials.

REFERENCES

1 Geret, V., Rahn, B.A., Mathys, R., Perren, S.M.: Quantitative Analyse der in vivo Gewebsverträglichkeit von Hydroxylapatite Ceros 80[R]. Hefte zur Unfallheilkunde, Heft 164, p. 75-76, 1983
2 Rahn, B.A., Neff, J., Leutenegger, A., Mathys, R., Perren, S.M.: Integration of synthetic apatite of various pore size and density in bone. In: P. Christel, A. Meunier, A.J. Lee, Biological and Biomechanical Performance of Biomaterials, Elsevier Science Publisher B.V., Amsterdam, p. 21-26, 1986
3 Geret, V., Rahn, B.A., Mathys, R., Straumann, F., Perren, S.M.: In vivo testing of tissue tolerance of implant materials: improved quantitiative evaluation through reduction of relative motion at the implant tissue interface. In: H. Uhthoff, Current Concepts of Internal Fixation of Fractures, Springer Verlag, p. 160-164, 1980
4 Capaul, C.: Prüfung eines Digitizercomputersystems zur quantitativen Auswertung von Gewebeelementen an Hand verschiedener Implantatmaterialien. Dissertation, Basel, 1982
5 Lardi, M.: Prüfung eines Digitizer-Mikrocomputersystems zur quantitativen Auswertung von Gewebeelementen: Zeitlicher Verlauf von Gewebsveränderungen um standardisierte Stahlimplantate. Dissertation, Basel, 1982
6 Perren, S.M., Geret, V., Tepic, M., Rahn, B.A.:
Quantitative evaluation of biocompatibility of vanadium free titanium alloys. In: P. Christel, A. Meunier, A.J. Lee, Biological and Biomechanical Performance of Biomaterials, Elsevier Science Publisher B.V., Amsterdam, p. 397-402, 1986

Biomaterials and Clinical Applications,
edited by A. Pizzoferrato, P.G. Marchetti, A. Ravaglioli and A.J.C. Lee
Elsevier Science Publishers B.V., Amsterdam, 1987 — Printed in The Netherlands

PRECLINICAL STUDIES USING A METHOTREXATE LOADED BONE CEMENT

E. DINGELDEIN[1], H. WAHLIG[1], A. METALLINOS[2], G. JOCHMANN[2], G. WEISSE[2] and Z. SIMANE[3]

[1]Department of Medical Microbiology
E. Merck, Frankfurter Straße 250, D-6100 Darmstadt, FRG

[2]Department of Toxicology
E. Merck, Frankfurter Straße 250, D-6100 Darmstadt, FRG

[3]Department of Clinical Chemistry
E. Merck, Frankfurter Straße 250, D-6100 Darmstadt, FRG

INTRODUCTION

Internal fixation in combination with bone cement is often the treatment of choice in pathological fractures due to sceletal metastases. The goal in palliative tumor surgery is pain relief and rapid mobilization of the patient together with decreased time of hospitalization.

In many cases complete tumor resection is not possible. Therefore in order to prevent recurrence and secondary loosening of the osteosynthesis during life period of the patient the bone cement was loaded with a cytostatic agent, which is locally released in high concentrations.

Palacos E flow a low viscous cement and Methotrexate were combined. Why Methotrexate?

1. Methotrexate is used in the treatment of bone metastases due to primary tumor of the breast, the bronchus and the prostate,
2. there is documented correlation between Methotrexate serum concentrations and side effects and
3. by Leucovorin treatment side effects can be abolished.

After Langendorff et al. (ref. 1) had demonstrated that Methotrexate containing bone cement was effective after local application in transplanted osteosarcoma in mice, we studied the correlation between the dose of Methotrexate in cement, its release in vitro as well as the resulting serum concentrations and the tolerance in animals after implantation of the various bone cement mixtures.

METHODS

The study was performed in 40 rabbits which were randomly assigned to 5 groups. Both femoral cavities were completely filled with one of the following bone cement versions containing different doses of Methotrexate, namely 0.63 (group 2), 1.25 (group 3), 5 (group 4) and 12.5 % (group 5) as well as plain cement as a control (group 1).

Release of Methotrexate was measured in vitro by elution of hardened bone cement cylinders (h 10 mm, Ø 25 mm) in pooled human serum over a time period of 80 days. The elution fluid was changed daily. Serum concentrations were measured at different time intervalls (0.5, 1, 2, 4, 6, 24 hours, 2, 4, 6, 8, 10 days, and thereafter twice weekly) starting after operation until the amounts of Methotrexate dropped below 0.03 μM, our lower detection limit. The assay methods used were enzyme immunological and radio immunological techniques.

Animals were controlled two times daily and weight was recorded twice a weeks.

Haematological and biochemical investigations were performed prior to surgery and 2, 5, 8 and 12 weeks after operation. After 8 weeks 4 animals out of group 1, 2 and 3 were sacrified and all remaining animals after 12 weeks. Histological investigations were performed with special interest in liver and kidneys. Both organs are known to be affected in long lasting high dose Methotrexate treatment in patients.

RESULTS

The release of Methotrexate from hardened bone cement proved to be clearly dose dependent. Doubling the loading dose led to two times increased concentrations. By using our standard elution technique 300, 700, 1400, 3000 and 8000 μM were measured on day 1. Elution curves ran in parallel until the 25th day when there was a distinct decrease in Methotrexate concentrations released from the cement containing 12.5 % Methotrexate (Figure 1).

Serum concentrations reached after implantation of the cement were considerably low, starting at 0.7 and 1.0 μM in two low dose groups (2 and 3). After 48 respectively 72 hours the concentrations dropped below 0.1 μM which is regarded as a toxic threshold in patients. In the two high dose groups (4 and 5) the highest concentrations were 3 and 9 μM at day 1 and remained above

0.1 μM until the 23rd and 30th day respectively (Figure 2).

Haematological findings revealed a decrease in Leucocytes, Erythrocytes and Hemoglobin and an increase in Reticulocytes in both high groups containing 5 % and 12.5 % Methotrexate in bone cement. Numbers of Leucocytes however returned to normal after Leucovorin treatment. A reversible decrease in AP was found in all treatment groups at 2 weeks and an increase of urea in the two high dose groups which returned to normal after Leucovorin treatment when the animals recovered.

Histologically 12 weeks after operation centrolobular atrophy and increased necrosis of hepatocytes of the liver were seen only in the high dose groups (4 and 5). Clinical survey of the animals showed severe diarrhea in group 5 and 4 starting 6 respectively 14 days after operation. This was reflected very clearly in the bodyweight curves. 4 animals in group 5 and 3 animals in group 3 died from Methotrexate toxicity. The remaining recovered after intensive treatment with Leucovorin. Bodyweight curves of animals treated with cements containing 0.63 and 1.25 % Methotrexate (low dose groups 2 and 3) ran parallel to the control group.

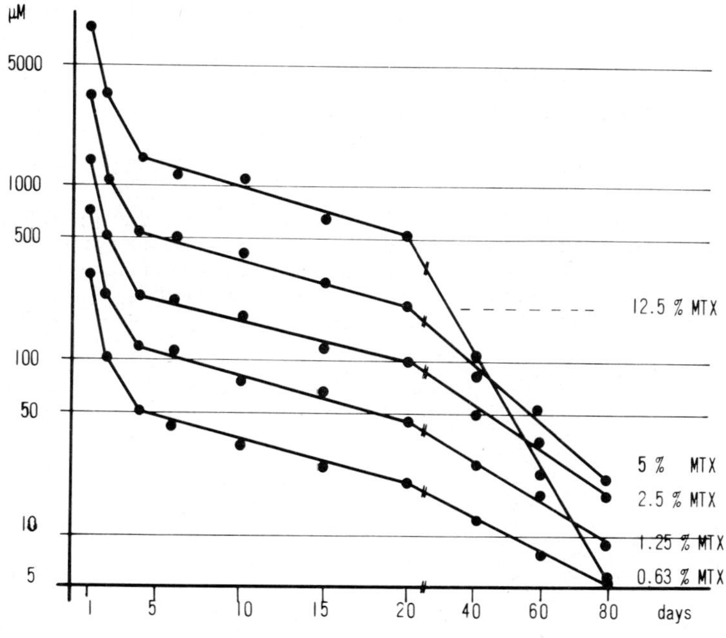

Fig. 1. Release of Methotrexate in vitro

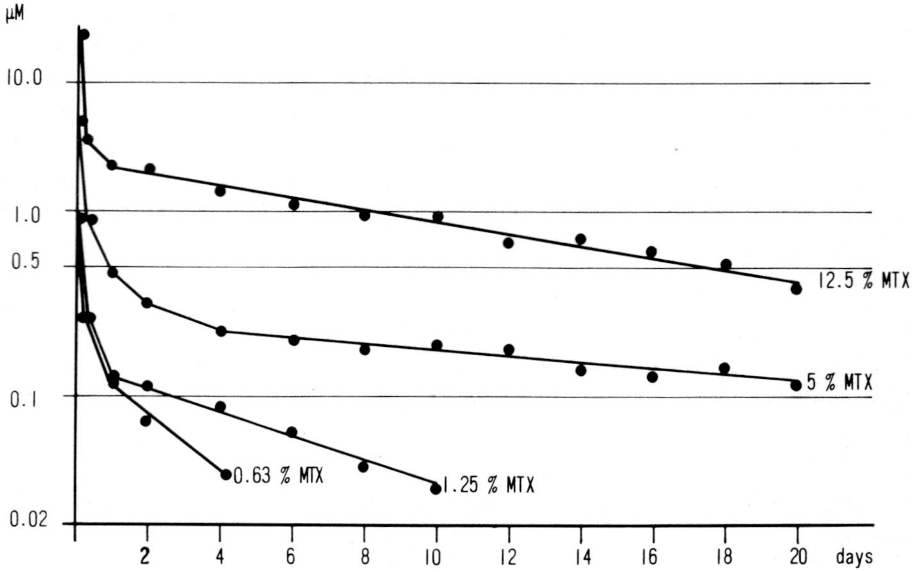

Fig. 2. Methotrexate Concentrations in Serum of Rabbits

CONCLUSION

Basing on these results for application in patients bone cement containing 0.63 % Methotrexate was chosen.

REFERENCE

1 H.-U. Langendorff, G. Delling, D. Sinekowicz, K. H. Jungbluth, Die chirurgische Therapie von Skelettmetastasen. Indikation, Möglichkeiten und Ergebnisse, 9. Symposium des Arbeitskreises für Osteologie "Deutsch-österreichisch-schweizerisch", 19. - 20. September 1985, Hamburg.

Biomaterials and Clinical Applications,
edited by A. Pizzoferrato, P.G. Marchetti, A. Ravaglioli and A.J.C. Lee
Elsevier Science Publishers B.V., Amsterdam, 1987 — Printed in The Netherlands

BIODEGRADABLE HOLLOW FIBER FOR THE CONTROLLED RELEASE OF DRUGS: A PRELIMINARY REPORT ON TISSUE REACTION.

J.M. SCHAKENRAAD[1], M.J.D. EENINK[2], J.A. OOSTERBAAN[1], J.FEIJEN[2], W.POTMAN[2], J. OLIJSLAGER[3], P.J. GREIDANUS[3], I. MOLENAAR[1] AND P. NIEUWENHUIS[1].

[1]Department of Histology and Centre for Medical Electron Microscopy, University of Groningen, Oostersingel 69/1-2, 9713 EZ Groningen (The Netherlands)

[2]Department of Biomedical Technology, Twente University, P.O.Box 217, 7500 AE Enschede (The Netherlands)

[3]Plastics and Rubber Research Institute TNO, P.O.Box 71, 2600 AB Delft (The Netherlands)

SUMMARY

Biodegradable hollow fibers of poly-L-lactic acid, measuring 1 cm in length and 0.7 mm external diameter were prepared to release drugs at a zero order rate for periods of at least nine months. To test this concept, the hollow fibers were filled with levonorgestrel suspended in castor-oil (approx. 500 ug per fiber), and after gamma sterilisation or alcohol sterilisation implanted subcutaneously in female AO/BN rats. The fibers were harvested at periods from 1 day to 2 months and evaluated for the reaction of surrounding tissues with the light and transmission electron microscope.The tissue reaction can best be described as a low turn-over foreign body granuloma;macrophages encapsulated the fiber and subsequently fibroblasts formed a loose sheath around the macrophage layer. Apparently macrophages stimulated capillary growth and subsequently fibroblasts deposited collagen in the intercellular matrix. The macrophages at the interface showed microvillous like membrane protrusions at the cell side not facing the polymer.

INTRODUCTION

Controlled release of drugs is a subject that has attracted much attention during the last decade. The drug administered must reach the target organ at the right concentration during an intended period of time. Many release devices have already been manufactured, but only recently biodegradable reservoirs are being applied. Several drugs are being considered for application in the biodegradable hollow fiber developed in our laboratories, e.g. cytostatica or progestagens. The site of fiber implantation can be chosen according to the target function: a fiber containing cytostatica can be placed into the centre of the tumour or close to a supplying bloodvessel, whereas a fiber containing hormones for contraception can easily be "injected" subcutaneously. Our hollow fiber concept aims at a zero order release of hormones for periods over nine months (ref. 1-2). Only after complete release of the drug the fiber should degrade. The zero order release of the drug guarantees a continuous and constant level in the peripheral blood. To test the hollow fiber concept we investigated the tissue reaction to the implanted foreign body, the effective release of drug after tissue encapsulation and the process of biodegradation. In this paper a preliminary study on tissue reactions will be reported; studies concerning fiber breaking strength and kinetics of drug release will be discussed in separate papers.

MATERIALS AND METHODS

Fibers. The hollow fibers were spun of poly-L-lactic acid (MW 150.000) using a "dry-wet" coagulation spinning process (ref. 1,2). The tube-in-orifice spinneret device contained an injection tube with an outside diameter of 0.6 mm, an inside diameter of 0.4 mm and an orifice diameter of 1.0 mm . The hollow fibers (Fig. 1) had a diameter of 0.7 mm, an internal diameter of 0.6 mm and a wall tickness of 0.05 mm. The fiber consisted of a porous body with a dense non-porous skin on both sides. The fibers were cut at a length of 1 cm, filled with levonorgestrel suspended in castor oil and heat-sealed at both ends. In vitro release studies (^{3}H-levonorgestrel) showed an average release rate of 3 ugr/day/cm fiber.

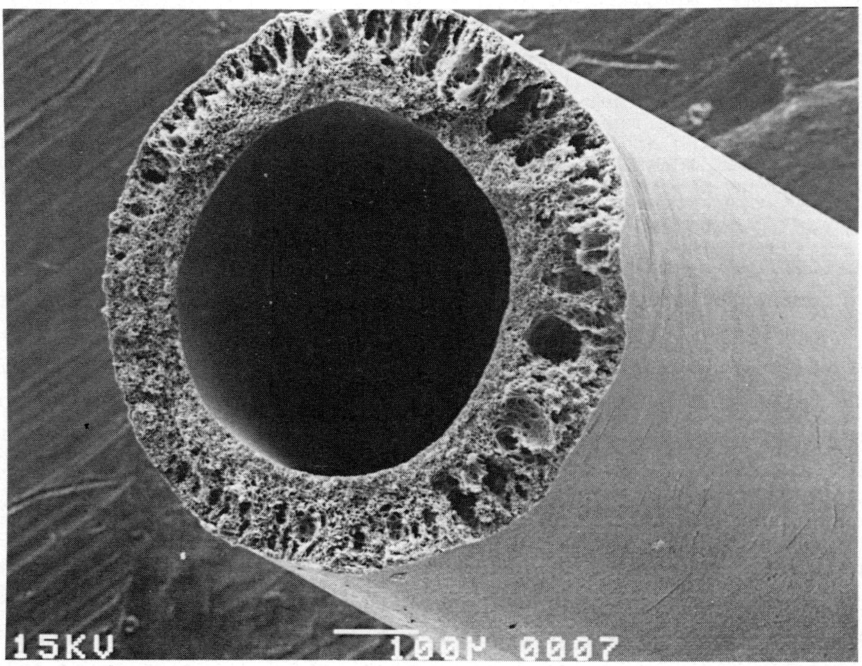

Fig. 1. Hollow fiber

Sterilisation. The fibers were either gamma-sterilised (2,5 Mrad) or alcohol sterilised and air dried.

Implantation. The fibers were implanted subcutaneously in female AO/BN rats of approximately 3 months of age weighing 200-250 grams. A specially adapted syringe (Fig. 2) was used for this purpose. The rat was shaved on its back which was subsequently alcohol sterilised.

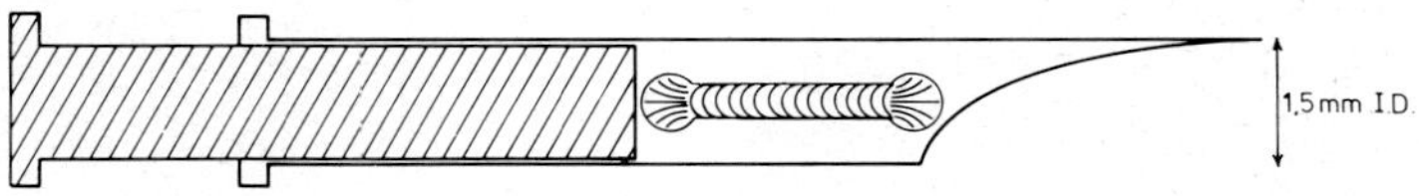

Fig. 2 Syringe used for injecting hollow fibers

Harvesting. At different harvesting times the rats were ether-anaesthetized and the fibers were collected including surrounding tissue. The fibers were immediately fixed in 2% glutaraldehyde in phosphate buffer (0.1 M, pH 7.4).

Tissue reaction. The fibers with adhering tissue were vibratomised perpendicular to their length in 300 um sections and postfixed with Karnovsky fixative. Dehydration was performed in an alcohol series followed by butyl-2,3 epoxypropylether. Subsequently the specimens were embedded in Epon 10:0. More contrast could be obtained after staining en bloc with 2% uranylacetate in 10% ethanol. Semithin sections (1 um) were cut, appropriate areas were selected for making ultrathin sections (50 nm), which were subsequently evaluated in a transmission electron microscope (002A-Akashi) at 60 kV. The 1 um sections were used for light microscopy after staining with toluidine blue.

RESULTS

At harvesting time the fibers could easily be found and removed without causing damage to the fibers. At day 1 macrophages and granulocytes had surrounded the fibers (Fig. 3). At day 7 a layer of macrophages had covered the fiber. These cells were very active as judged by the amount of mitochondria, endoplasmatic reticulum, lysosomes and Golgi-apparatus (Fig.4). The cell membrane contacting the fiber, closely followed the smooth contours of the polymer at a regular distance of approximately 100 nm, with occurrence of close contacts or focal adhesions. At day 30 this layer of macrophages was surrounded by a layer of fibroblasts and ingrowing

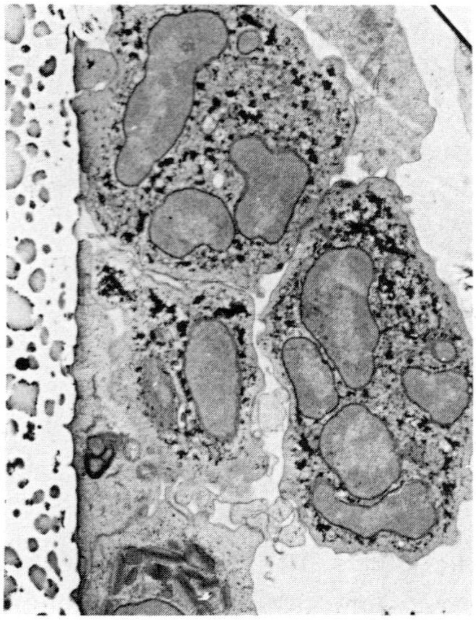

Fig. 3.

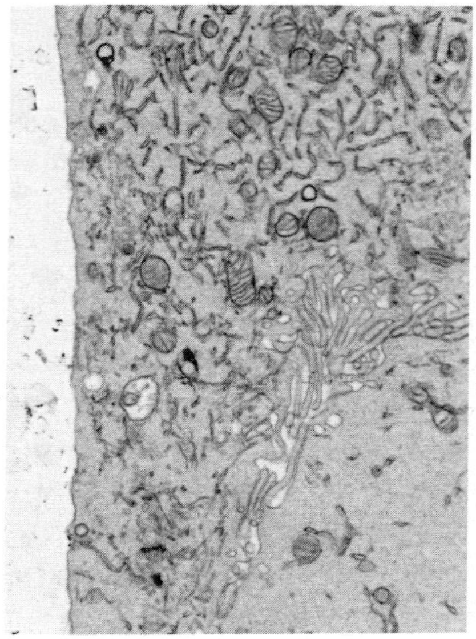

Fig. 4.

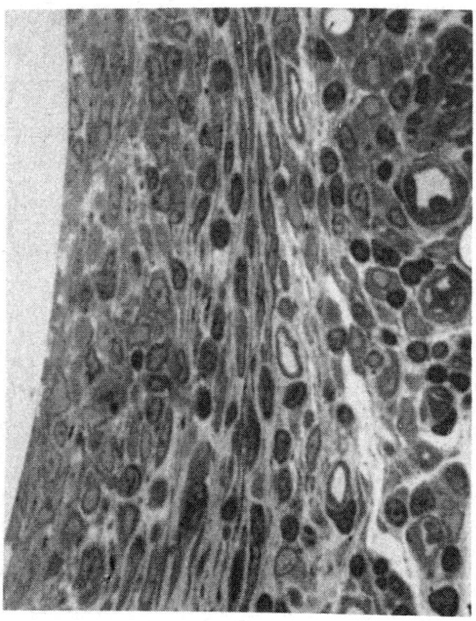

Fig. 5.

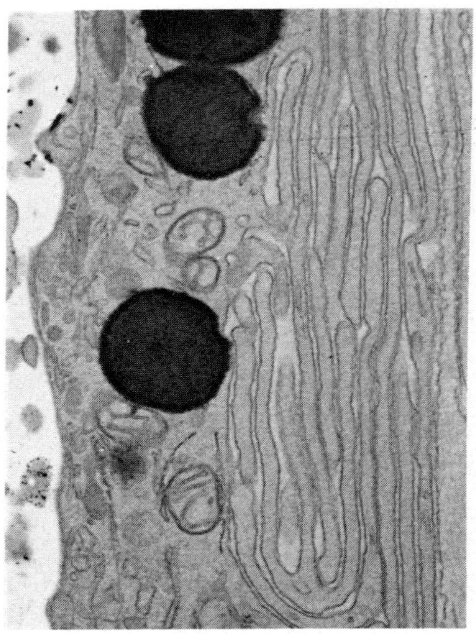

Fig. 6.

capillaries (Fig. 5). The macrophages at the cell-polymer interface showed a particular appearance of microvillous-like structures, sometimes interdigitating with neighbouring cells (Fig. 6). These villi were only observed at that cell side not facing the polymer. Very few giant cells could be observed. At day 60 the macrophage layer was still present, though flattened;the tissue reaction was not abundant and no inflammatory reactions were observed.

DISCUSSION

The results demonstrate that up till two months the implanted hollow fibers induced only a slight tissue reaction. The phenomenon of macrophages interpositioned between the polymer and the fibrous capsule resembles a very mild foreign body reaction. It might be expected that the fibrous capsule does not severely diminish the rate of drug release since capillaries, presumably attracted by macrophage angiogenesis factor, were invading the fibrous capsule. The tissue reaction can best be described as a low turn-over foreign body granuloma which is known to occur when the foreign body is non-toxic. The absence of lymphocytes at the polymer interface indicates that the poly-L-lactic acid does not elicit an immune response as has been postulated by Hirsh and Johnson (ref. 3) and Behling and Spector (ref. 4) for similar polymers .Since the surface contacting the cells was quite smooth, and the polymer did not rapidly degrade, we did not observe large amounts of foreign body giant cells (ref. 4).

The appearance of lamellopodial extensions are also described by Matlaga & Salthouse (ref. 5) and Salthouse (ref. 6) at the cell membrane not facing the polymer; these fingerlike projections often interdigitated with neighbouring cells. This phenomenon already occurred a few days after implantation. The function of these lamellopodia remains uncertain. Salthouse suggested (ref. 6) that these lamellopodia are involved in engulfing polymer debris and were indicative for macrophage activity. However,in our system no such proof is available, because the polymer to be engulfed is situated at the opposite side of the cell, we consider it a foreign body induced surface enlargement with yet unknown function. The activity of enzymes in the degradation process, and in our case of lactic acid dehydrogenase, has often been proven (ref. 3,5,6). The macrophage occupies a central role in woundhealing: control of fibroblast migration (ref. 7) and activity: secretion of lactate which stimulates collagen production by fibroblasts (ref. 8) (Fig. 7).

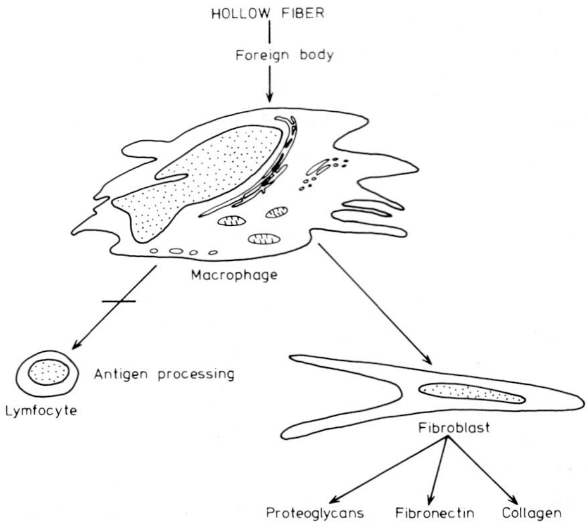

Fig. 7.

In conclusion: the functionality of the hollow fiber release concept seems satisfactory with respect to tissue reaction:only a slight foreign body reaction was observed.

REFERENCES

1 J.H.M. Albers, J.C. Rieke, J. Olijslager, P.J.Greidanus, M.J.D. Eenink and J. Feijen, Subdermal drug delivery with a biodegradable hollow fiber device, Proc.Int.Symp. Controlled Release Bioact.Mat., 11 (1984) 80-81.

2 M.J.D. Eenink, J.H.M. Albers, J.C. Rieke, J. Olijslager, P.J. Greidanus and J. Feijen, Biodegradable hollow fibers for the controlled release of drugs. Proc.Int.Symp. Controlled Release Bioact.Mat., 12 (1985) 49-50.

3 B.C. Hirsh and W.C. Johnson, Concepts of granulomatous inflammation, Int.J.Dermatol., 33 (1984) 90-100.

4 C.A. Behling and M. Spector, Quantitative characterization of cells at the interface of long-term implants of selected polymers, J. Biom.Mat.Res., 20 (1986) 653-666.

5 B.F. Matlaga and T.N. Salthouse, Ultrastructural observations of cells at the interface of a biodegradable polymer: Polyglactin 910, J.Biom.Mat.Res., 17 (1983) 185-197.

6 T.N. Salthouse, Some aspects of macrophage behavior at the implant interface, J.Biom.Mat.Res., 18 (1984) 395-401.

7 S.J. Leibovich and R. Ross, A macrophage-dependent factor that stimulates the proliferation of fibroblasts in vitro, Am.J.Pathol., 84 (1976) 501-513.

8 T.K. Hunt, W.B. Conolly, S.B. Aronson and P. Goldstein, Anaerobic metabolism and wound healing: a hypothesis for the initiation and cessation of collagen synthesis in wounds, Am.J.Surg., 135 (1978) 328-332.

Biomaterials and Clinical Applications,
edited by A. Pizzoferrato, P.G. Marchetti, A. Ravaglioli and A.J.C. Lee
Elsevier Science Publishers B.V., Amsterdam, 1987 — Printed in The Netherlands

POLYALKYLCYANOACRYLATE NANOCAPSULES AS DRUG CARRIERS : ADVANTAGE IN INSULIN TREATMENT OF STREPTOZOTOCIN-INDUCED DIABETIC RATS.

C. DAMGE , C. MICHEL , M. APRAHAMIAN , P. COUVREUR .

INSERM, Unité 61, Biologie Cellulaire et Physiopathologie Digestives, 3, avenue Molière, 67200-Strasbourg (France)

Laboratoire de Pharmacie Galénique et Biopharmacie, Université Paris XI, 5, rue Jean-Baptiste Clément, 92216-Chatenay-Malabry (France)

SUMMARY

Polyalkylcyanoacrylate nanocapsules composed of small spherical capsules, 220nm in diameter, have been used as a drug carrier for insulin. When administered subcutaneously in streptozotocin-induced diabetic rats, they prolong the therapeutic response of insulin. When administered intragastrically by force feeding, they normalize, for a prolonged period, hyperglycemia in fasted diabetic rats. Thus nanocapsules improve the efficiency of insulin and can be used for enteral administration of this hormone.

INTRODUCTION

During the last years, new drug delivery systems have been developed to utilize more effectively existing drugs and to minimize their unwanted toxic effects. Among these are polyalkylcyanoacrylate nanocapsules and nanoparticles constituted respectively by full polymeric spheres and empty polymeric capsules of 100 to 300 nm in diameter (refs. 1-2). These colloidal drug carriers are able to take over drugs by adsorption or encapsulation. They have been claimed to be biocompatible and biodegradable (refs. 3-4). Nanoparticles have been successfully applied to cytostatic drugs in "in vivo" cancer models (refs. 5-6) when administered parenterally. Nanocapsules have been shown to prolong the absorption rate of a lipophilic drug when administered intraluminally in the dog intestine (ref. 7) and to pass through the intestinal mucosa (ref. 8). The present work was designed to investigate further the advantage of the use of polyalkylcyanoacrylate nanocapsules as a drug carrier for insulin. Thus we attempted to treat streptozotocin-induced diabetic rats by the administration of encapsulated or non encapsulated insulin.

METHODS

1. Preparation of nanocapsules

Nanocapsules were prepared by an interfacial emulsion polymerization of isobutylcyanoacrylate according to Al Khouri et al (ref.2). A lipidic phase, containing 32 U of insulin (Umuline Ordinaire, Lilly France) and the monomer isobutyl-2-cyanoacrylate has been dissolved in ethanol and added under mechanical stirring to an aqueous phase containing a non ionic surfactant (0.25 %). An emulsion of oil-in-water was obtained and polymerization of the monomer occured at the surface of the lipidic droplets. The solvent was then partially evapourated in order to obtain a final volume of 12.5 ml. The nanocapsules suspension was purified by filtration and their size was estimated by laser light scattering.

The rate of encapsulation of insulin was estimated using methyl-^{14}C-methylated insulin as a tracor, nanocapsules being separated by sequential filtration on membranes with decreasing porosity.

2. In vivo studies

Diabetes was induced in male Wistar rats weighing 150 to 200 g by an intravenous injection of streptozotocin (65 mg/kg) in a citrate buffer at pH 4.5. The rats were left untreated for 15 days and were considered as diabetics when fasted glycemia was higher than 300 mg/100 ml.

The diabetic rats were then treated with encapsulated or free insulin, the therapeutic effect of insulin being estimated by a decrease of glycemia. Insulin was administered either subcutaneously or intragastrically.

Subcutaneous administration

22 diabetic rats were divided into 3 groups. Each group received subcutaneously normal saline (control group, n=7) or encapsulated insulin at the rate of 25 U/kg body weight (n=8) or free insulin at the same dose (n=7). The administrations were carried out by a single injection of a 10 ml volume/kg body weight. Blood was collected in non fasted animals at two-hour intervals after the injection for the first 24 hours, then at 32 and 50 hours.

Intragastric administration

16 diabetic rats were divided into two groups. Each group was subjected to a single intragastric administration of insulin loaded nanocapsules at the dose of 25 U/kg body weight (n=9) or normal saline for controls (n=7). These administrations were carried out by force feeding under a volume of 10 ml/kg body

weight. Blood was collected in fasted animals before and 2, 4, 6, 9, 13 and 15 days after administration.

RESULTS

Characterization of nanocapsules

Analysed by laser light scattering, the mean size of nanocapsules was 220 nm with 95 % in the range of 150 to 300 nm. Using labelled insulin as a tracer, the rate of encapsulation of insulin could be determined : nanocapsules were able to encapsulate 54.9 % of the initial amount of insulin. Thus, it was administered a total amount of 25 U/kg body weight of insulin in which only 13.7 U were encapsulated.

Effects of encapsulated insulin in diabetic rats

1. After subcutaneous administration

As illustrated in Figure 1, the glycemia of control diabetic rats varied between 400 and 600 mg/100 ml. The subcutaneous administration of nanocapsules induced a 60 % decrease of this glycemia ($p<0.001$) after the second hour. This low level was maintained for 20 hours. Control values were reached again 32 hours after the injection. Non-encapsulated insulin also depressed glycemia by 60 % ($p<0.001$) but this effect disappeared totally from the 8th hour after injection. Thus encapsulation of insulin prolongs its therapeutic effect for at least 12 hours.

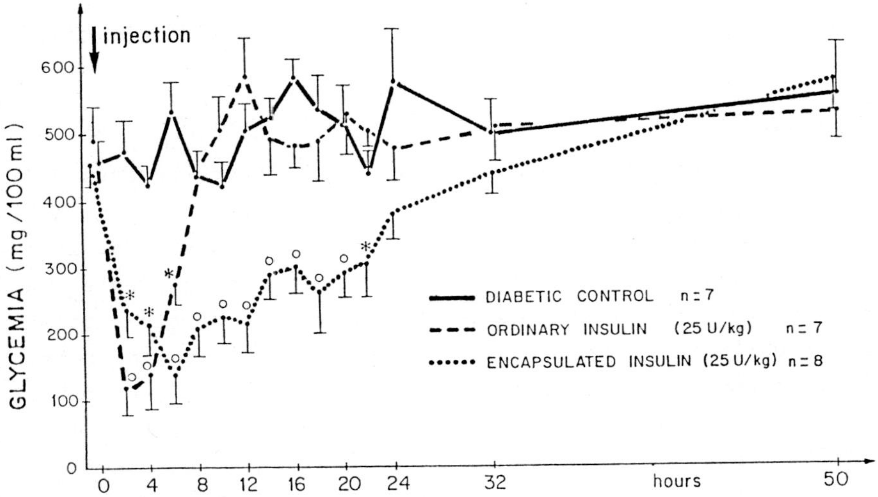

Fig. 1 : Effect of a single subcutaneous administration of insulin (encapsulated or ordinary) on glycemia in diabetic rats (* $p<0.01$; o $p<0.001$).

2. After intragastric administration

As represented in Figure 2, fasted glycemia in non-treated animals varied between 300 and 400 mg/100 ml. The intragastric administration of encapsulated insulin induced a 50 % decrease of glycemia ($p<0.001$) from the second to the ninth day after administration, control values being reached from the 13th day.

In consequence, the oral administration of insulin loaded nanocapsules markedly decreased glycemia in fasted streptozotocin-induced diabetic rats in which glycemia could be normalized. By comparison, in non-diabetic rats, fasted glycemia was comprised between 90 and 120 mg/100 ml.

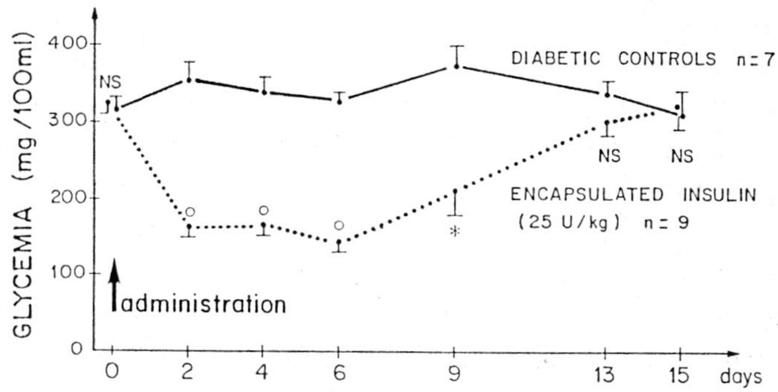

Fig. 2. : Effect of a single intragastric administration of encapsulated insulin on glycemia in diabetic rats (* $p<0.01$; o $p<0.001$).

DISCUSSION

This work indicates clearly that a new polymeric drug delivery system composed of polyalkylcyanoacrylate nanocapsules prolongs the therapeutic effect of insulin when administered subcutaneously. The immediate decrease of glycemia may be explained by the presence in the suspension of non encapsulated insulin while the long-term effect may be due to the release of insulin through nanocapsules.

In addition, our results show that insulin, administered per os in an encapsulated form, displays a significant physiological action. Indeed, a single administration of 13.7 U of encapsulated insulin per kg body weight normalizes glycemia within two days, this effect being maintained for the seven following days. These data suggest 1) that insulin may be protected in the intestinal lumen by encapsulation and 2) that insulin may be absorbed by the intestinal mucosa and remains biologically active.

In a previous work (ref. 8), we noted by electron scan microscopy of cryofixed and freeze-dried tissues, that nanocapsules were able to pass through the intestinal mucosa by a paracellular pathway and can be found in the vessels of the lamina propria. Thus it was suggested that at least a part of nanocapsules could attain portal blood after intestinal passage, as this pathway of insulin administration is the most physiological (ref. 9).

Finally, the question was to know how nanocapsules could release insulin. According to Leonard et al (ref. 3), polyalkylcyanoacrylates could be degraded under physiological conditions by hydrolysis, leading to the formation of formaldehyde and cyanoacetate. Another mechanism of degradation of polyisobutylcyanoacrylate has been proposed by Lenaerts et al (ref. 4). These authors suggest the existence of an enzymatic degradation by ester hydrolysis which could increase the hydrophilic properties of the polymeric chain and favor its elimination.

Progressive degradation of the polymer could also explain the progressive liberation of insulin by nanocapsules, leading to a prolonged therapeutic effect. It remains however unclear, why subcutaneous administration of nanocapsules immediately depressed hyperglycemia in diabetic rats while per os administration exhibits the same effect but only after two days.

In conclusion, our results demonstrate that biodegradable polymeric nanocapsules used as a drug delivery system can enhance the therapeutic response of insulin when administered subcutaneously and normalize hyperglycemia in fasted diabetic rats when administered per os. This long-term effect allows new possible developments in the treatment of diabetes to be considered.

ACKNOWLEDGMENTS

The authors wish to thank R. Kurtz and A. Hoeltzel for careful technical assistance. This work was supported by the "Conseil Régional Alsace" and by the "Ministère de la Recherche et de l'Industrie" (France). We are grateful to Dr. J.D. Heyl (Lilly France, Fegersheim) for the gift of Umuline and to Prof. M. Pinget for helpful advice and reviewing the manuscript.

REFERENCES

1. P. Couvreur, B. Kante, M. Roland, P. Guiot, P. Baudhuin, P. Speiser, Polycyanoacrylate nanoparticles as potential lysosomotropic carriers. Preparation and sorptive properties, J. Pharm. Pharmacol., 31 (1979) 331-332.
2. F.N. Al Khouri, L. Roblot-Treupel, H. Fessi, J.P. Devissaguet, F. Puisieux, Development of a new process for the manufacture of polyisobutyl cyanoacrylate nanocapsules, Int. J. Pharm., 28 (1986) 125-132.
3. F. Leonard, R.L. Kulkarni, G. Brandes, N. Nelson, J.J. Cameron, Synthesis and degradation of poly (alkylcyanoacrylates), J. Appl. Polym. Sci., 10 (1966) 259-272.
4. V. Lenaerts, P. Couvreur, D. Christiaens-Leyh, E. Joiris, M. Roland, B. Rollman, P. Speiser, Degradation of Poly (isobutylcyanoacrylate) nanoparticles, Biomaterials, 5 (1984) 65-68.
5. F. Brasseur, P. Couvreur, B. Kante, L. Deckers-Passau, M. Roland, C. Deckers, P. Speiser, Actinomycin D adsorbed on polymethylcyanoacrylate nanoparticles : increased efficiency against an experimental tumor, Eur. J. Cancer, 16 (1980) 1441-1445.
6. P. Couvreur, B. Kante, L. Grislain, M. Roland, P. Speiser, Toxicity of polyalkylcyanoacrylate nanoparticles II. : Doxorubicin-loaded nanoparticles, J. Pharm. Sci., 71 (7) (1982) 790-792.
7. C. Damgé, M. Aprahamian, G. Balboni, A. Hoeltzel, V. Andrieu, J.P. Devissaguet, Intérêt des vecteurs colloïdaux polymériques (nanocapsules) dans l'absorption intestinale. Etude expérimentale d'un traceur iodé chez le chien,
In : Proc. 4th Int. Conf. on Pharmaceutical Technology, Paris, France, June 3-5, 1986, (IV) 239-245.
8. M. Aprahamian, C. Damgé, W. Humbert, G. Balboni, V. Andrieu, J.P. Devissaguet, Les vecteurs colloïdaux polymériques franchissent-ils la barrière intestinale ?, In : Proc. 4th Int. Conf on Pharmaceutical Technology, Paris, France, June 3-5, 1986, (IV) 175-182.
9. A.M. Albisser, C.K. Botz, B.S. Leibel, Blood glucose regulation using an open-loop insulin delivery system in pancreatectomized dogs given glucose infusions, Diabetologia, 16 (1979), 129-133.

Biomaterials and Clinical Applications,
edited by A. Pizzoferrato, P.G. Marchetti, A. Ravaglioli and A.J.C. Lee
Elsevier Science Publishers B.V., Amsterdam, 1987 — Printed in The Netherlands

BIOACTIVE POLYMERS XLI. STUDIES IN VIVO ON CHLORAMPHENICOL RETARD RELEASING

Cr. SIMIONESCU, M. I. POPA and S. DUMITRIU
Polytechnic Institute of Jassy, 23 August 11, R-6600, Jassy (Romania)

SUMMARY

The release in vivo of chloramphenicol coupled on xanthan was studied in a dog. In the first stage, the chloramphenicol level in blood after the oral administration of the drug (a dose of 50 mg/Kg) was followed and then, after a week, the level on the xanthan - chloramphenicol product, containing an equivalent amount of antibiotic. Attaining the maximum concentration after 3 h from administration indicates the hydrolysis product of chloramphenicol - xanthan esteric bond to appear at the stomach level and the absorption to take place in the intestine.

INTRODUCTION

The synthesis of macromolecular prodrugs is a largely investigated field with the purpose of obtaining drugs coupled on natural or synthetic polymers by labile ionic or covalent bonds (refs. 1-4).

The major efforts in the development of new chemotherapeutic agents, up to a few years ago, were characterized by a narrowness of its concept involving the synthesis of new chemical entities and evaluation of their pharmacological activity. Today new and novel approaches are being explored not only in the discovery of new therapeutic agents, but more importantly new techniques are being investigated and developed, techniques that would permit the manipulation of drugs by getting them to targeted organs in the right amounts and at the right times.

In previous papers (refs. 5-8) some physico-chemical aspects of coupling of antibiotics - ampicilline, chloramphenicol, streptomycin, neomycin - on xanthan and carboxymethylcellulose derivatives were described.

The present paper aims at elucidating the mechanism of the in vivo action of chloramphenicol coupled on xanthan.

METHODS

Analysis of chloramphenicol in plasma

The chloramphenicol was analysed by high-pressure liquid

chromatography (HPLC), by using a Varian Model 5000 chromatograph provided with a MicroPak CN-10 column of 250 x 4.6 mm. The mobile phase was methanol - water (pH 2.5 with perchloric acid), 50/50 v/v at flow rate of 0.6 ml/min. The detection was performed in UV region, at 280 nm. The column temperature was maintained at 20°C.

200 µl serum were mixed with 200 µl acetonitrile for deproteinization. The mixture was centrifuged at 3500 r.p.m. for 3 minutes. 20 µl of supernatant liquid were then injected for analysis.

Study on chloramphenicol releasing

In vitro. To 45 ml of simulated (ref. 9) or natural gastric fluid , thermostated at 37° ± 0.5°C the chloramphenicol - xanthan product (150 mg polymers with 30% bound chloramphenicol) was added. The system was stirred at 30 r.p.m. Samples of 50 µl were taken at certain times, diluted in 500 µl acetonitrile and centrifuged at 3500 r.p.m. for 3 minutes. 20 µl of supernatant liquid were then taken and analysed by HPLC.

In vivo. A dose of 50 mg/Kg of free chloramphenicol (Cph) was administrated as tablets in a dog. Samples of plasma were collected at certain times, the serum separated and analysed by HPLC.

RESULTS AND DISCUSSION

The Cph was coupled on xanthan (Biozan R, HERCULES) in heterogeneous medium with diciclohexylcarbodiimide (DCI) as a catalyst.

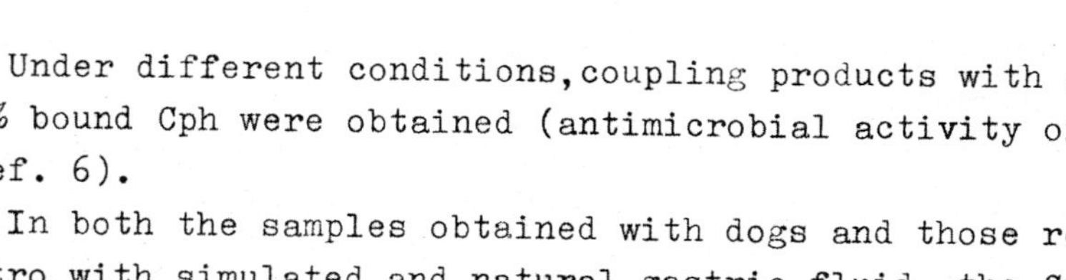

Under different conditions,coupling products with a content of 30% bound Cph were obtained (antimicrobial activity of 406 UI/mg) (ref. 6).

In both the samples obtained with dogs and those resulted in vitro with simulated and natural gastric fluid, the Cph released by hydrolysis was detected.

By comparing the distribution of the peaks in the standard serum (see Fig. 1a) and in the serum containing Cph (see Fig. 1b) the same positions are noticed, with no other metabolites. The chromatogram (see Fig. 1c) obtained with the serum of sample under study (from a dog to which Cph - xanthan was administered) contains instead an additional peak at 12.4 min, attributable to the metabolite composed from Cph and glucose.

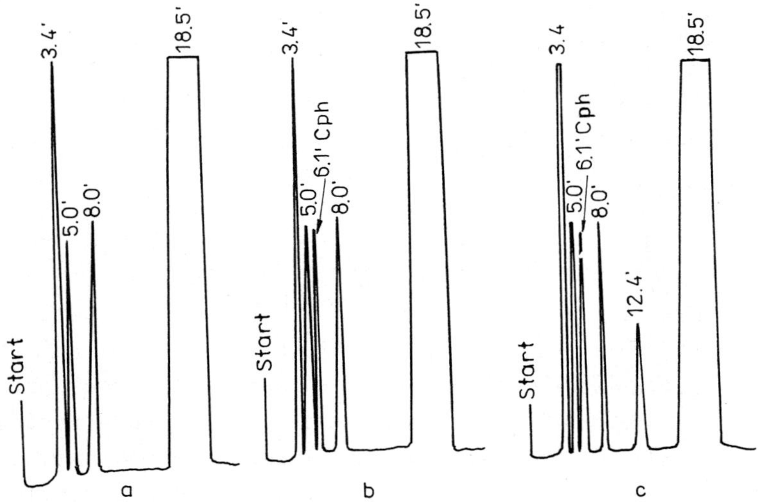

Fig. 1. Chromatogram of serum from a dog.
a - Standard serum;
b - Free Cph, oral dose of 50 mg/Kg;
c - Cph - xanthan, a dose with an equivalent Cph content.

In case of free Cph administered (see Fig. 2, curve 1), the concentration of antibiotic in serum passes through a maximum, decreasing then significantly.

For the Cph - xanthan <u>in vivo</u> (see Fig. 2, curve 2) the drug is split from the support, attaining a maximum concentration comparable to that of the free drug which remains about constant for 4 hours. If a new dose is given after 8 hours, the Cph content remains constant for 12 hours (see Fig. 2, curve 3).

The hydrolysis rates of Cph - xanthan product in the natural (see Fig. 3, curve 1) and simulated (see Fig. 3, curve 2) gastric fluid are noticed to be comparable, namely 82% and 79%, respectively, of the immobilized Cph released during 12 hours. Within the 2 - 10 hours range, the amount of Cph released is constant, of about 80 μg/h/ml serum.

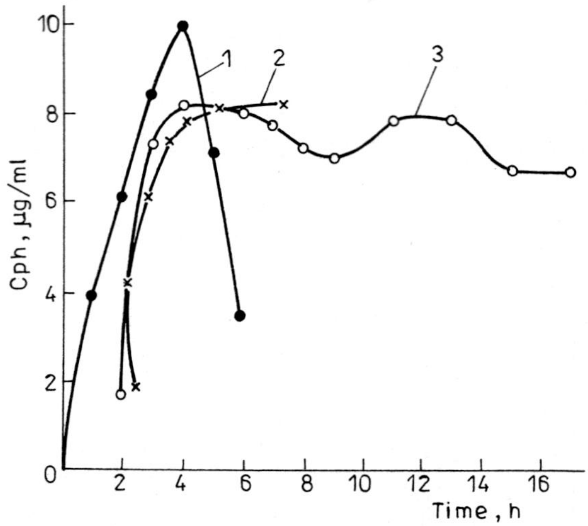

Fig. 2. Level of Cph in plasma. (1) Free Cph, a single oral dose of 50 mg/Kg. (2) Cph - xanthan, a single dose with an equivalent Cph content. (3) Cph - xanthan, as curve 2,but after administration of a new dose after 8 hours.

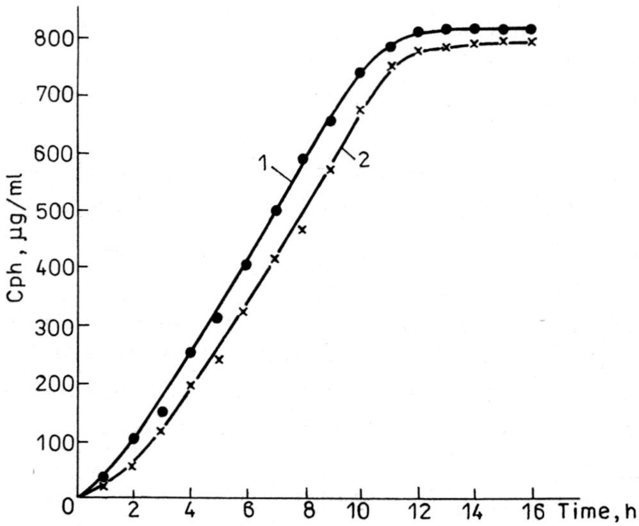

Fig. 3. Level of Cph in gastric fluid. (1) Natural gastric fluid. (2) Simulated gastric fluid.

CONCLUSIONS

The presence of Cph in the plasma of dog after the oral administration of Cph - xanthan attests the Cph releasing from the support by hydrolysis. Products of condensation of Cph with glucose formed by enzymatic hydrolysis of the macromolecular support also appear.

The administration in dog of two doses at 8 hours one after the other results in an attack concentration of Cph of 8 μg/ml in the plasma beyond the toxicity domain.

REFERENCES

1 Cr. I. Simionescu, S. Dumitriu, M. I. Popa and L. Denisova, Antibiotics immobilized on polysaccharides, Makromol. Chem. Suppl., 9 (1985) 179-187.
2 S. Dumitriu, M. Popa, C. Oniscu and M. Dumitriu, Bioactive polymers XXXIV. Cellulose derivatives as supports for enzymes and drugs immobilization, Cellulose Chem. Technol., 19 (1985) 601-607.
3 N. Ueno and M. F. Refojo, Ocular pharmacology of drug release devices, in: S. D. Bruck (Ed.), Controlled drug delivery Vol II Clinical applications, CRC Press, Inc. Boca Raton, Florida, 1983, pp. 89-109.
4 C. M. Samour, Polymeric drugs in the chemotherapy of microbial infections, in: L. G. Donaruma and O. Vogl (Eds.), Polymeric drugs, Academic Press, New York, 1978, pp. 161-184.
5 Cr. Simionescu and S. Dumitriu, Biologically active compounds immobilized on cellulose derivatives, in: E. Chiellini and P. Giusti (Eds.), Polymers in medicine. Biomedical and pharmacological applications, Plenum Press, New York, 1983, pp. 115-137.
6 Cr. I. Simionescu, M. I. Popa and S. Dumitriu, Bioactive polymers XXI. Coupling of chloramphenicol on Biozan R, Colloid & Polymer Sci., 263 (1985) 620-623.
7 S. Dumitriu and P. Cremonesi, Drug immobilization on natural polymers, Recent advances in chemotherapy, Proceedings of the 14th international congress of chemotherapy, Kyoto, University of Tokyo Press, 1985, pp. 243-244.
8 Cr. Simionescu, M. I. Popa and S. Dumitriu, Bioactive polymers XXXIII. Synthesis and evaluation of some pharmacological characteristics of chloramphenicol immobilized on Biozan R, Biomaterials, 7 (1986) 118-120.
9 A. J. Aguiar, L. M. Wheeler, S. Fusari and J. E. Zelmer, Evaluation of physical and pharmaceutical factors involved in drug release and availability from chloramphenicol capsules, J. Pharm. Sci., 57 (1968), pp. 1844-1850.

Biomaterials and Clinical Applications,
edited by A. Pizzoferrato, P.G. Marchetti, A. Ravaglioli and A.J.C. Lee
Elsevier Science Publishers B.V., Amsterdam, 1987 — Printed in The Netherlands

POSSIBLE ROLE OF PERFLUOROCHEMICAL PARTICLES AS DRUG DELIVERY AGENTS IN LIVER

S. CAIAZZA[1], C. FANIZZA[1] and M. FERRARI[2]

[1]Department of Ultrastructures and [2]Department of Organ and System Pathophysiology, Istituto Superiore di Sanità, Viale Regina Elena, 299 - 00161 Rome (Italy)

SUMMARY

Perfluorocarbons (PFCs), potential blood substitutes given their very high affinity for O_2 and CO_2, are stored mainly in liver. The available data on the solubility of different chemicals in PFC emulsions point out the possibility of their use as drug carriers to target organs. Many natural and synthetic substances as well as liposomes have been tested as hepatotropic drug carriers, but after many pre-clinical studies their future appears uncertain. Our data on the endocytosis of PFC particles by reticuloendothelial and parenchimal rat liver cells as well as by cultured rat hepatocytes underline the opportunity that second generation PFCs may be also checked as drug carriers and delivery agents, liver cells being the specific target.

INTRODUCTION

Perfluorochemical emulsions, chemically inert fluorinated compounds with high dissolving capability for O_2 and CO_2 (refs. 1-3) are potential blood substitutes with applications ranging from emergency surgery (ref. 4) and other conventional uses to cerebral and myocardial ischemia therapy (refs. 5, 6) and tumor radiosensitivity enhancement (refs. 7, 8).

Many in vivo studies have demonstrated that Fluosol 43 (FC-43) and Fluosol-DA 20% (FDA 20%), the most reliable blood substitutes respectively used in animal models and in humans, partially excreted by lung, kidney and skin, are accumulated and stored in reticuloendothelial cells of target organs (liver, spleen, lung) in which they may give rise to toxicity phenomena and morphological changes (refs. 9-11). Nevertheless, PFC particle localization in non-phagocytic cells such as hepatocytes has been reported (refs. 12, 13).

The in vivo and in vitro evidence of PC-43 particle uptake performed by rat hepatocytes we present, and the available data on the solubilization possibility of different chemicals in PFC emulsions, may suggest some considerations about a non-conventional biomedical use of such substances as drug carriers in liver.

MATERIALS AND METHODS

FC-43 (Green Cross Corporation, Osaka, Japan), supplied by Pfrimmer (Erlangen, West Germany), was prepared according to an established procedure (ref. 1).

Rats were injected in tail vein with 1-2 ml of FC-43 (equivalent to a clinical dose) and sacrificed after 24 hours.

BL8 hepatocytes from liver of male Fisher rats (ref. 14) were subcultured every three days in F14 medium with 10% foetal calf serum. 5×10^5 cells, seeded in 60 mm culture Petri dish were incubated to confluency at 37°C in 5% CO_2.

2×10^6 cells in monolayer per dish, exposed to 20% FC-43 emulsion (equivalent to a clinical dose) in culture medium, were incubated at 37°C for 15 minutes, 1 hour and 3 hours. Control cells were incubated for 3 hours.

Rat liver samples and isolated rat hepatocytes, prefixed in 2.5% glutaraldehyde in Millonig buffer pH 7.4 for 30 minutes and postfixed in 1% osmium tetroxide for 1 hour, were embedded in Agar 100 resin. Sections stained with uranyl acetate and lead citrate were examined with a Zeiss EM 10C electron microscope.

RESULTS AND DISCUSSION

In vivo FC-43 particles resulted to accumulate, as previously reported (ref. 10), in Kupffer cells as well as in hepatocytes (Fig. 1). In both the cell types particle localization pattern was identical, i.e. in vacuolizations and in lysosome-like structures often in paranuclear position.

In isolated rat hepatocytes FC-43 particle uptake was seen to occur after 3 hour incubation, particles being localized in lysosome-like structures (Fig. 2).

This finding underlines that hepatocytes "per se", as many eukariotic cells, retain the primitive function of phagocytosis that in vitro occurs soon after the exposition to FC-43. This aspecific PFC uptake could have interesting implications concerning their role in drug transport and release to target liver cells.

The problem of selective delivery of therapeuticals to cellular targets has received widespread attention in the last years. In particular, hepatotropic drug carriers have been investigated, such as lactosaminated human serum albumin (ref. 15), targetable soluble synthetic polymers (ref. 16), biodegradable polyacryl starch microspheres (ref. 17) as well as model colloidal carrier particles (ref. 18). Very attractive magnetic drug carriers (ref. 19), capable to adsorb a great number of drugs and degrade, have been developed since external magnetic guidance of intravascular particles has proved feasible. Moreover, much interest has been directed towards the use of liposomes which have been extensively studied as carriers of a number of drugs with tumoricidal effect on intrahepatic metastases (refs. 20, 21). Liposome differential uptake by hepatocytes and Kupffer cells has been also investigated, but after more than a decade of pre-clinical studies worldwide, the future of the liposomes as drug carriers appears uncertain (ref. 22), also given the toxicity of some of them (refs. 23, 24).

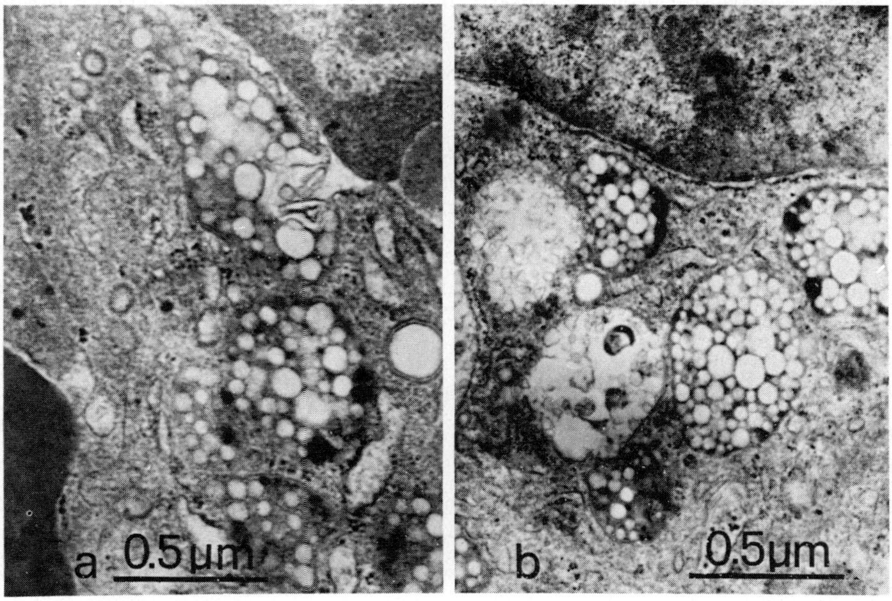

Fig. 1. FC-43 particles (a) in rat Kupffer cell and (b) in rat hepatocyte.

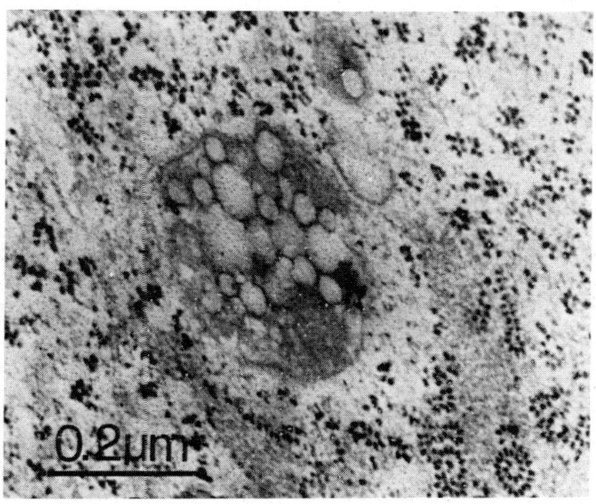

Fig. 2. FC-43 particles in cultured rat hepatocyte.

In this context, PFC particle clearance from the blood stream by means of Kupffer cells as wells as hepatocytes could open new perspectives in the field of selective drug release.

The mechanisms proposed for uptake into liver parenchimal cells of circulating carbon particles, some of which involve damage of hepatocyte membrane or a breakdown of the blood/hepatocyte barrier due to spillage of damaging enzymes from the Kupffer cells (ref. 25), seem not verified in the PFC-hepatocyte interaction. In our in vivo and in vitro experiments no cellular damage was noted at morphological level. Moreover, PFC particle uptake is perfomed by isolated hepatocytes "per se" and is not dependent on environmental influences.

As proposed for liposomes (ref. 26), intrahepatic distribution of PFC to hepatocytes could occur across sinusoid fenestrated endothelial layer whose pore size is about 0.1 um in diameter, that of PFC particle ideal for safe infusion being smaller than 0.1 um.

Conditions as suitable particle diameter, circulation time sufficient to allow particles to interact with target, controlled organ retention and excretion rate and statistically evaluated toxicity for target cells must be satisfied. Although little is known about solubilization of chemotherapeutic agents in PFCs, the exciting perspective of providing sinergic effects of oxygenation and chemicals, for instance in tumor therapy, is a more than sufficient stimulus for further studies.

In this framework new selected PFCs of suitable composition and dimensions (refs. 27, 28) might be also checked as drug carriers and delivery agents, liver parenchimal and Kupffer cells being the specific target.

ACKNOWLEDGEMENT

The authors would like to thank Dr. Orazio Sapora for cell culture facilities and helpful discussion.

REFERENCES

1 D.D. Dixon and D.G. Holland, Fluorocarbons: properties and syntheses, Fed. Proc., 34 (1975) 1444-1448.
2 R. Naito and K. Yokoyama, Perfluorochemical blood substitutes "FC-43" "Fluosol-DA 20% and 35%", The Green Cross Corporation, Vol. 5, Technical Information, Osaka, Japan, 1978, 1981.
3 M. Le Blanc and J.G. Riess, Artificial blood substitutes based on perfluorochemicals, in: R.E. Banks (Ed.), Preparation, properties, and industrial applications of organofluorine compounds, Chichester, Ellis Horwoord limited, 1982, pp. 83-138.
4 K.K. Tremper, A.E. Friedman, E.M. Levine, R. Lapin and D. Camarillo, The preoperative treatment of severely anemic patients with a perfluorochemical oxygen transport fluid, Fluosol-DA, N. Engl. J. Med., 307 (1982) 277-283.
5 J.A. Kusske, M.B. Pritz and K.K. Tremper, Perfluorochemical emulsions for the treatment of cerebral ischemia, Int. Anesthesiol. Clin., 23 (1985) 131-140.

6 M.B. Forman, S. Bingham, H.A. Kopelman et al., Reduction of infarct size with intracoronary perfluorochemical in a canine preparation of reperfusion, Circulation, 71 (1985) 1060-1068.
7 B.A. Teicher and C.M. Rose, Perfluorochemical emulsions can increase tumor radiosensitivity, Science, 223 (1984) 934-936.
8 J.J. Fischer, S. Rockwell and D.F. Martin, Perfluorochemicals and hyperbaric oxygen in radiation therapy, Int. J. Radiation Oncology Biol. Phys., 12 (1986) 95-102.
9 W.I. Rosenblum, M.G. Hadfield, A.J. Martinez and P. Schatzki, Alterations of liver and spleen following intravenous infusion of fluorocarbon emulsions, Arch. Pathol. Lab. Med., 100 (1976) 213-217.
10 T. Mitsuno, Y. Tabuchi, H. Ohyanagi and T. Sugiyama, Further studies on intake and retention of PFC substance of Fluosol-DA in RES in humans, Progr. Clin. Biol. Res., 122 (1983) 257-263.
11 L. Nanney, L.M. Fink and R. Virmani, Perfluorochemicals. Morphologic changes in infused liver, spleen, lung and kidney of rabbits, Arch. Pathol. Lab. Med. 108 (1984) 631-637.
12 M.L. Miller, R.E. Moore and L.C. Clark, Morphology and morphometry of the liver after infusion of perfluorochemical emulsions: an assessment of 19 selected compounds, in: Proceedings of the IVth International Symposium on perfluorochemical blood substitutes, Excerpta Medica, Amsterdam, 1978, pp. 81-97.
13 S. Caiazza, C. Fanizza and M. Ferrari, Fluosol 43 particle localization pattern in target organs of rats, Virchows Arch. A., 404 (1984) 127-137.
14 P.O. Seglen, Preparation of rat liver cells, Exp. Cell. Res., 74 (1972) 450-454.
15 L. Fiume, C. Busi and A. Mattioli, Lactosaminated human serum albumin as hepatotropic drug carrier. Rate of uptake by mouse liver, FEBS Letters, 146(1) (1982) 42-46.
16 R. Duncan, J. Kopecek, P. Rejmanova and J.B. Lloyd, Targeting of N-(2-Hydroxypropyl)methacrylamide copolymers to liver by incorporation of galactose residues, Biochem. Biophys. Acta, 755 (1983) 518-521.
17 P. Artursson, P. Edman, T. Laakso and I. Sjöholm, Characterization of polyacryl starch microparticles as carriers for proteins and drugs, J. Pharm. Sci., 73(11) (1984) 1507-1513.
18 L. Illum, N.W. Thomas and S.S. Davis, Effect of a selected suppression of the reticuloendothelial system on the distribution of model carrier particles, J. Pharm. Sci., 75(1) (1986) 16-22.
19 A. Ibrahim, P. Couvreur, M. Roland and P. Speiser, New magnetic drug carrier, J. Pharm. Pharmacol., 35 (1983) 59-61.
20 A. Gabizon, D. Goren, Z. Fuks, Y. Barenholz, A. Dagan and A. Meshorer, Enhancement of adriamycin delivery to liver metastatic cells with increased tumoricidal effect using liposomes as drug carriers, Cancer Res., 43 (1983) 4730-4735.
21 J.N. Weinstein and L.D. Leserman, Liposomes as drug carriers in cancer chemotherapy, Pharmac. Ther., 24 (1984) 207-233.
22 D.A. Tirrel, L.G. Donaruma and A.B. Turek, Macromolecules as drugs and carriers for biologically active materials, Ann. N.Y. Acad. Sci., 446 (1985).
23 E.A.H. Weereratne, G. Gregoriadis and J. Crow, Toxicity of sphingomyelin-containing liposomes after chronic injection into mice, Br. J. Exp. Path., 64 (1983) 670-676.
24 T.M. Allen and E.A. Smuckler, Liver pathology accompanying chronic liposome administration in mouse, Res. Comm. Chem. Pathol. Pharmacol., 50(2) (1985) 281-290.
25 J.W.B. Bradfield, H.R. Payne and D. Small, in: D.L. Knook and E. Wisse (Eds.), Sinusoidal liver cells, Elsevier Biomedical Press, Amsterdam, 1982, pp. 453-454.
26 G.L. Scherphof, J. Dijkstra, H.H. Spanjer, J.T.P. Derksen and F.H. Roedink, Uptake and intracellular processing of targeted and nontargeted liposomes by rat Kupffer cells <u>in vivo</u> and <u>in vitro</u>, Ann. N.Y. Acad. Sci., 446 (1985) 368-384.

27 J.G. Riess, Reassessment of criteria for the selection of perfluorochemicals for second-generation blood substitutes: analysis of structure/property relationships, Artificial Organs, 8(1) (1984) 44-56.
28 J.G. Riess, Principes du transport des gaz respiratoires par les émulsions de fluorocarbures. Avantages et limites. Indication potentielles, Communication au Colloque sur "Le globule rouge et autres transporteurs d'oxygène", Lyon, 1986.

Biomaterials and Clinical Applications, 661
edited by A. Pizzoferrato, P.G. Marchetti, A. Ravaglioli and A.J.C. Lee
Elsevier Science Publishers B.V., Amsterdam, 1987 — Printed in The Netherlands

MICROBIAL ADHESION AND MOLECULAR MECHANISMS IN BIOMATERIAL AND COMPROMISED TISSUE CENTERED INFECTION

A.G. GRISTINA, M.D., E. BARTH, M.D. and L.X. WEBB, M.D.
Section of Orthopedic Surgery, Bowman Gray School of Medicine, 300 South Hawthorne Road, Winston-Salem, North Carolina, U.S.A. 27103

SUMMARY

Our studies indicate that infections centered on biomaterials and compromised tissues are directed by characteristics of the substratum and by proteinaceous adhesins and extracapsular polysaccharides of bacterial origin. Bacterial slimes (polysaccharides) function in adhesion and aggregation and also blunt host defense mechanisms and antibiotics. Thus infections centered on nonliving or nonbiologic substrata persist until the "foreign body" is removed. Biomaterial and compromised tissue surfaces are not passive or inert vis a vis bacterial or tissue cells. Molecular phenomena at biomaterial surfaces direct initial adhesion and accelerate metabolic processes, resulting in microbial proliferation. Polymer substrata tend to favor colonization by Staphylococcus epidermidis and Pseudomonas aeruginosa, while metals and tissue are frequently colonized by Staphylococcus aureus. Such surfaces are more receptive to microbes when they have not been colonized and integrated by tissue cells. A suggested defensive strategy may be the precolonization of substrata by tissue cells. Antibiotics combined with the substratum should be effective in blocking infection as they are ideally located to interdict the onset of pathogenesis.

INTRODUCTION

The purpose of this communication is to discuss the relevant mechanisms in adhesion, biofilm-mediated, biomaterial-centered infections and osteomyelitis.

Adhesion to and colonization of substrata is a fundamental characteristic of the behavior of most bacteria and is the actual state of the majority of microbes in natural ecologies and in health or disease in man. Proliferating microcolonies of mixed organisms on surfaces in natural habitats form slippery films called "slime layers." When mixed with environmental debris, these thickened layers of slime or biofilm may form a biomass and are a ubiquitous feature of life-supporting environments (refs. 1-4).

ADHESION AND AGGREGATION IN DISEASE

The pathogenesis of biomaterial focused infections and osteomyelitis can best be understood in terms of microbial adhesion based on findings recently made in studies of bacterial ecosystems in nature and of bacterial behavior in certain tissue-centered diseases; as well as infections centered about biomaterials and foreign bodies. Insights derived from the mechanisms of prokaryocyte (bacterial) adhesion to surfaces are also relevant to tissue (eukaryotic) integration with biomaterial surfaces, to organ-specific metastases of neoplastic cells and to the ontogeny and the ultimate destiny of eukaryotic cells (ref. 3-10).

BACTERIAL ADHESION IN BIOMATERIAL CENTERED INFECTIONS

In 1963, studies by one of the authors suggested that internal fixation devices and dead bone provided a structural framework along which microorganisms (*S. epidermidis* and *S. aureus*) could colonize and propagate and that all foreign bodies or biomaterials tested caused a similar response (refs. 11,12). Subsequently, in 1972, Bayston and Penny described the excessive production of a mucoid substance as a possible factor in the colonization of Holter shunts by *S. epidermidis* (ref. 13). In 1976, surface effects and/or the sequestration of ions or metabolites from biometals and biomaterials were suggested as factors in the behavior of bacteria which colonized foreign bodies and biomaterials. It was noted that some reactive metals inhibited bacterial growth, but that growth was abundant adjacent to "inert" materials such as stainless steel, Vitallium, nylon and methylmethacrylate (ref. 14). Studies in 1979 first demonstrated bacterial adhesion and biofilm-mediated polymicrobial infections in tissue and internal fixation devices from infected surgical wounds (ref. 15-19). Reports in 1981 and 1982 indicated slime or biofilm-mediated colonization on plastic catheters by *S. epidermidis* (ref. 21, 22).

When nonliving substrata (biomaterial devices and some tissue transplants) are introduced into mammalian hosts, they may become favored sites for adhesive colonization, especially in the immunocompromised patient. For example, total joints or internal fixation devices, intravenous catheters, heart valves, vascular grafts, allografts, and almost all permanently or temporarily inserted transcutaneous or deep biomaterials may develop biofilm-mediated infections which are resistant to antibiotics and host defenses and tend to persist until the biomaterial or foreign body is removed (fig. 1)

ADHESION IN OSTEOMYELITIS

Recent EM studies of acute and chronic osteomyelitic bone specimens indicate that infecting organisms also use bone as a substratum for adhesive biofilm-mediated colonization (ref. 22). In addition to bone primarily involved in osteomyelitis, bone adjacent to biomaterial implants may be secondarily involved by contiguous spread from the infected joint space or colonized biomaterial (ref. 23,24).

Traumatized, ischemic, or devitalized bone secondary to fractures, bone grafts or allografts, as well as adjacent damaged tissues, may also act as infection-inducing foreign bodies.

MOLECULAR MECHANISMS IN ADHESION

Initial attachment (reversible nonspecific adhesion) is dependent on the general physical characteristics of the bacterium, the fluid interface and the substratum. Within effective range of these phenomena, initial attachment of bacteria may be partially predictable based on particle size, charge, and the

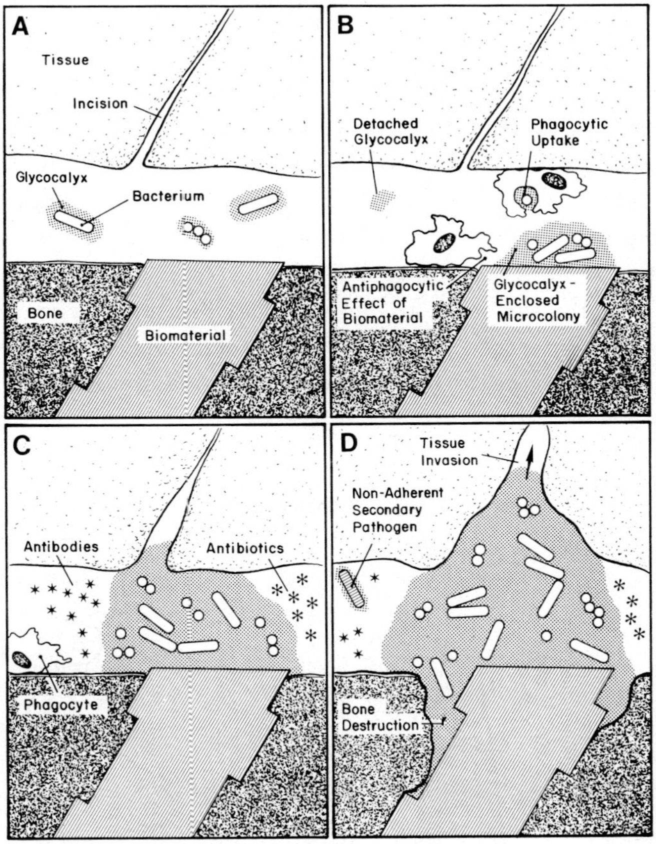

Fig. 1 Diagrammatic evolution of a cryptic infection associated with a prosthetic biomaterial. Initially, bacteria are introduced into the wound (A); they express their natural tendency to adhere (B) to an inert surface on which they are protected by the antiphagocytic effect of the biomaterial and on which they form as microcolonies within a biofilm that protects them from phagocytic uptake and from nonimmune antibacterial serum factors. When the bacterial microcolony has burgeoned to a greater size (C), the ion-exchange function of its glycocalyx affords a measure of protection from antibiotics and appears to protect the bacteria from both bactericidal and opsonizing antibodies. In the later stages of this infection (D), the pathogens may cause destruction of bone and other tissue changes, and the colonies may shed secondary pathogens that, being for some reason less adhesive, are not necessarily representative in numbers or types or pathogenicity of the adhesive colonies and may therefore confuse the diagnostic picture by dominating aspirates and other routine microbiologic samples. Reprinted with permission from Bacterial adherence and the glycocalyx and their role in musculoskeletal infection by A.G. Gristina and J.W. Costerton. Ortho. Clin. of N.A. 15 (1984) 517-535. Copyright 1984 by W.B. Saunders Company, Philadelphia, Pennsylvania.

relative hydrophobicity between the bacterium fluid phase and surface. Specific irreversible adhesion, which occurs after initial attachment, suggests time-dependent biosynthetic chemical processes which in part depend on specific protein adhesin-receptor interaction, as well as carbohydrate polymer synthesis. Exopolysaccharides are vital for subsequent cell-to-cell aggregation and the sequestration of nutrients from the substratum and adjacent milieu (refs. 1,8,22, 25-28).

The bacterial surface charge is negative, as are most substrata surfaces. However, isoelectric points of materials at the surface-liquid interface can vary with pH and tissue damage caused by surgery, trauma, and infection (refs. 29-31). Corrosion also alters pH and charge (ref. 31). The common charges of the microbe and substratum tend to repel each other, however van der Waals forces at the secondary minimum (approximately 10 nm) effectively position a particle or bacterium near the surface. At closer ranges repulsion is maximal until the primary minimum is entered (2-3 nm) where attraction occurs (ref. 8). New studies indicate that hydrophobic forces are exerted at distances as great as 15 nm,

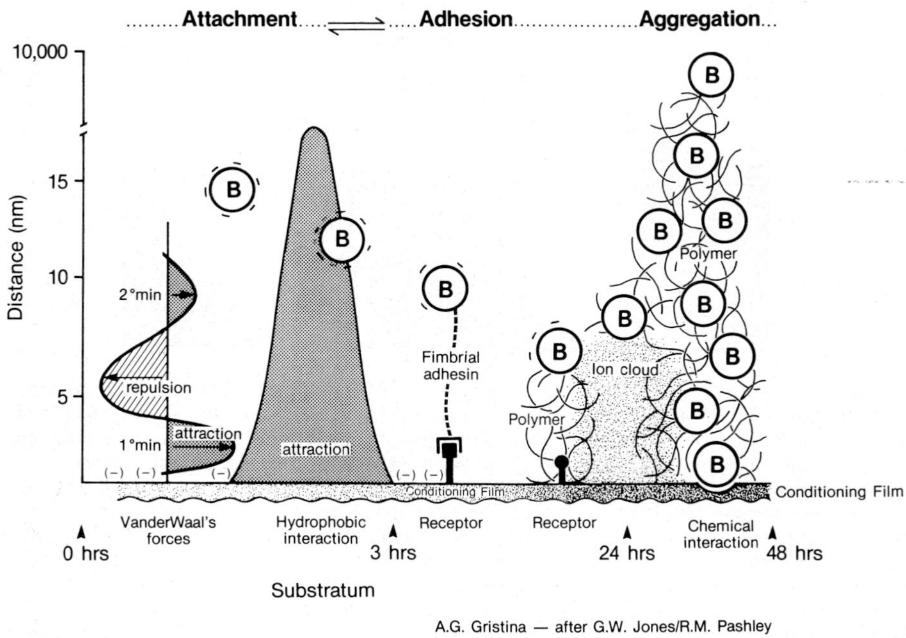

Figure 2. Molecular sequence in bacterial (B) attachment, adhesion and aggregation to substrata. Reprinted with permission from Biomaterial specificity, molecular mechanisms and clinical relevance of S. epidermidis and S. aureus infections in surgery by A.G. Gristina, et al. In: Proceedings of the Symposium on the Pathogenicity and Clinical Significance of Coagulase-negative Staphylococci, Heppenheim, Germany, in press. Copyright 1986 by Gustav Fischer Verlag, Stuttgart.

and at 8-10 nm are 10 to 100 times as great as van der Waals forces (ref. 26). Some degree of hydrophobicity exists for many bacteria and most surfaces (ref. 8, 32). Attractive hydrophobic interactions tend to overcome repulsion and position bacteria at the primary minimum (Fig. 2). When a bacteria is within 1 nm, or in surface contact, as demonstrated in the TEM preparation of S. epidermidis on the surface of a soft contact lens, it is conceivable that chemical bonding occurs (Fig. 3).

Subsequent to, or concomitant with, initial attachment, specific fimbrial adhesins and substratum receptors may interact if they are present in the particular biological system, as in bacteria-to-tissue cell pathogenesis (ref. 8).

THE BACTERIA

Generally, the bacteria involved are accepted pathogens such as S. aureus, P. aeruginosa or Escherichia coli. However, in immunocompromised patients, in association with particular substrata or under optimised conditions, selection of normally autochthonous bacteria or nonpathogens may occur.

The two most studied bacteria with regard to biomaterial-centered infections and osteomyelitis are S. epidermidis and S. aureus, respectively.

S. epidermidis, usually thought of as a nonpathogenic commensal human skin saprophyte, has emerged as a serious pathogen in biomaterial-related infections. Masur et al, and others have listed S. epidermidis as a leading cause of infection in prosthesis, shunts, and implants. Orthopedic reviews have also pointed

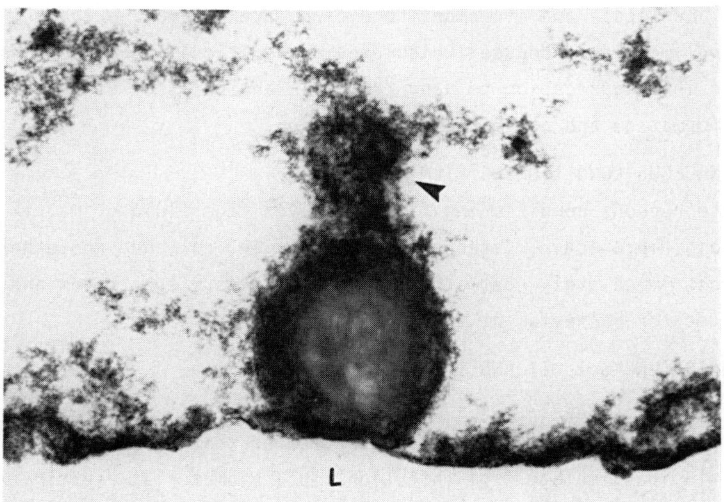

Figure 3. TEM of S. epidermidis (SE-360)(ruthenium-red stain) on the surface of soft contact lens (L). Note direct surface contact with a minimum of polysaccharide at contact interface and the aggregation of polysaccharides (arrow). Reprinted with permission from Biomaterial specificity, molecular mechanisms and clinical relevance of S. epidermidis and S. aureus infections in surgery by A.G. Gristina et al. In: Proceedings of the Symposium on Pathogenicity and Clinical Significance of Coagulase-negative Staphylococci. Heppenheim, Germany. Copyright 1986 by Gustav Fischer Verlag, Stuttgart.

out the pathogenic potential of S. epidermidis. Also disturbing is the fact that S. epidermidis is not only a significant biomaterial-associated pathogen, but is emerging as a leading organism in nosocomial infections, especially those in immunosuppressed patients (refs. 33-40).

S. aureus is the most common pathogen isolated in chronic osteomyelitis. Studies of adult osteomyelitis by Cierny have shown an incidence of polymicrobial infection approaching 75 percent (ref. 41). The most common pathogens were S. aureus, Pseudomonas species, Enterococcus species, S. epidermidis, and Streptococcus, Bacillus and Proteus species. Acute osteomyelitis also commonly involves S. aureus.

EXTRACELLULAR POLYMERS - THE "SLIME" AND BIOFILM

The exopolysaccharide "slime" produced by bacteria is probably one of the pivotal factors responsible for the behavior of biomaterial-centered infections. The complex exopolysaccharide acts an an ion exchange resin which enhances nutrition, moderates susceptibility to phagocytosis and response to antibodies, and functions in later stages of surface adhesion, aggregation and polymicrobial interaction. In general, exopolysaccharides are composed of neutral monosaccharides such as D-glucose, D-galactose, L-fucose, and L-rhamnose. They also contain amino sugars and sialic acid.

THE BIOFILM

Shortly after attachment and adhesion (3-4 hours or sooner), as growth and propagation accelerate and if colony conditions are optimal, extracellular polysaccharide polymers are produced which provide additional adhesion to surfaces and function in coaggregation to daughter cells and cells of other species in consortial formation and polymicrobial infection.

GLYCOPROTEINACEOUS CONDITIONING FILM

Glycoproteinaceous conditioning films, derived from fluid or matrix phases (which contain fibronectin, osteonectin, fibrinogen, collagen and other proteins), almost immediately coat a biomaterial or tissue substratum and provide receptor sites for bacterial or tissue adhesion.

RECENT STUDIES (PARTS I, II AND III)

I. Clinical Review (S. epidermidis and S. aureus)

Our review of the clinical literature indicates that S. epidermidis appears to be the principal isolate from infections in a biomaterials setting which contains polymers, and that S. aureus remains the predominant pathogen associated with metals, compromised tissues, surgical wounds, and osteomyelitis (refs. 35, 36, 42-48).

II. Direct Studies and Identification of Pathogenic Bacteria In Situ on Biomaterials

Clinical retrieval: Methods have been abridged. (For details, see ref. 45)

From 1979 through 1986, 171 specimens were retrieved, aerobically and anaerobically cultured. Selected specimens were examined by transmission and scanning electron microscopy.

Culturing techniques

For aerobic cultures. Biomaterials, bone, and tissue specimens were placed in 10 ml of phosphate buffered saline (PBS), pH 7.2. Bone and tissue specimens were homogenized in a tissue grinder. All specimens were sonicated for 5.5 minutes at 37°C. After "vortexing" for 30 seconds, the bacterial suspensions were serially diluted with PBS to a concentration of 10^{-6} and cultured on Schaedler's blood agar and chocolate blood agar plates at 37°C for 3 days (refs. 23,24,45).

For anaerobic cultures. Specimens were prepared similarly but in a CO_2-N_2 atmosphere. Dehority's broth was used instead of PBS. Dilutions were cultured on anaerobic blood agar plates for 10 days at 37°C within an anaerobic jar. (refs. 23,24,45).

Scanning Electron Microscopy (SEM)

Specimens were fixed in glutaraldehyde, dehydrated in ethanol, and critically point dried according to standard procedures. They were sputtered with an 100 A thick gold-palladium layer and examined in a Philips 501 scanning electron microscope (refs. 23,24,45).

Transmission Electron Microscopy (TEM)

Specimens were fixed in glutaraldehyde, dehydrated in ethanol, stained with ruthenium-red followed by OsO_4, dehydrated in propylene oxide, embedded in Epon resin and sectioned. The sections were then stained with uranyl acetate and lead citrate, stabilized with a 50 A thick carbon layer and examined in a Philips EM-400 scope (refs. 23,24,45).

Results: Direct Studies, Identification, Morphology, SEM and TEM

The review of our data at the Bowman Gray School of Medicine in the retrieval of 171 infected biomaterial specimens indicates that *S. epidermidis* predominates as an adhesive colonizer of polymers. *S. aureus* is the principal pathogen for metallic and compromised tissue substrata associated with surgical wounds, trauma and osteomyelitis.

III. Laboratory Studies

A. In vitro study (Methods). Methods have been abridged. (For details, see ref. 45).

Comparative colonization of the *S. epidermidis* [SE-360 strain (Yoshida)] and a clinical *S. aureus* strain (SA-WF1, retrieved from a biomaterial infection) was performed on standard-sized discs of Vitallium, 35 Multiphase Nickel Cobalt Chromium alloy, 316 stainless steel and polymethylmethacrylate (PMMA).

Results: Peak colonization time for all bacteria versus biomaterials combinations was 24 hours. S. epidermidis showed significantly greater preference for polymers than metals while the opposite was the case for S. aureus. The absolute maximum CFU/disc was found for S. epidermidis on PMMA (1.6×10^8 at 24 hours).

B. Colonization of hydrophilic contact lenses: S. epidermidis (SE-360) and P. aeruginosa (PA-WF1).(For methods, see ref. 45).

SEM and TEM of the bacteria-to-polymer interface revealed that the number of colonizing bacteria per lens of each strain did not differ significantly.

C. Energy Dispersive X-ray Analysis (EDXA): S. aureus (SA-WF1) and S. epidermidis (SE-360) on Polymer Surface. (For methods, see ref. 45).

Carbon, aluminum, chlorine, silicon, phosphorous, calcium and iron were found in the polysaccharide portion of the 8 microns thick bacterial film on the lens (fig. 4). S. epidermidis was more often proximate to the surface of the lens than P. aeruginosa. Both produced abundant polysaccharides which attached the

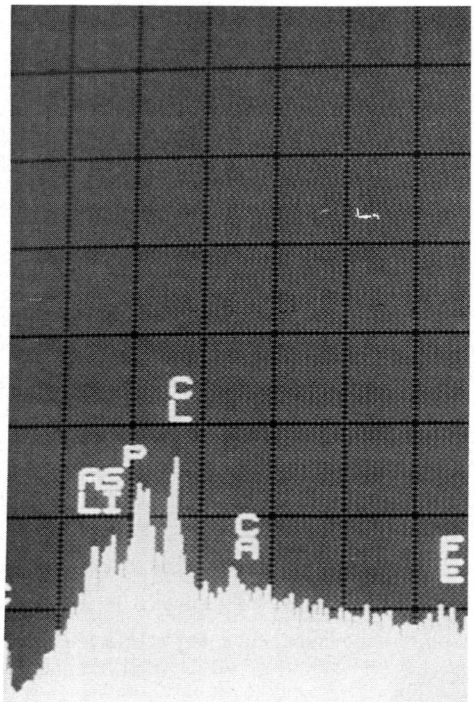

Figure 4. A representative scan of Energy Dispersive X-ray microanalysis of bacterial biofilm (SE-360) on a soft contact lens. Carbon (C), aluminum (AL), silicon (SI), chlorine (CL), calcium (CA) and iron (FE) were found and analyzed in sequential areas in 2 micron steps from the surface. Each area scanned measured 2 x 2 microns^2. Reprinted with permission from Biomaterial specificity, molecular mechanisms and clinical relevance of S. epidermidis and S. aureus infections in surgery by A.G. Gristina, et al. In: Proceedings of the Symposium on Pathogenicity and Clinical Significance of Coagulase-negative Staphylococci. Heppenheim, Germany. Copyright 1986 by Gustav Fischer Verlag, Stuttgart.

bacteria to the lens surface and to each other (fig. 3).

DISCUSSION

The Bacteria

S. aureus is frequently the major pathogen in biometal, bone and joint, and soft tissue infections, but is associated to a lesser degree with polymer-sited infections. *S. aureus* may also participate in concert with *S. epidermidis* and gram-negative organisms.

S. epidermidis by clinical studies shows a predilection to cause infection in association with biomaterial surfaces, especially when the biomaterial is a polymer or when a polymer is a component of a complex device. Our *in vitro* studies also verify preferential adhesion to the surfaces of polymers. Similar findings have recently been presented by other investigators (ref. 49). *S. epidermidis* is also a factor in polymicrobial infections associated with other substrata, such as metals, compromised bone and tissues; but in those cases it frequently augments or is augmented by other organisms.

SUBSTRATA AND SUBSTRATUM DISRUPTION

Substratum disruption (before or after bacterial colonization) caused by trauma, wear, corrosion, toxins, viral effects or bacterial mechanisms, establishes environmental conditions which natural selection has prepared microorganisms to opportunize (fig. 5). Polymer, metal, and compromised tissue fractions may be utilized directly within the bacterial envelope. For example, metal ions such as iron, magnesium, chromium, cobalt and others are available in trace or greater amounts, especially after corrosion. This process occurs to some degree even with more stable alloys such as stainless steel when they are scoured by wear, work or implantation.

On biomaterial surfaces within biofilm polysaccharide microzones, ions are shielded from host protein binding complexes (lactoferrin/transferrin) which lower ion concentration levels below those usually required by pathogenic bacteria. Iron is linked to virulence and inhibits macrophage function. Mg^{++} and Ca^{++} and other trace ions stabilize (via acidic groups) the complex polysaccharide polymers in gel formation, thereby enhancing both cell-to-cell and cell-to-surface adhesion and possibly increasing resistance to external antagonists. Some synthetic polymers, such as polyesterurethane and methylmethacrylate, contain esters which may be metabolized by *S. epidermidis*. Traces of aluminum and other substances may also be present from polymer manufacturing processes or contamination (fig. 4) (refs. 45, 50-54).

The presence of polymers in a prosthesis or the use of polymers alone appears to allow preferential colonization by *S. epidermidis*. Polymers in certain locations (the eye) appear to select for *P. aeruginosa* and *S. epidermidis*. When appropriate substrata are presented, the substratum in effect selects the organisms and if conditions are optimal, an infection results (ref. 45).

GENESIS AND PATHOGENESIS

Bacteria in natural habitats, certain tissue diseases, biomaterial-centered infections and osteomyelitis have a common survival mode based on adhesive colonization of substrata. Nutrition and resistance to host defenses and antibiotics are optimized by the biofilm. Within this biofilm, microzones of enhanced conditions may develop and the infection stabilizes or even spreads and characteristically, cannot be adequately treated until the substratum is removed. Thus, bacterial adhesion and its denominators direct the pathogenesis of osteomyelitis and bacterial infections.

DEFENSIVE AND THERAPEUTIC STRATEGIES

A novel defensive strategy may be to make biomaterial surfaces proadhesive to encourage rapid colonization by healthy tissue cells (endothelium, bone, soft tissue) which tend to resist colonization and infection and allow defense mechanisms to operate. It would be ideal if tissue colonization or integration was first in the "race for the surface" against microbes (refs. 45,55,56). Antiad-

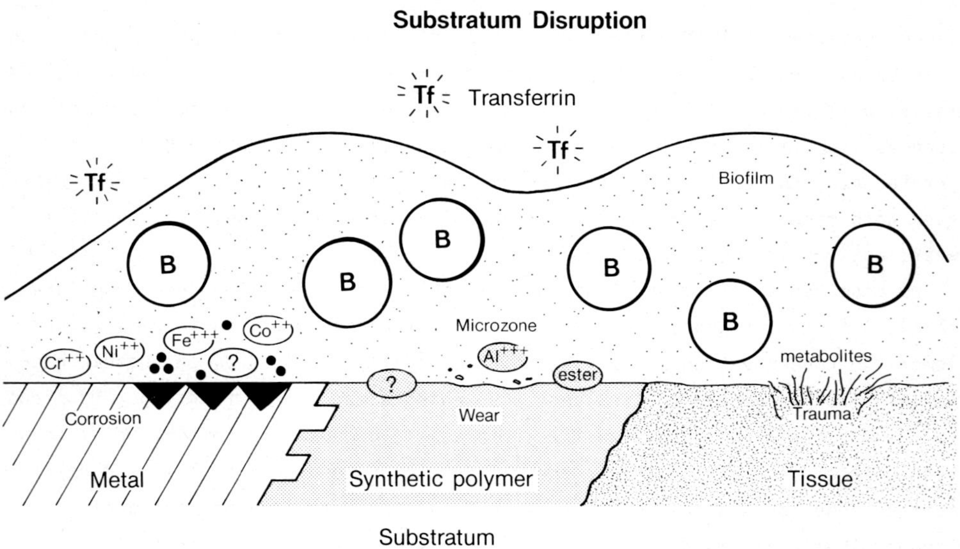

Figure 5. Surface disruption by wear, corrosion, trauma or bacterial mechanisms frees metabolites or ions which are then available to bacteria (B) within a biofilm microenvironment. Within the polysaccharide biofilm, metal ions required by pathogenic bacteria may be shielded from host protein binding complexes (tf). Reprinted with permission from Biomaterial specificity, molecular mechanisms and clinical relevance of S. epidermidis and S. aureus infections in surgery by A.G. Gristina et al. In: Proceedings of the Symposium on Pathogenicity and the Clinical Significance of Coagulase-negative Staphylococci. Heppenheim, Germany. Copyright 1986 by Gustav Fischer Verlag, Stuttgart.

hesive surfaces, though seemingly a clever approach and initially effective, are neutralized by conditioning films and, in effect, have already been defeated by an infinite number of experiments in nature. Antibiotics which interfere with bacterial polymer synthesis and adhesive mechanisms, which penetrate biofilm, or are delivered by the substratum should be effective. Blocking or saturating analogs are an appropriately sophisticated approach which should be studied and may provide an effective countermeasure (refs. 22,45,44,45).

In summary, microbes attach to surfaces as a natural life and survival mode. Foreign bodies or "inert biomaterials" provide passive or enhancing substrata for adhesion and both the biofilm and qualities of the substratum may frustrate countermeasures. The specific composition and surface qualities of various substrata may direct bacterial specificity. In effect, the substratum selects the bacteria. Microbial adhesion is fundamental in nature and in the pathogenesis of biomaterial and compromised tissue infection.

REFERENCES

1. M. Fletcher, Effect of solid surfaces on the activity of attached bacteria, in: D.C. Savage, M. Fletcher (Eds.), Bacterial Adhesion, Plenum Press, New York, 1985, pp. 339-362.
2. H.C. Jones, I.L. Roth, W.M. Sanders III, Electron microscopic study of a slime layer, J. Bacteriol., 99 (1981) 229-324.
3. J.W. Costerton, R.T. Irvin, K-J. Cheng, The bacterial glycocalyx in nature and disease, Ann. Rev. Microbiol., 35 (1981) 229-324.
4. J.W. Costerton, T.J. Marrie, K-J. Cheng, Phenomenom of bacterial adhesion, in: D.C. Savage, M. Fletcher (Eds.), Bacterial Adhesion, Plenum Press, New York, 1985, pp. 3-43.
5. J.D. Lopes, M. dos Reis, R.R. Brentani, Presence of laminin receptors in Staphylococcus aureus, Science, 229 (1985) 275-277.
6. I. Ofek, E.H. Beachey, General concepts and principles of adherence in animals and man, in: E.H. Beachey (Ed.), Bacterial Adherence, Chapman and Hall, New York, 1980, pp. 1-31.
7. G.D. Christensen, W.A. Simpson, E.H. Beachey, Adhesion of bacteria to animal tissues: complex mechanisms, in: D.C. Savage, M. Fletcher (Eds.), Bacterial Adhesion, Plenum Press, New York, 1985, pp. 279-305.
8. G.W. Jones, R.E. Isaacson, Proteinaceous bacterial adhesins and their receptors, Crit. Rev. Microbiol., 10 (1984) 229-260.
9. G.L. Nicolson, J.L. Winkelhake, Organ specificity of blood-born tumour metastasis determined by cell adhesion, Nature, 255 (1975) 230-232.
10. M.W. Kieran, B.M. Longnecker, Organ specific metastasis with specific reference to avian systems, Cancer Metastasis Rev., 2 (1983) 165-182.
11. A.G. Gristina, G.D. Rovere, An in vitro study of the effects of metals used in internal fixation on bacterial growth and dissemination, J. Bone Jt. Surg., 45 (1963) 1104.
12. A.G. Gristina, G.D. Rovere, An in vitro study of the effects of metals used in internal fixation on bacterial growth and dissemination, in: Book of Abstracts, 9th Annual Meeting of the Orthopaedic Research Society, Miami Beach, Florida, January 19-20, 1963, pp. 3-4.
13. R. Bayston, S.R. Penny, Excessive mucin production of mucoid substances in Staphylococcus SIIA: a possible factor in colonisation of Holter shunts, Dev. Med. Child Neurol., 14 (1972) 25-28.
14. A.G. Gristina, G.D. Rovere, H. Shoji, J.F. NIcastro, An in vitro study of bacterial response to inert and reactive metals and to methylmethacrylate, J. Biomed. Mater. Res., 10 (1976) 273-281.
15. A.G. Gristina, J. Kolkin, E. Leake, J.W. Costerton, M.J. Wright, Bacteria and their relationship to biomaterials, Book of Abstracts, First World Biomaterials Congress, Vienna, Austria, April 8-12, 1980, European Society for Biomaterials, Vienna, Austria, Kleinoffsetdruck Hoffmann, 1980, pp. 2.39.
16. A.G. Gristina, J.W. Costerton, E. Leake, J. Kolkin. Bacterial colonization of biomaterials: clinical and laboratory studies, Orthop. Trans., 4 (1980) 355.
17. A.G. Gristina, J.W. Costerton, E. Leake, J. Kolkin, M.J. Wright, Bacteria and their relationship to biomaterials, Orthop. Trans., 5 (1981) 332.
18. A.G. Gristina, J. Kolkin, Current concepts review: total joint replacement and sepsis, J. Bone Jt. Surg., 63A (1983) 128-134.
19. A.G. Gristina, J.W. Costerton. Bacterial adherence to biomaterials: the clinical significance of its role in sepsis, in: J.M. Anderson (Ed.), Biomaterials '84 Transactions: Second World Congress on Biomaterials, Vol. VII, Washington, D.C., April 27-May 1, 1984, Society for Biomaterials, 1984, pp. 175.
20. G.D. Christensen, W.A. Simpson, A.L. Bisno, E.H. Beachey, Adherence of slime-producing strains of Staphylococcus epidermidis to smooth surfaces, Infec. Immun., 37 (1982) 318-326.

21. G. Peters, R. Locci, G. Pulverer, Microbial colonization of prosthetic devices. II. Scanning electron microscopy of naturally infected intravenous catheters, Zentralbl. Bakter. Mikrobiol. Hyg. B., 173 (1981) 293-299.
22. A.G. Gristina, M. Oga, L.X. Webb, C.D. Hobgood, Adherent bacterial colonization in the pathogenesis of osteomyelitis, Science, 228 (1985) 990-993.
23. A.G. Gristina, J.W. Costerton, Bacterial adherence to biomaterials and tissue: the significance of its role in sepsis, J. Bone Jt. Surg., 67A (1985) 264-273.
24. A.G. Gristina, J.W. Costerton, Bacterial adherence and the glycocalyx and their role in musculoskeletal infection, Orthop. Clin. N.A., 15 (1984) 517-535.
25. E.H. Beachey, Bacterial adherence: adhesion-receptor interactions mediating the attachment of bacteria to mucosal surfaces, J. Infec. Dis., 143 (1981) 325-345.
26. R.M. Pashley, P.M. McGuiggan, B.W. Ninham, Attraction forces between uncharged hydrophobic surfaces: direct measurements in aqueous solution, Science, 229 (1985) 1088-1089.
27. J.H. Pringle, M. Fletcher, E.C. Ellwood, Selection of attachment mutants during the continuous culture of Pseudomonas fluorescens and their relationship between attachment ability and surface composition, J. Gen. Microbio., 129 (1983) 2557-2569.
28. M. Fletcher, Adherence of marine micro-organisms to smooth surfaces, in: E.H. Beachey (Ed.), Bacterial Adherence, Chapman and Hall, New York, 1980, pp. 345-374.
29. P.R. Rutter, F.B. Dazzo, E. Freter, D. Gingell, G.W. Jones, S. Kjelleberg, K.C. Marshall, H. Mrozek, E. Rades-Rohkohl, E.D. Robb, M. Silverman, S. Tylewska, Mechanisms of adhesion, in: K.C. Marshall (Ed.), Microbial Adhesion and Aggregation, Springer Verlag, Berlin, 1984, pp. 5-19.
30. J. Lyklema, Interfacial electrochemistry of surfaces with biomedical relevance, in: J.D. Andrade (Ed.), Surface and Interfacial Aspects of Biomedical Polymers, Vol. 1, Surface Chemistry and Physics, Plenum Press, New York, 1985, pp. 293-334.
31. D.C. Mears, Materials and Orthopedic Surgery, Williams and Wilkins, Baltimore, 1979.
32. A.H. Hogt, J. Dankaert, C.E. Hulstaert, J. Feijen, Cell surface characteristic of coagulase-negative staphylococci and their adherence to fluorinated poly(ethylenepropylene), Infec. Immun., 51 (1986) 294-301.
33. D.F. Bandyk, G.A. Berni, B.L. Thiele, J.B. Towne, Aortofemoral graft infections due to Staphylococcus epidermidis, Arch. Surg., 119 (1984) 102-107.
34. H. Masur, W.D. Johnson, Prosthetic valve endocarditis, J. Thorac. Cardiovasc. Surg., 80 (1980) 31-37.
35. S.H. Dougherty, R.L. Simmons, Infections in the bionic man: the pathobiology of infections in prosthetic devices, part 2, Curr. Probl. Surg., 19 (1982) 269-318.
36. F.D. Lowy, S.M. Hammer, Staphylococcus epidermidis infections, Ann. Intern. Med., 99 (1983) 834-839.
37. D.J. Winston, D.V. Dudnick, M. Chapin, G.H. Winston, R.P. Gale, W.J. Martin, Coagulase-negative Staphylococcal bacteremia in patients receiving immunosuppressive therapy, Arch. Intern. Med., 143 (1983) 32-36.
38. S. Pegram, H. Muss, C. McCall, R. Cooper, D. White, P. Richards, D. Jackson, J. Stuart, C. Spurr, J. Hopkins, R. Capizzi, A comparative study of moxalactam (M) vs. ticarcillin and tobramycin (TT) in febrile neutropenic cancer patients, Proc. of A.S.C.O., 3 (1984) 100.
39. R.H. Fitzgerald, The infected total hip arthroplasty, in: R.B. Welch (Ed.), Proc. 12th Open Scientific Meeting of the Hip Society, 1984, pp. 347-358.
40. K. Henderson, Infections associated with prostheses, shunts, and implants, in: T.T. Yoshikawa, A.W. Chow, L.B. Guze (Eds.), Infectious Diseases: Diagnosis and Management, Wiley Medical, New York, 1980, pp. 274-385.
41. G. Cierny, J. Mader, Adjunction local antibiotics in the management of contaminated orthopedic wounds, American Association of Orthopedic Surgeons 53rd Annual Meeting, New Orleans, Louisiana, February 20-25, 1986.

42. B. Sugarman, E.J. Young (Eds.), Infections Associated With Prosthetic Devices, Boca Raton, Florida, CRC Press, 1984.
43. D.D. Schmitt, D.F. Bandyk, A.J. Pequet, M.A. Malanzoni, J.B. Towne, Mucin production by Staphylococcus epidermidis: a virulence factor promoting adherence to vascular grafts, Arch. Surg., 121 (1986) 89-95.
44. A.G. Towers, Wound infection in an orthopedic hospital, Lancet, (1965) 369-371.
45. A.G. Gristina, C.D. Hobgood, E. Barth, Biomaterial specificity, molecular mechanisms and clinical relevance of S. epidermidis and S. aureus infections in surgery, in: Proceedings of the Symposium on Pathogenicity and Clinical Significance of Coagulase-negative Staphylococci, Heppenheim, Germany, June 10-14, 1986, Gustav Fischer Verlag, Stuttgart, 1986, in press.
46. S.A. Green, M.J. Ripley, Chronic osteomyelitis in pin tracks, J. Bone Jt. Surg., 66A (1984) 1092-1098.
47. R.H. Fitzgerald, P.J. Kelly, Infections in the skeletal system, in: R.L. Simmons, R.J. Howard, A.I. Henricksen (Eds.), Surgical Infectious Diseases, Appleton-Century-Crofts, Norwalk, Connecticut, 1982, pp. 1005-1028.
48. J.R. Patrinely, K.R. Wilhelmus, J.M. Rubin, J.E. Key, Bacterial keratitis associated with extended wear soft contact lenses, C.L.A.O. J., 11 (1985) 234-236.
49. K.Merritt, G.E. Turner, Adherence of bacteria to biomaterials, Abstract, 11th Annual Meeting of the Society for Biomaterials, San Diego, California, April 25-28, 1985.
50. L.X. Webb, A.G. Gristina, R.T. Myers, A.R. Cordell, C.D. Hobgood, J.W. Costerton, Inhibition of bacterial adherence by antibacterial surface pretreatment of vascular prostheses, J. Vasc. Surg., 4 (1986) 16-21.
51. H.W. Paerls, Influence of attachment on microbial metabolism and growth in aquatic ecosystems, in: D.C. Savage, M. Fletcher (Eds.), Bacterial Adhesion, Plenum Press, New York, 1985, pp. 363-400.
52. M.R.W. Brown, P. Williams, The influence of environment on envelope properties affecting survival of bacteria in infections, Ann. Rev. Microbiol., 39 (1985)527-556.
53. I.D. Robb, Stereo-biochemistry and function in polymers, in: K.C. Marshall (Ed.), Microbial Adhesion and Aggregation, Springer Verlag, Berlin, 1984, pp. 39-49.
54. P.R. Rutter, B. Vincent, Physiochemical interactions of the substratum, microorganisms, and the fluid phase, in: K.C. Marshall (Ed.), Microbial Adhesion and Aggregation, Springer Verlag, Berlin, 1984, pp. 21-38.
55. A.G. Gristina, E. Barth, L.X. Webb, Microbial adhesion and biofilm in the pathogenesis of biomaterial centered infections and osteomyelitis, in: R.B. Gustilo, R.P. Gruninger, P.K. Peterson (Eds.), Current Concepts in the Management of Musculoskeletal Infections, in press, W.B. Saunders Company, Philadelphia, Pennsylvania, 1986.
56. A.G. Gristina, E. Barth, L.X. Webb, Microbes, metals and other nonbiological substrata in man: substratum and substrate factors in infection, in: R.B. Gustilo, R.P. Gruninger, P.K. Peterson (Eds.), Current Concepts in the Management of Musculoskeletal Infections, in press, W.B. Saunders Company, 1986.

Biomaterials and Clinical Applications,
edited by A. Pizzoferrato, P.G. Marchetti, A. Ravaglioli and A.J.C. Lee
Elsevier Science Publishers B.V., Amsterdam, 1987 — Printed in The Netherlands

MICROBIOLOGY OF POROUS HYDROXYLAPATITE IMPLANTS IN HUMAN PERIODONTAL OSSEOUS DEFECTS

RAMAGLIA L.*,SBORDONE L.*,LENCI F.*,GULLETTA E.**,AMATO G.**,KENNEY E.B.***

*University of Naples,2a Fac. Med. e Chir.,Istituto di Discipline Odontostomatologiche,Italy
**University of Naples,2a Fac. Med. e Chir.,Cattedra di Microbiologia,Dip. di Biologia e Patologia Cellulare e Molecolare,Italy
***U.C.L.A.,School of Dentistry,Sec. of Periodontics,USA

SUMMARY

A microbiological survey of the effect of known periodontal pathogens on the reconstructive therapy of complete interradicular bone loss in human lower molars implanted with granular porous hydroxylapatite has been carried out.Microbiological samples in 7 experimental and 7 control sites have been taken from the deepest furcation lesion prior to and during the surgery;the same sites have been resampled 6 months later,immediately prior to a control surgical reentry procedure.Samples have been analyzed with darkfield microscopy and with non-selective and selective for BPB,Ha,Capno,Fn,Ec cultural anaerobic techniques.Results suggest that the failure of reconstructive therapy of implanted furcations is associated with high levels of periodontopathic indicator bacteria,indicating a correlation between the outcome of the surgical procedure and the recolonization of the major periodontal pathogens.

INTRODUCTION

Periodontitis (P.D.) is associated with bacterial infections of a chronic nature which lead to ongoing destruction of the periodontium and affect the outcome of the therapy.Apparently there are certain microorganism,Black Pigmented Bacteroides (BPB) mainly B.intermedius (Bi) and B.gengivalis (Bg),Hemophilus actinomycetemcomitans (Ha),Capnocytophaga spp.(Capno),Eikenella corrodens (Ec),Fusobacterium nucleatum (Fn) and oral Spirochetes,which have a high degree of correlation with the disease and are related to active tissue damage (refs. 1-2).The progression of P.D. determines in many cases defects of the supporting bone and in multi-rooted teeth these areas of bone destruction are most frequently located in the area of furcations.Regenerative procedures involving the use of different biomaterials are currently used to replace the lost supporting tissue (refs.3-4).

Therefore the present study has been undertaken in order to monitor if the presence and/or the rapid recolonization of known periodontal pathogens could affect the outcome of the reconstructive therapy of complete interradicular bone loss (class III furcation involvement) in human lower molars implanted with a granular porous hydroxylapatite (HA).

MATERIALS AND METHODS

Patient selection and experimental design

Subjects selected for this study were 7 adult male or nonpregnant female affected by Adult Periodontitis and with at least two class III periodontal furcation involved lower molars.After 4 weeks from the conclusion of a comprehensive course of initial therapy,patients were surgically treated with a standard modified Widman flap in order to expose the furcation defects.Immediately prior to the surgical phase,gingival inflammation (G.I.) and plaque levels (Pl.I.) were assessed.At the same time,following the removal of supragingival plaque,a microbiological sample of subgingival flora was taken by using a periodontal curette (Morse 00).During the surgery a second microbiological sample from the exposed furcations was taken using a calcium-alginate wrapped barbed broach.Following this sampling,one furcation was randomly selected as experimental site and implanted with a granular porous HA (Interpore 200 R;mash:400-625 u);the other furca (with no implant) served as control site.All patients received standard postoperative care and were placed on a regular course of maintenance therapy.Six months postsurgery,two patients returned for the reentry surgical procedure.At this time,the clinical parameters were repeated and a subgingival microbiological sample was taken with a curette from the same site sampled presurgery.

Microbiological procedure

Subgingival plaque samples were dispersed into 1 ml of PRAS Ringer's solution and aliquots of 0.1 ml of dispersion were processed for whole plaque Gram staining and darkfield microscopy.Serial ten-fold dilutions of the sample dispersion were performed and aliquots of 0.1 ml of appropriate dilutions were plated onto non-selective,selective and elective media.After plating,media were incubated at 35 °C for 4-7 days in 85%N_2,10%H_2,5%CO_2,and examined for the presence of colonies typical of the species sought;10 representative colonies,where possible,were subcultured until pure and speciated or confirmed on the basis of a selective series of tests including colony morphology,aerotolerance,Gram staining and biochemical tests.The non-selective medium contained a base of Trypticase Soy Agar and 5% defibrinated sheep blood (TSA-SB),and a commercially available TSA-SB (BBL) was used as elective medium for the isolation of members of the genus Capno.These species were identified and speciated according to Socransky et al. (ref.5).The selective media of Walker et al. (refs.6-7) were employed for the enumeration of Fn and Ec.The selective medium of Mandell and Socransky (ref.8) and the selective medium of Slots (ref.9) permitted the enumeration of Ha.The selective medium of Zambon et al. (ref.10) was used for the isolation of BPB.Speciation was based on methods of Holdeman et al. (ref. 11).Bacterial cells darkfield microscopy counts were performed at 1000x magnification according to Listgarten and Hellden (ref. 1).

RESULTS

In tables 1 and 2 are reported the percentages of indicator bacteria of predominant cultivable subgingival microflora in experimental and control sites prior to and during the surgery.The bacterial species isolated by means of selective media in the 14 sampled sites are BPB ss. gingivalis and intermedius,Ha,Capno sp.,Fn and Ec.Approximately 1/3 of sites sampled presurgery shows the presence of all the above mentioned bacteria.However every furcation presents at least one of such species in percentage significantly associated with deep periodontal lesions.Wherever recovered,BPB account for the major part of predominant cultivable subgingival microflora ranging from 4% to 38%.Samples taken during the surgical procedure following granulation tissue debridement and open flap root planing in the furcation area,show non-recoverable levels of indicator bacteria in all but three sites in which Bg,although reduced comparing to presurgery levels, is still present in significant percentage count respectively of 15.4%,12.5% and 8%.Two patients returned 6 months postsurgery for the reentry surgical procedure and in table 3 are reported the percentages of indicator bacteria of predominant cultivable subgingival microflora in experimental and control sites prior to this reentry procedure.Comparing the data regarding the pre,intra and postsurgery samples both in experimental and control sites,it is evident that a recolonization of periodontopathic indicator species has occured.Particularly BPB seem to have a recolonization potential greater than other known periodontal pathogens;in fact they are recovered in percentages higher than those found presurgery,especially

Patient	site	B.g.				B.i.				H.a.			
		Pre		Intra		Pre		Intra		Pre		Intra	
		%	(ni)	%	(ni)	%	(ni)	%	(ni)	%	(ni)	%	(ni)
I	46*	21.2	(11)	-	(-)	11.5	(6)	-	(-)	0.35	(18)	-	(-)
	47	18.6	(8)	-	(-)	11.6	(5)	-	(-)	0.27	(12)	-	(-)
II	36	21	(21)	8	(3)	-	(-)	-	(-)	0.3	(13)	-	(-)
	46*	22	(22)	15.4	(2)	16	(16)	-	(-)	-	(-)	-	(-)
III	47*	26	(13)	-	(-)	12	(6)	-	(-)	0.54	(27)	-	(-)
	48	4.3	(1)	-	(-)	-	(-)	-	(-)	0.8	(19)	-	(-)
IV	46	-	(-)	-	(-)	-	(-)	-	(-)	1.5	(19)	-	(-)
	47*	-	(-)	-	(-)	-	(-)	-	(-)	0.15	(5)	-	(-)
V	46*	13.5	(5)	12.5	(1)	5.4	(2)	-	(-)	0.13	(5)	-	(-)
	36	-	(-)	-	(-)	-	(-)	-	(-)	-	(-)	-	(-)
VI	46*	34.8	(8)	-	(-)	-	(-)	-	(-)	-	(-)	-	(-)
	47	34.3	(12)	-	(-)	-	(-)	-	(-)	-	(-)	-	(-)
VII	46*	4	(2)	-	(-)	-	(-)	-	(-)	12	(6)	-	(-)
	47	-	(-)	-	(-)	-	(-)	-	(-)	0.75	(3)	-	(-)

B.g.=Bacteroides gingivalis
B.i.=Bacteroides intermedius
H.a.=Hemophilus actinomycetemcomitans

*=implanted site
ni=number of isolates

Patient	site	Capno.				F.n.				E.c.			
		Pre		Intra		Pre		Intra		Pre		Intra	
		%	(ni)	%	(ni)	%	(ni)	%	(ni)	%	(ni)	%	(ni)
I	46*	0.33	(17)	-	(-)	3.1	(19)	-	(-)	0.55	(13)	-	(-)
	47	0.44	(19)	-	(-)	3.4	(15)	-	(-)	0.54	(14)	-	(-)
II	36	0.4	(18)	-	(-)	3.2	(19)	-	(-)	0.5	(12)	-	(-)
	46*	10	(10)	-	(-)	3.5	(11)	-	(-)	0.6	(16)	-	(-)
III	47*	0.5	(1)	-	(-)	3.4	(10)	-	(-)	0.7	(19)	-	(-)
	48	0.8	(19)	-	(-)	2.5	(16)	-	(-)	0.51	(15)	-	(-)
IV	46	-	(-)	-	(-)	-	(-)	-	(-)	0.6	(13)	-	(-)
	47*	-	(-)	-	(-)	3.5	(4)	-	(-)	0.5	(16)	-	(-)
V	46*	0.32	(12)	-	(-)	2.6	(7)	-	(-)	0.65	(14)	-	(-)
	36	0.04	(2)	-	(-)	2.5	(1)	-	(-)	0.51	(15)	-	(-)
VI	46*	0.04	(1)	-	(-)	3.3	(16)	-	(-)	0.9	(19)	-	(-)
	47	-	(-)	-	(-)	3.2	(18)	-	(-)	0.84	(17)	-	(-)
VII	46*	-	(-)	-	(-)	3.5	(8)	-	(-)	0.6	(13)	-	(-)
	47	-	(-)	-	(-)	3.2	(7)	-	(-)	0.53	(14)	-	(-)

Capno.=Capnocytophaga
F.n.=Fusobacterium nucleatum
E.c.=Eikenella corrodens

*=implanted site
ni=number of isolates

Tables 1-2.Percentages of indicator species of predominant cultivable subgingival flora in experimental and control sites pre and intra-surgery.

in the sites in which they were still present in the intrasurgery sample (sites 46 and 36,patient II).However one furca shows only two recolonizing periodontopathgens:Capno and Fn.The recolonization pattern tested with cultural technique is confermed by darkfield microscopy counts.These microbiological results match with the clinical evidence of the failure of reconstructive therapy in the experimental sites implanted with granular porous HA.

Patient	site		pre-surg.		intra-surg.		post-surg.	
			%	(ni)	%	(ni)	%	(ni)
I	46*	B.g.	21.2	(11)	-	(-)	38.5	(50)
		B.i.	11.5	(6)	-	(-)	-	(-)
		H.a.	0.35	(18)	-	(-)	0.7	(9)
		Capno.	0.33	(17)	-	(-)	5.4	(70)
		E.c.	0.55	(13)	-	(-)	3.7	(21)
		F.n;	3.1	(19)	-	(-)	3.7	(21)
	47	B.g.	18.6	(8)	-	(-)	-	(-)
		B.i.	11.6	(5)	-	(-)	-	(-)
		H.a.	0.27	(12)	-	(-)	-	(-)
		Capno.	0.44	(19)	-	(-)	15	(150)
		E.c.	0.54	(14)	-	(-)	-	(-)
		F.n.	3.4	(15)	-	(-)	3.1	(10)
II	36	B.g.	21	(21)	8	(3)	46.6	(140)
		B.i.	-	(-)	-	(-)	-	(-)
		H.a.	0.3	(13)	-	(-)	-	(-)
		Capno	0.4	(18)	-	(-)	0.1	(30)
		E.c.	0.5	(12)	-	(-)	-	(-)
		F.n.	3.2	(19)	-	(-)	-	(-)
	46*	B.g.	22	(22)	15.4	(2)	66.6	(4)
		B.i.	16	(16)	-	(-)	-	(-)
		H.a.	-	(-)	-	(-)	-	(-)
		Capno.	10	(10)	-	(-)	0.16	(1)
		E.c.	0.5	(16)	-	(-)	0.5	(14)
		F.n.	3.5	(11)	-	(-)	3.2	(10)

B.g.=Bacteroides gingivalis
B.i.=Bacteroides intermedius
H.a.=Hemophilus actinomycetemcomitans
Capno.=Capnocytophaga
E.c.=Eikenella corrodens
F.n.=Fusobacterium nucleatum
* =implanted site
ni =number of isolates

Table 3.Percentages of indicator species of predominant cultivable subgingival flora in experimental and control sites pre,intra and six mos. post-surgery

DISCUSSION

Microbiological data have shown that 4 weeks following the conclusion of a comprehensive course of initial therapy,including oral hygiene instruction and reinforcement,known periodontal pathogens are still recovered in the subgingival plaque sampled from complete furcation lesions.The presence of these bacteria could be due either to an incomplete removal because of technical difficulties to perform a proper root planing in the furcation area,or to an unusual rapid recolonization.On the contrary data concerning intrasurgery samples show the complete elimination from the furcation area of periodontopathic bacteria by means of an open flap root planing,proving the need of a surgical treatment for the furcation lesions.At the same time our results suggest that the failure,6 months postsurgery,of reconstructive therapy of class III furcation involvements in human lower molars implanted with granular porous HA,could be due to a rapid recolonization of known periodontal pathogens which have prevented the connective tissue proliferation within the HA porous system and the consequent bone regeneration.On the other hand we could also assume that the esfoliating implant material has prevented the formation of a new dento-gingival attachment and has,consequently,recreated a deep periodontal pocket rapidly colonized by indicator periodontopathic bacteria acting only as lateral spreaders of a preexisting lesion and not as etiological agents.

REFERENCES

1 Listgarten M. and Hellden L.,Relative distribution of bacteria at clinically healthy and periodontally diseased sites in humans,J. Clin. Periodontol.,5 (1978) 115
2 Dzink J.,Tanner A.,Haffajee A,Socransky S.,Gram negative species associated with active destructive periodontal lesions,J.Clin. Periodont.,12 (1985)648
3 West T. and Brustein D.,Freeze-dried bone and coralline implants compared in the dog,J. Periodontol.,56 (1985) 348
4 Kenney E.,Sa Ferreira J.,Dimitrijevic T.,Carranza F.Jr.,Bone formation within porous hydroxylapatite implants in human periodontal defects,J. Periodontol.,57 (1986) 76
5 Socransky S.,Holt S.,Leadbetter E.,Tanner A.,Savitt E.,Hammond B., Capnocytophaga new genus of gram negative gliding bacteria.III.Physiological characterization,Archs. Microbiol.,122 (1979) 29
6 Walker C.,Ratliff D.,Muller D.,Mandell R.,Socransky S.,Medium for selective isolation of F. nucleatum from human periodontal pockets,J. Clin. Microbiol. 10 (1979) 844
7 Walker C.,Tanner A.,Smith C.,Socransky S.,Selective medium for Eikenella corrodens,J. Dent. Res.,57 (A) (1978) 961
8 Mandell R. and Socransky S.,A selective medium for Actinobacillus actinomycetemcomitans and the incidence of the organism in Juvenile Periodontitis,J. Periodontol.,52 (1981) 593
9 Slots J.,Selective medium for isolation of Actinobacillus actinomycetemcomitans,J. Clin. Microbiol.,15 (1982) 606
10 Zambon J.,Reynolds H.,Slots J.,Black pigmented bacteroides spp. in the human oral cavity,Infect. Immun.,32 (1981) 198
11 Holdeman L.,Cato E. and Moore W.,Anaerobe Laboratory Manual,4th Edn.,V.P.I. and Blacksburg State University,Virginia,1977

Biomaterials and Clinical Applications,
edited by A. Pizzoferrato, P.G. Marchetti, A. Ravaglioli and A.J.C. Lee
Elsevier Science Publishers B.V., Amsterdam, 1987 — Printed in The Netherlands

THE REMOVAL OF THE PROSTHESIS (GIRDLESTONE PROCEDURE) FOR INFECTED CEMENTED TOTAL HIP REPLACEMENT: A CLINICAL EVALUATION OF 67 CASES.

P.G.MARCHETTI, R.BINAZZI, L.D'ELIA, A.MORONI and A.TONI

ORTHOPAEDIC DEPT., UNIVERSITY OF BOLOGNA, ISTITUTO ORTOPEDICO RIZZOLI, BOLOGNA

SUMMARY

We have reviewed 67 patients (45 females and 22 males) operated on between 1970 and 1983, with cemented total Hip replacement and in whom the removal of the prosthesis became necessary for deep infection.
In 23 cases (34%) the infection became evident in the immediate post-op, 42 cases (63%) showed signs of subacute infection within the first 3 months and 2 cases (3%) became infected more than 3 months after the operation.
In 20 cases (30%) surgical debridment of the wound was attempted prior to removing the prosthetic components, without any success.
The average follow up was 4 years (range 6 months-12 years). We could not evaluate the results with the usual scoring systems used for routine total Hip replacements and we had to review the Charnley's and Harris' scores.
In our series we had 26 good results (39%), 11 fair (16%) and 30 poor (45%). We believe that wide soft tissue destruction produced by deep infection has undoubtedly been the major cause of failure of the Girdlestone procedure in septic Hip replacements.
Early removal of septic prostheses avoids further extension of the infection, enhancing a rapid recovery when associated with intensive antibiotic therapy and preparing the ground (in younger patients) for a successive reimplantation.

INTRODUCTION

Loosening may be due either to septic or aseptic mechanism, both of which require different surgical treatments. There are three possible solutions:

1) Resection arthroplasty or the Girdlestone procedure
2) Girdlestone procedure plus local additional surgery

3) Total or partial revision surgery

Much controversy exists regarding the use of resection arthroplasty as definite solution for septic prosthetic loosening. For instance, the Girdlestone resection is thought by Anderson (1) to cause unaccetable instability; while other such as Calandruccio (2) has better opinion of this procedure, stating that, after Girdlestone, the Hip is usually stable enough to permit a satisfactory gait with a cane, with a good range of motion and minor pain. In our experience we seldom had to face patients primarly treated with the simple implant removal requiring later on a major Hip surgery.

As usual the Girdlestone procedure involves both advantages as well as disadvantages. It is certainly an advantage to limit surgery to the prosthesis removal as this procedure is fast and simple, reduces blood loss(occasionally being a major problem for this kind of surgery), reduces the risk of a new or persisting septic inflammatory reaction and it may well be a definitive solution permitting a fair Hip function.

Nevertheless some younger patients may not appreciate the leg length discrepancy (often more than 3 cm.) complaining at the need of the heel pad on their shoes. Even the fact of limping and the limitations of activities, with the need of at least a support may be the reason for some complaints.

In our opinion a Girdlestone procedure is mainly designed to control infection or to relieve pain without restoring normal function: obviously, this is a limitation wich restricts the indications of this surgery.

For septic loosening the resection procedure is the treatment of choice, either as a definitive solution or as a temporary one, waiting for a future prosthetic implant. Severe bone stock deficiency makes revision surgery technically difficult and poorly liable. Elderly patients and those with compromised general condition are also obvious selections. Diabetes is for us a controindication for a major reconstruction, because of the higher infectionrisk. Finally we think that the patients should be honestly told about the risks of revision surgery.

MATERIAL AND METHODS

Between 1970 and 1983 we removed 127 total Hip prostheses in 123 patients. All the prostheses removed were cemented. Of the 104 cases reviewed, 37 were aseptic. In the remaining 67 Hips with septic loosening: 23 cases showed evidence of infection in the immediate post-operative period; 42 displayed signs of subacute infection in the first three months and in two cases infection appeared much later. In 20 Hips surgical debridment was performed before removing the prosthetic component, without any success.

The surgical technique and the after treatment are quite different in septic and aseptic cases. In aseptic loosening a complete removal of the femoral or pelvic cement is not needed. We didn't find any significant difference among aseptic cases with or without cement remaining after surgery. In septic loosening , maintaining that femur dislocation has to be performed without any major stress, it is mandatory to obtain a complete removal of cement and of the granulation tissue surrounding the implant.In nine patients out of the sixty seven septic cases (13%), a draining fistula persisted for 15- to 36 months after implant removal. Five patients had additional surgical debridment after the Girdlestone procedure.

After surgery septic patients were maintained in plaster for four to six weeks. In these cases a continuous suction- irrigation with antibiotics and antiseptic solution was carried out for about twenty days. We found the use of passive motion immediately after the removal of the plaster cast very useful in these patients, both for the Hip and the Knee. After two to four days of passive motion and active exercise we encourage the progressive weight bearing with deambulatory support and later on with crutches; a temporary heel pad is chosen to make leg length approximately equal. After 8 to 10 days adjustment is made to the heel pad height on the basis of a standing pelvis X-rays.

To evaluate Girdlestone treated patients we reviewed the Charnley's and Harris' score evaluation systems, giving a considerable emphasis to pain, walking,daily activities and joint motion. (Tab. 1) 74% of the 104 patients declared themselves satisfied. While the dissatisfied group always corresponded to bad clinical results, four cases among the satisfied group presented a negative score. Subjective evaluation of satisfaction was then considered to define the lower borderline of fair evaluation.

RESULTS

Results are then considered referring to the prosthetic loosening aetiology. (Tab.2) None of the aseptic losening treated with Girdlestone resection present bad results, while none of the septic ones are classified as excellent. Even if aseptic cases performed positively, it could be pointed out that aseptic loosening is not a proper indication for the resection arthroplasty. In our experience a very severe bone stock deficiency in aged patients lead us to perform the Girdlestone procedure in these cases. The results for septic loosening are strikingly different: in fact 45% of them didn't improve at all, and only 39% could be evaluated as having good results. Going deeper into results we found a significant relation between pain and joint mobility (Tab.3): the greater the range of movement the better the results as referred to pain.

Relation between clinical results and age is also performed, splitting the cases in two groups: patients aged sixty or less versus patients older than

CLINICAL AND FUNCTIONAL PARAMETERS

1. PAIN	6.painless	4-5.bearable	1-2-3.unbearable
2. WALKING			
a. Limping...........................	1.slight		0.severe
b. Supports..........................	2.one crutch	1.two crutches	0.unable to walk
c. Distance..........................	2.+300 meters	1.only at home	0.unable
3. DAILY ACTIVITIES			
a. Stairs............................	2.without sup.	1.with sup.	0.unable
b. Use of means of transportation.....	1.possible		0.impossible
c. Sitting...........................	2.any chair	1.high chair	0.impossible
d. Wearing shoes......................	2.easily	1.difficultly	0.unable
4. MOTION................................	5.good	3-4.satisf.	1-2.unsatisf.

TABLE 1

sixty years. Summarizing the results one out of three younger patients presents a bad results versus only one out of ten for the older patients.

CONCLUSION

None of the resection arthroplasty in aseptic cases shows a bad result, while none of the septic loosening shows an excellent overall result.

CLINICAL RESULTS

	EXCELLENT	GOOD	FAIR	BAD
SEPTIC	-	39%	16%	45%
ASEPTIC	33%	21%	46%	-

TABLE 2

	MOTILITY		
	GOOD	FAIR	BAD
ABSENT	69%	29%	-
MILD PAIN	12%	50%	31%
SEVERE PAIN	19%	21%	69%

TABLE 3

The soft tissue destruction produced by acute and deep infection is the major cause of failure of Girdlestone procedure in septic Hip replacement. Early removal of septic prosthesis avoids any further extension of the infection enhancing a rapid recovery when associated with intensive antibiotic therapy and preparing the ground for prosthetic revision surgery in younger patients. Adjuvant surgery to Girdlestone procedure is not felt of any use. Only cobra plate Hip arthrodesis may be indicated in younger patients with aseptic loosening. Early, but not immediate Hip mobilization is considered of vital importance in order to avoid formation of scar tissue causing painful ankylosis.

REFERENCES

L.D. Anderson, Campbell's operative orthopaedics: Infections,in: Edmonson-Crenshaw (Ed.), Mosby, St. Louis, i980 p.1070

R.A. Calandruccio,Campbell's operative orthopaedics: Arthroplasty, in: Edmonson-Crenshaw (Ed.), Mosby, St. Louis, 1980, p.2242

Biomaterials and Clinical Applications,
edited by A. Pizzoferrato, P.G. Marchetti, A. Ravaglioli and A.J.C. Lee
Elsevier Science Publishers B.V., Amsterdam, 1987 — Printed in The Netherlands

MICROBIAL CONTAMINATION DURING VASCULAR SURGERY

L. PRATELLI[1], T. CURTI[2], F. FIORI[1], S. STEA[1], G. CIAPETTI[1], O. PARAGONA[2], D. CAVEDAGNA[1], M. RODIO[2].

[1]Centro di Ricerca per la Biocompatibilità dei Materiali da Impianto, Istituto Ortopedico Rizzoli, Bologna, Italia.

[2]Cattedra di Chirurgia Vascolare, Policlinico S. Orsola, Bologna, Italia.

SUMMARY

The most feared complication of vascular reconstructive surgery is infection involving a prosthetic arterial substitute.

To show the presence of any microrganism at the time of the implantation of the vascular graft, sterile swabs were employed to obtain material before and after the operation for microbiological investigations. In this first series of cases, no bacterial growth was observed in the tested samples.

INTRODUCTION

The infection of a vascular graft is a most catastrophic complication for both the patient and the surgeon.

The true incidence of prosthetic graft infection has remained remarkably unchanged for nearly 20 years,varying from 1% to 6% (Refs. 1-3).

The percentage of the infection is influenced by various factors including the anatomic location of the graft and the use of peri-operative prophylactic antibiotics. Many Authors have found the highest incidence in the inguinal portion of the graft. The nature of the prosthetic material implanted also affects the incidence of graft infection (Ref. 4).

The majority of prosthetic graft are probably infected at the time of their implantation.

The possible sources of contamination might be

a) improper sterilisation of surgical instruments or of the

prosthesis itself;

b) infected arterial wall;

c) intestinal transudate;

d) infected lymph glands;

e) concurrent infection of the body;

f) contact of the prosthesis with the skin.

Staphylococcus aureus is the most common pathogen, but there is an increasing incidence of graft infection due to gram-negative bacteria or mixed infection involving both aerobic and anaerobic organisms.

Early graft infections generally appear in the inguinal area and involve organisms of high virulence (Staphylococcus aureus, Pseudomonas, E. coli).

Graft infections that present later tend to involve organisms of low virulence, i.e. Staphylococcus epidermidis (Ref. 5).

The aim of our work was to verify the presence of bacterial contamination in the operating theatre during surgery.

METHODS

A bacterial examination was carried out on 160 samples taken from 20 patients who underwent aorto-bifemoral by-pass graft following aorto-iliac occlusive disease.

None of the patients showed signs of concurrent infections at the time of the operation, and all were disinfected locally with antiseptic solutions.

The samples were taken at the time of the operation using sterile swabs, from the left and right inguinal lymphatic nodes where the femorals were isolated, as well as from the inside of the aorta and from the peri-aortic tissues (Fig. 1).

After the implantation, when the tissues were no longer to be exposed to possible environmental contamination, swabs were again taken from the left and right inguinal lymphatic nodes and from the peri-aortic tissues.

The sampling was completed by taking a sample from the aorto-prosthesis suture (Fig. 2).

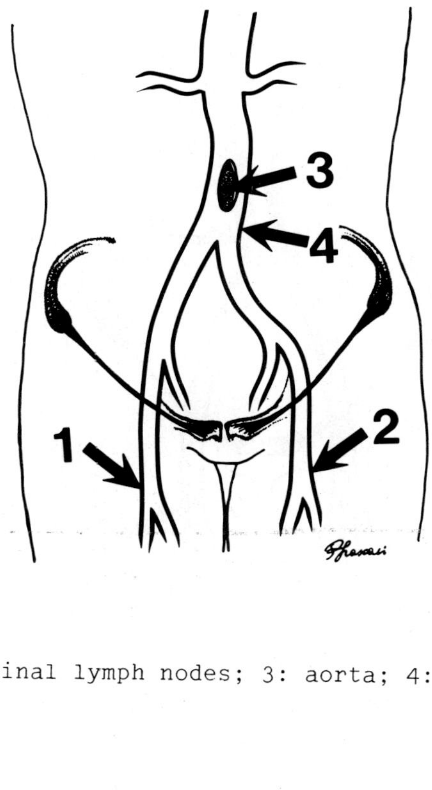

Fig. 1 1,2: inguinal lymph nodes; 3: aorta; 4: peri-aortic tissue

Microbiological investigations were carried out on the samples collected in this way, in order to detect the presence of any germs, whether aerobic or anaerobic.

These examinations included the preparation of cultures in both solid and liquid mediums in aerobic, microaerophilic and anaerobic environments.

The samples were defined as sterile if there was no growth after 48 hours in the cultures in the aerobic environment and

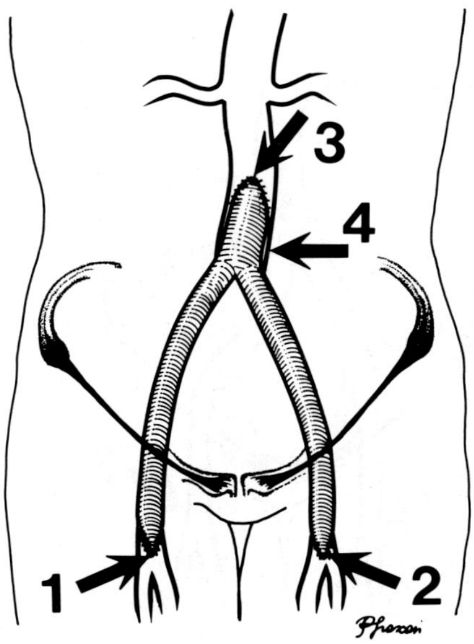

Fig. 2 1,2: inguinal lymph nodes; 3: aorto-prosthesis suture;
4: peri-aortic tissue.

after 7 days for the cultures in anaerobiosis (Fig. 3).

Samples collected with sterile swabs	Samples collected with sterile swab for anaerobes
AEROBIC CULTURE:	ANAEROBIC CULTURE:
Tripticase Soy Broth Blood-agar plates Mc Conkey plates Saboraoud plates	Thioglycollate Broth Schaedler agar plates

Incubation for
48 hrs to 7 days

Fig. 3

RESULTS and CONCLUSION

All the bacteriological examinations we carried out gave negative results, since no growth of bacteria occurred.

However, it is not yet possible to make a definitive judgement on intra-operative contamination, considering the limited number of cases examined in this work. Nevertheless, the levels of hygiene adopted have been shown to be efficient in the cases examined: no clinically evident infection developed in the immediate post-operative period. Moreover none of the patients examined showed clinical signs of infections within six months of the operations.

This type of research, if carried out systematically, could be of use in pinpointing the cases in which contamination has actually occurred during surgery.

These patients could be considered a category at risk of infection and could therefore receive long-term antimicrobial therapy, considering the seriousness of the evolution of an infection affecting a subject who has undergone vascular graft.

Furthermore, the patient will be followed in the long term, in order to document any late infections that might arise. The appearance of such infections would lead to take into consideration other causes of infection of the graft, different from microbic contamination during surgery.

REFERENCES

1 E.D. Szilagyi, R.F. Smith, J.P. Elliott, M.P. Vradecic, Infection in arterial reconstruction with synthetic grafts, Ann. Surg., 1976 (1972) 321-329.
2 A. Stella, V. Loperfido, T. Curti, Le complicanze infettive nella chirurgia, in: Atti Società Italiana di Chirurgia, Roma, Italia, Ottobre 10-15,1976, p.p. 833-838.
3 W.G. Liekweg, L.J. Greenfield, Vascular prosthetic infections: collected experience and results of treatment, Surgery, 81 (3) (1977) 335-338.
4 J. Goldstone, W.S. Moore, Infection in vascular prostheses, Ann. J. Surg. 128 (1974) 225-232.
5 J. Goldstone, Infection in vascular grafting: pathogenesis, prevention and treatment, in: S.H. Skotnicki (Ed.), Proc. Symposium on recent Advances in Vascular Grafting, Nijmengen, The Netherlands, April 26-28, 1984, p.p. 207-215.

Biomaterials and Clinical Applications,
edited by A. Pizzoferrato, P.G. Marchetti, A. Ravaglioli and A.J.C. Lee
Elsevier Science Publishers B.V., Amsterdam, 1987 — Printed in The Netherlands

IN VITRO BACTERIAL PHAGOCYTOSIS OF MACROPHAGES AFTER CONTACT WITH BIOMATERIALS

L. PRATELLI, G. CIAPETTI, S. STEA, C. TARABUSI, A. PIZZOFERRATO.

Centro di Ricerca per la Biocompatibilità dei Materiali da Impianto, Istituto Rizzoli, Bologna, Italia.

SUMMARY

To investigate the cell-biomaterial interaction, the Authors developed an experimental model where macrophages, after remaining in contact with "extracts" of different biomaterials, are challenged with a bacterial suspension of Staphylococcus aureus. In such a way the residual ability of macrophages, which have been previously exposed to biomaterials, to phagocytose bacteria is measured.

INTRODUCTION

The particles that are generated by wear and corrosion from an implanted orthopaedic prosthesis are usually cleared of tissue macrophages by means of the phagocytic mechanism. However, when wear is excessive the particles accumulate and the local defense mechanisms can be hampered. Such a decrease in the defense processes can then foster the onset of the so-called "late infection" (1).

Experimental study of prosthetic infection often investigates the effects of the prosthetic material to be implanted in the living body.

Bacterial phagocytosis by the macrophages is one of the defense mechanisms with which the organism reacts (2).

The aim of this work is to see if, and to what extent, a biomaterial may influence such a defense mechanism.

METHODS

In order to study the phagocytosis of bacteria by the macrophages exposed to biomaterials we used: mouse peritoneal macrophages challenged with extracts of biomaterials and a suspension of Staphylococcus aureus.

After collecting peritoneal fluid from Swiss mice, the macrophages are "purified" by adherence to Petri dishes at 37°C for 1 hour (3). Then, purified macrophages are further incubated for 24 hours with 2 ml biomaterial-extracts prepared following ASTM recommendations.

The tested materials are used in orthopaedic surgery and they include: alumina, stainless steel, and carbon resin composite. The effect these materials have on the macrophages was compared to that of copper.

The extracts were obtained by putting for 5 days the powder of the materials in the same culture medium used to grow macrophages.

Macrophages that had not been placed in contact with biomaterials were used as a control.

By examining the cells by light microscopy, the index of phagocytosis and the phagocytic index of the macrophages have been determined, so allowing an evaluation of the effect of biomaterials on phagocytosis.

RESULTS

The phagocytic index can be evaluated by light microscopy in a reproducible way when the number of staphylococci phagocytized fluctuates between 1 and 6, and the index of phagocytosis can be evaluated when the number of phagocytizing cells is more than 10%.

The incubation period of macrophages and staphylococci was chosen in order to satisfy these conditions. A series of experiments was carried out with periods of incubation of 5, 15, 30, 60 and 120 minutes.

The number of phagocytizing macrophages (index of phagocytosis) ranges from 2% at 5 minutes to 79% at 120 minutes (Fig. 1).

The phagocytic index of the macrophages, that is to say the number of staphylococci phagocytized by a single cell, tends to increase with the incubation time.

The condition when there is the maximum number of phagocytizing cells, that is to say when there is a maximum number of macropha-

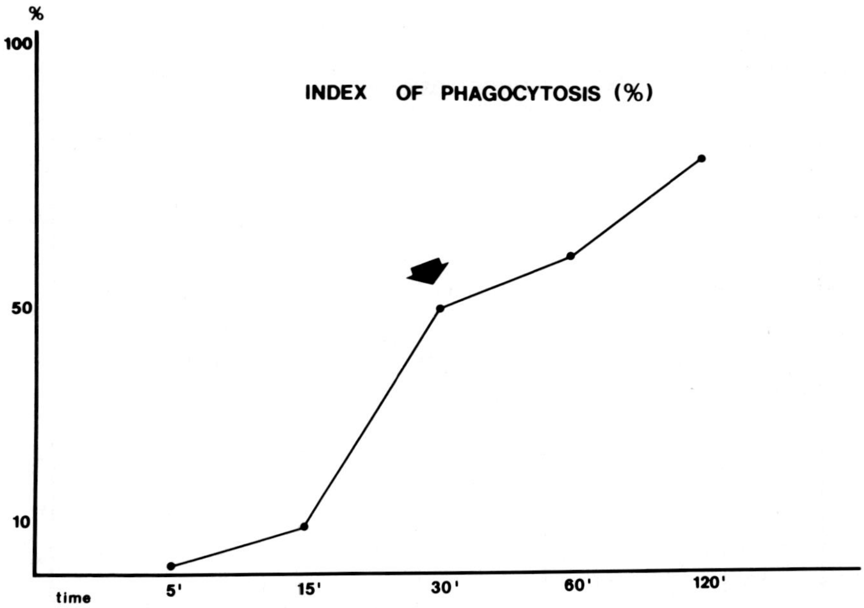

Fig. 1

phages that have phagocytized a number of staphylococci not greater than 6, occurs after 30 minutes of contact (Fig. 2).

This is the best ccndition for microscopic examination.

The percentage that indicates the index of phagocytosis is on the right of the ordinate axis. The value of this index at different times is shown with the dotted line.

The number of cocci phagocytized per cell, i.e. the phagocytic index, varies from 0 to more then 20 cocci per macrophage. "Classes of frequency" have been determined within this range, that is to say 1-6, 7-12 etc.,are shown on the left of the ordinate axis. The small circles represent the number of cells that contain that given number of staphylococci.

After 30 minutes of contact with the staphylococci the index of phagocytosis is only slightly more than 50% for the control ma-

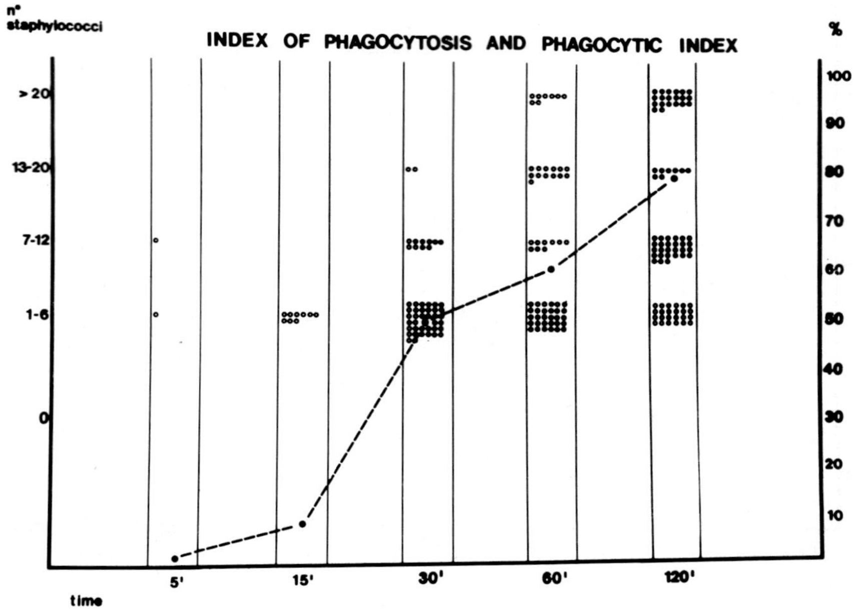

Fig. 2

crophages, whose morphological appearance is shown in Fig. 3.

The macrophages exposed to the aqueous extracts of stainless steel and carbon do not present statistically significant variations in the index of phagocytosis, while those exposed to alumina seem to have an inhibited capacity for phagocytosis. The reduction in phagocytosis of the cells exposed to copper is striking; this is not surprising since it is renowned for its toxicity.

The phagocytic index of the macrophages exposed to the different extracts of the biomaterials shows very little difference from the control.

The exception to this is copper where only 4% of the macrophages phagocytize 1 to 6 cocci.

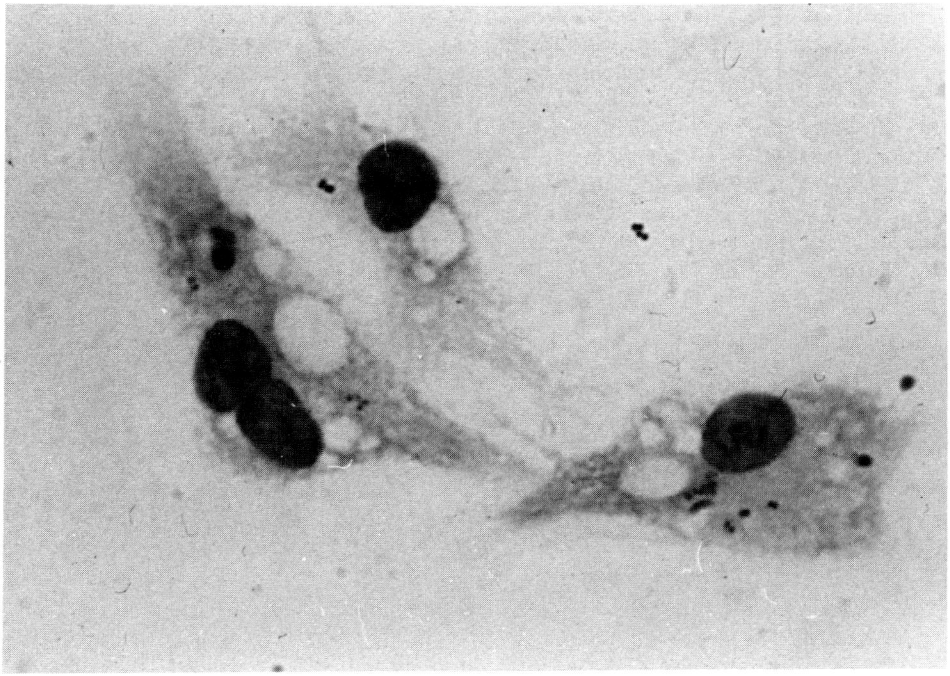

Fig. 3

CONCLUSIONS

In conclusion we can say that the extracts of alumina, stainless steel and carbon-resin composite do not noticeably hamper the phagocytosis of the macrophages. Therefore, at least in our experience, they do not negatively influence the defense mechanisms of macrophages against any possible bacterial contamination of the implant while other materials have been shown to be able to modify such mechanisms (4).

In our hands copper, which is quite toxic, alters the cells so that their phagocytic properties are almost completely inhibited.

REFERENCES

1 H.G. Willert and M. Semlitsch, Reaction of the articular capsule to artificial joint prostheses, in: D.F. Williams (Ed.), Biocompatibility of Implant Materials, Sector Publishing Limited, London, 1976, pp. 40-48.
2 B.J. Zeligs, Bactericidal and fungicidal assay, in: H.B.

Herscowitz, H.T. Holden, J.A. Bellanti, A. Ghaffar (Eds.), Manual of Macrophage Methodology, Marcel Dekker Inc., New York and Basel, 1981, pp. 271-280.
3 A. Pizzoferrato, A. Vespucci, G. Ciapetti, C. Sangiorgi, Mouse peritoneal macrophages modifications after alloplastic materials inoculation, in: Trans. Eight Annual Meeting of the Society for Biomaterials, Orlando, Florida (U.S.A.), April 24-27, 1982, 29.
4 T. Rae, A study on the effects of particulate metals of orthopedic interest on murine macrophages in vitro, J. Bone Joint Surg., 57B (1975) 444-447.

Biomaterials and Clinical Applications,
edited by A. Pizzoferrato, P.G. Marchetti, A. Ravaglioli and A.J.C. Lee
Elsevier Science Publishers B.V., Amsterdam, 1987 — Printed in The Netherlands

INTERACTIONS BETWEEN S. EPIDERMIDIS ISOLATED FROM CATHETER INFECTIONS AND MEDICAL GRADE POLYURETHANE

B. JANSEN, F. SCHUMACHER-PERDREAU, G. PETERS and G. PULVERER

Hygiene Institute, University of Cologne, Goldenfelsstr. 19 - 21,
5000 Koeln 41, FRG

Summary

The adhesion of two S. epidermidis strains (KH 11 and KH 6) onto the polyetherurethanes TUFTANE and BIOMER in phosphate buffer saline and in a chemically defined growth medium was investigated. The more hydrophobic strain KH 6 adhered stronger to both polymers in each of the two media, stressing the importance of hydrophobic bonding in the adhesion process. Incubation of the strains together with the polymers for a period up to 30 days in buffer led to altered properties of the strains, especially in the case of KH 11: surface hydrophobicity increased, reactivity with the lectin Con A was lost, urease activity and quantitative changes in the SDS-page pattern of extracellular proteins were observed. Strains incubated together with the polymers in the growth medium exhibited no changes. Physicochemical investigations including contact angle measurement, differential thermoanalysis and ATR-infrared spectroscopy of the polymers after incubation with the bacteria revealed no drastic changes.

INTRODUCTION

S. epidermidis is the most common causative organism of catheter infections. Several studies have been performed on the adhesion of these bacteria to polymer substrates which is regarded as the first step of infection (ref.1-3). The aim of our study was to investigate interactions between well-characterized S. epidermidis strains isolated from catheter infections and polyetherurethanes. This type of polymer was chosen since (i) polyetherurethanes are increasingly used as catheter materials and (ii) they can be manufactured without low-molecular additives. The adhesion behaviour of two strains, KH 11 and KH 6, to the polyetherurethanes TUFTANE and BIOMER was studied in nutrient-free phosphate buffered saline (PBS) and in a chemically defined growth medium (CDM). To determine in how far an extended contact between polymer and bacteria could affect the bacterial and polymer properties, the strains were incubated with the polymers for periods up to 30 days either in buffer or in CDM. The bacteria were investigated for possible changes of their biochemical, physiological and surface properties. To measure any influence of the bacteria on the polyetherurethanes (e. g. degradation of polymer chains), the polymers were examined by several physicochemical methods including contact angle measurement, differential thermoanalysis and ATR-infrared spectroscopy.

MATERIAL AND METHODS

Characterization of the strains

S. epidermidis strains KH 11 and KH 6 were characterized according to the scheme of KLOOS and SCHLEIFER (ref.4) and with a set of 28 biochemical reactions (API-Staph system, BIOMERIEUX, France). The surface properties of the strains were measured with the salt aggregation test (SAT, ref. 5), the xylene test (ref.6) and by contact angle measurements of thin bacterial layers on cellulose acetate membranes (ref.7). The bacterial surface free energy was calculated from the water contact angle using the equation-of-state approach (ref. 8). The reactivity with lectins from Concavalis (Con A) and from Lens culinaris and with Poly-L-Lysine and Polybrene was tested in slide agglutination.

Extracellular products were obtained by growing the strains over a cellulose acetate membrane on BHI agar (Oxoid); 1 mg of dry weight substance was separated in SDS-electrophoresis.

Characterization of the polymers

Polyetherurethanes TUFTANE (B. F. Goodrich, USA) and BIOMER (Ethicon, USA) were supplied as films of 400 and 200 µm thickness, respectively. Both polymers are composed of 4-4'di-isocyanato diphenylmethane and poly(tetramethylene glycol). To remove residual solvents or other low molecular compounds, they were first extracted in ethanol for 24 h and then in water for 48 h. They were sterilized by gamma-irradiation at a dose of 2.5 Mrad.

Contact angle measurements were performed using a Lorentzen + Wettre goniometer; the surface free energy of the polymers was calculated from their water contact angles (ref. 8). Differential thermoanalysis in the range of 25 - 600 ^{o}C was done using a DTA-instrument from Mettler, Switzerland. ATR-infrared spectra of the polymer surfaces were recorded with a Nicolet 20 DXB Fourier Transform infrared spectrometer taking 150 scans per sample.

Characterization of the suspension media

Surface tensions of PBS and CDM were measured with an interfacial tensiometer (Krüss GmbH, FRG) at room temperature.

Adhesion assay

Polymer discs (d = 6 mm) were incubated in bacterial suspensions of KH 11 or KH 6, either in PBS or in CDM at room temperature for various periods up to 3 h. Bacterial concentration was approximately 2 x 10^8 colony forming units (CFU)/ml in all experiments. The polymers were then washed 5 times with PBS to remove loosely attached bacteria. Adenosine triphosphate (ATP) of the adhered bacteria was extracted with 100 µl of 2.5 % trichloroacetic acid and diluted with 400 µl TRIS-EDTA buffer (pH 7.75). An aliquot (50 µl) was mixed with 400 µl TRIS-EDTA buffer, 200 ul of ATP monitoring reagent (LKB Wallac, Finland) was added and the amount of ATP measured in a luminometer (LKB 1251, Wallac, Finland). The number of adhered bacteria was calculated from a standard curve. Mean values of five measurements per polymer sample were taken as final result.

Incubation of KH 11 and KH 6 with TUFTANE or BIOMER

TUFTANE or BIOMER sheets (4 x 4 cm) were incubated in bacterial suspensions containing KH 11 or KH 6 in PBS in a concentration of ~ 10^8 CFU/ml. Parallel experiments with the strains incubated only in PBS were performed as control. The survival of the bacteria in the nutrient-free media was followed by measuring the colony forming units by plating and the optical density of the suspension. The experiments were run until no bacterial growth could be detected in the suspensions and on the polymers. Viable cells isolated from the suspensions and from the polymers in the late stage of the experiment were subcultured and analysed with the methods described above. The polymers were analysed after ultrasonic cleaning.

Similar experiments were performed using the growth medium CDM with a starting inoculum of ~ 10^6 CFU/ml. After 2 days, a concentration of ~ 10^8 CFU/ml was measured which was stable until the end of the experiment after 30 days. Isolated bacteria and polymers were examined in the same manner already described.

RESULTS

The strains KH 11 and KH 6 were classified according to KLOOS and SCHLEIFER (ref. 4) as *S. epidermidis* sensu stricto. Differences in their biochemical and physiological behaviour are listed in table 1.

KH 6 proved to be the more hydrophobic strain as determined by three different methods(table 2).

TABLE 1

Biochemical and physiological differences between KH 11 and KH 6

	Arginine-Dehydrolase activity	Urease activity	Slime production	Susceptibility to penicillin G + ampicillin
KH 11	+	-	++	+
KH 6	-	+	(+)	-

TABLE 2
Surface hydrophobicity of KH 11 and KH 6 determined by different methods and calculated surface free energy of the strains

	SAT	Binding to xylene (%)	water contact angle (^{o})	surface free energy (dyn/cm)
KH 11	3.2	40	14.1	67.9
KH 6	1.4	80	46.5	61.1

Different reactivity patterns were obtained with lectins Con A and Lens culinaris and with Poly-L-Lysine and Polybrene (table 3).

TABLE 3
Reactivity with lectins and with Poly-L-Lysine and Polybrene (slide agglutination test)

	Con A	Lens culinaris	Poly-L-Lysine	Polybrene
KH 11	+	-	+	+
KH 6	-	-	+	-

The water contact angles of TUFTANE and BIOMER were measured to 77.1^{o} and 78.9 ^{o}, respectively; the surface free energies were 41.9 dyn/cm (TUFTANE) and 39.2 dyn/cm (BIOMER). The liquid surface tensions of PBS and CDM were 72.4 dyn/cm and 72.3 dyn/cm.

Fig. 1 shows the results of the adhesion of the two S. epidermidis strains KH 11 and KH 6 to the polyetherurethanes in PBS. KH 6 adhered stronger to both polymers than KH 11. Almost no differences were found in the adhesion of the individual strains to the different polymers. Similar results were obtained in CDM (not shown).

No viable cells could be detected either in the buffer supensions or in the control after 18 days incubation for KH 6 and after 27 days for KH 11. The properties of these strains were similar to those of the original strains. However, both strains could be cultivated from the polymers after a longer period (KH 6: 20 days, KH 11 > 30 days). They showed the following alterations:

1) KH 11: The reactivity with Con A was lost;this property could be regained after 20 passages on blood agar. The surface hydrophobicity increased from 40 % to > 90 % binding to xylene. The ability to produce acid from glucose and mannose was reduced and urease activity appeared. Quantitative changes in the SDS-page pattern of extracellular proteins were observed .

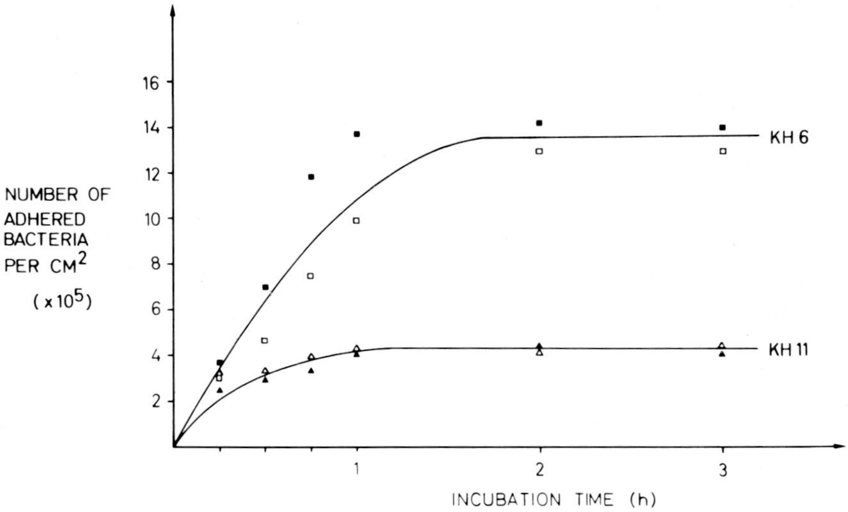

Fig. 1: Adhesion of KH 11 and KH 6 to TUFTANE (▲●) and BIOMER (△o) in PBS

2)KH 6: An increase in surface hydrophobicity from 80 % to > 90 % binding to xylene was the only observed difference.

The incubation performed in CDM instead of PBS revealed no changes of the strain properties in comparison with the original strains.

The analysis of the polymers TUFTANE and BIOMER performed after the end of the incubation period led to the following results: No detectable weight loss was observed. A slight increase in water uptake and in surface hydrophilicity was measured (the water contact angles decreased from 77.1^0 and 78.9^0 for the original polymers to ~ 72^0). Differential thermoanalysis showed a shift of the beginning of polymer decomposition to lower temperatures (TUFTANE: 232^{0}C → 225^{0}C, BIOMER: 204^{0}C → 196^{0}C). The ATR-FTIR spectra revealed no shift in the wave-numbers of characteristic polyetherurethane absorption bands; also no changes in the relative intensities of the urethane absorption and the polyether absorption could be observed.

DISCUSSION

The adhesion behaviour of *S. epidermidis* strains KH 11 and KH 6 to the polyetherurethanes TUFTANE and BIOMER stresses the role of hydrophobic bonding in the adhesion process. The more hydrophobic strain KH 6 adheres stronger to both polymers than the more hydrophilic strain KH 11. The adhesion of a single strain to the different polymers is similar; since both polymers have almost the same surface free energies, no differences in adhesion should be expected according to the thermodynamical model of Absolom et al. (ref. 9). This holds also for the adhesion performed in CDM instead of PBS. CDM has the same liquid surface tension as PBS, and no differences in the adhesion behaviour of the strains in the different media are observed.

The incubation of the strains with polyetherurethanes was performed in buffer and in a chemically defined growth medium. The buffer medium was chosen to establish an environment in which the polymers were the only possible nutrient source. The quantitative changes in the extracellular protein pattern of the strains isolated from the polymers could indicate an adaptation of bacterial metabolism to the new environment. The appearance of urease activity and the decrease in acid production from glucose and mannose further demonstrate a possible change in metabolism. The prolonged polymer contact leads to changes in bacterial surface properties as shown by a loss of Con A reactivity and an increase in hydrophobicity, supporting our assumption of specific interactions between polymer and bacteria.

Regarding a possible degradation of polymer chains caused by the bacteria,the appearance of urease activity is probably the most interesting observation. We assume that the presence of the polyetherurethanes with their urethane (-NH-CO-O) and urea (-NH-CO-NH)-groups induce urease activity. Our physicochemical analysis of the polymers could not directly detect a cleavage of urethane- or urea bonds by the bacteria; however we cannot totally exclude a bacterial degradation, since the applied methods were probably not sensitive enough to detect minor changes. Investigations of the polymers with more sensitive tools like mass spectrometry and Electron Spectroscopy for Chemical Analysis (ESCA)are in progress.

REFERENCES

1 G. D. Christensen, W. A. Simpson, W. A. Bisno, E. H. Beachey, Infect.Immun., 37 (1982) 318.
2 A. H. Hogt, J. Dankert, J. A. de Vries, J. Feijen, J. Gen. Microbiol., 129 (1983) 2959 - 2968.
3 A. Ludwicka, B., Jansen, T. Wadström, L. M. Switalski, G. Peters, G. Pulverer,in: S. W. Shalaby (Ed.) Polymers as Biomaterials, Plenum Publ. Corp.1984, 241 - 255.
4 W. E. Kloos, K. H. Schleifer, Int. J. Syst. Bacteriol., 25 (1975), 62 - 79.
5 M. Lindahl, A. Faris, T. Wadström, S. Hjertend, Biochim. Biophys. Acta, 677 (1981) 471 - 76.
6 M. Rosenberg, D. Gutnick, E. Rosenberg, FEMS Microbiol Lett., 9 (1980), 29 - 33.
7 C. J. van Oss, C. F. Gillman, J. Reticulo-endothel. Soc., 12 (1972) 497.
8 A. W. Neumann, R. J. Good, C. J. Hope, M. Sejpal, J. Coll. Interf. Sci. 49 (1974), 291 - 304.
9 D. R.Absolom, F. V. Lamberti, Z. Polikova, W. Zingg, C. J. van Oss, A. W. Neumann, Appl. Environm. Microbiol. 46 (1) (1983), 90 - 97.

Biomaterials and Clinical Applications,
edited by A. Pizzoferrato, P.G. Marchetti, A. Ravaglioli and A.J.C. Lee
Elsevier Science Publishers B.V., Amsterdam, 1987 — Printed in The Netherlands

INFECTION AT THE SITE OF IMPLANTS WITH VARIOUS MATERIALS AND ORGANISMS

K. MERRITT

Department of Biomedical Engineering, Case Western Reserve University
Cleveland Ohio, 44106, (U.S.A.)

SUMMARY

Infection at the site of an implanted material is a major reason for unsatisfactory performance of a device. It is well known that the presence of a foreign body increases the risk of infection by reducing the number of organisms required to establish an infection. Our studies indicate that the type of material is not very important in determining the risk of infection. The organisms involved may be very important in determining the risk of infection. Studies on infection associated with implanted materials and devices need to consider what organism or organisms are likely to cause infection at the site and these organisms should be used in establishing device or material safety.

INTRODUCTION

The use of sutures to close wounds was associated with a high risk of infection and prompted early studies on factors involved in infections at the site of foreign materials. It was demonstrated that it took 10^6 Staphylcoccus aureus organisms to establish an infection in normal human skin and only 10^2 organisms to cause an infection when a piece of suture was present at the site. Work on suture site infections was then extended to include studies on the chemical nature of the suture material (ref. 2) and the configuration of the suture (ref. 3). The infection risk was greatest when natural materials (provoking a strong inflammatory response) formed into multifilament strands were used. It was also shown that patients with a strong inflammatory response resulting from an allergic response to the suture material had a higher risk of infection than did the patients who were not allergic to the suture material (ref. 4). These findings have been very important in the design of devices for use in the body and have led to the use of inert, biocompatible materials. The materials used, the device used, and the implant sites involved are numerous.

The organism generally used in the studies on infection at implant sites has been *Staphylococcus aureus*. This is a common contaminant of the skin and nasopharynx and frequently causes infection following surgical procedures (ref. 5). However as the investigations of infection at various sites were evaluated, it became apparent that *S. aureus* was not always the most frequent cause of infection and that both the implant and the site had a major effect on the organism involved. It was soon discovered, beginning with studies on the teeth, that bacteria often would adhere to materials (ref. 6). Thus studies were begun on the ability of a variety of organisms to adhere to different materials. This includes various streptococci for dental materials, and coagulase negative staphylcocci (related to S. aureus but not as virulent, and biochemically quite different)(ref. 7-9). It is presumed that infection at the site of biomaterials may be associated with bacterial adherence. The studies presented here examine infection rates at the sites of different biomaterials and infection rates when various types of organisms are used.

METHODS

Implants: Stainless steel, Co-Cr alloys, titanium, alumina, polyethylene, and a polyester based resin.

Organisms: S. aureus, S. epidermidis (A) (which is adherent to polystyrene (ref 7)), S. epidermidis (NA) (which is not adherent to polystyrene), and Proteus mirabilis.

Animals: Balb C mice, 20-25 gms, either sex and golden hamsters, 110-150 gms, either sex, were used for these studies.

Surgical procedure: The animals were anaesthetized with sodium pentobarbital at a dose of 72 mg/kg. The back was shaved and disinfected with betadine, and a small incision was made over the regions of the left and the right pelvis using scissors. A tube with a trochar was then inserted through the incision and advanced subcutaneously to the region of the shoulder. The trochar was removed, leaving the tube in place. The implant was then inserted into the tube and driven out the end of the tube near the shoulder using the trochar. The tube and trochar were then carefully removed leaving the implant in the subcutaneous space. Each animal received 2 implants, one on the left and one on the right spaced at least 2 cm apart.

Injection of organisms: Organisms were grown in trypticase soy broth or nutrient broth for 18-24 hours. The organisms were then centrifuged, washed with saline, and resuspended to a Klett reading of 100 (Klett-Summerson Photometer). This is approximately 10^7 organisms per ml. The organisms were then diluted in saline until the appropriate concentration for each organism (10^4 to 10^7 per ml) was reached.

Evaluation of infection: The animals were sacrified 5 days after the injection of the organism. The implant sites were examined for visual signs of infection and then the implant and surrounding tissue was explanted aseptically. This implant with tissue was ground in saline and glass beads and plated for bacterial culture. An implant site with 100 or more organisms grown from the site was considered infected. The data from the bacterial culture are the ones included in the tables.

RESULTS

In this series of experiments, various types of implants were inserted into mice. Staphylococcus aureus was then injected into the implant site. Various doses of organisms were used and the dose that would cause infection in approximately 50% of the animals (ID_{50}) was determined. The data shown in Table 1 indicate that the dose is similar for all the materials with no statistically significant differences. A similar study was undertaken in the hamster using 3 materials and 3 organisms. Again the dose of a particular organism required to establish an infection was about the same for all materials. The doses of the different organisms was quite different. It is of interest to note that the Staphylococcus epidermidis strain chosen for these experiments was a nonadherent strain and yet it caused infection in these animals.

TABLE 1
Dose of organisms resulting in infection at 50% of the sites.
Comparison of different materials.

	Mouse	Hamster		
	S. aureus	S. aureus	Proteus	S. epidermidis (NA)
steel	10^5	10^4	10^5	10^6
Co-Cr	10^5			
Titanium	10^5			
Alumina	10^6	10^4	10^5	
polyethyl	10^6			
polyester		10^4	10^5	10^6
silk suture	$<10^2$	$<10^2$		

Studies were then undertaken to investigate the infection rate when only one type of organism was used and to compare this to the infection rate when two different organisms were used.

TABLE 3
Infection rates with stainless steel implants in the hamster using S. aureus, S. epidermidis, and Proteus alone and together.

S. aureus	Proteus	S. aureus + Proteus	S. epi	S. epi + Proteus
10^4= 30%	10^4=30%	10^4 + 10^4= 90%	10^5=40%	10^4+10^4=90%

The infection rate is much greater when the two organisms are mixed together. The dose of 10^4 plus 10^4 = 2x 10^4, not 10^8. A dose of 2x10^4 when the organisms are given alone does not alter the infection rate signficantly from that with 10^4. Thus the mixture of two different organisms at the site of an implant can markedly alter the risk of infection.

Since bacterial adherence is postulated to be important in development of infection at the site of an implant, tests were done to compare adherence of the S. epidermidis strains and the Proteus to the implant materials stainless steel, titanium, and various polymers. The Proteus did not adhere markedly to any of the materials. The adherent strain of S. epidermidis adhered more to the materials than did the nonadherent strain and both adhered more than did the Proteus. The adherence to the polymeric materials is approximately 10 times that to titanium. The adherence to titanium is approximately 10 fold that to stainless steel.

Since there was a large difference in adherence, it was decided to undertake some studies on infection and adherence. Two different studies were done. The first was to implant the stainless steel and then inject the organisms into the implant site 2 weeks later. The second was to immerse the material in a solution of the organism for 60 minutes, rinse it in saline to dislodge nonadherent organisms, and then implant it. The results shown in table 3 indicate the ability of both the adherent and the nonadherent S. epidermidis to cause infection at the site of the implant under both conditions. The infection data with the immersed samples is surprising since it would be anticipated that in a solution of 10^6 organisms only 100 organisms of the adherent strain would adhere to the implant and even fewer of the nonadherent strain would be present. Thus it apparently requires only a few organisms on the implant to develop an infection at the site.

TABLE 3
Adherence and infection using an adherent (A) and a nonadherent strain (NA) of Staphylococcus epidermidis.

	Infection with injected organisms		Infection from immersed materials	
	S. epi (A)	S. epi (NA)	S. epi (A)	S. epi (NA)
106	12/20	10/20	8/8	8/8
105			8/8	16/16
104			8/8	4/4

DISCUSSION

The presence of a foreign body does decrease the number of organisms required to establish an infection and thus increases the risk of infection. The nature of the material has little effect as long as it is biocompatible. In our studies the highest risk of infection was with suture with little difference in infection rate when stainless steel, cobalt-chromium alloys, titanium, dense ceramic, polyethylene, and polyester were used. This is in agreement with the study of Petty et al demonstrating that polymethyl methacrylate (PMMA) polymerizing in vivo and thus having some toxicity had a higher risk of infection than did the other inert materials such as stainless steel, titanium, polyethylene (ref 10). The question of organisms to use for testing is an important issue. The standard organism used is S. aureus. However our studies and others, especially the study reported by Petty et al (ref 10) indicate the appropriateness of using other types of organisms. The four organisms suggested would be S. aureus, a coagulase negative staphylococcus that is known to be adherent, a coagulase negative staphylcoccus that is non adherent, and a gram-negative enteric organism such as E. coli or Proteus. If the implant is being inserted into a site that has polymicrobial contamination such as the oral cavity, open fractures, and intestinal surgery, the four organisms should be used alone and all 4 together. If the implant is to be used in a location that is supposedly clean as in orthopaedic total joint replacement or vascular surgery, then the organisms need to be assessed separately.

How do we model the problem of infection at the site of implants so that we can minimize the risk to human patients? S. aureus is a virulent organism that causes infection at comparatively low doses (this study and ref 11). The gram negative organisms are virulent organisms causing infection at higher doses than S. aureus but at lower doses than the coagulase negative staphylococci. These two organisms given together result in a very high infection rate with low doses. Many of these infections can be prevented with the appropriate use of prophylactic antimicrobial agents but exacerbated by the inappropriate use of antimicrobial agents. Infection with coagulase negative staphylococci is a more difficult study to approach. High doses of these organisms are required in order to establish an infection at the site of an implant. Infection with these organisms is almost entirely limited to implant sites. It is believed that the ability of some of these organisms to adhere to implants is related to their ability to cause infection (ref. 7-9). Thus infection with these organisms may be related more to material properties than is infection with nonadherent organisms. However the data in our studies does not convince us yet that an adherent strain is any more infective than is a nonadherent strain. The coagulase negative staphylococcus used in ref 10 was not defined as adherent or nonadherent and high doses were required. Further careful studies are needed with these four organisms and candidate materials to study the relationship of bacterial adherence, material properties, and infection in order to minimize the risk of infection in patients with implants.

REFERENCES

1. S.D. Elek and P.D. Conen, The virulence of Staphylococcus pyogenes for man. A study of the problem of wound infections. Br. J. Exp. Pathol. 38 (1957) 573-576.
2. J.W. Alexander, J.Z. Kaplan, and W.A. Altemeier, Role of suture materials in the development of wound infections. Ann. Surg. 165 (1967) 192-195.
3. R.F. Edlich, P.H. Panek, G.T. Rodeheaver, J.D. Kurtz, and M.T. Edgerton, Surgical sutures and infection: A biomaterial evaluation. J. Biomed. Mater. Res. 8 (1974) 115-126.
4. L.C. Getzen and G.A. Jansen, Correlation between allergy to suture material and postoperative wound infections. Surgery 60 (1966) 824-827.
5. S.J. Jay, Nosocomial infections. Med. Clinics of N.A. 67-6 (1983) 1251-1277.
6. S.E. Mergenhagen and B. Rosan, Molecular Basis of Oral Microbial Adhesion, American Society for Microbiology, Washington, D.C. 1985.
7. G.D. Christensen, W.A. Simpson, J.J. Younger, L.M. Baddour, F.F. Barrett, D.M. Melton, and E.H. Beachley, Adherence of coagulase negative staphylococci to plastic tissue culture plates: A quantitative model for the adherence of staphylococci to medical devices. J. Clin. Microbiol. 22 (1985) 996-1006.
8. A.G. Gristina and J.W. Costerton, Bacterial adherence and the glyococalyx and their role in musculoskeletal infection. Orthop. Clinic. N.A. 15 (1984) 517- 535.
9. A.G. Gristina and J.W. Costerton, Bacterial adherence to biomaterials and tissue J. Bone Joint Surg. 67A (1985) 264-273.
10. W. Petty, S. Spanier, J.J. Shuster, and C. Silverthorne, The influence of skeletal implants on incidence of infection. Experiments in a canine model. J. Bone Joint Surg. 67A (1985) 1236-1244.

ACKNOWLEDGEMENTS

I would like to thank Karen Rittle for her help in some of the experiments. Supported in part by NIH AM 35908

Biomaterials and Clinical Applications,
edited by A. Pizzoferrato, P.G. Marchetti, A. Ravaglioli and A.J.C. Lee
Elsevier Science Publishers B.V., Amsterdam, 1987 — Printed in The Netherlands

ALLERGIC REACTIONS TO MATERIALS USED IN PROSTHETIC SURGERY

Katharine Merritt

Department of Biomedical Engineering, Case Western Reserve University
Cleveland, Ohio, 44106, (USA)

SUMMARY

It is estimated that at least 15% of the normal human population is allergic to metal as manifested by skin testing with metal salt solutions. The allergy develops from contact with jewelry, metal salt solutions or corroded metals in the workplace, or by contact with cookware and other activities of daily living. Prosthetic devices implanted into patients are often made of the same materials to which the patients are allergic and there is concern about the role of allergy in the failure of these devices to function appropriately. It is well documented that allergic reactions to components of the device materials have necessitated the premature removal of various devices but that the percentage of the population that has such reactions is extremely small. The problem in individual patients needs to be recognized and the magnitude of the problem in the entire population needs to be kept in perspective. Allergic reactions to acrylics and other polymeric materials are less common than allergy to metals but the possibility of reactions in patients with prosthetic devices remains a concern.

INTRODUCTION

The immune response is an important defense mechanism responsible for protecting us against infection by micro-organisms. However in some instances the immune system in eliminating a foreign substance that might of itself cause no harm, releases a variety of soluble substances that provoke a strong inflammatory response and thus inadvertently causes harm to the host. This is generally referred to as an allergic reaction. The actual mechanism of this allergic reaction varies from substance to substance (ref. 1). The metallic ions nickel, cobalt, and chromium are among the most frequent causes of allergy. This allergy is generally caused by the contact of the metal ion as a salt or a corrosion product with the skin of the indvidual. The metal ion combines with skin proteins and becomes an allergen. This response is referred to as contact dermatitis because it results from skin contact and the reaction is manifest in the skin. The actual percentage of the population sensitive to metals varies probably reflecting life styles in different countries or different regions and ethnic backgrounds. The estimates would indicate that about 15% of the population is sensitive to nickel, 8% sensitive to chromium, with the sensitvity to cobalt not studied as thoroughly but probably similar to that of nickel (ref. 2-3). With sensitivity to these metals so common, concern has been raised about the possibility of sensitivity reactions to implanted materials occurring because of a reaction to a component of the material.

This question raises several questions. The first one is: Do metal ions enter the body from an implanted material? This question has generated alot of discussion and scientific investigation. The answer to this question is an unequivocal yes. This is important since the sensitivity reaction develops not to the implant itself but to the metal released from the implant into solution. This release may be as metal ions or as metal cell or metal protein complexes. Whether the metals are released as metal ions or organo-metallic complexes is important for the electrochemistry of corrosion mechanisms. The important point from the immunologic point of view is that the metal is released and capable of binding to cells and proteins and thus able to stimulate the immune response. Thus for simplicity the release will be referred to as metal ions indicating that particular metal is in solution and not part of the bulk material or particle of metal. Numerous studies have shown that immersion in salt or protein solutions will result in metal ions being released into solution (ref. 4-5). It is also apparent in studies on retrieved implants that there has been wear and corrosion and loss of metal into the body (ref 6). Thus development of allergic reactions is possible.

The second question is whether or not there is something peculiar about the environment in the skin that results in a contact dermatitis but that such a reaction cannot develop in the deep tissue. There is not agreement on the answer to this question but in general the answer is that such a reaction can occur in any deep tissue that has the necessary components: antigen processing and presenting cells, T and B lymphocytes, and a lymphatic and vascular supply (ref. 7). There does not seem to be anything unique in the immunologic reaction of the skin but it is also apparent that there are tissues that are "immunologically privileged" and either do not have the necessary components or give different responses. These tissues are of concern for the investigator considering implants in these tissues. These tissues include portions of the eye, portions of the brain, and may include the bone marrow and the oral cavity. Thus any discussion of allergic reactions to prosthetic devices must include considerations of the type of material, the type of device, the wear and corrosion potential of the device in its ultimate application, and the tissue into which the device is placed

The concern about allergic reactions to metallic implants was stimulated by the studies on patients who were apparently reacting to total hip replacements (ref. 8-9). These were metal articulating with metal prostheses and the problem of loosening and pain was associated with the presence of a metal allergy as manifest by skin testing (thus a contact dermatitis). Subsequent studies on patients receiving metal articulating with plastic total hips has indicated patients with metal sensitivity but no evidence that there was a metal sensitivity reaction to the device (ref. 10-11). Thus at this time it is recognized that the metal-metal total joints pose a problem for the allergic patient and that there is no evidence that there is a problem with the metal-plastic devices. The concern in total joint surgery now resides with the use of the biological fixation devices requiring tissue ingrowth and bony fixation. These devices are of the metal-plastic type but there is extensive bone-metal and tissue-metal contact. Will this cause a problem?

The analysis of patients with fracture fixation devices has indicated that allergic reactions to these implants do occur and that the reaction is to a variety of fixation devices including plates, screws, rods, and pins (ref. 1). The reactions are manifest in a variety of ways including inflammation, pain, skin rashes and evidence of implant loosening or bone resportion. In most cases, the fracture has healed or almost healed by the time the allergic reaction has developed and signs and symptoms are manifest. Thus removal of the device is generally of little consequence and relieves the problem. Thus it seems to be accepted by the orthopaedic community that allergic reactions to implants can occur and that with the exception of reactions to total joint replacements, the consequences of such reaction are minimal.

Similar thoughts are given to many other implants causing such reactions. Reactions to metal sutures, infusion needles, and surface electrodes occur (ref 1), but again the device can be removed and easily replaced. With the increasing use of implanted stimulating devices with many tiny electrodes implanted into bone and into muscles, allergic reactions may become important since removal and replacement of the electrodes will not be simple. Other surgical specialities such as otolaryngology and neurology may also be faced with problems if metallic implants are placed into immunologically functional tissue.

The other major speciality, in addition to orthopaedic surgery, where metallic implants are being used and where the issue of metal sensitivity reactions is important is in the field of dentistry. The bulk of dental materials are inserted into the oral cavity so as to be in contact with the oral cavity and the buccal and gingival mucosa rather than embedded in tissue. The oral cavity has some unique immunologic characteristics which need to be considered in addressing the issue of metal sensitivity (ref. 12). The major questions from the immunological side are : Can substances in the mouth actually stimulate a new immune response? Are the necessary immunologic components of antigen processing cells, antigen presenting cells, and the necessary trafficking of T and B cells present? Do the substances in the mouth activate an immune response that has already developed? Do the substances in the mouth stimulate immune responses that have a reaction manifest in other parts of the body (ie is there systemic activation)? Do substances in the mouth depress the specific immune system resulting in immunologic unresponsiveness to this antigen? Should we take advantage of this capacity for unresponsiveness? Since we do not know the answers to the first questions on immunologic activation, the answer to the last question is that we should not try an alter a response that we do not know much about. We may get exactly the opposite result from that anticipated.

It is the general assumption that implants inserted into the tissue in oral surgery, such as tempero-mandibular joints, tooth root replacements, and fracture fixation devices are in contact with tissue similar to that observed in orthopaedic surgery and that the same rules apply. However this has never actually been documented and some studies similar to those being undertaken in patients with orthopaedic implants should be undertaken in dental patients with implants embedded in the tissue. Sensitivity reactions to dental implants in the oral cavity have been reported and are in many cases well documented (ref. 13-14).

What are the consequences of allergic reactions to metallic implants? The reactions are usually manifest as the signs of inflammation with pain and swelling being the major complaints of the patients. The long term consequences include alterations in the risk of infection, general toxicity reactions, overstimulation of the phagocytic responses of host cells with accumulation of superoxide and other oxidative intermediates with subsequent toxicity and extensive bone resorption.

A great deal of work has been done on the role of allergic reactions in the failure of metallic implants to function as intended. However major questions remain including the question of how to test for sensitivity and how to test for sensitivity reactions. The use of in vitro testing with peripheral blood for the production of a lymphokine such as migration inhibition factor or lymphocyte transformation factor is safer for the patient than is skin testing (ref. 1, 15-16) but is not accepted by the medical community for three basic reasons: (1) the in vitro testing procedures, although easy to do, are limited to a few centers, (2) there is enough variation from laboratory to laboratory in the details of the technique (especially concentration of metals) that standard protocols will be difficult to produce unless a large enough market for the tests is present so that development of test kits is worthwhile, (3) the skin test is the "standard" of the community and results of in vitro tests are not accepted by some physicians and the insurance companies. Although the skin test is the acceptable test, there are many problems with it. The first problem is the possibility of causing sensitivity with repeat testing, the second problem is convincing the dermatologist or allergest to include the appropriate metals into the testing protocol (ref 17), and the third is the misuse of the test by the surgeon. The skin test needs to be done with metal salts in the appropriate concentration as an epicutaneous or subcutaneous application (ref 18-19). Skin tesing with the device or a piece cut from the device is misleading and inappropriate. There is still discussion as to whether metal salts or corrosion products should be used for both skin testing and in vitro assays. To date the only available safe and efficacious test material is the metal salt solution.

There are still many basic studies to be undertaken on the problem of metal sensitivity. One of the major ones remaining concerns the safety of the alternatives. We know that nickel, cobalt, and chromium cause allergic reactions and are toxic. Can we say that vanadium, aluminum, titanium as well as all the metals used in dental procedures are safe? (ref 13,14,17). We need proof that something is better before abandoning others. Allergy to textiles occurs,but in lower frequency,and the reaction is usually to the components and not the polymer (ref 21-22). The rules of testing are similar to that for metals. The risk benefit ratios are the important factors in deciding whether or not to use a device and whether or not to substitute another material. A patient who has reacted to a previous implant is likely to react to another implant of the same material. Other than that, we cannot predict who is likely to have an allergic reaction necessitating premature device removal.

Studies on the major questions on allergic reactions to materials used in prosthetic surgery continue. The topics of implant corrosion and release and transport of metals, the use of in vitro testing for sensitivity and toxicity, sensitivity reactions to polymeric materials, and general considerations of foreign body reactions, inflammatory reactions and host defense mechanisms are the subject of other papers in this conference. This is an active area of investigation and there are many studies yet to be done.

REFERENCES

1. K. Merritt and S. Brown, Hypersensitivity to metallic biomaterials, in:D.F. Williams (Ed), Systemic Aspecits of Biocompatibility, CRC Press, Boca Raton, Fla. 1981, II: 33-48.
2. E.J. Rudner, W.E. Clendenning, E. Epstein, A.A. Fisher, O.F. Jillson, W.P. Jordan, N. Kanof, W. Larsen, H. Maibach, J.C. Mitchell, S.E. O'Quinn, W.F. Schorr, M.B. Sulzberger, The frequency of contact dermatitis in North America 1972-1974, Contact Dermatitis 1 (1975) 277-280.
3. L. Peltonen, Nickel sensitivity in the general population, Contact Dermatitis 5(1979) 27-32.
4. M.H. Samitz and S.A. Katz, Nickel dermatitis hazards from prostheses, Br. J. Dermatol. 92 (1975) 287-289.
5. J. Black, Systemic effects of biomaterials, Biomaterials 5 (1984) 11-18.
6. J.P. Simpson, V. Geret, S.A. Brown, K. Merritt, Retrieved fracture plates: implant and tissue analysis, in: A. Weinstein, D. Gibbons, S. Brown, W. Ruff (eds) Implant Retrieval: Material and Biological Analyses, NBS, Washington, D.C. SP 601 (1981) 395-422.
7. J.D. Bos and M.L. Kapsenberg, The skin immune system: its cellular constituents and their interactions. Immunology Today 7 (1986) 235-240.
8. M.K.D. Benson, P.G. Goodwin, and J. Boostoff, Metal sensitivity in patients with joint replacement, Br. Med. J. 4 (1975) 374-375.

9. M.W. Elves, J.N. Wilson, J.T. Scales, and H.B.S. Kemp, Incidence of metal sensitivity in patients with total joint replacements, Br. Med. J. 4 (1975) 376-378.
10. R. Duetman, T.J. Mulder, R. Brian, and J.P. Nater, Metal sensitivity before and after total hip arthroplasty, J. Bone Jt. Surg. 59 (1977) 862-864.
11. A.H. Waterman and J.J. Schrik, Allergy in hip arthroplasty, Contact Dermatitis 13 (1985) 294-301.
12. L.R. Eversole, Allergic stomatitides, J. Oral Med. 34 (1979) 93-102.
13. K. Merritt, Biochemistry/Hypersensitity/Clinical Reaction in: B.R. Lang, H.F. Morris, M.E. Razzoog (eds). International Workshop on Biocompatibility, Toxicity, and Hypersensitivity to Alloy Systems used in Dentistry, Ann Arbor, 1986.
14. A. Hensten-Pettersen, Dermatitis and dental materials, Contact Dermatitis 7 (1981) 174-175.
15. J.E. Clausen, Cell migration inhibition in agarose, in: N.R. Rose and H Friedman (eds), Manual of Clinical Immunology, ASM, Washington, D.C. 1976, pp. 101-105.
16. M.W. Elves, Transformation in the presence of metals of lymphocytes from patients with total joint prostheses, J. Pathol. 122 (1977) 35-38.
17. L.A.J. Van Loon, P.W. van Elsas, Th. van Joost, and C.L. Davidson, Test battery for metal allergy in dentistry, Contact Dermatitis 14 (1986) 158-161.
18. T. Fischer and H. Maibach, Aluminum in Finn chambers reacts with cobalt and nickel salts in patch test materials, Contact Dermatitis 12 (1985) 200-202.
19. J.E. Wahlberg and E. Wahlberg, Skin irritancy from nickel sulfate and test patches, Contact Dermatitis 13 (1985) 224-225.
20. T. Fischer and I. Rystedt, False-positive, follicular and irritant patch test reactions to metal salts, Contact Dermatitis 12 (1985) 93-98.
21. K.L. Hatch and H.I. Maibach, Textile fiber dermatitis, Contact Dermatitis 12 (1985) 1-11.
22. B.W. Boom and L.M.J. van Driel, Allergic contact dermatitis to epoxy resin in infusion sets of an insulin pump, Contact Dermatitis 12 (1985) 280.

Biomaterials and Clinical Applications,
edited by A. Pizzoferrato, P.G. Marchetti, A. Ravaglioli and A.J.C. Lee
Elsevier Science Publishers B.V., Amsterdam, 1987 — Printed in The Netherlands

AN IN VIVO MODEL FOR QUANTIFICATION OF METAL ION RELEASE AND TRANSPORT

S.A. BROWN, K. MERRITT, L.J. FARNSWORTH, and T.D. CROWE

Department of Biomedical Engineering, Case Western Reserve University
Cleveland Ohio, 44106, (U.S.A.)

SUMMARY

An accelerated corrosion method has been developed which permits calculation of ion release rates from implants in vitro and in vivo, for comparison with measurements of metal ion concentrations in the in vitro solutions, as well as in blood and urine. The results demonstrate that Faraday's law can be used to calculate the amount of metal ion release. Release rates are in proportion to alloy composition. Urine excretion levels of nickel are equal to the amount released, most of the cobalt is excreted. The excretion of chromium represents a small percentage of the amount released in vivo. Chromium released in saline has a valence of +3, a combination of +3 and +6 are released in serum and in vivo.

INTRODUCTION

A number of approaches have been taken to study corrosion and metal ion release from implants. Electrochemical methods have been utilized in a number of studies to measure corrosion rates in vivo (refs.1-2). However, these studies have not related the corrosion rates with the release and transport of corrosion products. Ferguson et al (ref. 3) implanted solid metal cylinders in muscle in rabbits and demonstrated that metal ions are released and transported in vivo. In studies with metal powders, Black and co-workers (refs. 4-5) have shown that metal ion concentrations in blood components and urine indicate significant nickel release which is not in proportion to the alloy composition. Chemical analysis of tissues adjacent to implants as well as analysis of hair and urine from humans have also shown significant amounts of metal ion release (ref. 6). While these studies have measured release, the amount or rate of release and transport in various compartments has not been correlated with the actual corrosion rates.

The objectives of the present study were to to develop a method of accelerating corrosion of implant specimens in vitro and in vivo, and to use weight loss and corrosion current measurements to calculate the amount of metal ion release. Because of the biological activity of chromium with a valence of +6 (refs. 7-9) the correlation between the measured and calculated metal ion data using Cr+3 and Cr+6 was examined to determine the valence of chromium release. The relationship between release rates, blood levels and excretion rates can thus be established.

METHODS

A PAR 363 potentiostat was used to apply fixed anodic potentials relative to a saturated calomel electrode (SCE) to the test specimens for 30 or 60 minutes. A Linear strip chart recorder was used to record the corrosion current. Current recordings were integrated to determine total charge (Q). Potentials were maintained at 500 mV or 750 mV relative to a saturated calomel reference electrode. The specimens used were 4 mm 316L stainless steel rods (13.69% Ni, 17.25% Cr, 2.08% Mo), 4 mm cast Vitallium nails (0.41% Ni, 28.03% Cr, 5.48% Mo), and 3.2 mm F-75 rods with 25 mm coated with 200 um beads (Bio-Vac,Southfield MI). The solid rods were cut in 30 mm lengths and were sanded to 600 grit within 1 hour of exposure of a 25 mm length to the test environment. The porous coated rods were passivated as per F-86. Implants were ultrasonically cleaned, dried and weighed on a Mettler AE-163 microbalance before and after each experiment to determine weight loss.

In vitro experiments were conducted with the test specimens inserted through a silicone rubber gasket in the bottom of the test chamber. The in vitro test solutions were 35 ml of 0.9% NaCl and a 10% solution of calf serum (GIBCO) in saline. A luggin probe was used as a salt bridge to the reference electrode. Stainless steel counter electrodes were inserted directly into the test solutions in vitro.

In vivo experients were performed with the test specimens placed subcutaneously in the back of Syrian hamsters anaesthetized with pentobarbital (7.2mg/100g). The rods were inserted through a small incision in lower back. A saline soaked cotton sponge was used as a bridge for in vivo experiments. The abdomen of the hamsters were shaved and they were placed on the stainless steel counter electrode which had been coated with electrode paste. In one series, porous coated rods were implanted for 10 days prior to initiation of the corrosion experiment. All hamsters were maintained on water and food ad lib. They were housed individually in metabolic cages for collection of pretest 24 hour urine samples and for 3 or 4 days after an experiment for collection of 24 hour samples.

Chemical analysis of individual saline, serum and urine samples was performed by graphite furnace atomic absorption spectroscopy (GFAAS) with a Perkin Elmer 2380 and a HGA-400 furnace. Samples were diluted as necessary with nitric acid. The data have been corrected for background levels of the individual elements.

The weight loss and metal ion release were also calculated using Faraday's Law which states that the amount of weight loss (W) of a pure metal is equal to the total charge (Q), times the atomic weight (M), divided by the valence (n), and Faraday's constant (F):$W=QM/nF$. To correct for alloy composition, proportionality coefficients were calculated. The number of electrons transfered for each element is equal to the percentage of the element in the alloy (P), times its valence (n) and Avogadro's number (N), divided by its atomic weight (A): (PnN/A). The total charge transferred is equal to the sum of the elemental contributions. The fraction of charge associated with each element is therefore: f=(PnN/A)/(sum of all PnN/A's). The weight of the individual element released was then equal to fQM/nF. A valence of the elements used in the calculations were: Ni=2, Co=2, Fe=2, Mo=3 and Cr=3 and 6.

Weight loss of stainless steel and concentration of metals in solutions were measured directly and are presented as mean value with standard deviation in parentheses. Average values are presented for metal ion release calculated from weight loss, and for weight loss and metal ion release calculated from Faraday's law using +3 and +6 for the valence of chromium. The comparisons between measured and calculated data are expressed as percent recovery (100 x measured/calculated).

RESULTS AND DISCUSSION

The measured and calculated weight loss data for 6 stainless steel rods in saline, 5 in 10% serum and 6 in vivo are shown in Table 1. These data indicate that the weight loss of stainless steel at 500 mV for 30 minutes in saline is greater than in serum (69%, p<.001) and greater than in vivo (65%, p,.005). The differences between serum and in vivo were not statistically significant. These results demonstrate the opposite effect of serum on accelerated corrosion that we observed at 5 volts (10).

Calculations of weight loss with Faraday's law indicate that with chrome +3, the measured weight loss in saline of 1.85 milligrams was 101% of the calculated value of 1.83. With Chromium +6, the value in saline was statistically different from the measured value, indicating that chromium release in saline is not as +6. There is very close agreement for the calculated values in serum and in vivo using chromium +3. The differences in serum and in vivo are not significant, and thus the form of release in these environments is equivocal.

The measured and calculated values for nickel release from stainless steel in saline, serum and 4 days of urine are shown in Table 2. The calculations based on weight loss indicate somewhat less was recovered than predicted. The calculations based on Faradays law indicate a low recovery rate with chromium +3 and a high recovery rate with chromium +6. None of these differences are statistically significant, and therefore it is not clear which valence is correct. It should be noted that the recovery rate in urine is very close to that in vitro and is in proportion to alloy composition.

Analysis for chromium in saline and serum from stainless steel shown in

Table 3 showed a similar close agreement between measured and calculated values using weight loss and chromium +3. The chromium value with +6 in saline is significantly different, again indicating +3 release in saline. The Cr+3, +6 differences in serum are equivocal. However, only 7 to 9 percent of the calculated in vivo release of chromium was excreted in four days. Based on the in vitro data and the calculations for nickel and weight loss, it can be assumed that the release of chromium was close to calculations. Therefore, chromium was not being excreted in proportion to its release but was being stored in the animal tissues.

Table 4 shows the total charge and measured and calculated values for nickel release from 6 vitallium rods in saline, 6 in serum, 7 in vivo, and 1 in vivo that had a very high corrosion current. These were tested for 30 minutes at 500 mV (SCE). Excluding the high corrosion specimen, the data show very high release of nickel compared to the calculated levels. However, the measured values are very close to the detection limits of the machine; 0.68ug/35ml is equal to 19 ppb. The calculated values (.02 ug/35ml = 0.5ppb) are well below the detection limits. The release from the one in vivo sample was very close to predictions using chromium +6.

Table 5 shows the measured and calculated values for cobalt and chromium from solid vitallium rods. The values are quite reasonable although chromium is low in saline and in vivo. The one in vivo specimen fits well with calculations for cobalt and, like stainless steel, indicates low chromium excretion.

Preliminary results with porous coated F-75 rods are presented in Table 6. The table shows the total charge and calculated percent recovery rates for weight loss and metal ion release from 2 rods in saline and 4 in vivo at 500 mV (SCE) for 30 minutes and 3 rods in saline and 7 in vivo held at 775 mV (SCE) for 60 minutes. There are two sets of in vivo data. In the first group (4 animals) the potential was applied within 5 minutes of insertion, in the "implant" group (3 animals) the specimens were implanted for 10 days prior to the experiment.

The results at 500 mV are similar to those seen with solid vitallium at 500 mV; very high nickel release and low chromium. At 775 mV, in saline the weight loss, nickel, and cobalt are close to calculated, chromium is low. The data are closer with chrome +6. In both in vivo groups, the nickel release was reasonable. It is clear that some cobalt and most of the chromium are not being excreted. It is not clear as to whether Chromium +3 or chromium +6 gives the more accurate results.

In conclusion, the method permits the calculation of metal ion release from weight loss and charge with stainless steel. Chrome release in saline is as +3, and probably a combination of +3 and +6 in serum and in vivo. As with the injection of salts, nickel from in vivo corrosion is excreted, chromium is not. Chromium is in the red cells and the tissues (refs. 8-9).

With Cobalt-chromium-molybdenum alloy, nickel release seems high when the levels are near the level of detection. When the corrosion rate is high enough to accurately measure current and metal ion concentrations, release is in proportion to alloy composition, chrome release may be as +6. Nickel is excreted while chromium is stored.

TABLE 1

Weight loss of solid stainless steel rods as measured, and calculated values and percent (100 x meas/calc) based on total charge measurements.

Solution	MEASURED (mg)	CALCULATED Cr+3		CALCULATED Cr+6	
Saline	1.85(.34)	1.83	101%	*1.46	127%
10% serum	0.58(.57)	0.55	105%	0.44	132%
In Vivo	0.62(.23)	0.58	107%	0.46	135%

* p<.05 significantly different

TABLE 2

Nickel in solutions from solid stainless steel rods as measured, calculated from weight loss and charge, and percent recovery.

solution	MEASURED (ug)	CALCULATED -Wt.loss-		--Cr +3--		--Cr +6--	
saline	221(103)	253	87%	249	89%	198	112%
10% serum	57(37)	79	72%	75	76%	60	95%
in vivo	73(35)	85	86%	78	94%	62	118%

TABLE 3

Chromium in solutions from solid stainless steel rods as measured, calculated from weight loss and charge, and percent recovery.

solution	MEASURED (ug)	CALCULATED -Wt.loss-		--Cr +3--		--Cr +6--	
saline	341(45)	319	107%	314	109%	*251	136%
10% serum	89(83)	100	89%	95	94%	76	117%
in vivo	7(4)	*107	7%	*99	7%	*79	9%

* p<.005 significantly different

TABLE 4

Total charge and nickel release from solid Vitallium rods as measured and calculated from charge, and percent recovery.

SOLN	CHARGE (Coul)	MEASURED (ug)	CALCULATED ---Cr+3---		---Cr+6---	
saline	.021(.005)	.68(.45)	.02	3400%	.01	6800%
serum	.029(.005)	.17(.05)	.03	567%	.02	850%
in vivo	.026(.003)	.63(.28)	.02	3150%	.02	3150%
1 in vivo	5.005	3.20	4.57	70%	3.04	105%

TABLE 5

Cobalt and chromium release from solid Vitallium rods as measured, as calculated from charge, and percent recovery.

soln	MEASURED (ug)		CAL RELEASE				CAL %			
			Cr+3		Cr+6		Cr+3		Cr+6	
	Co	Cr	Co	Cr	Co	Cr	Co	Cr	Co	Cr
sal	5.1(2.6)	.6(.2)	3.5	1.5	2.5	1.1	147%	41%	205%	57%
ser	9.7(4.9)	.8(.2)	4.9	2.1	3.5	1.5	197%	40%	275%	55%
vivo	4.1(0.9)	.9(.3)	4.3	1.8	3.1	1.3	96%	50%	134%	70%
1 vivo	949	98	836	354	599	254	114%	28%	159%	38%

TABLE 6

Total charge, and percent recovery of weight loss and metal ions from porous coated F-75 rods.

	CHARGE	Cr+3 WL	Cr+3 Ni	Cr+3 Co	Cr+3 Cr	Cr+6 WL	Cr+6 Ni	Cr+6 Co	Cr+6 Cr
500 mV:									
saline	.08(0)	403	604	92	42	562	906	128	59
in vivo	.15(.1)	98	1335	41	38	137	2003	57	53
775 mV:									
saline	1.70(.2)	83	180	73	44	116	270	102	61
in vivo	1.60(.4)	80	129	40	21	112	193	56	29
implant	4.59(1.4)	--	59	40	24	--	89	55	33

ACKNOWLEDGEMENTS

This work was funded in part by USPHS NIH grant AM-35590. Donation of the porous coated F-75 specimens by Bio-Vac, Inc. is gratefully acknowledged.

REFERENCES

1 S. Steineman, Corrosion of surgical implants, in: G. Winter, J. Leray, K. de Groot (Eds.), Evaluation of Biomaterials, Wiley, Chichester, 1980, pp. 1-34.
2 S.A. Brown and J. Simpson, Crevice and fretting corrosion of stainless steel plates and screws, J. Biomed. Mater. Res., 15, (1981) 867-878.
3 A.B. Ferguson, Jr., Y. Akahoshi, P.G.Laing, and E.S. Hodge, Characteristics of trace ions released from embedded metal implants in rabbits, J. Bone Joint Surg. 44A (1962), 317-322.
4 J.L Woodman, J. Black and S.A. Jiminez, Isolation of serum protein organometallic corrosion products from 316LSS and HS-21 invitro and invivo, J. Biomed. Mater. Res. 18 (1984) 99-114.
5 A. Koegel and J. Black, Release of corrosion products by F-75 cobalt base alloy in the rat, J. Biomed. Mater. Res. 18 (1984) 513-522.
6 R. Owen, G. Meachim and D.F. Williams, Hair sampling for chromium content following Charnley hip arthroplasty, J. Biomed. Mater. Res. 10 (1976) 91-99.
7 S.J. Gray and K. Stirling, Tagging of red cells and plasma with radioactive chromium, J. Clin. Invest. 29 (1950), 1604-1613.
8 K. Merritt, S.A. Brown and N.A. Sharkey, The binding of metal salts and corrosion products in vitro, J. Biomed. Mater. Res. 18 (1984) 1005-1015.
9 K. Merritt, S.A. Brown and N.A. Sharkey, Blood distribution of nickel, cobalt and chromium following intramuscular injection into hamsters. J. Biomed. Mater. Res. 18 (1984) 991-1004.
10 S.A. Brown and K. Merritt, Electrochemical corrosion in saline and serum, J. Biomed. Mater. Res. 14 (1980) 173-175.

Biomaterials and Clinical Applications,
edited by A. Pizzoferrato, P.G. Marchetti, A. Ravaglioli and A.J.C. Lee
Elsevier Science Publishers B.V., Amsterdam, 1987 — Printed in The Netherlands

QUANTITATIVE EXPRESSION OF T-LYMPHOCYTE SURFACE ANTIGENS IN CHRONIC DIALYSIS PATIENTS

S. STEFONI, A. NANNI COSTA, S. IANNELLI, L.C. BORGNINO, T. D'ATENA, M.P.SCOLARI, V. BONOMINI

Department of Nephrology and Dialysis, S.Orsola University Hospital,via Massarenti 9, 40138 Bologna, Italy

SUMMARY

The blood components of uremic patients on artificial substitution therapy come in close contact with foreign materials for more than 600 hours a year. The possible effects of various dialysis membranes on patients' lymphocytes were studied considering those cells from a dual point of view: as key elements of the immune system and as representating a cellular biological system; in particular, the present study deals with the quantitative expression of specific glicoproteic antigens (T3,T4,T8) placed on the surface of T-lymphocytes. Recent studies have pointed out the role of T3, T4 and T8 molecules in recognition of foreign antigens and in immune response. The fact that these molecules are only faintly expressed on the lymphocyte surface may help to explain the pathogenesis of the acquired immunodeficiency detectable in dialysis patients.

Biocompatibility evaluation of artificial materials currently used in dialysis treatment

The blood components of uremic patients on artificial substitution therapy come in close contact with foreign materials for more than 600 hours a year. These repeated extracorporeal circulations may modify the reactivity of the various blood component both directly through chemical, biophysical and mechanical interactions and indirectly by transmission of the message of the contact with the foreign surface .

Proper evaluation of biocompatibility and clinical tolerance of biomaterials currently used in chronic dialysis is therefore becoming more and more important, and entails a complex appraisal extending beyond the usual hematochemical parameters. Studies should concern both acute and chronic aspects of hemocompatibility, while the tests used should investigate both humoral and cellular parameters (1).

In this paper we examine the possible action of various dialysis membranes on the lymphocyte populations, considered from a dual point of view: as key elements of the immune system and as representating a cellular biological system (2).

Lymphocyte impairement in chronic dialysis patients

Chronic renal failure is characterized by an acquired immunodeficiency which involves marked changes in humoral and cellular immunity (3,4); the high incidence of infections, enhanced graft tolerance, a reduced tumor surveillance and cutaneous anergy are some of the main clinical expressions of such impairment(5,6) .

The immunopathogenetic mechanisms of these alterations are still unclear, despite the various factors claimed as responsible , such as uremic toxins, malnutrition, blood transfusions, piridoxyne deficiency, continuous disruptions of the mucocutaneous barrier between host and environment,etc.(7). One possible cause of the immunological abnormalities among patients on artificial substitutive therapy might be their cyclical and repeated contacts with the various artificial membranes and materials currently used for chronic hemodialysis (8) .

The present study deals with the evaluation of the quantitative expression of specific glicoproteic antigens (T3,T4,T8) placed on the surface of T-lymphocytes. These rather sophisticated analyses are now possible thanks to the availability and employment of new technologies such as flow cytometry(9) and monoclonal antibodies in clinical research.

PATIENTS AND METHODS

The study included 31 patients on RDT,18 males and 13 females, ranging in age from 17 to 64 years (mean 43±10), free from any intercurrent disease,who had been on chronic treatment for at least 1 year (mean duration 53±18 months) .

Three different groups have been considered : Group 1) 15 patients on dialysis with cuprophan membrane (CU); Group 2) 8 patients with polyacrylonitrile membrane (PAN); Group 3) 8 patients on a combined hemodialysis/hemoperfusion treatment with activated charcoal coated by a methacrilate membrane(CH)(10). Data from 15 normal subjects were used as controls .

Separation of lymphocytes Peripheral blood lymphocytes were separated from freshly heparinized blood on a Ficoll-Hypaque gradient (Pharmacia,Uppsala,Sweden) by centrifugation. Mononuclear cells were collected from the plasma gradient interface, washed twice in Hanks Balanced Salt Solution and resuspended in RPMI 1640 culture medium(Gibco,Paisley,Scotland) .

T-cell subsets analysis The assessment of the various T-lymphocyte subsets was performed using murine monoclonal antibodies specific for T3, T4 and T8 T-lymphocyte membrane bound antigens, originally described (11) as marker for total T cells (OKT3-Ortho Diagnostic System, Raritan, USA), T-helper/inducer cells (OKT4), T-suppressor/cytotoxic cells (OKT8): a 0,2 ml of the mononuclear suspension (1 X 10^6 cells/ml) was added to 2 ul of fluorescein isothiocyanate-tagged monoclonal antibody and allowed to react at 4°C for 30 minutes .

Surface antigen expression Lymphocytes were analyzed on a Spectrum III laser beam Cytofluorograph and distinguished according on their forward and right angle scatter properties (12). For each sample an histogram was obtained showing the fluorescence patterns of the selected lymphocytes:the average intensity and the percentage of positive cells were determined according to a fixed threshold .

Statistical analysis was performed according Student's "t test" for unpaired data

RESULTS AND DISCUSSION

The density of the considered membrane-bound antigens (T3,T4 and T8) on cellular surface are virtually the same in cuprophan, charcoal and polyacrylonitrile treated patients (Fig.1); T3 density (Fig.2) is slightly reduced if compared to normal subjects, while T4 and T8 expression are significantly lower in dialysis patients ($p<0.001$) independently from the substitutive treatment.

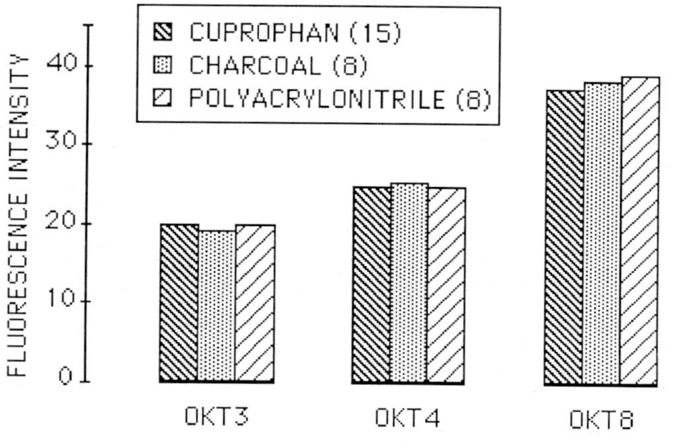

Figure 1:

Surface antigen expressions in chronic dialysis patients treated with different substitutive techniques.

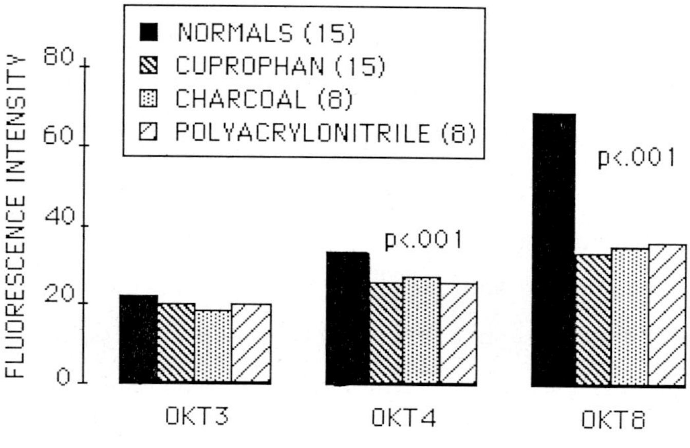

Figure 2:

Surface antigen expressions in chronic dialysis patients; comparison with normal subjects

According to these findings we can suppose that in chronic renal failure the intensity of fluorescence staining after reaction with OKT4 and OKT8 monoclonal antibodies is poor, depending on the reduce density of the corresponding surface antigens.

Recent studies have pointed out the role of T3, T4 and T8 molecules in recognition of, and immune response to, foreign antigens. In fact T-lymphocytes recognize self and foreign (non self) antigens by means of the association between an individual antigen and the membrane-bound products of the Major Hystocompatibility Complex (MHC). This "dual" recognition is important for the activation of both cytotoxic and immunoregulatory T-cells.

Various structures situated on the T-cell membrane are involved in these processes (14) : a) the individual T receptor (Ti), b) a trimolecular glicoproteic complex named T3, which is strictly connected to Ti and transmits the signal for activation through the cell membrane, and c) two further glicoproteins termed T4 and T8 , required to facilitate recognition of and binding to the target antigens ; T4 recognizes MHC-class II molecules (Ia-related), T8 MHC-class I molecules (HLA-A,B,C).

If our preliminary results are confirmed, suggesting as they do that these molecules are only faintly expressed on the lymphocyte surface,they may help to explain the pathogenesis of the acquired immunodeficiency found in dialysis patients.

ACKNOWLEDGMENTS

Supported in part by a Grant (1985) from Ministero della Pubblica Istruzione

REFERENCES

1 S. Stefoni, A. Nanni Costa, G. Liviano D'Arcangelo, M. Biavati, S. Iannelli and V. Bonomini, Biocompatibility of charcoal hemoperfusion.Effects of long term treatment on lymphocytes characteristics and function, Int. J. Art. Organ 1986, in press.

2 S. Stefoni, A. Nanni Costa, M.P. Scolari, L. Colì and V. Bonomini, DNA content and surface antigen characteristics of T-cell subsets in chronic dialysis patients. Flow cytometry analysis, In L.C. Smeby, S. Jorstad, T.E.Wideroe eds. Immune and

Metabolic Aspects of Therapeutic Blood Purification Systems. Karger, Basel,1986 ,pp. 168-174.

3 J. Traeger, J.L. Touraine, J. Navarro,J. Freyria and P. Contreras, Immunodeficiency in chronic renal insufficiency. In: Robinson BHB, Hawkins JB, eds. EDTA Proceedings, vol XVII, Pitman Press, Bath, 1980, pp. 375-382

4 T. Kunori, I. Fehrman, O. Ringdén and E. Moller, In vitro characterization of immunological responsiveness of uremic patients. Nephron 26 (1980) 234-239.

5 M.A.Watson, D.N.H. Hamilton, J.D. Briggs, S.G. Macpherson and D. Tsakiris, Cell mediated immunity during RDT and the outcome of transplantation. In: Robinson BHB, Hawkins JB, Davison AM, eds. EDTA Proceedings vol XVII, Pitman Press, Bath,1981, pp. 387-393.

6 P.I. Konrad and B.S. Husberg, The immunosuppressive effect of experimentally induced uremia. Nephron 38 (1984) 183-187.

7 D.A. Casciato, L.P. McAdam, J.D. Kopple, R. Bluestone, L.S. Goldberg,P.J. Clements and D.W. Knutson, Immunologic abnormalities in hemodialysis patients: improvement after pyridoxine therapy. Nephron 38 (1984) 9-16.

8 S.E. Goldblum and W.P. Reed, Host defences and immunologic alteration associated with chronic hemodialysis. Ann. Int. Med. 93 (1980) 597-613.

9 R.A. Hoffman and W.P. Hansen, Immunofluorescent analysis of blood cells of flow cytometry. Int. J. Immunopharmac. 3 (1981) 249-254.

10 S. Stefoni, L. Coli', G.Feliciangeli, M.P. Scolari and V. Bonomini V, Combined hemodialysis/hemoperfusion treatment reduces the weekly hours of treatment in chronic uremia. Int. J. Artif. Organs 4 (1981) 186-191.

11 P.C. Kung, M.A. Talle,M.E DeMaria, S. Butler, J. Lifter, G. Goldstein, Strategies for generating monoclonal antibodies defining human T lymphocyte differentiation antigens. Transpl. Proc., 12 (Suppl.1), (1980) 141-145.

12 G.Stelzer, K. Mc Leish, R Lorden and S. Watson, Alterations in T lymphocyte subpopulations associated with renal allograft rejection. Transplantation, 37, (1984) 261-266.

13 O. Acuto and E.L. Reinherz, The human T-cell receptor. Structure and function. N. Eng. J. Med., 312, (1985) 1100-111

14 E. Reinherz, S. Meuer, S. Schlossman,The delineation of antigen receptors on human T lymphocytes. Immunology Today 4 (1983) 5-8

Biomaterials and Clinical Applications,
edited by A. Pizzoferrato, P.G. Marchetti, A. Ravaglioli and A.J.C. Lee
Elsevier Science Publishers B.V., Amsterdam, 1987 — Printed in The Netherlands

METAL IONS LEVELS IN ORGANIC FLUIDS OF PATIENTS WITH Co-Cr-Mo ALLOY HIP PROSTHESES

G. GUALTIERI[1], I. GUALTIERI[1], S. GAGLIARDI[1], U.E. PAZZAGLIA[2], C. MINOIA[2] and L. CECILIANI[2]

[1]Seconda Clinica Ortopedica e Prima Divisione Istituti Ortopedici Rizzoli Bologna, Italy.

[2]Istituto di Clinica Ortopedica Università di Pavia, Pavia, Italy.

ABSTRACT

Metal ions levels were measured in urine and plasma of 17 patients who received a Co-Cr-Mo alloy total hip replacement 7-15 years before.

INTRODUCTION

The Co-Cr-Mo alloy has demonstrated to be the best in term of wear and corrosion among the materials used in prostheses.

The importance given to metal release from the implant is supported by the risk of toxicity, of sensitivity to the metals as a possible cause of loosening and carcinogenecity (refs. 1, 2, 3, 4,5, 6, 7, 8).

So far, few long term studies have been performed on the dosage of metal ions in organic fluids of patients with orthopaedic implants .

The following research was undertaken to assess the levels of metal ions in patients with Co-Cr-Mo alloy total hip replacement and a follow up of 7-15 years.

METHODS

17 clinically successful prostheses were studied.

The patients underwent a total hip arthroplasty 7-15 years ago at Istituto Ortopedico Rizzoli in Bologna.

In 15 cases a Mueller Co-Cr-Mo alloy prosthesis was applied articulating against a RCH-1000 polyethylene socket.

In 2 cases a Mc Kee Farrar prosthesis whith a metal socket was used.

The population includes males and females from 45 to 80 years of age, with an average age of 68.3 years.

Both patients' occupation in the past 30 years and the presence of industries near the place of residence have been carefully in investigated in the anamnesis.

Alcohol and tobacco consumption and drugs taken in the last two years were recorded. The following pathologies were specifically researched: hemophilia, thalassemia, Wilson's disease, diabetes, liver disease, kidney disease and heart diseases.

The patiens underwent general and local physical examination with a hip roentgenogram (both frontal and lateral views).

Blood was drawn using a polyethylene syringe and a 5 ml. test tube with sodium heparin. For every patient a test tube of whole blood was refrigerated at +5 °C, while another was centrifugated at about 2500 R.P.M. at room temperature and the plasma pipetted and stored at -20 °C till six hours before beginning the analysis.

Urine samples were taken using plastic containers decontaminated with a 10 per cent nitric acid water solution and repeatedly washed with bidistilled water.

Analytical determinations were performed with two atomic absorbtion spectrophotometers (Perkin Elmer model 5000 and 603 equiped respectively with HGA500 and HGA76B).

The determination of cobalt in urine was improved using a digestion procedure (wet ashing with nitric and sulfuric acid). The ashed solution was adjusted to pH 3.5 and the cobalt was extracted with ammonium pyrrolidine dithiocarbamate/ methil-iso-buthylketon(ref. 9).

Plasma samples were dried in a low temperature asher and resoluted with diluted nitrc acid. A microaliquot of the organic layer (methyl-iso-butilthyketon) or in HNO_3 was analyzed by electrothermal atomic aborption spectrometry.

Chromium determination in plasma and urine was performed following the method of guthrie et al.(ref. 10). Partially modified for the utilized equipment.

Manganese determination in blood and urine was performed utilizing both the method of Ross & Gonzales (ref. 11) and the extractive procedure with sodium diethyldithicarbamate methil-iso-buthylketon (ref. 12).

The determination of molybdenum in plasma and urine was performed utilizing the method of Baert et al (ref. 13).

Skin sensitivity to the alloy metals was investigated utilizing epicutneous tests with the following as aptens: a 2 per cent solution of $CoCl_2$; a 0.5 per cent solution of $K_2Cr_2O_7$; a 2 per cent solution of $MnCl_2$. A trained dermatolo-

gist read the skin test after 48 hours.
The control population consists of individuals male and female, with no record of prostheses or other metallic implant. They are all resident in Lombardia and have not been professionally exposed to the metal tested. This population is similar to the first in age and it is formed by apparently healthy individuals. Plasma and urine samples were collected from april 1982 until november 1983 with same procedures formerly reported; only individuals with normal values of glucose and plasmatic lipids were included in the control group.

RESULTS

This population of Co-Cr-Mo alloy prostheses may be considered clinically successful as assessed by both interview and physical examination. All the patients had a good functional recovery following surgery which was then maintained for 7-15 years until the time of this research.

The results of Co, Cr, Mo and Mn determination in plasma and urine of the patients with Mueller total hip replacement are reported in Tab. 1 where they have been compared to a control population.

Statistical analysis with Student's test has been carried out and significant increases in levels of Co and Cr in urine and of Cr in plasma have been found in prostheses population.

Metal ions values in plasma and urine of the two Mc. Farrar,metal on metal, total hip replacement are reported in the same table; they are in the same range of values of metal on plastic prostheses.

There is no correlation between prostheses with osteolysis around the cement and the highest levels of metal ions in plasma and urine inside the population.

Skin sensitivity tests to Co, Cr and Mn were negative in 15 patients; 2 did not return for the control appointment.

DISCUSSION

Levels of Cobalt in urine and Chromium in both plasma and urine of the prostheses population are significantly higher than in controls.

Differences of Molybdenum and Manganese are not significant.

These results are not unexpected because Cobalt and Cromium are the major constituent of the Co-Cr-Mo alloy (approximately 65% and 30%), while Molybdenum and Manganese represent only 5% and 1% respectively.

Tab. 1 Cobalt, Chromium, Molybdenum and Manganese levels in biological fluids ° of 15 patients with Co-Cr-Mo alloy prostheses and controls. Values of two patients with metal on metal McKee-Farrar prosthesis are also reported

Metal and biological matrix	* Control Population average ± S.D. (μg/l)	Patients with Co-Cr-Mo alloy prostheses average ± S.D. (μg/l)	P	Patients with metal on metal McKee-Farrar prostheses (μg/l) n=2	
Co_{pl}	0.5 ± 0.3 (n=28)	0.72 ± 0.58 (n=15)	n.s.	0.8	0.5
Co_u	0.5 ± 0.2 (n=36)	0.86 ± 0.37 (n=15)	$P < 0.01$	1.05	0.4
Cr_{pl}	0.5 ± 0.1 (n=310)	1.63 ± 0.45 (n=15)	$P < 0.01$	1.80	1.5
Cr_u	0.6 ± 0.2 (n=70)	1.84 ± 0.54 (n=15)	$P < 0.01$	1.35	1.7
Mo_{pl}	less than 1γ/1 (n=28)	less than 1γ/1 (n=15)		less than 1γ/1	
Mo_u	less than 1γ/1 (n=28)	less than 1γ/1 (n=15)		1.1	0,85
Mn_b	9.0 ± 0.1 (n=20)	6.99 ± 0.97 (n=15)	n.s.	7.0	6.0
Mn_u	1.2 ± 0.4 (n=136)	1.26 ± 0.6 (n=15)	n.s.	0.96	0.75

° pl=plasma b=blood u=urine

The observed levels of metals in Co-Cr-Mo alloy prostheses population do not represent a toxic hazard for the patients however they are a index of ions release from the metallic implant and of the probable accumulation in other organs.

Urine Chromium levels in this population are considerably lower than in professionally exposed groups, where the urinary excretion of Chromium is usually used for biological monitoring of workers exposed to water soluble Chromium (VI).

In prostheses population Chromium is released from the implant surface or from particles formed by wear and it seems likely that it consists almost exclusively of metallic or trivalent Chromium since no possibility exists in vivo of oxidation to hexavalent Chromium ions.

Tumor induction has been observed in industrial workers, following exposure to hexavalent Chromium (VI), but not to the trivalent ion (Cr III).

Since the large number of total hip replacements so far performed the observation of tumors at the site of a prosthesis is a rare event and the few cases reported may be coincidential; in any of them definite evidences of tumor induction by metal ions has not been presented.

Skin sensitivity to Co-Cr-Mo alloy metals, expecially Cobalt has been considered a possible test to demonstrate allergicreactions to the constituents of the implant, which eventually may lead to loosening (ref. 14).

Skin sensitivity was not observed in the studied population, even after a long-term exposure to the alloy metals.

REFERENCES

1 M.R. Elves, J.N. Wilson, J.T. Scales and H.B.S. Kemp, Incidence of metal sensitivity in patients with total joint replacement, Br. Med. J. 4, 1975 376-378.
2 E.M. Evans, M.A.R. Freeman, A.J. Miller and B. Vernon-Roberts, Metal sensitivity has a cause of bone necrosis and loosening of the prostheses in total joint replacement, J. Bone Joint Surg. 56 (B) (1974) 626-642.
3 L. Langlais, M. Postel, G.P. Berry, Y. Le Carpentier and B.J. Weill, L'intolerance aux débris d'usure dés prosthéses. Bilan immunologique et anatomopathologique de 30 cas, Int. Orthop. 4, (1980) 145-153.
4 S. Uchida, S. Yoshino, M. Doi and H. Kudo, Side effects of prosthetic materials on the human body, Int. Orthop. 3, (1980) 285-291.
5 J.C. Heath, M.A.R. Freeman and S.A.V. Svanson, Carcinogenic properties of wear particles from prostheses made in Co-Cr alloy, Lancet (I) (1971) 564-566.
6 G. Kazantzis, Role of cobalt, iron, lead, manganese, mercury, platinium,seleniu and titanium in carcinogenesis, Environ. Health Perspect 40 (1981) 143-161.

7 B.S. Oppeneimer, T.S. I. Danishefsky and A.P. Sout, Carcinogenic effect of metal in rodentes, Cancer. Res. (16) (1956) 439-441.
8 T. Norseth, The carcinogenecity of chromium, Environ.Health Perspect 40 (1981) 121-130.
9 Y. Ichikawa, Y. Kusaka, and S. Goto, Biological monotoring of cobalt exposure based on cobalt concentration in blood and urine, Int. Arch. Occup. Environ Health 55 (1985) 269-276
10 B.E. Guthrie, W.R. Wolf and C. Veillon, Backgroun correctionand related problems in the determination of chromium in urine by graphite furnace atomic absorption spectrometry, Anal. Chem. 50 (1978) 1900-1905.
11 R.T. Roos and J.G. Gonzales, Direct determination of trace quantities of manganese in blood and serum samples using selective valorizationand graphite tube reservoir, Bull. Environ. Contam. Toxicol 12 (1974) 470.
12 C. Minoia and A. Cavalleri Determinazione dei metalli in tracce nel laboratorio chimico tossicologico La Goliardica Pavese Pavia (1983)
13 Baert, Cornelis and Moste, Molybdenum in human blood, Clin. Kim. Acta 68 (1976) 355-356.
14 M.K.D. Benson, P.G. Goodwin and J. Brostoff, Metal sensitivity in patients with joint replacement arthroplasties, Br. Med. J. 4 (1975) 374-375.

Biomaterials and Clinical Applications,
edited by A. Pizzoferrato, P.G. Marchetti, A. Ravaglioli and A.J.C. Lee
Elsevier Science Publishers B.V., Amsterdam, 1987 — Printed in The Netherlands

VIBRATION SPECTRA AND BIOCOMPATIBILITY OF 4 ARTIFICIAL DRUM MEMBRANE MATERIALS

D. BAKKER[1], C.A. VAN BLITTERSWIJK[1], W.L.C. RUTTEN[2], J.G.BOTS[3], J.H. KUIT[3], W.TH. DAEMS[4] and J.J.GROTE[1]

[1]ENT Department, University Hospital, Leiden (The Netherlands)
[2]Biomed. Engineering Division, Twente University of Technology, Enschede (The Netherlands)
[3]Department of Chemical Technology, Twente University of Technology, Enschede (The Netherlands)
[4]Laboratory for Electron Microscopy, Leiden University, Leiden (The Netherlands)

SUMMARY

Vibration spectra were obtained and *in vitro* biocompatibility was studied for two silicon rubbers, a polyether polyester copolymer, and a polyether urethane.

Membrane vibration patterns, measured with a SQUID-magnetometer, showed that all tested biomaterials vibrated with greater amplitudes than the human drum membrane. In order to study biocompatibility, rat middle ear explants and epithelium were used in three *in vitro* tests. In contrast with the results of the (1) morphological test, which did not discriminate between the various biomaterials, the (2) quantitative test and the (3) simulation test for long-term *in vivo* exposure to body-fluid indicated better biocompatibility for the polyether urethane and the polyether polyester copolymer when compared with both silicon rubbers. Explant and epithelium morphology were studied using scanning and transmission electron microscopy, and X-ray microanalysis.

INTRODUCTION

In developing a total alloplastic middle ear prosthesis (TAM)* (ref. 1) an artificial drum membrane is necessary for proper acoustical functioning and for the attachment of the ossicular chain to the hydroxyapatite canal wall of the prosthesis. Therefore the need exists for a biocompatible elastomer with mechanical properties comparable to those of the human drum.

The bulk-material of the TAM is porous hydroxyapatite. This ceramic showed good biocompatibility, both with implantation studies and *in-vitro* using middle ear explants and epithelium (ref. 2). In long-term clinical studies hydroxyapatite proved to be successful (ref. 3).

To study the biocompatibility of several candidate drum materials tissue culture tests were used in order to obtain both rapid results and a quantification of biocompatibility (ref. 4). These *in vitro* tests comprised a quantitative and a morphological test based on proliferative activity and morphology respectively

*The following abbreviations are used throughout this study:
PECF; pseudo extracellular fluid; PVC: polyvinyl chloride; SEM and TEM: scanning and transmission electron microscopy; TAM: total alloplastic middle ear; TCPS: tissue culture polystyrene

of tissue cultured on the biomaterials, and a simulation test of long-term *in vivo* exposure of a given biomaterial to body-fluid. Rat middle ear epithelium and explants were used for tissue culture (ref. 5). The simulation test was according to Homsy (ref. 6).

MATERIALS AND METHODS

The following biomaterials were used: the silicon rubbers Silastic^r, and Dow Corning^r MDX-4-4210 Clean Grade Elastomer, a polyether urethane (Estane^r 5714 F1), and a poly(ethylene oxide-hydantoin) / poly(tetramethylene terephtalate) segmented polyether polyester copolymer (ref. 7). All biofilms were 100 - 125 µm thick.

For vibration measurements the SQUID-magnetometer set-up and biomaterial preparation were used as described by Rutten et al. (refs. 8,9). The human drum membrane served as a control.

Rat middle ear mucosa explants and epithelium were obtained and cultured as described elsewhere (ref. 5). Growth curves of serial cultures are based on cell counts in 30 mm Costar^r culture dishes after 1,3,6,10 and 14 days. Dishes with and without (control) a biofilm were UV-sterilized prior to use. To simulate long-term *in vivo* exposure to body-fluid, equal quantities of the various polymer specimens and PVC (cytotoxic control) were heated in a 115 ^oC pseudo extracellular fluid (PECF) for 48 hr. Further, aliquot portions of PECF from a given experiment and PECF (biomaterial free when heated, control), were used to prepare the nutrient-mediums for serial cultivation on tissue culture polystyrene (TCPS) (ref. 6). All mediums were sterilized by passing through a .22 µm Millipore filter. Biomaterials used for the morphological tissue culture experiment and the simulation test were cleaned with 70% ethanol and copiously rinsed in distilled water, air dried and steam-sterilized. Explants and epithelium were studied after 10 days of cultivation. Routine scanning and transmission electron microscopy and X-ray microanalysis were carried out in accordance with Van Blitterswijk et al (ref. 2).

RESULTS

Vibration measurements

Fig. 1 shows the displacement-rms-amplitude versus frequency for the human drum membrane and the four biomaterials. The human drum membrane vibrated with amplitudes of about 2000 Å. The 4 biomaterials had maximum amplitudes of about 20000 Å. Fig. 1 has been taken from ref. 9 with minor changes.

Biocompatibility

A quantitative analysis.

The growth curves of the epithelial cells serially cultured on the 4 biomaterials and TCPS were sigmoidal of shape (Fig. 2). After one day the number of cells on TCPS was greater than on the 4 biomaterials. However, cell numbers on three of the tested biomaterials more or less equalled that of TCPS at day 14. An exception to this was the smaller number of cells on Elastomer. When the complete growth curves were considered a Wilcoxon two sample test showed that epithelial cells proliferated significally less on Elastomer when compared to the other tested biomaterials and TCPS.

B Epithelium morphology

Middle ear explants attached to all biomaterials, and explants always showed outgrowth of epithelium (Fig. 3). Electron microscopy revealed that on all tested biomaterials and TCPS, the morphology of explant and epithelium closely resembled that of normal middle ear mucosa. Flat polygonal and ciliated epithelium was seen on all studied materials (inset of Fig. 3).

As revealed by transmission electron microscopy (TEM) epithelial outgrowth on the 4 biomaterials and TCPS predominantly consisted of flat polygonal cells comprising a flattened nucleus, rough endoplasmic reticulum, ribosomes, and a Golgi apparatus. Cells had varying quantities of microvilli. Scanning electron microscopy (SEM) showed that most ciliated cells in the outgrowth had a primary cilium, but ciliated epithelium was also seen with normal and altered cilia.

Rat middle ear epithelium serially cultured on the various biomaterials and TCPS was flat with a morphology comparable with that of outgrowth epithelium.

C Simulation of long-term in vivo exposure

The morphology of rat middle ear epithelium cultured in control-medium was comparable with that of epithelium cultivated in routinuously used medium. The confluence and morphology of epithelium cultured in the simulation mediums of polyether urethane and polyether polyester copolymer resembled that of cells cultured in the control medium (and thus of normally serially cultured cells).

Cells cultured in Silastic^{r}- and Elastomer-medium often showed deviating morphology. A fair number of cells were not flat. Furthermore culture dishes were not confluent. Particularly cells exposed to the Silastic^{r}-medium showed inclusions (Fig. 4a). Inclusions with prominent membranes (arrowheads in Fig. 4a) were seen in cells cultured in the mediums of both silicon rubbers. In case of Silastic^{r} such cells also contained electron-dense inclusions (arrows in Fig. 4a). The largest inclusion measured about 1.2 μm x .6 μm the smallest measured no more than .2 x .2 μm. X-ray microanalysis showed that these inclusions contained silicon (Fig. 4b).

DISCUSSION

The SQUID-magnetometer set-up, which detects displacement amplitudes of 1 nm has been successfully used for middle ear research (ref. 8). In Fig. 1 it is seen that all biomaterials vibrated with greater amplitudes than the human drum membrane. After the implantation of the TAM-prosthesis, damping of the vibration amplitudes of the biomaterials is a possible consequence of tissue overgrowth and contraction. Biomaterials, which vibrate with amplitudes comparable with or lesser than the human drum membrane, might vibrate with unfavourable smaller amplitudes after implantation.

Rat middle ear epithelium and explants were investigated by Van Blitterswijk et al. (ref. 5), and contributed to the study of the *in vitro* biocompatibility of hydroxyapatite (ref. 2). For all tested biomaterials the morphology of the rat middle ear epithelium, whether part of an explant, growing out of an explant, or serially cultured can be compared with normal middle ear mucosa and epithelium growing out or cultured on TCPS, respectively. The morphological variability of epithelium that is seen (number of microvilli, presence of cilia) is also found in the rat middle ear and in specimens on TCPS (ref. 5).

The quantification of epithelial growth revealed that proliferative activity was significantly less on Elastomer when compared with the other tested biomaterials and TCPS. The best substrate for attachment was TCPS, as indicated by the greatest number of cells on this material after one day of cultivation. After one day cell densities on the studied biomaterials were more or less equal. The fact that after 14 days on all biomaterials except Elastomer epithelial cell density just about equalled that on TCPS suggests that not only cell/substrate adhesion is responsible for the overall lesser proliferative activity on Elastomer, but also cell behaviour on this biomaterial in culture. The latter is related to the nature of the synthetic substratum (ref. 10).

The simulation test of long-term *in vivo* exposure of biomaterials to bodyfluid was introduced by Homsy, who showed that for a number of materials cell migration and morphology corresponded well with the presence of several chemical structural groupings in the PECF, as detected by infrared spectro-photometry (ref. 5). Epithelium cultured in mediums prepared with PECF in which Silastic^{r} and Elastomer had been heat-exposed showed morphological abnormalities when compared with normal serially cultured epithelium. This was in contrast with cells grown in the polyether urethane- and the copolymer-medium.

Intracellular silicon is suggestive for endocytosis by the epithelium of material derived from Silastic^{r}. After preparing the nutrient mediums for tissue culture all mediums were sterilized by passing through a .22 µm Millipore filter. Inclusions of greater size than .2 x .2 µm are suggestive for an accumulative process.

To sum up, all biomaterials vibrate with greater amplitudes than the human drum membrane. On behalf of the results of the three *in vitro* tests (quantitative, morphological, and simulation) the polyether urethane and the polyether polyester copolymer possess better biocompatibility than the silicon rubbers Silastic^{r} and Elastomer. For final conclusions concerning the biocompatibility of these biomaterials, and in order to correlate results of in vitro and in vivo tests, extensive implantation studies in rats are being performed.

Acknowledgements: The authors are greatly indebted to Mrs. P.v.d.Hoek, Mr. B. v.d. Lans, Mr. J.J.Beentjes, Mr. L.D.C.Verschragen. These investigations were supported by the Netherlands Technology Foundation (STW).

REFERENCES

1. J.J.Grote, Tympanoplasty with calciumphosphate, in: J.J.Grote (Ed.), Biomaterials in Otology, Proc. 1st Int. Symp. Biomats, Otol., Leiden, The Netherlands, April 21-23, 1983, Martinus Nijhoff Publishers, Boston, 1984, pp. 274-280.
2. C.A. van Blitterswijk, W.Kuijpers, W.Th. Daems, and J.J.Grote, Epithelial reactions to hydroxyapatite: An in vivo and in vitro study, Acta Otolaryngol (Stockh.), 101 (1986) 231-241.
3. J.J.Grote and C.A. van Blitterswijk, Reconstruction of the posterior auditory canal wall with a hydroxyapatite prosthesis, Ann. Otol. Rhinol. Laryngol. 95, 2,2, Suppl. 123 (1986) 6-9.
4. T.Rae, A review of tissue culture techniques suitable for testing the biocompatibility of implant materials, in: G.D.Winter, J.L. Leray, and K. de Groot (Eds.), Evaluation of Biomaterials, John Wiley & Sons Ltd., 1980, pp. 289-293.
5. C.A. van Blitterswijk, M.Ponec, G.N.P. van Muijen, M.C.Wijsman, H.K.Koerten, and J.J.Grote, Culture and characterization of rat middle ear epithelium, Acta Otolaryngol. (Stockh.), 101 (1986) 453-466.
6. C.A.Homsy, Bio-compatibility in selection of materials for implantation, J. Biomed. Mater. Res., 4 (1970) 341-356.
7. P.C.Mody, G.L.Wilkes, and K.B.Wagener, Structure-property relationships of a new series of segmented polyether-polyester copolymers, J. Appl. Pol. Sci., 26 (1981) 2853-2878.
8. W.L.C.Rutten, M.J.Peters, C.J.Brenkman, H.Mol, J.J.Grote, and L.C.van Marel, The use of a SQUID magnetometer for middle ear research, Cryogenics, Sept. (1982) 457-460.
9. W.L.C.Rutten, C.A. van Blitterswijk, C.J.Brenkman, and J.J.Grote, Vibrations of natural and artificial middle ear membranes measured by a SQUID-magnetometer, in: H.Weinberg, G.Stroink, and T.Katila (Eds.), Biomagnetism, Theory and Applications, Pergamon Press, New York, 1985, pp. 461-465.
10. M.J.Lydon, and C.S.Clay, Substratum topography and cell traction on sulphuric acid treated bacteriological-tradeplastic, Cell Biol. Int. Rep., 9,10 (1985) 911-921.

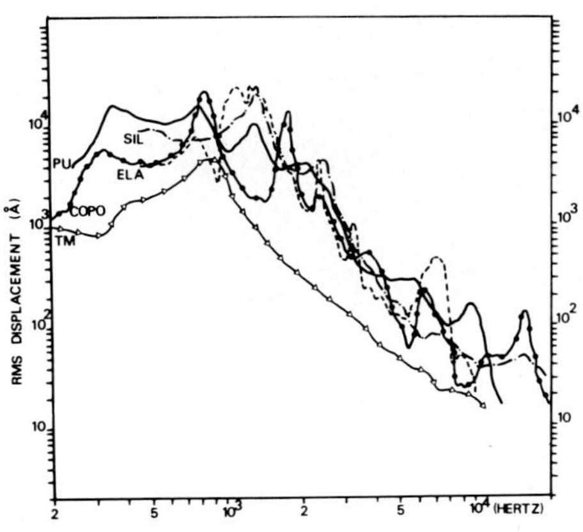

Fig. 1
Vibration spectra. Stimulation sound level was 80 dB SPL.
TM = human drum membrane;
COPO = the copolymer;
PU = the polyether urethane;
ELA = Elastomer; SIL = Silastic^{r}.

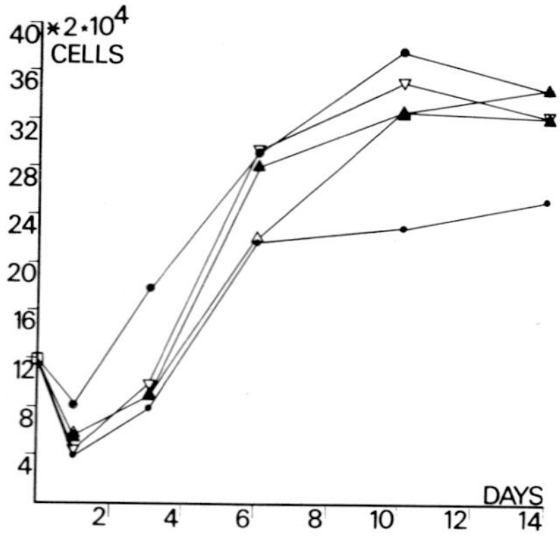

Fig. 2

Growth curves. (●) tissue culture polystyrene; (△) the copolymer; (▲) the polyether urethane; (▽) Silastic; (•) Elastomer.

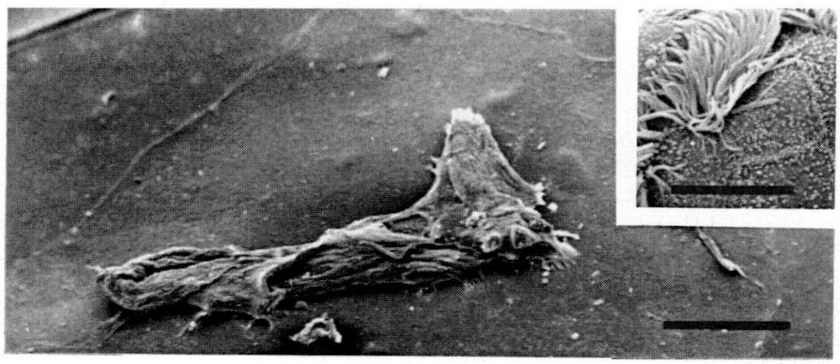

Fig. 3
Scanning electron micrograph of middle ear mucosa explant with epithelial outgrowth on copolymer. Bar = 900 µm. Inset: Ciliated epithelium of an explant on Silastic^{r}. Bar = 10 µm.

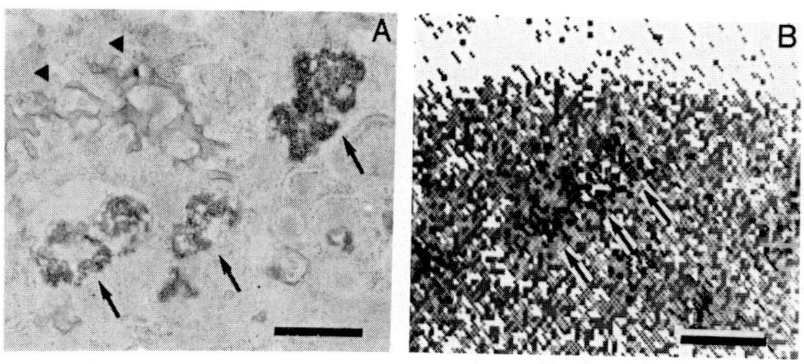

Fig. 4a
Transmission electron micrograph of epithelium cultured in Silastic-medium. Note the electron-dense inclusions (arrows , arrowheads). Bar = .6 µm.

Fig. 4b X-ray mapping for silicon. Cells were cultured in Silastic-medium. Arrow point to silicon-containing inclusions, which are comparable to the arrow inclusions of Fig. 4a. Bar = 1.2 µm.

Biomaterials and Clinical Applications,
edited by A. Pizzoferrato, P.G. Marchetti, A. Ravaglioli and A.J.C. Lee
Elsevier Science Publishers B.V., Amsterdam, 1987 — Printed in The Netherlands

TISSUE REACTION TO ALUMINA POWDER INJECTED INTO THE JOINTS OF A PIG

G. GUALTIERI[1], I. GUALTIERI[2], N. BETTINI[2], G. CIAPETTI[3], S. STEA [3],
A. PIZZOFERRATO[3] and G. GALLETTI[4].

1 Seconda Clinica Ortopedica, Istituti Ortopedici Rizzoli, Bologna, Italy.
2 Prima Divisione, Istituti Ortopedici Rizzoli, Bologna, Italy.
3 Laboratorio di Patologia Clinica, Istituti Ortopedici Rizzoli, Bologna, Italy.
4 Istituto di Chirurgia Sperimentale, Università di Bologna, Italy.

ABSTRACT

In order to evaluate the biological response to alumina powder we used a pure powder of Al_2O_3 and experimental animals. We put alumina powder into the elbow and nock joint cavities of experimental animals. Then we sacrificed the animals and started macroscopic and microscopic investigation. This study has proved a significant level of biocompatibility for this material.

INTRODUCTION

Our experience in the field of arthroprosthetic hip surgery began in 1969.

We started using metal-metal coupling arthroprostheses, then the metal-plastic (polyester-polyethylene) types.

Finally from 1977 we also began to implant ceramic-ceramic low friction prostheses (ref. 1).

The implantions have always been fixed with acrylic cement.

The high number of patients undergoing surgery and above all reoperated for the removal of the arthroprostheses led us draw some considerations about the failure of this surgery.

Apart from mechanical errors and infection, our experience led us to regard the wear of the materials forming the neojoint as the main cause of failure of this operation.

The wear, due to abrasion in the metal-plastic types, brings about the formation of debris which gives rise to an intolerance reaction (of the allergic-toxic type), subsequently granulation tissue (refs. 2-3).

The granulation tissue consequently gives rise to the resorption of the bone and the mobilization of the implant (ref. 4).

The chemical and physical characteristics of the debris, their surface, shape and size and their chemical composition condition the macrophagic response (ref. 5).

It was precisely for the above reason that from 1977 onwards we also began to make use of cemented ceramic-ceramic friction arthroprostheses.

This choice was based on the physical and chemical characteristics of the material and on the fact that ceramic is subject to very low wear.

This has been established a large number of experiments among which we mention Boutin's, in which ceramic-ceramic coupling arthroprosthesis showed slight wear for up to 600 hours in the step simulator; this wear then completely stopping between 600 and 2100 hours (ref. 6).

However the evaluation of the response when the amount of powder present in the joint is high was lacking in our exeperience.

In order to evaluate the biological response to alumina powder we put the same into the joint cavity of the elbow and nock of experimental animals.

METHODS

We made use of alumina powder and experimental animals in this experiment.

The alumina powder used by us was a highly reactive powder to sinter at a high density even at relatively low temperatures (1500°-1600°C).

From a chemical point of view it was pure Al_2O_3 powder.

A diafrattometric test revealed that this powder contained a high proportion of alpha Al_2O_3, with a tendency toward hexagonal "habitus" grains, distributed in a relatively narrow tridimensional spectrum (0.2-1 micron).

The powder showed high hardness and a microstructure with remarkably uniform granulometry.

The experimental animals were male pigs, about six months old and weighing between 70 and 85 kilograms.

Before placing the powder in the joint, we sterilized the former in ethylene oxide in order not to alter its characteristics in any way.

Under general anesthesia, we carried out an internal para-rotular incision at the level of the nock and at the level of the elbow we carried out a medial incision; after having incised the skin, sub-skin and joint capsule, we reached the joint plane.

The powder was placed into the cavity making sure that it did not spread out of the joint.

Then suture of the capsule and reconstruction of the anatomical planes were carried out.

The post-surgery course was regular: the pigs did not have a temperature; they did not lose weight and started eating regularly again on the second day.

The surgery healed in a period of about 10 days following the first operation; in one case only slight reddening occured, involving a delay of 5 days in healing of the wound.

For our convenience we named the four pigs A, B, C and D.

The amount of alumina placed in each joint was 1 gram in pig A, 0.50 grams in pigs B and D, and 0.25 grams in pig C.

The animals were sacrificed after a period of more than two months.

At this point we started the macroscopic and microscopic investigation of the joint in which the powder had been placed.

RESULTS

From a macroscopic point of view the joints appeared quite normal: the synovia did not show lesions in any way likely to suggest damage caused by alumina; in fact, the small hemorrhages found therein have been taken as a sign of the trauma caused by the operation.

Again from a macroscopic point of view the joint cartilage appeared free from lesions and standard in colour.

Microscopic examination revealed almost intact synovial membrane without any signs of phlogistic reaction (Fig. 1).

In some areas of the periarticular tissue the powder was phagocytosed by histiocytes.

In other areas of the connective tissue the intra and extracellular spaces were infiltrated by powder, the nuclei of the fat cells were also surrounded by foreign material.

There were no lesions caused by powder in the muscular tissue.

The alumina was found dispersed in the tissue, in some areas accumulated in masses of varying dimensions; there was no evidence of tissue reaction in this case either (Fig. 2).

Finally, the synovial villi seemed to be intact.

Eosinophiles were rare in the tissue and were found in only one of the experimental animals.

DISCUSSION

On the whole,the alumina tested, under the experimental conditions involved in our research,showed no noticeable signs of intolerability and toxicity.

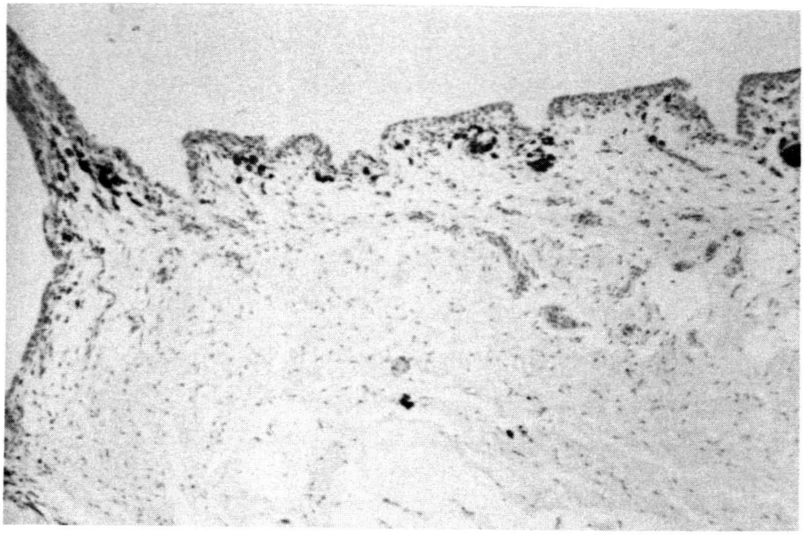

Fig. 1

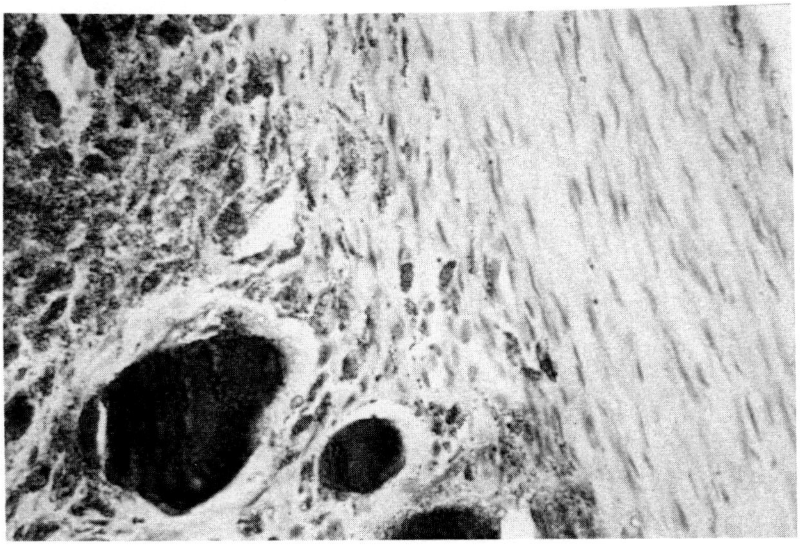

Fig. 2

REFERENCES

1 L. Gui and G. Gualtieri, Risultati sulle prime 50 artroprotesi d'anca fissate con cemento acrilico, Arch. Ortop. Reum., 94(3) (1981) 7-20.

2 U. Pazzaglia, La reazione da corpo estraneo nelle protesi totali d'anca, Min. Ortopo., 34 (1983) 57-62.

3 L. Ranieri, A. Pizzoferrato, A. Toni and S. Stilli, Reazione dei tessuti periarticolari ai prodotti di usura del polietilene ad alta densità, C.O.M., 65 (1979) 1-11.

4 F. Greco, L. De Palma and A. Santucci, La risposta dei tessuti periarticolari al polietilene nelle artroprotesi d'anca, Min. Ortop., 36 (1985) 951-956.

5 L. Gui, A. Pizzoferrato, L. Ranieri and I. Gualtieri, Reazione tessutale articolare e para-articolare negli impianti protesici, LXII Congr. (S.I.O.T.) 4 (2) (1978) 215-217.

6 P. Boutin, Arthroplastie totale de la hanche par prothese en alumine frittèe. Etude experimèntale et premieres applicationes clinique, Rev. Chir. Orthop., 58 (1972) 229-246.

Biomaterials and Clinical Applications,
edited by A. Pizzoferrato, P.G. Marchetti, A. Ravaglioli and A.J.C. Lee
Elsevier Science Publishers B.V., Amsterdam, 1987 — Printed in The Netherlands

IS THERE A HOMOLOGY OR A SPECIES SPECIFITY OF BONE GELATINE`S ACTIVE FRACTION ?

J.M. RUEGER, K. WAGNER, H.R. SIEBERT, A. PANNIKE.

Unfallchirurgische Klinik, Zentrum der Chirurgie, Universitaetsklinik Frankfurt, Theodor Stern Kai 7, 6000 Frankfurt am Main. Leiter: Prof. Dr. med. A. Pannike.

SUMMARY

Bone gelatine, a bone matrix extract of diaphyseal cortical bone, is osteoinductive and osteostimulative in allogeneic implantation. It is unclear, whether active bone gelatine can be extracted out of cortical bone of every species. Our aim is to use xenogeneic bone gelatine as a bone replacement material in traumatologic surgery. To investigate in their osteoinductive and osteostimulative properties, nude rat bone gelatine, sheep -, dog -, rabbit - and human - bone gelatine was implanted ortho - and heterotopically in Spraque - Dawley rats. Only nude rat bone gelatine was highly active in osteoinduction and osteostimulation, due to the close proximity of the nude - and the Spraque - Dawley - rat strains, while the other bone gelatine preparations showed only little effects. A constant lymphoplasmacellular reaction to the xenogeneic protein complexes reduced there activity markedly or even to nil. Without further extraction or modifications of its antigenicity xenogeneic bone gelatine can not be used as a bone replacement material.

INTRODUCTION

Bone gelatine, an antigenetic active, acellular bone matrix extract, protein complex, of diaphyseal cortical bone (ref. 1) is active in osteoinduction, i.e. osteogenesis after heterotopic implantation (muscle), and osteostimulation, i.e. enhanced bone formation and repair after orthotopic implantation(bone), after allogeneic implantation in rats. Purification of bone gelatine results in bone morphogenetic protein (BMP) (ref. 2), which is a controlling factor of bone repair in fracture healing (ref. 3, 4). The implantation of extraction products of bone gelatine as well as of BMP leads to a decrease in the incidence and total yield of ectopically induceable bone (ref. 5) after heterotopic implantation while their activity in osteostimulation after orthotopic implantation can not be demonstrated convincingly (ref. 6).

Our aim is to use bone gelatine, probably in combination with a calcium-phosphate compound, either beta-tricalciumphosphate or hydroxyapatite (ref. 7), as a bone replacement material for autogenous cancellous bone in traumatologic or orthopedic surgery. Since we do want to use xenogeneic bone gelatine (availability of human bone gelatine on a large scale would be difficult) a problem arises out of the fact that implantation of allogeneic bone gelatine in rats, mongrel dogs and sheep leads to a moderate lymphoplasmacellular reaction, whereas xenogeneic implantation (human bone gelatine -- S.D.-rats, human bone gelatine -- mongrel dogs) (ref. 8) elicits a massive reaction with adverse effects on the osteoinductive and osteostimulative potency of bone gelatine. To avoid the above mentioned decrease of activity of extraction products of bone gelatine and BMP as well as the adverse lymphoplasmacellular reaction to xenogeneic material one would have to reduce bone gelatine`s immunogenicity or use bone gelatine of a species with an acceptable biologic activity and low antigenicity.

Since it remains unclear whether active bone gelatine can be extracted out of diaphyseal cortical bone of every species, we investigated the potency of bone gelatine of five different species by implantation in Sprague-Dawley rats.

METHODS

In 45 Sprague-Dawley rats, three to four months old, body weight between 250 and 400gr, eight 50mg aliquots of the bone gelatine preparation of one species were implanted in six muscle pouches of the rect. abd. muscle as well as in two bilateral diaphyseal femoral drill holes (2 X 3mm).

Materials were implanted for 7, 21, 42, 60 and 90 (sheep and nude rats only) days. An intravital tetracyclin double labelling 14, 13 (if applicable) and two and one days prior to sacrifice was carried out. Explants were evaluated by xeroradiography of the native whole femurs and abdominal musculature, light- and fluorescent microscopy of micro-sections of undecalcified PMMA embedded specimen after Masson-Goldner, v. Kossa and Methylgreen-Pyronin stainings. The micro - sections of the femurs were subjected to histomorphometry (ref. 9).

Bone gelatine was extracted according to Urist 1973 (ref. 1).

Dog bone gelatine: diaphyseal cortical bone of adult mongrel dogs, femurs, tibiae.

Sheep bone gelatine: diaphyseal cortical bone of adult sheep, femurs.

Rabbit bone gelatine: diaphyseal cortical bone of adult rabbits, femurs, tibiae.

Nude rat bone gelatine: diaphyseal cortical bone of adult nude rats, two to three months old, femurs, tibiae.

Human bone gelatine: diaphyseal cortical bone of the unfractured femur of a late adult motorvehicle accident trauma victim.

Particle size after sieving for all bone gelatine preparations was 400-800 μm.

RESULTS

Heterotopic Implantation

Except for the nude rat bone gelatine implantations only scattered induced bone did develope. Overall incidence as well as yield of ectopically induced bone was low. There was a decrease of the osteoinductive activity of the different bone gelatine preparations following the line: rabbit - human - dog - sheep bone gelatine, with no visible induction at all in the latter implants.

After seven days of implantation in none of the preparations any bone or cartilage formation was demonstrable. There was an extensive lymphoplasmacellular reaction except for the nude rat bone gelatine implants, with the most intense reaction after the implantation of sheep bone gelatine.

After 21 days histologically the implanted bone gelatine particles seemed to be packed more closely with vessels in direct contact to the implants. All materials were surrounded by a fibril rich connective tissue capsule. In some of the implants (never in sheep) vital bone with scattered osteocytes, osteoid seams and osteoblasts with very few osteoclasts did develope. This vital bone was either detectable inside of a large or inbetween very closely packed smaller bone gelatine particles. Only in human -, dog - and rabbit - bone gelatine implants chondrocytes with matrix formation (metachromasia on methylgreen - pyronin stainings) were visible. The intensity of the lymphoplasmacellular reaction was unchanged after 21 days.

After 42 and 60 days the histologic appearance of the implanted materials and their elicited effects remained the same. There was neither an increase in the amount of induced bone, osteoblast and osteoclast activity nor a decrease in the intensity of the lymphoplasmacellular reaction. The formation of bone marrow inside the induced patchy bony islands was never, despite close contact to nearby vessels, demonstrable. Remnants of the implanted bone gelatine particles were visible until the end of the observation period.

In nude rat implants after 21 days there were vital bony ossicles with bone marrow formation. Small remnants of bone gelatine particles seemed to be remineralised with osteoblast activity on their surfaces. After 42 days the interior of the ossicles was filled with fatty marrow, osteoblast activity on the inner surface of the bony ring and some osteoclasts on its outside. After 60 and 90 days histologic appearance remained the same except for a decrease in the osteoblast activity. A lymphoplasmacellular reaction was never visible.

Orthotopic implantation

Probably due to biomechanical reasons after 21 days in all implants a stabiliser and support of trabecular bone developed between the edges of the drill - hole and the opposite cortical bone. In the nude rat group peripheral particles of the bone gelatine implants were partly incorporated into this support with osteoblasts on those surfaces that were directed towards the medullary cavity. In this group after 42 days the cortical defects were filled and bridged by trabecular bone with the formation of a secondary marrow cavity. The cup like trabecular-bone support was detached from the opposite corticalis. At 60 days the femoral cavity was recanalised with no bone gelatine particles visible inside of the femurs. At 90 days the former drill-holes were indistinquishable except for the secondary marrow cavities.

In none of the other implants, regardless of the time, a filling of the cortical defects or a recanalisation of the medullary cavities of the femurs did occur. In every species group large remnants of the implanted bone gelatine preparations remained visible, surrounded by scar tissue, until the end of the observation period. The lymphoplasmacellular reaction, obvious in all implants already after seven days, remained intense until 60 days after implantation.

Histomorphometry

(Cortical defects only)

Volume density bone (V_V %)	7d	21d	42d	60d
Nude rat BG	9.17	18.48	15.32	27.32
Rabbit BG	11.11	13.75	15.28	19.63
Human BG	12.04	13.75	14.26	14.26
Dog BG	10.79	10.65	17.09	21.44
Sheep BG	11.49	9.49	13.94	22.18
Controlls	16.21	25.61	15.74	11.44

Vol. dens. osteoid (V_{VOS}%)	7d	21d	42d	60d
Nude rat BG	0.42	2.04	0.61	1.07
Rabbit BG	0.37	0.60	0.33	0.65
Human BG	0.24	0.84	0.51	0.24
Dog BG	0.23	0.47	0.28	0.51
Sheep BG	0.56	0.09	0.33	0.46
Controlls	0.33	0.42	0.14	0.19

Total surface resorption density (HT %)

	7d	21d	42d	60d
Nude rat BG	1.72	2.89	1.58	2.27
Rabbit BG	2.01	1.04	1.24	0.56
Human BG	5.32	3.16	2.66	1.12
Dog BG	2.07	1.59	1.05	1.81
Sheep BG	1.43	1.60	1.17	0.85
Controlls	1.42	1.33	0.83	2.36

DISCUSSION

Despite the fact that there seems to be a homology of bone inductive factors (ref. 10, 11) and the excellent clinical results with only demineralised xenogeneic bovine matrix (ref. 12), partly purified bone matrix, i.e. bone gelatine, in our experiment was only active when implants of a closely related species to the host were used. In the other implants the probably exertable effects were overrode by the immunologic reaction to the foreign protein complexes. The further extraction of bone matrix with the isolation of growth factors (ref. 13), so called matrix derived factors (ref. 14) or chemotactic factors (ref. 15) might finally result in a better understanding of the regulation of bone formation and resorption but are no immediate solution to the problem of finding a suitable bone replacement material. In view of the dubious results of BMP as a bone replacement material reduction of the antigenicity of bone gelatine could lead to the developement of a clinically applicable bone replacement material.

REFERENCES

1 M.R. Urist, Iwata, H. et al. Bone morphogenesis in implants of insoluble bone gelatine. Proc. Nat. Acad. Sci. USA, Vol 70, 12, Part 1, (1973), 3511.
2 M.R. Urist, Huo, Y.K. et al. Purification of bovine bone morphogenetic protein by hydroxyapatite chromatography. Proc. Nat. Acad. Sci. USA 81. (1984) 371.
3 M.R. Urist, DeLange, R.J. et al. Bone cell differentiation and growth factors. Science 220, (1983), 680.
4 M.A. Parfitt. The cellular basis of bone remodelling. Calcif Tissue Int 36 (1984) 37.
5 M.R. Urist, Lietzte, A. et al. Beta-Tricalciumphosphate delivery system for bone morphogenetic protein. Clin Orthop Rel Res. No 187 (1984), 277.
6 O.S. Nilsson, Urist, M.R. et al. Proceedings 31st annual ORS, Las Vegas (1985) 107.
7 J.M. Rueger, Siebert, H.R. et al. Observation on bone formation sequence elicited by the implantation of bone gelatine together with calciumphosphate compounds.Biological and Biomechanical Performance of Biomaterials, ed. P. Christel, A. Meunier, A.J.C. Lee. Elsevier Science Publishers (1986), 45.
8 J.M. Rueger. Unpublished material
9 G. Delling. Endokrine Osteopathien. Veröffentlichungen aus der Pathologie. Heft 98. Fischer Verlag 1975, Stuttgart.
10 T.K. Sampath, Reddi, A.H. Homology of bone inductive proteins. Proc. Nat. Acad. Sci. USA Vol 80, (1983), 6591.
11 N. Muthukumaran, Sampath, T.K. et al. Comparison of bone inductive proteins of rat and porcine bone matrix. Biochem Biophys Res Com Vol 131, No 1 (1985) 37
12 J. Glowacki. Personal communication.
13 J.R. Farley, Baylink D.J. Purification of a sceletal growth factor. Biochemistry Vol 21, No 14 (1982), 3502.
14 T.K. Sampath, DeSimone D.P. et al. Extracellular bone matrix derived growth factor. Exp Cell Res 142 (1982), 460.
15 M. Somerman, Hewitt, A. Z. et al. identification of a bone matrix derived growth factor. Calcif Tissue Int 35 (1983), 481.

Biomaterials and Clinical Applications,
edited by A. Pizzoferrato, P.G. Marchetti, A. Ravaglioli and A.J.C. Lee
Elsevier Science Publishers B.V., Amsterdam, 1987 — Printed in The Netherlands

HISTOMORPHOMETRICAL AND ROENTGENOLOGICAL EVALUATIONS OF BONE REACTIONS TO CEMENTLESS NIOBIUM FEMORAL STEMS IN DOGS

F. Gottsauner-Wolf[1,2], P. Dallant[2], G. Pflüger[3], H. Plenk Jr.[2], F. Grundschober[2], and S. Schider[4]

[1]Orthopaedic University Clinic, Garnisongasse 13, A-1090 Vienna

[2]Bone & Biomaterials Res.Lab., Histological-Embryological Institute, University of Vienna, Schwarzspanierstraße 17, A-1090 Vienna

[3]Orthopaedic Department, HERA-Hospital, Löblichgasse 14, A-1090 Vienna

[4]Metallwerk PLANSEE GmbH, A-6600 Reutte/Tirol

(Austria)

SUMMARY

The bone reactions to cement-free implanted, surface grooved niobium femoral stems in unilateral total hip-joint replacements ofbeagle dogs were evaluated after periods ranging from 2 to 33 months.

Bimonthly X-ray check-ups were analysed subjectively and using a morphometrical method. From the 13 dogs, 5 developed radiolucent seams and periosteal bone formations after 4.5,14,17,and 31 months respectively, and these were found loose at sacrifice. Also in the remaining 8 stable stems, a decrease of the apparent zones of bone-implant contact was observed after 12 months of implantation. Only in one case of loosening a subsidence of the stem could be measured.

For the histomorphometrical analysis microradiographs were used, prepared from cross ground sections through femurs and implants in the proximal, mid, and distal stem region. Longitudinal sections and microradiographs were made also from the proximal end and the stem's tip. Using a microcomputer and a digitizing tablet, different parameters of the implant-related bone reactions were quantified by a specially developed programme. New spongy bone formed implant contacts in all 3 regions at random, and while the overall bone mass decreased after 12 months of implantation no significant changes in trabecular structure could be observed around the stable stems. However, a periosteal bone formation occured also adjacent to the stable implants,but disappeared until about 12 months. It can be concluded from this evaluation that a merely spongy bone anchorage of these cementless stems develops until 12 months and can withstand functional loading up to 3 years in the dog despite some decrease in bone mass.

INTRODUCTION

The bone reactions to cementless implanted joint endoprostheses are influenced by a variety of factors. In order to compare the influences of material and/or design of the prosthesis, the clinical and in particular the roentgenological evaluation will not prove sufficient. Experimental studies can be evaluated histomorphologically in addition, but the subjectivity inherent to both these methods of evaluation can at least partly overcome by morphometrical techniques. It is the aim of this study to prove the usefulness of such self-developed techniques in the evaluation of an animal experiment(ref. 1).

MATERIAL AND METHODS

In the animal experiment, a surface-grooved femoral stem was implanted without using bone cement as part of an unilateral total hip-joint replacement in 13 beagle-dogs (ref. 1). During observation periods ranging from 2 to 33 months, the dogs were allowed to move freely on a farm, and monthly alternating clinical and roentgenological check-ups and a sequential fluorochrome labelling were performed. After sacrifice, the retrieved femurs with the stems were embedded in methylmethacrylate and cut into cross sections in analogous proximal, mid, and distal regions of the stem, and into frontal longitudinal sections of the proximal and distal ends. For this study only the corresponding microradiographs were evaluated.

On the 2-monthly X-rays, apparent bone to implant contact areas and the subsidence of the stem were measured after introducing a correction factor for the varying projection of the implant in the radiographs, and the appearence of radiolucent seams around the stem and of periosteal bone formations was recorded.

So far, only the microradiographs corresponding to cross sections of the 8 stable implants were histomorphometrically analysed. Using a microcomputer (EPSON QX-16) and a digitizing tablet, a specific programme was developed on the basis of previous work (ref. 2). The perimeter of the implant was first digitized, and then its position in the medullary cavity and the surrounding old and new spongy bone, the cortical bone, and periosteal bone formations if present. A computer outprint of the microradiograph in Fig.1 can be seen in Fig. 2 with all the values for the different parameters. These values were partly pooled for the presentation of results in Figs. 3-6, but no statistical evaluation could be performed because of the low number of cases at the same observation periods. The same applies to the data obtained from a structural analysis of the old and new spongy bone formations around the implants, where volume density and a ratio of perimeter/area of the trabeculae were calculated(see Fig.5) Similar programmes for the evaluation of the longitudinal sections through the distal and proximal end of the stems are under development.

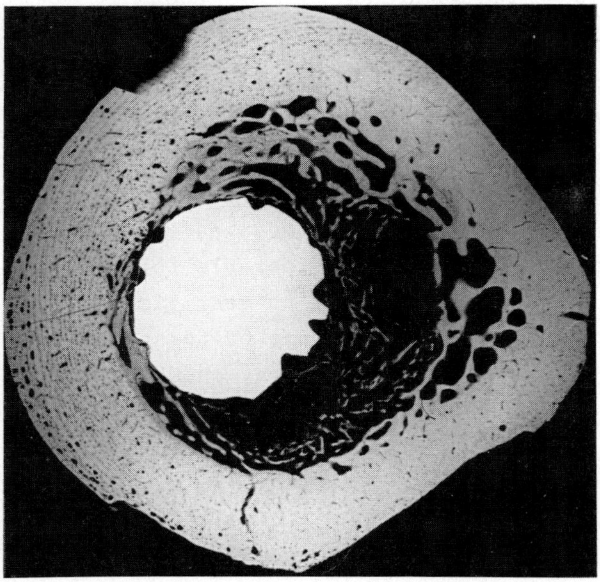

Fig.1. Micradiograph of a cross section through the mid region of a canine femur with a niobium stem, 6.5 months p.impl.(4.5 x)

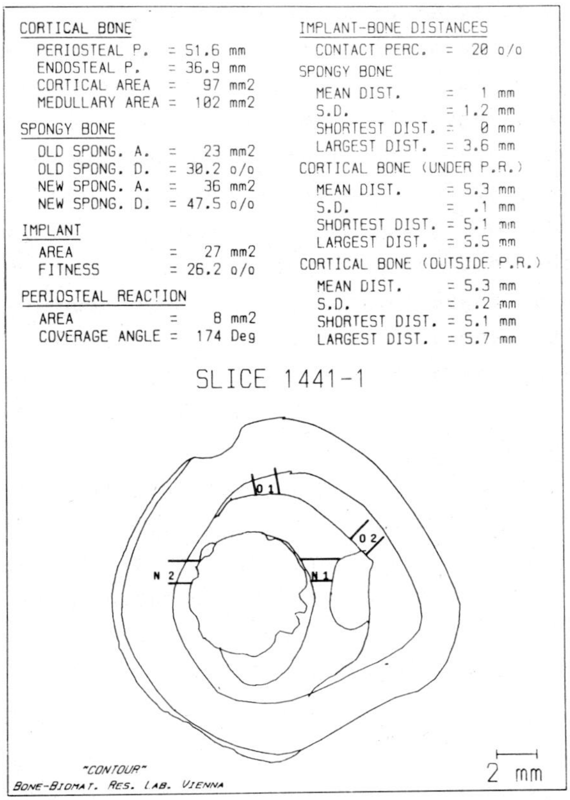

Fig.2. Computer-outprint of the evaluation of Fig.1 and the fields for spongy bone structure analysis(O and N).

RESULTS

Roentgenological Evaluation

On the X-rays, the implanted stems seemed in good position with only the tip in close juxtaposition to the diaphyseal cortex of the femur. When measuring apparent bone to implant contact areas,a slight decrease of these areas was recorded in course of time. However,only when distinct radiolucent seams developed around the stems in 5 dogs after 4.5, 14, 17, and 31 months, this was accompanied by the formation of periosteal new bone, leading to considerable thickening of the femur. All these stems were found loose at sacrifice. A subsidence of the stem could only be measured in one of these cases, where the brusque abduction of the leg at the X-ray check-up had eventually caused the fracture of the bone ingrowth fixation of the stem, as could be confirmed by the histomorphological evaluation.

Histomorphometrical Evaluation

The analysis of the position of the stem and its fitness(i.e. the space it filled in the medullary cavity)showed that the implants were first mainly hold in place by the bone structures in the proximal, trochanteric region, while secondary stability was achieved by ongrowth and ingrowth into the surface grooves of new spongy bone also distally. As can be seen on Fig.3, there was considerable variation, but appreciable amounts of new spongy bone formed in all 3 regions of the stem over the whole observation period of 33 months. However, a slight decrease and a more steady state becomes visible after 12 months, and this can be also shown when the values for the 3 regions are pooled (see Fig.4), even mainly on the costs of old spongy bone.On the other hand, the structural analysis of these new spongy bone formations did not reveal any significant changes (Fig. 5). Finally, periosteal bone formations could be detected also in juxtaposition ofthe stable stems, but seemed to disappear from distally to proximally until 12 months after implantation (Fig. 6).

In contrast, spongification of cortical bone and growing periosteal bone formations were observed around loosened stems, but these are not evaluated morphometrically so far. There seems to exist also a difference in the amount and structure of the bone formations at the tip of stable and loosened stems which also awaits analysis and quantification by a similar computer-software programme.

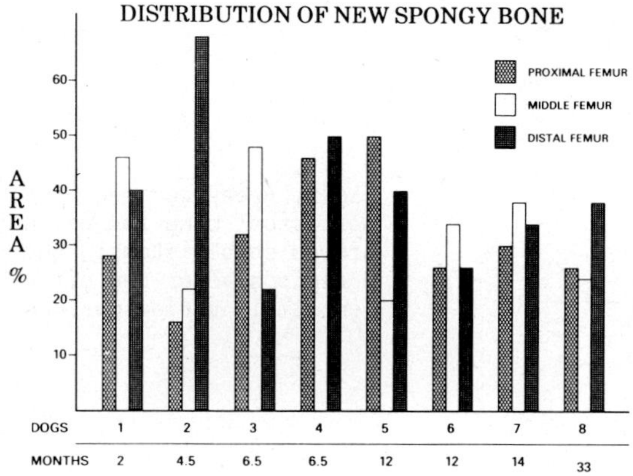

Fig.3. Distribution of new spongy bone(% of medullary area)in the 3 regions of the femoral stem after the different implantation periods.

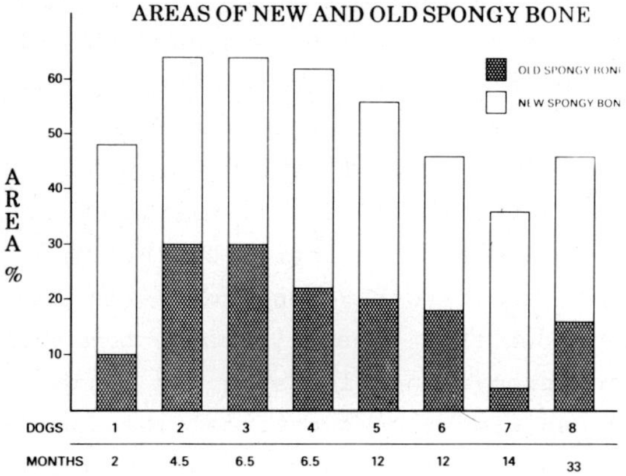

Fig.4. Total areas of the medullary cavities filled with new and old spongy bone (regions pooled)after the different implantation periods.

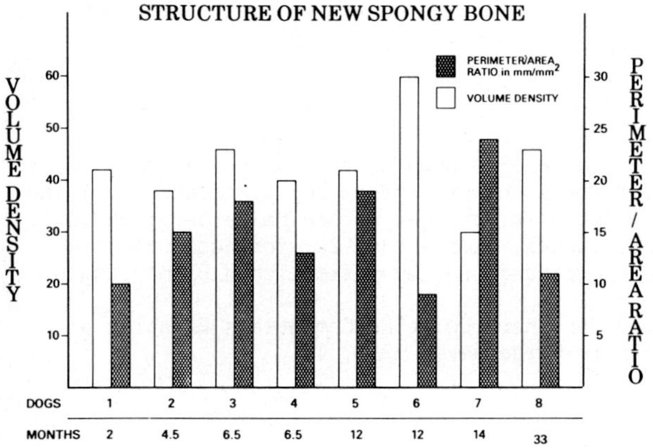

Fig.5. Structure of new spongy bone(regions pooled) around the femoral stem implant after the different implantation periods.

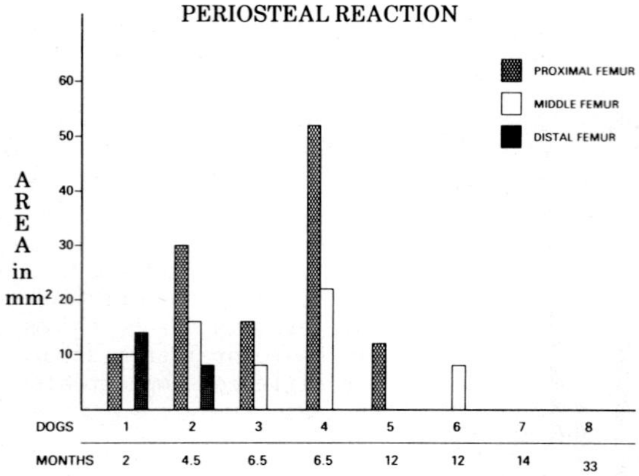

Fig.6. Areas covered by a periosteal bone formation around stable stemsin the 3 regions after the different implantation periods.

DISCUSSION AND CONCLUSIONS

The subjective roentgenological evaluation could only detect major changes of the bone structure around the implants which consequently led then to loosening. The simple morphometrical method applied did, however, give some indication of the time course of the overall bone reaction, and could detect the one severe subsidence of a stem.

The newly developed computerized histomorphometry, on the other hand, seems to yield suitable data for the analysis of bone reactions to heavy loadbearing implants which are to be anchored by the skeleton itself. A further extension of the software-programme is in progress. For this study it could be shown that a merely spongy bone anchorage of the cementless, surface-grooved niobium stem was established after about 12 months and can withstand functional loading up to 3 years in the dog. The diminution of anchoring bone structures, however, and the one case of accidental fracturing this anchorage gives us cause for concern in view of the critical period for the cementless fixation of endoprostheses (ref.3).

REFERENCES

1 H.Plenk Jr.,G.Pflüger,S.Schider,N.Böhler,F.Grundschober, The current status of uncemented tantalum and niobium femoral endoprostheses,in: E.Morscher(Ed.),The Cementless Fixation of Hip Endoprostheses,Springer,Berlin-Heidelberg,1984,174.
2 P.Dallant,A.Meunier,P.S.Christel,L.Sedel, Semi-automatic micro-computerized image -analysis applied to bone microstructure quantification,J.Biomed.Engin., in press.
3 E.Morscher, Introduction I, in: E.Morscher (Ed.),The Cementless Fixation of Hip Endoprostheses, Springer, Berlin-Heidelberg, 1984, 1.

Biomaterials and Clinical Applications,
edited by A. Pizzoferrato, P.G. Marchetti, A. Ravaglioli and A.J.C. Lee
Elsevier Science Publishers B.V., Amsterdam, 1987 — Printed in The Netherlands

SURGICAL APPLICATION OF BIODEGRADABLE FILMS PREPARED FROM LACTIDE-ε-CAPROLACTONE COPOLYMERS

T. NAKAMURA,[1] S. HITOMI,[1] T. SHIMAMOTO,[2] S,-H. HYON,[2] Y. IKADA,[2] S. WATANABE,[2] Y. SHIMIZU[2]

Chest Disease Research Institute, Kyoto University[1]
53 Kawara-cho, Shogo-in, Sakyo-ku, Kyoto 606, JAPAN

Research Center for Medical Polymers and Biomaterials, Kyoto University[2]

SUMMARY

The objective of this study was to prepare biodegradable films with adequate flexibility and mechanical properties and to apply them for the prevention of postoperative pleural and pericardial adhesion. We synthesized copolymers with various compositions from L-lactide, D,L-lactide and ε-caprolactone and determined their resulting changes in molecular weight, morphology, and mechanical properties. The glass transition temperature (Tg) of each of these copolymers was lower than 50 °C.

In mongrel dogs a 3-cm piece of the parietal pleura was excised and the pleural defect was covered with film (200 μm thickness) prepared from D,L-lactide: ε-caprolactone copolymer with a proportional composition of 80:20.

A 2 x 2 cm^2 piece of the pericardium was also excised and the defect was closed with a patch of film prepared from the same copolymer 20 μm in thickness. At 2 weeks, 1 month and 2 months the dogs were killed and examined.

For any of these periods no adhesion was seen between the lung and the thorax wall where the parietal pleura had been excised. The films had maintained their morphological forms until 1 month after application.

At 2 months the film patched on to the defect in the pericardium had changed into new membranous tissue. Between this renewed membrane and the heart no adhesion was observed.

Key Words : poly-lactic-acid, poly-caprolactone, bioabsorption, postoperative adhesion

INTRODUCTION

Polylactide(PLA), polyglycolide(PGA), and their related copolymers are promising materials for implantation in the human body. At present, bioabsorbable fibers made from these polymers are widely used clinically as suture materials.

We have been studying the characteristics of bioabsorbable films made of PLA, PGA and their copolymers. However, because lactide, glycolide homopolymers and their copolymers have a high Tg, films made from them are too stiff and rigid in the body at body temperature. Consequently, they stimulate adjacent tissues cause inflammation there, and because of their stiffness they tend to be easily torn from the needle hole made by the suture.

In order to solve these problems, we synthesized more flexible bioabsorbable films from copolymers of D,L-, L-LA and ε-caprolactone(CL) with various compositions and examined their degrees of degradation in vitro and in vivo.

In an attempt to examine the possibility of preventing the postoperative pleural and pericardial adhesion that makes reoperation dangerous, these copolymer films were implanted in the pleural cavity and also used for pericardial patching in dogs. The subsequent tissue reaction, especially the influence of the copolymers on the natural healing of adjacent tissue was then determined.

MATERIAL

P-D,L-LA, poly-ε-caprolactone and their copolymers with various compositions were prepared by bulk ring-opening polymerization of the monomers at 190 °C in vacuo using stannous octoate as a catalyst at 0.03wt% of monomer.

P-L-LA, poly-CL and their copolymers were also prepared with the same method. (Fig. 1)

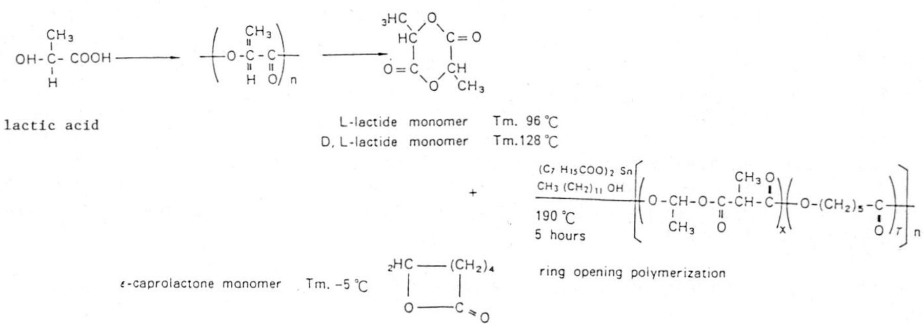

Fig. 1

The polymerization products were dissolved in chloroform, followed by precipitation with methanol to remove the unreacted monomers. Films were prepared by methylene chloride solution casting on a glass plate and then sterilized with E-O gas.

METHODS

In vitro degradation tests were performed using films measuring 30 x 5 x 1 mm^3 in PBS (pH 7.4) at 37 °C in order to follow the changes occuring in their molecular weight, morphology and mechanical properties.

In vivo test: four mongrel dogs (weight 7-15 kg) were anesthetized with

Kethalar and Rompun (10 mg/kg and 1.0 mg/kg, respectively) i.m. and then incubated. Positive-pressure ventilation was maintained with a respirator. A left thoracotomy was then made at the eighth intercostal space. Two parts of the parietal pleura (each ϕ 3 cm) were excised from the underlying muscle with an electric coagulator to form a pleural defect area. One part of the pleural defects was covered with film (200 μm thickness) prepared from the D,L-LA : CL copolymer (80:20 mol composition).

The film was fixed at four or five places with 4-0 Proline suture thread. Another part was left uncovered as a control. Then, a 2-cm piece of the pericardium was excised anterior to the left phrenic nerve. This defect was patched with a film 20 μm thick made from the same D,L-LA : CL copolymer. The margine of the film was sutured with five or six 4-0 Proline interrupted stitches. The left lung was reinflated and the chest closed. The dogs were subsequently killed at 2 weeks, 1 month and 2 months postoperatively.

At autopsy, the chest wall and the pericardium were excised *en bloc* and tissue reactions were histopathologically examined. The changes in the molecular weight and mechanical properties of the films were also measured. The morphological changes observed with SEM. One dog was not killed, so that a long-term evaluation could be made.

RESULTS

(*in vitro*)

Weight and molecular weight loss for D,L-LA : CL copolymer films in the *in vitro* test are shown in Fig.2, while the results of the *in vitro* test for L-LA : CL copolymer films are given in Fig.3.

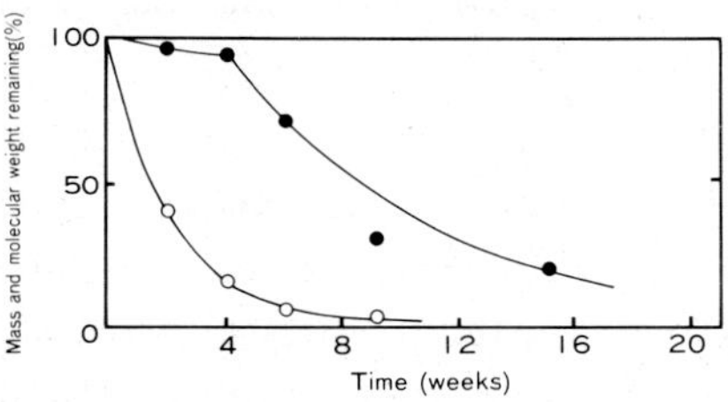

Fig.2 Mass and molecular weight loss for D,L-lactide-ε-caprolactone copolymer(D,L-lactide mole 84%) as a function of hydrolysis time. Open mark;molecular weight, Closed mark;mass

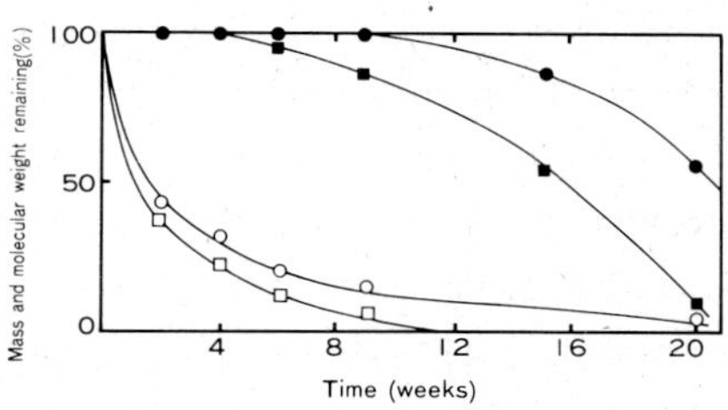

Fig.3 Mass and molecular weight loss for L-lactide -ε-caprolactone copolymers as a function of hydrolysis time.
(○):L-lactide mole 88% (□):L-lactide mole 65%
Open marks;molecular weight, Closed marks; mass

For both types of copolymer films, molecular weights were reduced rapidly from the beginning of immersion in PBS. Weight changes were not marked by 4 weeks for D,L-LA : CL copolymers and by 8 weeks for L-LA : CL copolymers. From those times marked weight changes were observed for both types of copolymer and by 20 weeks the weights of the films had become almost zero.

(<u>in vivo</u>)

The mechanical properties and morphological changes in the films which covered the pleural defects are shown in Table 1.

Table I <u>in vitro</u> EVALUATION OF THE FILMS OF D,L-LA-ε-CL COPOLYMER (200 μ)

Implantation time	gross out look	$\overline{M}w$	Tensile Strength	Elongation ($\Delta L/L$)	Tg
0	clear film	100,000	1.67 kgf/mm^2	509 %	39 ℃
2 weeks	white speck film	55,000	4.98 kgf/mm^2	150 %	39 ℃
1 Month	white opaque film	32,000	4.56 kgf/mm^2	15 %	37 ℃
2 Months	white compact mass	4,200	–	–	–

The film 200 μm in thickness retained their original form at the place of fixation for one month. At 2 months, each film had become transformed into a small compact mass and slipped out into the pleural cavity.

At no time within 2 months were we able to observe any adhesion between the area of the pleural defect covered by the film and the lung, while in contrast the defects which were not covered with the films adhered to the lung.

By SEM the surfaces of the films were seen to be flat and no change was observed under the surface by 2 weeks. And at 1 month, however, small waves were seen on the surface, and the inside of each film appeared homogeneous. (Fig.4) At 2 months, the film had become a small compact mass, the surface of which was irregular and the interior of which showed a porous structure when observed at areas which had cracked. Histopathological examination at 2 weeks revealed one layer of flat cells apparently mesothelial in origin in several areas of the pleural defect. At 2 months, after the film had slipped down, a layer of sequential flat cells, presumably replaced mesothelium, was seen in the area of the pleural defect. (Fig.5.)

The pericardial defect patched with the film 20 μm in thickness was replaced at 2 months with thin membranous tissue, in which the remnants of the degraded film were seen. No adhesion between this membrane and the heart observed. (Fig.6.) Histopathologically the replaced membrane was thin connective tissue and on the pericardial side, a single layer of mesothelial cells had reformed. (Fig.7.)

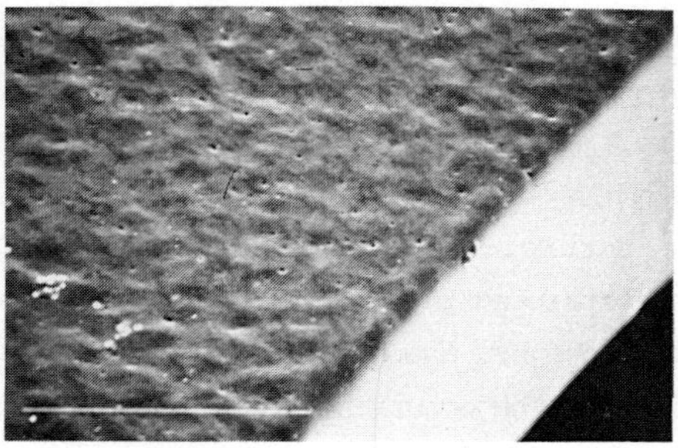

Fig.4 SEM of the aurface and the edge of the film one month after implantation. (Scale bar=100 μm)

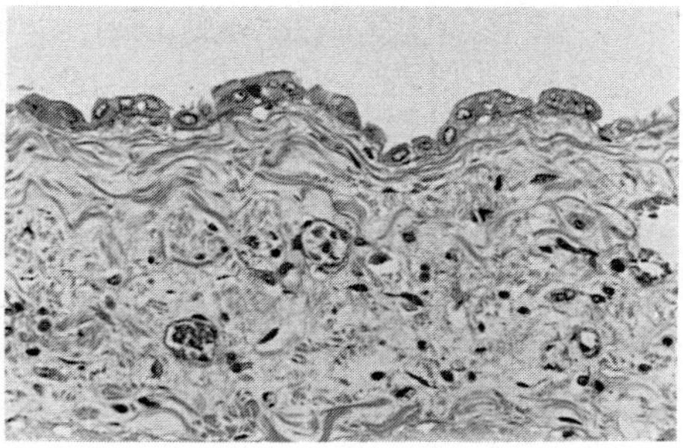

Fig.5 Replaced mosothelium in the area of the pleural defect at 2 months

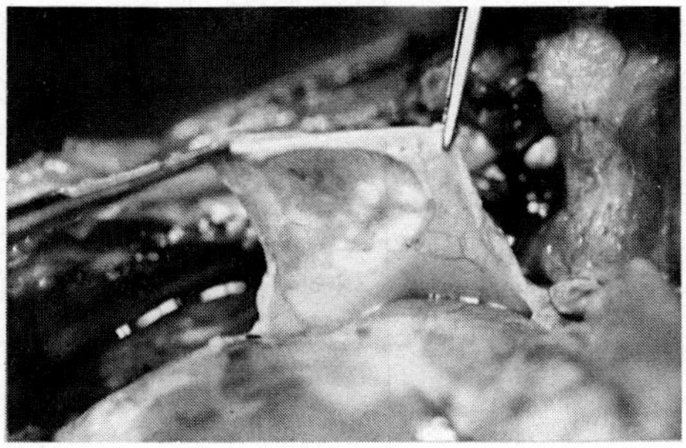

Fig.6 Replaced membranous tissue at the pericardial defect at 2 months.

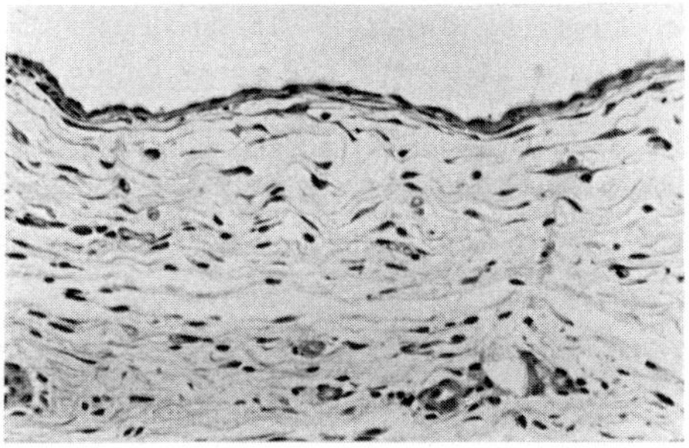

Fig.7 Replaced membranous tissue on the pericardial side at 2 months.

DISCUSSION

The question of preventing postoperative adhesion which makes reoperation dangerous has become an important problem as reoperations are frequently performed especially in cardio thoracic surgery.[1)]

Adhesion occurs at the space where ischemic, inflammatory, or serosally injured defective tissue comes in direct contact with another tissue. Therefore, in order to prevent adhesion, wounded tissue must be keep separated from surrounding tissue until the injured tissue heals and the serosa recovers.

We have been considering the use of biodegradable films for application as adhesion-preventing membranes. The properties essential for on ideal adhesion-preventing membrane are : (1) it must cause minimal inflammatory reaction and not interfere with the healing process of adjacent wounded tissue, (2) it must retain its form until the injured tissue has repaired itself, and (3) it must be easy to handled during the operation, and be elastic and flexible enough for fixation to the injured tissue with sutures. As both the pleural and pericardial spaces contain body fluids, any membranes used there should be absorbed in an aqueous environment through hydrolysis without attack by lysosomal enzymes.

We have been investigating the bioabsorption of films made of PLA, PGA and their copolymers and have found that these polymers have good biocompatibility and cause minimal inflammation during their degradation. However, films made from these polymers are too rigid and fragile, so that they tend to be easily torn from the needle hole made by the suture. In order to improve the mechanical properties of such films, those containing plasticizer (TRIACETIN) or PGA fiber-reinforced films were evaluated.[2] However, adequate results could not be obtained because of their rapid breakdown and the occurrence of inflammation.

The homo polymer of ε-caprolactone is a hydrophobic polyester with a glass transition temperature (Tg) of -60 °C and a melting temperature (Tm) of about 63 °C which degrades in the body slowly.[3] Compared with L-LA : CL copolymers, D,L-LA : CL copolymers degraded faster and showed an earlier weight loss. Through evaluation of the degradation behavior of the copolymer in vitro, we consider the D,L-LA : CL copolymer (composition, 80:20 mol%) to be adequate for use as an adhesion-preventing membrane. The films used in this in vivo test had sufficiently adequate mechanical properties so as not to be torn from the needle hole, and we were able to fix them easily onto the thorax wall with the sutures. Indeed, as long as the smooth films remaine between the two tissues, adhesion is not observed. However, Oppenheimer and co-workers have reported that a non-absorbable film, regardless of its material, causes a high frequency of malignant tumor.[4] As for the resorption rate, since healing of the pleural mesothelium is very fast, a period of one month might be sufficient for prevention of adhesion in the pleural cavity. In the in vivo experiment in the pleural cavity no adhesion was seen in the defective pleural areas covered with the films. In contrast, in the non- covered defect, adhesion to the lung was seen from the beginning of observation at 2 weeks.

For the pericardial defect we used thin films of this copolymer for pericardial patching. At 2 months the film was absorbed and replaced by new connective tissue membrane at that site. This thin film might thus act as a scaffolding for regrowth of the host connective tissue.

REFERENCES

1) Meus P.J, Wernly J.A, Campbell C.D, Takanashi Y., Pick R.L, Qui Zhao-kun, Replogle R.L, Long-term evaluation of pericardial substitutes, J. Thor. card. surg. 85, 54-58, 1983.

2) Nakamura T., Shimizu Y., Ikada Y., Hyon S.-H., Biodegradable Polymers and their in vivo Effects(4), Prep. Jap. Soc Biomater. 7th, 171-172, 1985.

3) Pitt C.G., Chasalow F.I., Hibionada Y.M., Klimas D.M., Schindler A., Aliphatic Polyesters. I. The Degradation of Poly(ε-Caprolactone) In Vivo, J. Appl. Polym. Sci., 26, 3779, 1981.

4) Oppenheimer B.S., Oppenheimer E. T., Danishefsky I., Stout A.P., Eirich R., Further Studies of Polymers as carcinogenic Agents in Animals, Can. Res. 15 333-340, 1955.

Biomaterials and Clinical Applications,
edited by A. Pizzoferrato, P.G. Marchetti, A. Ravaglioli and A.J.C. Lee
Elsevier Science Publishers B.V., Amsterdam, 1987 — Printed in The Netherlands

BEHAVIOR OF DIFFERENTLY STERILIZED ALLOGENIC LYOPHILIZED CARTILAGE IMPLANTS IN DOGS

K. WANGERIN, R. EWERS, and A. BUMANN
Department of Oral and Maxillo-Facial Surgery,
Christian-Albrechts-University Kiel (West-Germany)

SUMMARY

The behavior of beta-propriolactone-sterilized, radiation-sterilized and gas-sterilized lyophilized cartilage implants was investigated histologically after various times up to 328 days. Beta-propriolactone-sterilized lyophilized cartilage implants were completely resorbed after 230 days and had only undergone partial osseous substitution. The radiation-sterilized lyophilized cartilage implants behaved in the same way after 125 days. Despite partial resorption of the gas-sterilized lyophilized cartilage after 328 days, we found form-constant behavior and complete bony substitution of the absorbed regions in each case.

INTRODUCTION

There are divergent views in the literature on the value of lyophilized cartilage as an implant material. Unfortunately, the data on the lyophilization procedure, type of sterilization, and the behavior of the implant in its cartilage, bony or soft-tissue bed is often imprecise or incomplete. Blackstone (1) reported 1948 that his lyophilized implants for experimental augmentation of the alveolar ridge had already ossified after a period of 130 days. In 1966, Nasteff (2) concluded after using lyophilized cartilage for augmenting the alveolar ridge that the implant had been converted into connective tissue under the influence of its new function. Sailer (3) reported 10-20% implant resorption after clinical use of these alloimplants for 12 years. According to Eitschberger et al. (4) lyophilized gamma-sterilized cartilage implants showed bone induction and hardly any resorption. Sailer reported once more in 1983 on reconstruction of an alveolar defect with allogenic and xenogenic lyophilized cartilage in an animal experiment. He found ossification and calcification after a period of 240-260 days; these calcified areas changed into lamellar bone. Resorption was already pronounced after 23 days in both types of implant, but was replaced by intense remodeling of bone. The highly different findings on the behavior of lyophilized cartilage in various transplant beds led to the question of whether different kinds of sterilization have an influence on resorption, calcification and ossification of these implants. The purpose of this study was to attempt to answer this important question.

MATERIALS AND METHODS

Implantation of allogenic lyophilized cartilage was performed on three inbred adult beagle dogs. Under anesthesia, pieces of rib cartilage 1cm long were removed from another animal, freed of perichondrium and stored in hypertonic NaCl solution up to the time of lyophilization. Freeze-drying was carried out by the company Braun-Melsungen AG.

The lyophilized implants were variously sterilized in the following ways:

1) Sterilization with 1% betapropriolactone solution in accordance with the Zurbuchen technique (5), during the entire conservation period.
2) Gamma-ray sterilization by a single exposure to 2,500 rads.
3) Gas sterilization with ethylene oxide for 48 hours.

Afterwards, two 1cm long lyophilized cartilage preparations of each type were allogenically implanted in each experimental animal. The bony portions of the host's ribs served as the implant beds. After reflection of the periosteum the implants were used either to replace a resected portion of the rib or were placed on a cancellous bed after creation of a box-shaped osteotomy. Multi-hole miniplates and miniscrews were used for fixation. At intervals of 125, 230 and 328 days, one experimental animal each was perfused. The uncalcified hard tissue was sectioned according to the saw-polish technique of Donath and Breuner (6) with the modification of Kestel and Ewers (7). The preparations were stained with van Gieson stain.

RESULTS

Betapropriolactone-sterilized lyophilized cartilage

After 125 days, these implants were largely resorbed in the boxshaped implant bed and had undergone osseous substitution. There was considerable parallel loss of the prominent parts of the implant raised above the level of the cortical plate (Fig. 1). The new bone formation in the triangular cavity under the raised periosteum on both sides between the bony surface and the lyophilized cartilage was a striking feature. The interposed implant had also been largely resorbed. Neosynthesis of the cortical structures at the superior and inferior cortical plate was found with lamellar and reticular bone regions and nonabrupt transition in the osteotomy region. Whereas the rib contour had been restored away from the plate, a depression of the superior cortical plate in the form of a trough, and limited to the implant bed, was observed.

Complete resorption of the lyophilized implants inserted in the rib was found after 230 days. Osteoneogenesis had occured up to the level of the rib cortex with a relative thickening of the cortex and rarefaction of the spongiosa. Complete resorption and bony substitution with pronounced depression of the cortex near to the fixation plate was observed in the interposed implant. Doubling of the width of the cortex was found in the adjacent regions (Fig. 2).

After 328 days, the region of the boxshaped cartilage implants was identified only on the basis of the osteosynthesis screw which had been left behind, and which was surrounded by bone at its tip. Only the cortex far away from this screw appeared to be thickened. In the interposed implant region, there was still a thickening of the inferior cortical plate.

Radiation-sterilized lyophilized cartilage

After 125 days, these implants had already been completely resorbed in the boxshaped beds with only partial osseous substitution and shallow widening of the bony structures near the screw. Subperiostal lamellar bone formation had also occured in the triangular cavities. The interposed lyophilized cartilage was completely replaced with cortical and spongy bone and likewise displayed a trough-shaped depression in the cortex near to the fixation plate.

After 230 days, the implants inserted into the rib were totally resorbed. They had been only partly substituted by bone and this led to a loss of form of the prominent parts of the implant. A slight bony elevation was seen only around the osteosynthesis screw. Complete resorption of the lyophilized cartilage in the interposed bed was likewise observed. Bony substitution with normal cancellous regions, thinning of the superior cortical plate and typical trough formation and cortical osteoneogenesis distant to the plate, with doubling of the thickness of the rib, were also seen.

After 328 days, the osteoneogenesis with shallow elevation of the bony structures around the osteosynthesis screw was typical for these implants in the boxshaped bed. Near to the screw threads, trabecular thickening and formation of periostal bony lamellae were found around the tip of the screw. Reformation of the cortex and doubling of rib diameter was characteristic of the radiation-sterilized interposed implants (Fig. 3).

Gas-sterilized lyophilized cartilage

The implants in the excavated bed showed constancy of form after 125 days with preservation of the portion projecting above the level of the rib cortex. Layer-like remodeling of the implant with peripherally preserved cartilage structures, a broad zone of calcification in the middle and a basal spongy substitution of the same width were likewise seen, as well as periosteal osteoneogenesis in the triangular cavities (Fig. 4).

The interposed lyophilized cartilage had also maintained its form. The resorbed areas were all replaced with cortical or spongy bone. Distant from

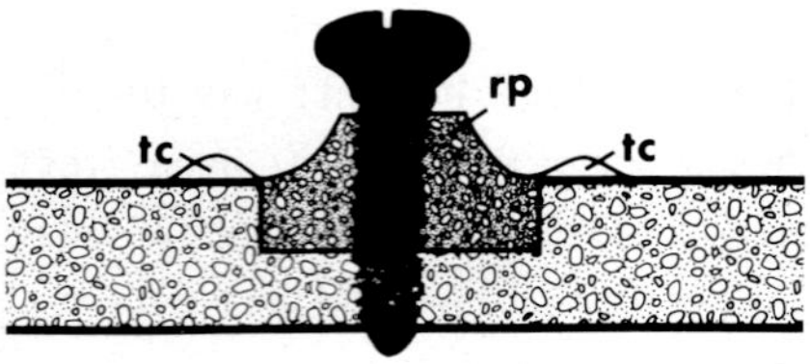

Fig. 1: Betapropriolactone-sterilized lyophilized cartilage implant in a box ostectomy after 125 days. Diagram showing resorption pattern (rp) and area of new bone formation in the distal triangular cavity (tc).

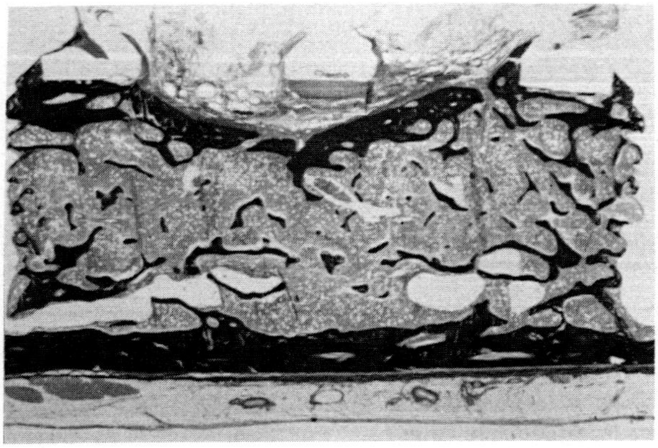

Fig. 2: Photomicrograph at 230 days showing loss of form and complete absorption of the betapropriolactone-sterilized lyophilized cartilage (x5).

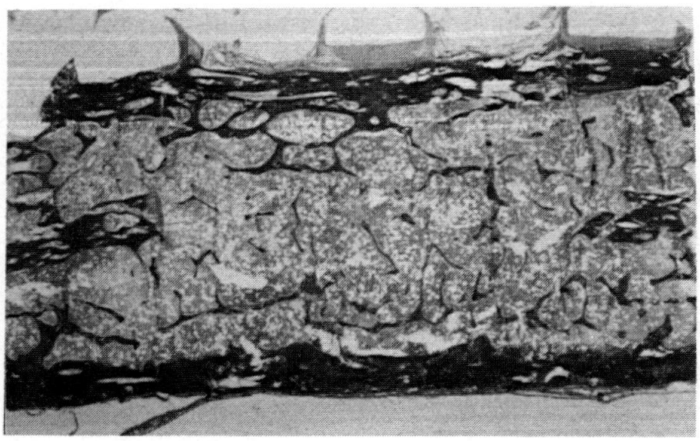

Fig. 3: Photomicrograph showing complete resorption of the radiation-sterilized lyophilized cartilage interposed after rib resection after 328 days (x5).

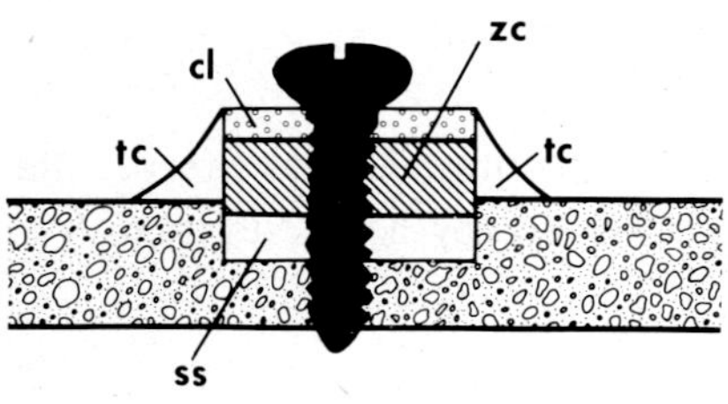

Fig. 4: Diagram showing constancy of form and characteristic triple layering of the gas-sterilized lyophilized cartilage implant at 125 days (cl=cartilage layer,zc=zone of calcification,ss=spongy substitution,tc=triangular cavity).

the fixation plate, pronounced periosteal bone apposition was found with development of additional cortex, spongy remodeling of the original rib and widening of its diameter.

After 230 days, in the gas-sterilized implants placed within the rib, the form was found to be almost constant with only slight resorption of the edge. There was bony filling of the triangular cavities and a characteristic three-layered structure. Whereas the peripheral cartilaginous implant layer remained roughly the same width, the middle zone of calcification had decreased in favor of the basal zone of osseous substitution. Small droplets of cartilage or of calcification could still be found in the interposed lyophilized implants; these were surrounded by cancellous trabeculae resembling a frame. Far away from the plate, periosteal osteoneogenesis has occured with doubling of the width of the rib.

Even after 328 days, the embedded cartilage implants showed constancy of shape. The characteristic triple layering and the bony triangulations hardly showed any alteration compared to the findings after 230 days (Fig. 5).

The interposed implants had a completely preserved cartilage border with zones of calcification in the superior cortical plate. In the inferior cortical plate islets of residual cartilage surrounded by trabeculae and doubling of the cortex were seen (Fig. 6).

CONCLUSION

These experiments show that the kind of sterilization influences the behavior of lyophilized cartilage in the implant bed.

It follows from these findings that the use of lyophilized cartilage implants must be managed in a different fashion than has been the case so far. If stability is required from the implant, and if it is bedded on the spongiosa or interposed in the bone, then it is advantageous to use gas-sterilized lyophilized cartilage. This might be the case in maxillofacial surgery when, for example, the stability after Le Fort I osteotomy with maxillary prepositioning can be ensured by insertion of gas-sterilized lyophilized cartilage between the pterygoid process and the maxillary tuberosity, or in an otomandibular dysostosis case, when the bony defects in the region of the maxilla or mandible can be permanently restored by gas-sterilized lyophilized cartilage fixed with osteosynthesis plates. If implant resorption is desired, with simultaneous bony substitution, radiation-sterilized or betapropriolactone-sterilized lyophilized cartilage should be used. This might be the case when filling the lumen after extirpation of large cysts in the jaw.

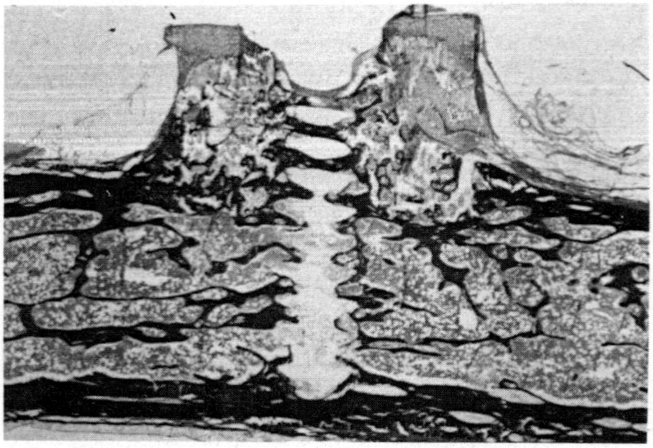

Fig. 5: Photomicrograph showing at 328 days the characteristic triple layering of the gas-sterilized lyophilized cartilage inserted in rib defect (x5).

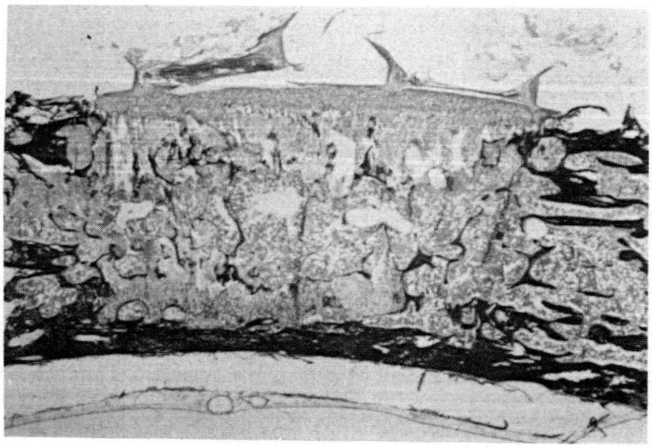

Fig. 6: Photomicrograph of the interposed gas-sterilized cartilage showing the residual implant and new bone formation in the center of the implant and at the lower border after 328 days (x5).

ACKNOWLEDGEMENT
Financial support was obtained from the Deutsche Krebshilfe, Bonn, Grant M 45/84/Wa 1.

REFERENCES

1 C.H. Blackstone, M.L. Parker, Rebuilding the resorbed alveolar ridge, J Oral Surg 14, (1948), 283
2 D. Nasteff, Klinische Beobachtungen über lyophilisiertes Gewebe in der wiederherstellenden Kiefer- und Gesichtschirurgie, Österr Z Stomat 63, (1966), 172
3 H.F. Sailer, Experiences with the use of lyophilized bank cartilage for facial contour correction, J maxillofac Surg 4, (1976), 149
4 E. Eitschberger, C. Gammert, W.D. Heine, Über das histologische Verhalten von Knorpel (Amboßgelenkpfanne) im Mittelohrraum nach unterschiedlicher Konservierung, HNO 25, (1977), 419
5 P. Zurbuchen, A.J. Held, M. Spirgi, Les homogreffons de cartilage lyophilisés et leur apllication en chirurgie stomatologique, Schw Mschr Zahnheilk 69, (1959), 703
6 K. Donath, G. Breuner, A method for study of undecalcified bones and teeth with attached soft tissues, J Oral Path 11, (1982), 318
7 M. Kestel, R. Ewers, Die systematische Aufarbeitung von Hartgewebsschnitten. -Eine Kombination von drei Methoden, Acta Medica Austriaca 12, Suppl. 32, (1985), 17

Biomaterials and Clinical Applications,
edited by A. Pizzoferrato, P.G. Marchetti, A. Ravaglioli and A.J.C. Lee
Elsevier Science Publishers B.V., Amsterdam, 1987 — Printed in The Netherlands

IN VITRO ASSESSMENT OF THE BLOOD COMPATIBILITY AND MECHANICAL PROPERTIES OF MEMBRANE BIOMATERIALS

J.M. COURTNEY,[1] M. TRAVERS,[1] D.L. MWANIKI,[1] J.P. PAUL,[1] G.D.O. LOWE[2] and C.D. FORBES[2]

[1]Bioengineering Unit, University of Strathclyde,106 Rottenrow,Glasgow G4 ONW (UK)

[2]University Department of Medicine, Royal Infirmary, 10 Alexandra Parade, Glasgow G31 2ER (UK)

SUMMARY

In vitro assessment procedures have been used to investigate the blood compatibility and mechanical properties of membrane biomaterials. Blood compatibility was studied in terms of the effect of regenerated cellulose (Cuprophan 150 PM), modified cellulose and a hydrogel on platelet adhesion, platelet aggregation and complement activation in the absence and presence of the anticoagulant heparin. The relevance of the assessment procedures was demonstrated by detection of the improved blood compatibility of modified cellulose in comparison with data relating to clinical use of cellulose. Measurements made with the hydrogel confirmed the need to take into account platelets lost to aggregate formation when determining in vitro platelet loss. The advantage of multiparameter assessment was exemplified by the low platelet response to the hydrogel compared with its influence on the complement system. The mechanical properties of Cuprophan 150 PM and acrylonitrile - sodium methallyl sulphonate copolymer (AN69S) were considered from the point of view of their integrity after processing for reuse. AN69S had higher values of breaking load and elongation at break than Cuprophan 150 PM in both membrane axes and, in comparison to Cuprophan 150 PM, was minimally affected by treatment with sodium hypochlorite.

INTRODUCTION

For the specification of standards for materials to be used as implants or in extracorporeal circuits, it is necessary to formulate in vitro methods of assessment. With respect to membrane biomaterials, in addition to the essential property of permeability, it is necessary to take into account the properties of blood compatibility and mechanical strength (ref.1).

To the accepted advantage of basing blood compatibility evaluation on multiparameter assessment (ref.2) there has been added the awareness of avoiding a narrow perspective (ref.3). This supports the view that an assessment of membrane blood compatibility should acknowledge that the blood response to a membrane may involve the haemostatic and complement systems and that membranes are normally used in association with antithrombotic agents. Therefore, we have added to our procedures for monitoring the platelet response to membranes (ref.4) a technique for determining the influence of membranes on the complement system. This article describes the effectiveness of the procedures in distinguishing between a standard haemodialysis membrane, a recently developed membrane and a hydrogel control material.

It has been long recognised that standards for the mechanical strength of a membrane must take account of the physical procedures in its manufacture and incorporation in a dialysis unit. However, recent years have seen an increasing interest in haemodialysis membrane reuse as a possible means of overcoming the leucopenia and complement activation occurring with regenerated cellulose membranes (ref.5). This has led to the need for assessment procedures to evaluate membrane integrity prior to reuse after processing with cleaning agents. This article describes the application of a mechanical testing protocol to haemodialysis membranes before and after contact with sodium hypochlorite and the suitability of this protocol for predicting membrane performance during clinical reuse.

MATERIALS AND METHODS

Polymers Investigated

Measurements were made with the following flat sheet materials :

regenerated cellulose Cuprophan 150 PM (Enka AG)
modified cellulose (Enka AG) with modification achieved by substitution of hydroxyl groups by diethylaminoethyl groups (ref.6)
poly (ethylene oxide) - based hydrogel supplied by Professor N.B. Graham, Dept. of Pure and Applied Chemistry, University of Strathclyde (ref.7)
acrylonitrile - sodium methallyl sulphonate copolymer AN69S (Sandoz Hospal)

Blood - Material Contact

The test cell for the examination of flat sheet materials and the method for achieving blood - material contact have been described previously (refs.4,8). Essentially, blood contacts two sheets of the test material of exposed area 46 cm^2, in a test cell which is oscillated at 150 cycles/min. Prior to examination membranes were stored in distilled water for a period of 24 hr to accomplish plasticiser removal.

In this investigation, oscillation was at room temperature and samples were withdrawn at 3,6 and 9 min. Materials were examined in the absence of anticoagulants and in the presence of heparin (1 IU/ml).

Platelet Response

The influence of materials on platelets was expressed in terms of the following (refs. 4,9) :

1. Platelet adhesion in the absence of platelet aggregates.
2. The tendency of the material to induce platelet aggregates.

Blood, obtained in each case from a healthy donor, was added to ethylenediaminetetraacetic acid (EDTA) and to an EDTA - formalin mixture in order to providefour platelet counts :

E_N Platelet count in normal blood added to EDTA

EF_N Platelet count in normal blood added to EDTA - formalin

E_T Platelet count in EDTA for blood after material contact

EF_T Platelet count in EDTA - formalin for blood after material contact

Platelet adhesion (PA) was obtained from $PA = (E_N - E_T)/E_N$

The contribution of circulating platelet aggregates to platelet loss (CAC) was obtained from $CAC = (E_T - EF_T)/E_N$

After addition of blood to EDTA or to the EDTA - formalin mixture, platelet counts were measured in whole blood using an Ultra - Flo 100 whole blood platelet counter (Clay Adams, New Jersey, USA) using the standard technique for that instrument (ref.10).

Complement Activation

The extent of complement activation was determined by measurement of the concentration of complement component C3a using a C3a des Arg radioimmunoassay kit (Upjohn Diagnostics, Kalamazoo, MI, USA).

Mechanical Testing

Membranes were washed with distilled water at 37°C for 30 min and then immersed in isotonic saline at 37°C for 1 hr. To simulate the effect of processing for reuse, membranes were agitated in 1% sodium hypochlorite solution at room temperature for 10 min and then washed with distilled water. In the case of repeated treatment, membranes were stored in distilled water at room temperature for 72 hr before additional contact with sodium hypochlorite. Membranes for control tests were stored in distilled water at room temperature for 12 days after removal from the saline.

Tests were made on waisted (dumb-bell) specimens subjected to uniaxial tension at a crosshead speed of 50 mm/min. All tests were performed on an Instron Model 11 - 95.

RESULTS

Blood Compatibility

Results for PA, CAC and C3a concentration obtained after 6 min blood - membrane contact with Cuprophan 150 PM, modified cellulose and the hydrogel are given in Table 1.

Mechanical Properties

For Cuprophan 150 PM and AN69S, changes in breaking load are shown in Figure 1. Results for elongation at break are given in Table 2.

TABLE 1

Blood changes after 6 min blood-membrane contact (mean values, n = 7).

Membrane	Anticoagulant	PA %	CAC %	C3a g/ml
Cuprophan 150 PM	none	4.38	42	4000
Cuprophan 150 PM	heparin	9.08	74	660
Modified Cellulose	none	4.90	12	216
Modified Cellulose	heparin	-	-	400
Hydrogel	none	1.60	10	560
Hydrogel	heparin	-	-	-

TABLE 2

Mean percentage elongation at break for membranes stored in distilled water (unprocessed) and treated 4 times with sodium hyprochlorite solution (processed) (Mean values, n = 11).

Membrane	Longitudinal Axis		Transverse Axis	
	Unprocessed	Processed	Unprocessed	Processed
Cuprophan 150 PM	31.60	11.96	179.56	73.56
AN69S	89.49	76.18	678.36	623.09

DISCUSSION

The measurements of blood response indicate the potential benefit of the in vitro procedures to membrane development in that the comparable performance for regenerated cellulose and modified cellulose with respect to platelet response and the superiority of modified cellulose over cellulose with respect to complement activation are consistent with ex vivo (ref.11) and clinical (ref.12) investigations.

The platelet adhesion and platelet aggregate studies made with the hydrogel demonstrate the possibility of obtaining platelet adhesion lower than that of haemodialysis membranes. The low platelet response with the hydrogel is supported by measurements of β thromboglobulin release made with that polymer (ref.13).

The results also indicate the possible misinterpretation which could stem from assigning platelet loss entirely to platelet adhesion and failing to take into account platelets lost to aggregate formation. In addition, the advantage of multiparameter assessment is clearly demonstrated by comparison of the low platelet response of the hydrogel with the influence of that polymer on the complement system.

The testing of membrane mechanical properties reveals the much greater influence of sodium hypochlorite cleaning on Cuprophan 150 PM than on AN69S. In this respect, the data support the reported increase in incidence of membrane rupture during reuse of dialysers containing regenerated cellulose membranes (ref.14).

REFERENCES

1 J.M. Courtney, J.D.S. Gaylor, M. Holtz and H. Klinkmann, Polymer membranes, in: G.W. Hastings and P. Ducheyne (Eds.), Macromolecular Biomaterials, CRC Press, Boca Raton, 1984, pp. 143-180.

2 J.D. Andrade, D.L. Coleman, P. Didisheim, S.R. Hanson, R. Mason and E. Merrill, Blood - materials interactions - 20 years of frustration, Trans. Am. Soc. Artif. Intern. Organs, 27 (1981) 659 - 662.

3 S. Murabayashi and Y. Nosé, Biocompatibility : Bioengineering aspects, Artif. Organs 10 (1986) 114-121.

4 M. Travers, J.M. Courtney, J.P. Paul, J.T. Douglas, G.D.O. Lowe and C.D. Forbes, In vitro assessment of the platelet response to haemodialysis membranes, in : P. Christel, A. Meunier and A.J.C. Lee (Eds.), Biological and Biomechanical Performance of Biomaterials, Elsevier, Amsterdam, 1986, pp. 281 - 285.

5 C. Woffindin, S.R.D. Johnson, N.A. Hoenich, M. Quereshi and D.N.S. Kerr, Membrane - induced neutropenia, in : J.P. Paul, J.D.S. Gaylor, J.M. Courtney and T. Gilchrist (Eds.), Biomaterials in Artificial Organs, Macmillan, London, 1984, pp. 64 - 71.

6 H. Klinkmann, D. Falkenhagen and J.M. Courtney, Biomaterials and biocompatibility in hemodialysis, Contr. Nephol, in press.

7 N.B. Graham and M.E. McNeill, Hydrogels for controlled drug delivery, in : J.P. Paul, J.D.S. Gaylor, J.M. Courtney and T. Gilchrist (Eds.), Biomaterials in Artificial Organs, Macmillan, London, pp. 141 - 151.

8 S.K. Bowry, J.M. Courtney, J.T. Douglas and C.R.M. Prentice, Utilization of the platelet release reaction in the blood compatibility assessment of polymers, Biomaterials, 5 (1984) 289 - 292.

9 S.K. Bowry, C.R.M. Prentice and J.M. Courtney, A modification of the Wu and Hoak method for the determination of platelet aggregates and platelet adhesion, Thromb. Haemostas., 53(1985) 381 - 385.

10 H.J. Day, E.B.S. Young and M.B.S. Helfrich, An evaluation of a whole blood platelet counter, Amer. J. Clin. Pathol., 73 (1980) 588 - 593.

11 D. Falkenhagen, G. Zinner, U. Falkenhagen, P. Ahrenholz, M. Holtz, E. Behm, H. Klinkmann, T. Bosch and H.J. Gurland, A modified cellulose (MC) membrane with improved biocompatibility, Artif. Organs 9A (1985) 74.

12 B. Schmidt, P.C. Spencer, T. Bosch, W. Samtleben and H.J. Gurland, Ex vivo biocompatibility evaluation of a new modified cellulose (MC) membrane, Artif. Organs 9A (1985) 77.

13 M. Travers, J.M. Courtney, J.T. Douglas, C.D. Forbes, G.D.O. Lowe, D. Falkenhagen and H. Klinkmann, Hemodialysis membranes and the platelet release reaction, Artif. Organs, in press.

14 T.L. Pollard, B.M.S. Barnett, J.W. Eschbach and B.H. Scribner, A technique for storage and multiple re-use of the Kiil dialyzer and blood tubing, Trans. Am. Soc. Artif. Intern. Organs 13 (1967) 24 - 28.

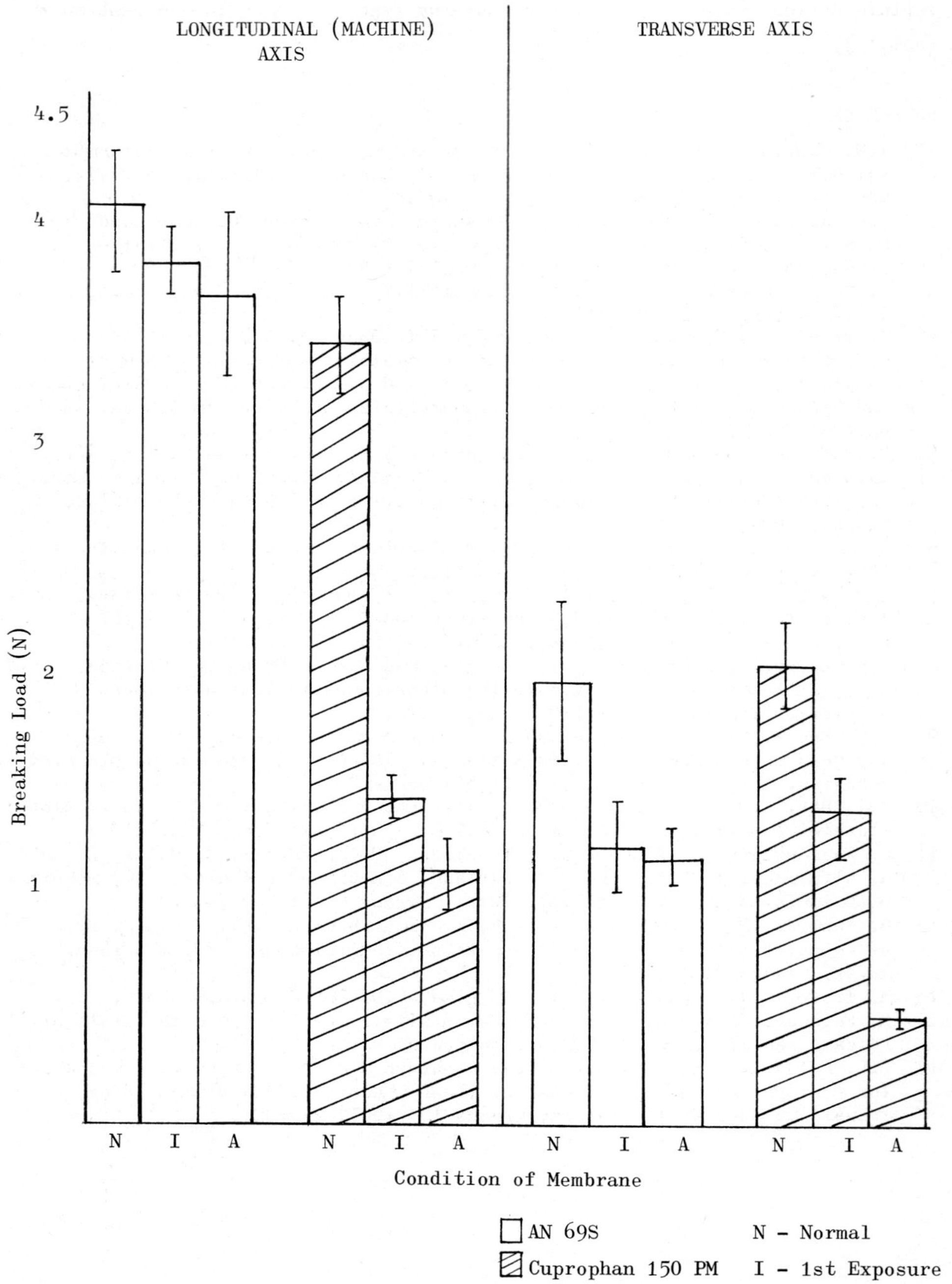

Fig. 1. Effect of 1% sodium hypochlorite (bleach) treatment on mechanical properties of the haemodialysis membranes (n = 11)

Biomaterials and Clinical Applications,
edited by A. Pizzoferrato, P.G. Marchetti, A. Ravaglioli and A.J.C. Lee
Elsevier Science Publishers B.V., Amsterdam, 1987 — Printed in The Netherlands

STANDARD FOR HARD TISSUE EVALUATION

H. Plenk Jr.

Bone & Biomaterials Research Laboratory, Histological-Embryological Institute, University of Vienna, Schwarzspanierstraße 17, A-1090 Vienna, AUSTRIA.

SUMMARY

In this presentation the currently available techniques and methods for the evaluation of hard tissues containing implants are reviewed. Based mainly on the authors own experiences a recommendation is given as to what can be regarded as standard requirements and procedures, what are special methods, only available in special laboratories and only to use for more basic investigations, and what are substandard techniques which do not or not fully provide the necessary informations about the reaction of the hard tissues to implants.

Besides improvements of roentgenological techniques for the non-invasive in-vivo evaluation, the preparation of microscopical sections containing the implants in situ within undecalcified hard tissues is a general prerequisite. After plastic embedding, all the techniques such as polyfluorochrome sequential labelling, polarization microscopy, and microradiography can be employed on ground sections, and sufficient cellular details are visible even on 100 µm thick sections, provided adequate fixation and appropriate surface staining. Only after taking full advantage of all these techniques, electron microscopy (TEM, SEM, Microprobe Analysis) should be used, in the best way in combination with the light mocroscopical methods.

A selection of the most recent publications on this matter is presented in the references.

INTRODUCTION

The hardness of bone and teeth is mainly due to the impregnation of the organic matrix constituents with mineral salts. A standard for the morphological evaluation of hard tissues is, therefore, incomplete, if their mineral content(and structure) is not preserved. Demineralization will also considerably reduce the existing armamentarium of methods for evaluation. In addition, the techniques for specimen preparation without demineralization allow for keeping in situ implants of even greater hardness than that of hard tissues. So, the interface between a well preserved tissue and the implant can be kept intact for a morphological evaluation, and these methods are also applicable for soft tissue implants.However, in this regard it must be emphasized that a material or implant, which is intended to be used in contact with hard tissues, should preferably be tested in this future environment. It could be shown with materials such as calciumphosphate ceramics that these more or less degradable materials are only compatible with bone, while in soft tissues they elicit a considerable foreign body response. Thus, the compatibility of a material should only be stated in respect to a certain tissue, i.e. tissue compatibility, and not with the more general term "bio-compatibility". Especially with bone the prefix "bio" refers to the very complex functional interactions which keep this tissue alive, and a bone implant has to match these functions to be tolerated, or even"integrated". Naturally, this makes the testing procedures more complicated, and in the following presentation the currently available methods are reviewed and estimated according to the personal experience of the author. Key references are presented at the end.

DISCUSSION OF METHODS

The main tool for intravital and non-invasive investigations of hard mineralized tissues is still roentgenology. However, it should be possible to better standardize the contrast of the radiographs for the sake of comparison. Fine grain X-ray films such as for mammography should be used together with appropriate filters to improve the resolution of structural details. To avoid overprojection an orthograde beam course is mandatory, and while computerized tomography is surely a constantly improving method, the pantomography used routinely in dentistry provides only substandard documentation of the bone reaction to a dental implant. Much better is computerized densitometry of good radiographs. So far also bone scintigraphy can not provide more than a rough estimate of the remodelling activity around an implant area due to lack of resolution.

The intravital application of fluorochromes has become an indispensable method to monitor bone remodelling activity over a longer period of time. Thanks to the pioneer work of the Laboratory for Experimental Surgery in Davos, Switzerland, this method has become routine in many laboratories all over the world (ref.1). However, it requires that the implant area can be evaluated histomorphologically without decalcification.

The investigation of hard tissues retrieved post mortem or ex vivo (biopsy specimen) requires first of all adequate fixation. Only if mechanical testing is performed first, the substandard method of cryopreservation (freezing) should be tolerated. In such a specimen the cellular details will never be well preserved and the penetration with embedding media will be impaired, but after mechanical testing (pull-out or better push-out test) the interfacial region will not be adequately preserved anyway. As a comment about so-called non-loaded or better, since such a condition is impossible in a loadbearing tissue like bone, not-functionally-loaded skeletal implants, this method of test should be restricted to more basic investigations, employing then the whole array of standard and special methods. However, not only for such advanced studies, but also for routine experiments the fixation by perfusion is preferable to sole immersion of the specimen in the fixative. This former method can also be used for the application of dyes to make the vascular supply of bone visible (microangiography, see ref.1).

The preparation of sections for the microscopical investigation ofhard tissue specimens should avoid in any situation the removal of the implant, at least before embedding has preserved the surrounding and interfacial tissues. Implant removal, decalcification, and routine histological techniques have to be regarded as substandard. The only seemingly more elaborate techniques of plastic embedding and the preparation of undecalcified ground and microtome sections is already a routine in many laboratories, and information about it (see ref. 1) and training possibilities are available in many places. So, there should be no excuse for wasting money and efforts in an investigation which is not properly evaluated. Specific emphasis should be given to the so-called "glueing-sawing-grinding-techniques" which provide the full versatility of techniques on the light and electron microscopical level. In this context, the sole application of scanning electron microscopy to the analysis of bone and other tissue reactions is critisized because it yields only results which are inferior to a subtle light microscopical evaluation. However, there is no question about the suitability of the microprobe analytical methods which depend on the scanning mode of electron microscopy.

The methods discussed here are summarized in Table 1 and 2.

REFERENCES

1 H.Plenk Jr., The microscopic evaluation of hard tissue implants, in: D.F.Williams (Ed.), Techniques in Biocompatibility Testing, Vol. I,Chapter 3, CRC-Press, Boca Raton, 1986.
2 G.H.Bourne (Ed.), The Biochemistry and Physiology of Bone, Vol. 1-4, 2nd ed., Academic Press,New York, 1971-1976.
3 D.J.Simmons and A.S.Kunin (Eds.), Skeletal Research: An Experimental Approach, Vol. 1-2, Academic Press, New York, 1979, 1983.
4 M.R. Urist (Ed.), Fundamental and Clinical Bone physiology, Lippincott, Philadelphia, 1980.
5 C.Anderson, Manual for the Examination of Bone, CRC-Press,Boca Raton,1982.

TABLE 1: HARD TISSUE IMPLANT EVALUATION

Recommended Methods:	STANDARD	SPECIAL	Substandard
IN VIVO	RADIOGRAPHY	*Morphometry	
		*Computerized Tomography(CT)	Pantomography(Dentistry)
		*Computerized Densitometry	
			Bone Scintigraphy
	FLUOROCHROME LABELLING	Autoradiography	
POST MORTEM EX VIVO		MECHANICAL TESTING	
	FIXATION		Cryopreservation
	* Immersion -	* Perfusion -	
	SPECIMEN RADIOGRAPHY		
	IMPLANT IN SITU		Implant Removal
			Decalcification
	PLASTIC EMBEDDING		Wax Embedding
	SECTION PREPARATION		
	* GLUEING-SAWING-GRINDING-TECHNIQUES		
	** HEAVY DUTY MICROTOMY	ULTRAMICROTOMY	Routine Microtomy

TABLE 2: HARD TISSUE IMPLANT EVALUATION

MICROSCOPICAL METHODS:	STANDARD	SPECIAL	Substandard
	STAINING		
	*SURFACE STAINING OF GROUND SECTIONS	*ENZYME HISTOCHEMISTRY	
		*IMMUNE HISTOCHEMISTRY	
	LIGHT MICROCOPY	*Computerized Morphometry	
	* BRIGHT FIELD		
	* POLARIZATION		
	* FLUORESCENCE		
	MICRORADIOGRAPHY		
		ELECTRON MICROSCOPY	
		* TEM	
		* SEM	* SEM *
		* MICROPROBE ANALYSIS	

Biomaterials and Clinical Applications,
edited by A. Pizzoferrato, P.G. Marchetti, A. Ravaglioli and A.J.C. Lee
Elsevier Science Publishers B.V., Amsterdam, 1987 — Printed in The Netherlands

STANDARD TESTS FOR SOFT TISSUE EVALUATION

D. F. WILLIAMS[1]

[1]Institute of Medical and Dental Bioengineering, University of Liverpool, P. O. Box 147, Liverpool (England)

SUMMARY

The following comments provide a basis for the discussion on standard tests for the evaluation of the host response to biomaterials in respect of soft tissues. The paper refers to the rationale for standardisation of testing, the difficulties of interpreting the data and the dangers of extrapolating from one set of standard conditions to different clinically-relevant conditions.

INTRODUCTION

Biocompatibility has been defined as the ability of a material to perform with an appropriate host response in a specific situation (ref. 1). Obviously a critical part of the biocompatibility phenomenon is the host response itself, which is the reaction of a living system to the presence of a material, and in order for us to determine the biocompatibility characteristics of a material in any specific situation, we need to assess, descriptively or quantitatively, this host response.

The host response will contain elements of localised and systemic effects. Standard test methods have been described in relation to the latter, for example acute systemic toxicity tests, but these largely arise from conventional toxicology and will not be considered here. With respect to the localised host response, it is necessary to define the specific location and, therefore, the precise nature of the tissues in question. Leaving aside blood compatibility, it is usual to distinguish between hard and soft tissue responses in this respect. The hard tissue response is dealt with elsewhere (ref. 2) and this discussion concentrates on the role of standard test methods for the evaluation of soft tissue biocompatibility.

THE RATIONALE FOR THE EVALUATION OF THE SOFT TISSUE RESPONSE

It is necessary at this point to comment on the reasons for conducting assessments of biocompatibility in general and the soft tissue host response in particular. At least four quite separate reasons may be identified, two of which are specific to product development and two of which are more universal in their intentions.

First, the assessment of the soft tissue response may be included as part of the screening procedure for the assessment of the overall safety of candidate biomaterials, or occasionally configurations of biomaterials. Indeed, it is usual, if not required by statutory or voluntary regulations, for anyone engaged in product development that involves new materials to undertake some form of soft tissue evaluation as a major component of this screening procedure, whatever the intending application and ultimate tissue location. Thus, candidate materials for intrabony, intraocular, periodontal, transcutaneous, intravascular or other specific sites will usually be evaluated in a simple subcutaneous or intramuscular experiment.

Secondly, and also related to product development, in-use tests may have to be performed in which the test conditions duplicate the clinical situations as closely as possible and especially where the test site involves contact with those tissues involved in the eventual application.

These two different types of test, being directly related to product development, are largely designed to provide go - no go answers, especially the screening tests. They do not generally provide a great deal of scientifically valid knowledge about the mechanisms that are involved. There is, therefore, a need for test methods that are able to provide a model system for studying basic mechanisms in biocompatibility. The reasons for any response may then be explored and attempts made to modify them or the devices in order to improve the soft tissue response.

Fourthly, there is the one reason which is perhaps most closely related to the purpose of standard tests in general and that is the requirement for basic data with which to write material specifications. Standards organisations in several countries have been engaged in writing specifications for certain classes of biomaterials, such as titanium alloys, stainless steels, high density polyethylene and alumina. These standards include compositional specifications and minimum mechanical property requirements. In order for reasonable and meaningful specifications to be established, it is necessary to be in possession of data on the effect of compositional or structural variations on performance. This is relatively easy to do in the case of composition and structure-property relationships in areas of mechanical properties and corrosion but it is becoming increasing evident that composition and structure-property relationships with respect to the host response are equally important. This data is far more difficult to obtain and the need to undertake this type of evaluation, and to provide standard test methods and protocols for this purpose is becoming more urgent.

The need for standardisation of the test procedures varies with each of these reasons and these will be discussed below. A few general comments, however, will be given first.

THE PARADOX OF BIOCOMPATIBILITY AND STANDARDISATION

In the above section an analogy was made with testing mechanical properties and using this data for material specifications. Materials scientists have long recognised that experimental conditions influence mechanical behaviour so that test conditions stipulate strain rates, temperatures, specimen sizes, surface treatments, precise stress systems and so on. Present knowledge is such that the influence of these variables on performance is reasonably well understood and data from standard test procedures is predictive, within a reasonable degree of certainty, of service performance.

Let us look, however, at the situation with the testing of the host response and the use of this data to provide material specifications or to serve as a basis for decision taking. The host response is a key factor in biocompatibility and is controlled by very many variables. These we may describe under three headings, the material variables, the host tissue variables and the system variables.

Bearing in mind that the local host response is a compromise between inflammation and repair processes, it will be controlled by the manner with which the biomaterial can elicit, or promote, inflammation, and the extent to which the biomaterial can modify fibroblastic proliferation and fibrogenesis. These themselves can be mediated via a range of material variables which include bulk chemistry, surface chemistry, specimen size and shape, surface topography, rate of corrosion or degradation, the physical and chemical nature of corrosion and degradation products and surface energy.

In relation to the host tissues, their response will naturally depend on their own structure but also on the species involved, the age, general health, pharmacological status, sex, previous history and so on. On top of this there are system variables, relating to the tissue-implant system and including the degree of attachment of one to the other (or conversely the relative movement between the two), the stress distribution within the system and the surgical technique.

If all of these variables contribute to the development of the local host response, the predictive nature of any one test system or model must be very limited. Superimposed on this we have the vexed questions of biological variability and idiosynchratic behaviour. It is a lesson that materials scientists often find difficulty in learning that animals, when used as a model for studying biological responses are themselves so unpredictable. Even with a tight control on all those variables mentioned above, and with one single material being tested in one animal model, different results can be obtained with different animals purely because of intrinsic biological variability. As if large standard deviations were not sufficient, we also find all too frequently the idiosyncratic behaviour from some animals which yield extraordinary results and lessen confidence.

To talk, therefore, of standardisation in biocompatibility testing, is almost a contradiction of terms. It is a paradox that if we are to make any progress in generating data for the basis of understanding biocompatibility we need to control and standardise our experiments as much as possible but yet standards for biocompatibility in general, and of the host response in particular, are largely inappropriate. It is for this reason that whilst we can have biocompatibility, defined previously, as a phenomenon, we do not have biocompatible materials; a material may elicit an appropriate host response in one situation, but that cannot qualify that material to be called 'biocompatible' since an inappropriate host response might be seen in another situation, in which case it would be 'bio-incompatible'. The greatest danger of conducting standard tests, especially screening tests, for soft tissue evaluation, is that the achievement of a pass-grade or high rating in the test is often seen as the qualification required to become 'biocompatible'.

THE INTERPRETATION OF DATA FROM STANDARD TESTS

The other major difficulty with the establishment, or performance of standard tests for the soft tissue response relates to the acquisition and interpretation of data. Returning to the analogy with mechanical property testing, the end point of, say, a uniaxial tensile test is absolutely clear; a specimen is strained in tension, the load is continuously and accurately measured and from the output of load cell and extensometer, together with details of specimen size, the parameters of Young's Modulus, proof of yield strength, U.T.S. and ductility can be calculated. This is entirely objective, quantitative, parametric data that is reproducible and easily handled by statistical methods if necessary.

Now examine the method of data acquisition and handling for biocompatibility testing. The ASTM standard practice for the assessment of compatibility of non-porous polymeric materials for surgical implants with regard to the effect of materials on tissues (ref. 3) states "compare the amount of tissue reaction adjacent to the test implant to that adjacent to a similar location on the control implant in regard to thickness or scar, presence of inflammatory or other cell types, not normally present at the site, presence of particles detectable by polarised light, and such other indications of interaction of tissue and material as might occur with the actual material under test. Note any evidence of neoplasia or tissue degeneration".

Clearly the assessment of biocompatibility does not lend itself to objective, parametric data but rather to subjective observations which are very difficult to compare across the spectrum of variables already mentioned.

Even greater difficulties arise when attempts are made to adopt scoring criteria and handle the data statistically. The ASTM standard practice for testing biomaterials for primary skin irritation (ref. 4) refers to a scoring system for test and control sites in which erythema, for example, is graded as:

no erythema	0
very slight erythema (barely perceptible)	1
well-defined erythema (pale-red in colour)	2
moderate to severe erythema (red and area well defined)	3
severe erythema (beet redness to slight eschar formation)	4

Erythema and edema scores for six animals are added up in respect of observations at 1 hr, 24 hr and 48 hr and an average primary irritation index calculated.

There are inherent dangers in this type of approach. First it relies on reproducibility between observers, or within one observer over a period of time and it is unlikely that such reproducibility can be assured.

Secondly, and more importantly, the handling of the data in this way is only valid for parametric data but is inappropriate for non-parametric grades or rankings. Thus to have a series of numbers on a scale of 0 to 4, to represent a variable and to add them up and divide by the number of observations to produce a mean is only valid if there is a linear relationship between the number itself and the significance of the event. When a parameter is actually measured, for example tensile strength, it is quite in order to calculate mean values, since a value of 1000 MPa is quite clearly double the value of 500 MPa. There is no reason to suppose, however that a well-defined erythema, with a score of 2 is twice as bad as a very slight erythema with a score of 1, or twice as good as a severe erythema with a score of 4. It may be that an exponential rating system is more appropriate.

Thus it is very important to avoid the use of parametric statistical analysis to demonstrate that one material is better or worse than another on the basis of non-parametric data.

SCREENING TESTS

It is undeniable that if screening tests are desirable to investigate candidate biomaterials, then standardisation of the test procedures is a worthwhile goal. In comparison with all other methods of evaluating host responses, it is the soft tissue procedures that have received most attention because of their relative simplicity and relevance. All of the recognised collections of standard test procedures that have been published, for example A.S.T.M. (ref. 5), B.S.I. (ref. 6), U.S.P. (ref. 7) and F.D.I. (ref. 8) include tests for the evaluation of either or both the responses to subcutaneous or intramuscular implantation.

The true value of these procedures is that they specify the precise conditions under which the evaluation should be made with reference, for example, to specimen size, shape, sterilisation method, implantation procedure, animal species, tissue location, experimental duration and so on. Provided the severe limitations mentioned above in respect of the assessments of the response are borne in mind, the development of these standard screening tests is to be welcomed.

IN-USE TESTS

Reflecting the concern that the response does vary with the conditions, it is a wise, and often required step for a material or device that has been cleared by a screening procedure to be subjected to an in-use test where the conditions more realistically represent those that will be encountered in the anticipated application. Examples include the assessment of the response of muscle to porous coated tips of pacemaker electrodes under conditions of stimulation, the response of the dura to cranial implants, the response of nerve tissue to neural prostheses and of dental pulp to *in situ* curing dental restorative materials.

Clearly standard tests are far less practical in this type of experiment since there may well be unique variables within each system. It is equally important here to recognise the limited predictive ability of even the best-controlled in-use test, for every animal model will be different in some respect from clinical reality. In particular we have to take into account the considerable difference in age or maturity between the average laboratory animal and clinical patient and the probable, but as yet indeterminate, species differences. There is also a concern over the duration of the experiments. As the requirements for longevity with implantable devices become more demanding, so it becomes necessary to test for long term biocompatibility, but the ability to do so in animal models at reasonable cost is very limited.

MODEL SYSTEMS

Scientifically the more interesting reasons for carrying out host response studies relate to the use of knowledge gained in increasing our understanding of biocompatibility. Almost by definition, and certainly because of the individualistic nature of the experimentalists, standardisation is again somewhat impractical here. Certainly the adoption of some procedural guidelines would be very valuable. The real difficulty, however, which has implications in the other areas mentioned above, lies in the fact that mechanisms in biocompatibility are so varied that it is impossible to devise universal experimental methods to account for all types of material and all types of soft tissue.

Returning once again to the analogy with mechanical property testing, this problem has already been encountered and has resulted in different modalities of testing to account for the various classes of material. Thus the use of uniaxial tensile tests at moderate strain rates has proved quite acceptable for the charaterisation of elastic and plastic properties of metallic materials, but is far less applicable in the case of the infinitely more brittle ceramics and the viscoelastic polymers. Basic information on these latter materials is therefore derived from other test procedures.

In studying the development of the soft tissue response, we are primarily studying changes in cellular activity and tissue architecture. If we know precisely what parameters of this activity and architecture are important, we do not need to worry about the nature of the material in order to determine the extent (and acceptability) of that host response. We might, for example, be able to measure a parameter of inflammatory cell activity (related to histamine, serotonin or prostaglandin activity perhaps) and/or fibrogenesis and use them as markers, and reproducible markers of biocompatibility.

Unfortunately this is not what happens since there are so many ways in which materials can mediate the host response and searching for and measuring one marker of inflammation or repair in one system may be highly inappropriate with another. The histochemical determination of enzymes as a marker of the metabolic activity in the soft tissues adjacent to an implant may be entirely satisfactory with an "inert" polymer which itself has no direct influence on enzymes, but may be inappropriate with metals which would conceivably interact with those marker enzymes and, in fact, could actually exert their most significant effect on the local tissue via inhibition of enzyme activity. This certainly points to the caution needed when applying standard test procedure over a wide range of biomaterials and clinical situations.

CONCLUDING REMARKS

These comments are not meant to serve as a criticism of standard test methods that have been written; there is a clear need for the establishment of standards or guidelines relating to the procedures for assessing biocompatibility in general and the local response in particular. What we must avoid, however, is an undue reliance on the objectivity of these methods and the tendency to extrapolate for a set of test conditions to quite different clinical conditions.

REFERENCES

1. European Society for Biomaterials, Consensus Conference on 'Definitions in Biomaterials', Chester 1986. Proceedings to be published by Elsevier Science Publishers.
2. H. Plenk, Standards for hard tissue evaluation. This volume.
3. A.S.T.M., Standard Practice for Assessment of Compatibility of Nonporous Polymeric Materials for Surgical Implants with Regard to Effect of Materials on Tissue. Standard F469-78, 1978 A.S.T.M. Philadelphia.
4. A.S.T.M., Standard Practice for Testing Biomaterials in Rabbits for Primary Skin Irritation. Standard F719-81, 1981. A.S.T.M. Philadelphia.
5. A.S.T.M., Annual Book of ASTM Standards, section 13, 1985. A.S.T.M. Philadelphia.
6. British Standards Institution, Evaluation of Medical Devices for Biological Hazards, Part 2. Method of testing by Tissue Implantation. BS 5736: Part 2: 1981. British Standards Institution, London.
7. United States Pharmacopeia, 20th Revision 1980, Section 661 "Containers". p. 948 U.S. Pharmacopeial Convention Inc. Rockville, Maryland.
8. Federation Dentaire International, Commission on Dental Materials, Instruments, Equipment and Therapeutics. Recommended standard practices for biological evaluation of dental materials. Int. Dent. J. 30, 140, 1980.

Biomaterials and Clinical Applications,
edited by A. Pizzoferrato, P.G. Marchetti, A. Ravaglioli and A.J.C. Lee
Elsevier Science Publishers B.V., Amsterdam, 1987 — Printed in The Netherlands

NON-DESTRUCTIVE STRUCTURAL ANALYSIS FOR NON-METALLIC BIOMATERIALS.

A. BERTOLUZZA

Istituto Chimico "G. Ciamician" - Cattedra di Chimica e Propedeutica Biochimica - Facolta' di Medicina e Chirurgia, Via Selmi 2, Bologna (Italy) Centro di Studio Interfacolta' sulla Spettroscopia Raman - Universita' di Bologna (Italy).

SUMMARY.

The applications of a non-destructive and non-invasive structural technique can make a new and meaningful contribution to the study of biomaterial standards at a molecular level. A suitable and promising technique is Raman-laser spectroscopy, which has the above-mentioned properties and also is not limited by the physical state.

Raman-laser spectroscopy applications to different classes of biomaterials are reported, considering vitreous, ceramic and composite materials, carbon fiber and organic polymers. Results on the application of this technique before and after implantation of some biomaterials are also discussed.

The success of a prosthesis is related on the one hand to the biomaterial properties in the different working stages, on the other to the biomaterial-tissue interaction.

Therefore, we can make a new and meaningful contribution to the study of biomaterial standards generally by using instrumental, non-destructive and non-invasive techniques suitable for the structural characterization of the biomaterial at the different working stages and after explantation.

For some years we have been using the Raman laser spectroscopy, a vibrational technique, for the study of biomaterials and their applications.

This tool consists of a laser source emitting coherent and monochromatic radiations generally in the visible region. The incident radiation activates the "structural centers" of the sample and is scattered with a frequency which is lower, (or higher), of a vibrational quantum with regard to the exciter line frequency. The scattered radiations are analyzed by a spectrometer and recorded as a spectrum of bands from which one can detect either the frequencies or the intensities due to the vibrational modes of the "structural centres" of the sample. A characterization of the sample structural centres can be obtained by the analysis of the band frequencies and intensities.

The sample can be in different states: solid, liquid or gas; hence the technique is more widely applicable as compared with other techniques which are limited by the physical state. Moreover, no preliminary sample treatment is required which involves structural perturbations.

The use of this technique in the study of a soft contact lens (ref. 1) in its different working stages and after explantation from a rabbit eye (ref. 2) in a pathological state, exemplifies the potentiality of the technique.

The lens is essentially formed by poly-HEMA, that is 2-hydroxymethyl-methacrylate which, with the methacrylate family, is a typical example of a polymeric organic material. In Fig. 1 the a and b spectra are referred to the blank and to the dry lens obtained from the blank without purification. The spectra show not only the typical bands of poly-HEMA, but also the more typical bands at 1640 and 1405 cm^{-1} due to stretching C=C and bending $=CH_2$ vibrations of the monomer. The monomer is not permissible to be present in the final state owing to its high reactivity; it has to be removed by appropriate treatment. The c and d spectra refer to finished lens, hydrated and dried, respectively. In these spectra the monomer bands are absent, but at the same time, compared to the previous spectra, some modifications are discernible regarding the relative intensities and positions of some bands due to water influence.

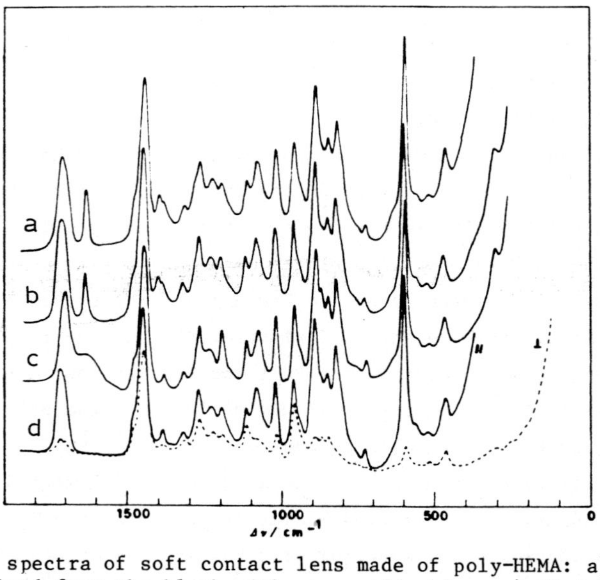

Fig. 1. Raman spectra of soft contact lens made of poly-HEMA: a) blank; b) dry lens obtained from the blank without purification; c) finished hydrated lens; d) finished dried lens.

Finally, Fig. 2 shows the spectrum of the lens explanted after 7 days from a rabbit eye, where a serious pathological state was observed. In this spectrum, the band at 1640 cm^{-1} due to the C=C stretching mode is superimposed on a wide fluorescence band. Afterwards, the formation of monomeric centers due to polymer biodegradation can be seen.

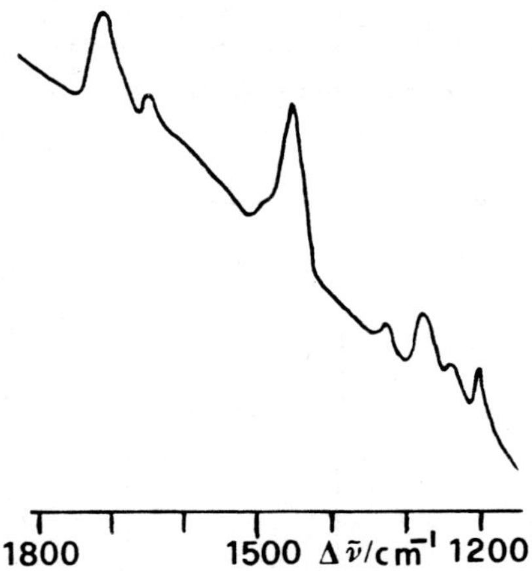

Fig. 2. Raman spectrum of soft contact lens made of poly-HEMA after 7 days from implantation in rabbit eye (phlogosis signs).

The Raman applications to the structural study of biomaterials are manifold; in the following some examples will be shown, subdividing the biomaterials into vitreous, ceramic composite materials and carbon fibers. An example has already been given of the Raman applications to organic polymers.

Vitreous materials

Two vitreous matrices are essentially used to obtain coatings for orthopedic prostheses with higher mechanical properties: SiO_2(v), vitreous silica and $Ca(PO_3)_2$(v), calcium metaphosphate glass.

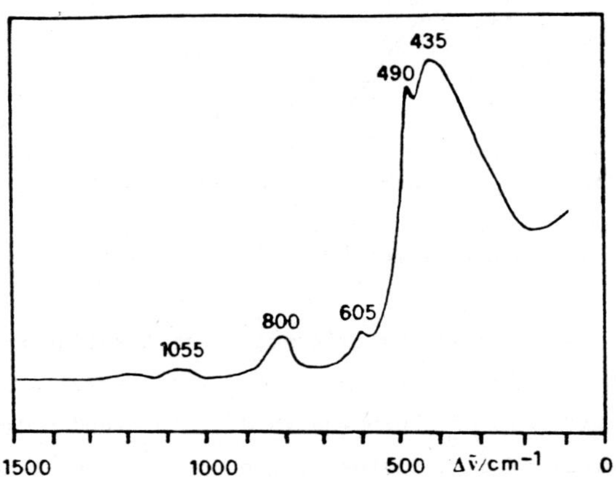

Fig. 3. Raman spectrum of SiO_2 (v), vitreous silica.

The Raman spectrum of vitreous silica is shown in Fig. 3. From this spectrum we can detect a three-dimensional structure formed by SiO_4 groups ordered within a short range only; in such a structure the oxygen atoms are prevalently localized between two silicon atoms with a widely scattered angular distribution. Moreover, the typical "defect bands", are present at about 600 and 500 cm^{-1} due to partially opened Si-O-Si bonds and to isolated structures of four membered rings of SiO_4 tetrahedra, respectively (ref. 3).

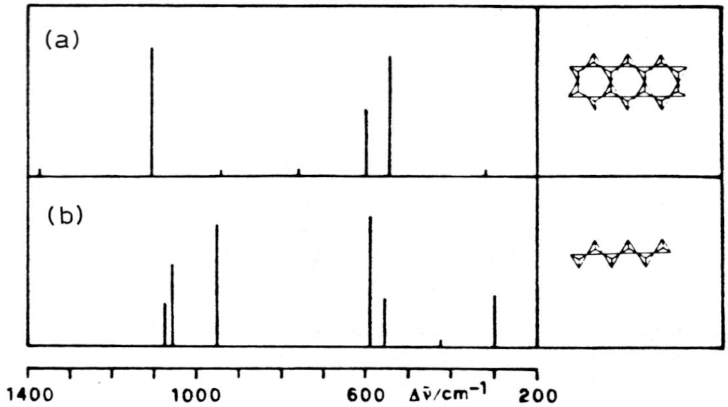

Fig. 4. Raman spectra of alkaline or alkaline earth silicate glasses with different basic oxide content: a) 0.3; b) 0.5.

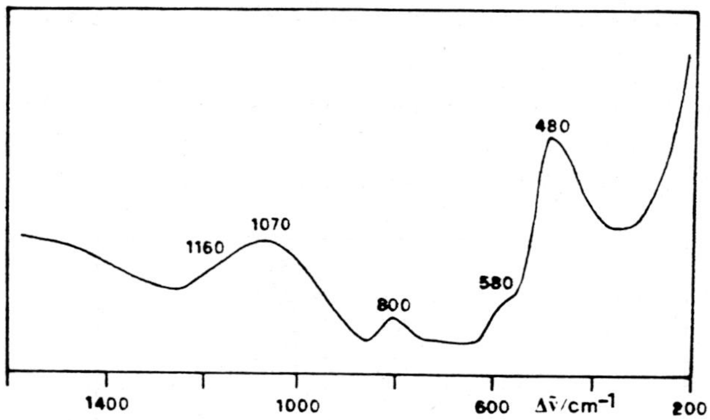

Fig. 5. Raman spectrum of S 85 bioglass.

When vitreous silica is added, by melting, to an alkaline or alkaline earth oxide, or both, the Raman spectrum of the glass is changed as shown in Fig. 4. When the molar ratio of the oxide is 0.3, independently of the oxide, a Raman spectrum typical of disilicates can be obtained, that is a structure prevalently formed by hexagonal condensed rings of SiO_4 groups in which one oxygen atom for every group is not bridged. The analogy between the Raman spectrum of the glasses and that of crystalline disilicates confirms this result. When the molar ratio of the basic oxide corresponds to 0.5, the Raman spectrum of the glass prevalently shows the polycondensed trend typical of metasilicate, that is of linear structures of SiO_4 groups in which two oxygen atoms in every SiO_4 group are not bridged.

On the basis of these results, we can characterize the structure of vitreous materials made up of $SiO_2(v)$. For example, in Fig. 5, the Raman spectrum of the S 85 bioglass, recently studied by us, is shown; from this spectrum, the typical structure of disilicate can be seen.

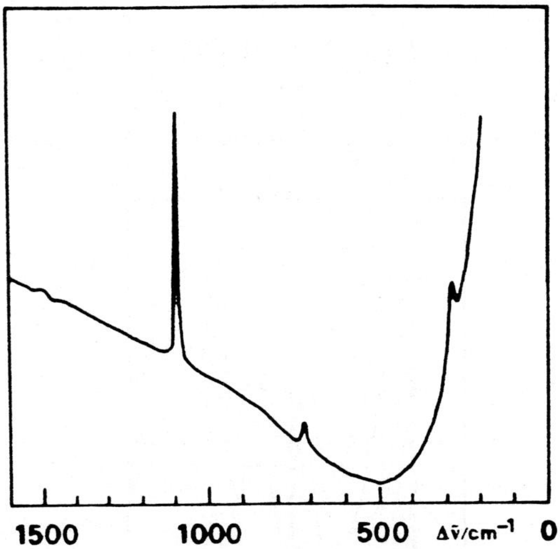

Fig. 6. Raman surface spectrum of KRV1 17 glass.

Fig. 6 shows the surface spectrum of KRV1 17 glass, derived from an Hench glass by enriching it with CaO and Na_2O, maintained in physiological solution for 9 months (ref. 4). In Fig. 7 we give the surface spectrum of an analogous glass, AKRA 17, after explantation from the femur of a rabbit in which a metallic rod coated with the glass was implanted (ref. 4). In the first case, the Raman spectrum clearly shows the superficial formation of a species with carbonate structure; in the second, on the contrary, it shows a bony growth structure in which one can detect either the bands of the inorganic phase or those of the organic bone matrix.

As regards the class of glasses made of calcium metaphosphate the Raman laser spectroscopy can give useful information (ref. 5).

Fig. 8 shows the spectra of calcium metaphosphate glass $Ca(PO_3)_2$ and of calcium oligophosphate $xCaO.P_2O_5$ glasses obtained by melting mixtures of calcium metaphosphate and hydroxyapatite so that the molar ratio x does not exceed the value 1.65, the limit value for the vitreous state.

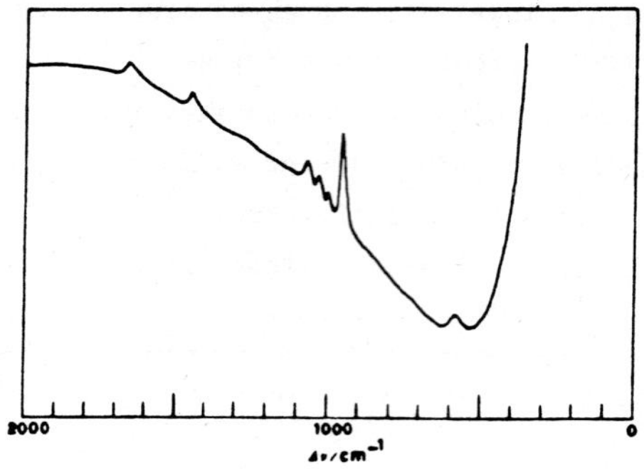

Fig. 7. Raman surface spectrum of AKRA 17 glass.

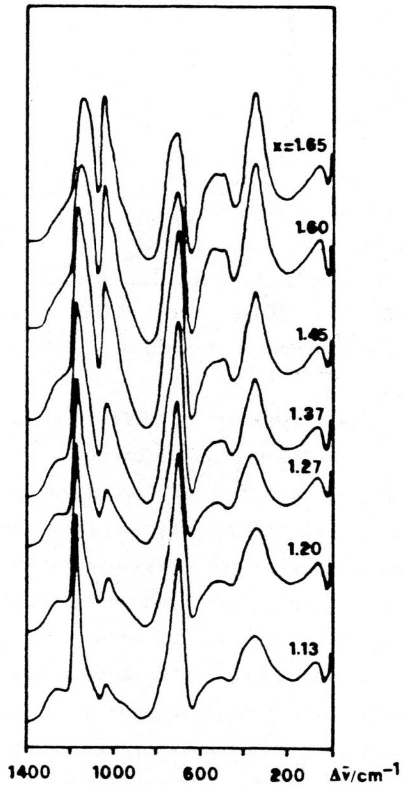

Fig. 8. Raman spectra of calcium metaphosphate $Ca(PO_3)_2$ glass and calcium oligophosphates x $CaO.P_2O_5$ glasses.

The lower value of the molar ratio for the samples examined is not 1 (the ideal value corresponding to vitreous calcium metaphosphate), but 1.13 owing to a slight loss of P_2O_5 during the glass melting.

It is known that the calcium metaphosphate has an indefinite polymeric linear structure of PO_3 unities mutually interacting with oxygen bridges and with a non-bridged oxygen available for cation. Oligophosphates, on the contrary, always have a linear structure with average chain length n depending on the x molar ratio between calcium oxide and phosphorous oxide, according to the formula

$$x=\frac{\bar{n}+2}{\bar{n}}$$

In this case the Raman spectroscopy makes it possible not only to characterize the oligophosphate glass structure, but also to show, from a structural point of view, the polymeric degradation due to calcium oxide as regards the indefinite polymeric structure of calcium metaphosphate.

In the Raman spectrum (Fig. 8), the strong bands at 1175 and 695 cm^{-1} are attributable to symmetrical stretching vibrations of PO_2^- and of P-O-P groups, respectively. As molar ratio x is increased, significant changes are observed for these bands and for other new ones. In particular, we can observe a progressive intensity lowering of the 1175 cm^{-1} band and the appearance of a new strong band at 1140 cm^{-1} in the spectrum of the glass with x=1.65. Likewise, the intensity of the band at 695 cm^{-1} decreases and a new component appears at 710 cm^{-1}. These changes in the spectra are in agreement with a structural breakdown of the polyphosphatic chains and with the formation of oligomers with a lower average chain length, n, related to x by the above mentioned formula. Moreover, the breakdown of the polyphosphatic chains, as x increases, gives rise to the formation of $PO_3^=$ terminal groups. The presence of these groups can be deduced by the appearance in the spectra of a band between 1020 and 1040 cm^{-1}, which intensifies as x increases.

Ceramic materials .

Aluminium oxide and the titanium oxide are two most important orthopedic biomaterials. Other oxides, as for example zirconium oxide, have recently been used.

In nature, aluminium oxide can exist in different states, such as α modification, known by the name corundum, γ modification (really, several "metastable" phases) and as β modification, which really is a non-stoichiometric aluminate with a low content of basic oxide.

The Raman spectrum of a corundum monocrystal obtained by different laser light polarization orientation is described in the literature (ref. 6). The alumines are also described; in particular, the sodium one shows a typical spectrum between 950 and 200 cm^{-1}. At very low frequencies, two bands, at 100 and 60 cm^{-1}, appear; these are known as cationic bands and they can be considered as due to traslational modes of the cation in the oxide structure (ref. 7).

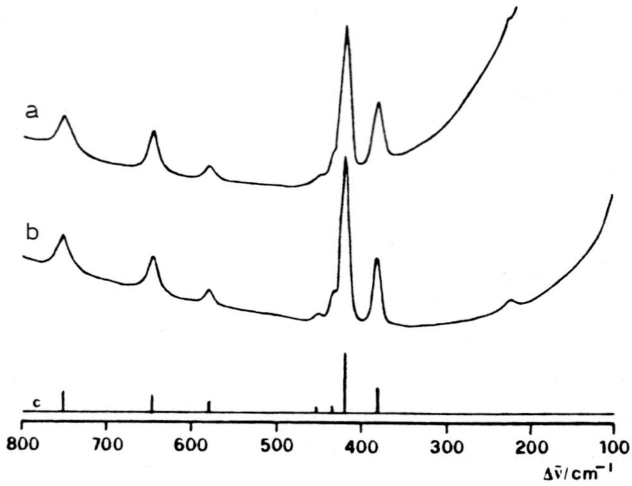

Fig. 9. Raman surface spectra of a Al_2O_3 cup: a) external surface after two years from implantation; b) inner surface obtained by dissecting the cup; c) α-Al_2O_3, corundum.

We have studied alumina as biomaterial for different orthopedic prostheses. In particular, in Fig. 9, the Raman surface spectra of a cup made of 99.7% pure alumina after 2 years from implantation (spectrum a) and of the inner surface obtained by dissecting the same cup (spectrum b) are reported. The spectra are coincident with that of the polycristalline α-Al_2O_3, corundum (spectrum c). The Raman spectrum of the prosthesis did not show any superficial modification attributable to changes from aluminium oxide interacting with tissues. In fact, the spectrum of the prosthesis inner surface confirms the chemical stability of this material.

Titanium dioxide exists in two main modifications: rutile and anatase (Fig. 10). The two forms have packed octahedron structures, but with different Ti-O distances (ref. 8). The Raman spectra are clearly distinguishable: in this case as well, the technique shows its ability to characterize this ceramic prosthesis material in a non-destructive way.

Finally, zirconium dioxide can exist in 3 polymorphic modifications: the monoclinic, the tetrahedric, obtained by heating the monoclinic modification up to 1100°C, and the cubic, obtained by further heating up to 2000°C. Amorphous ZrO_2 can also be obtained. The Raman spectra of these three modifications are also clearly distinguishable (ref. 9).

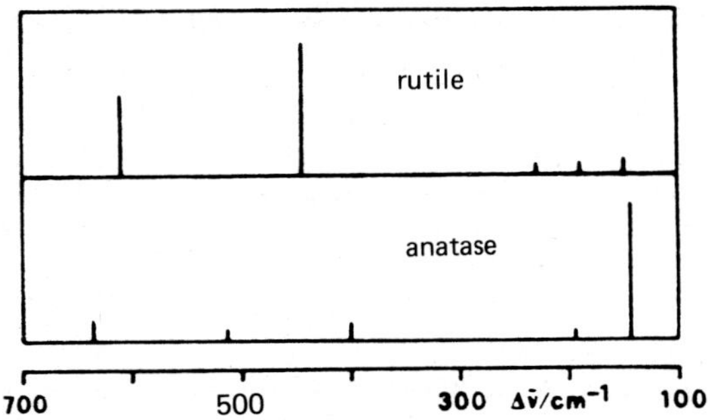

Fig. 10. Raman spectra of the two main polymorphic forms of TiO_2.

Composites .

As examples of the use of Raman spectroscopy for the structural study of composites, the Raman results of a composite made of TiO_2 anatase, ZrO_2 monoclinic and PbO initially mixed in the ratio 0.53:0.47:1, are reported (ref. 10). By sintering at 750°C, the combined spectrum of PbO and $PbTiO_3$ appears; at 1100°C a tetragonal $Pb(Zr_{0.53}Ti_{0.47})O_3$ structure is been from the spectrum; at 1260°C the structure changes towards the rombohedral one.

Carbon fibers .

Carbon-carbon materials can also be studied with good results using Raman spectroscopy. These materials are made of carbon fibers immersed in a carbon matrix, and they have different mechanical properties (high or low modulus of elasticity) in relation to the structural organization of the carbon.

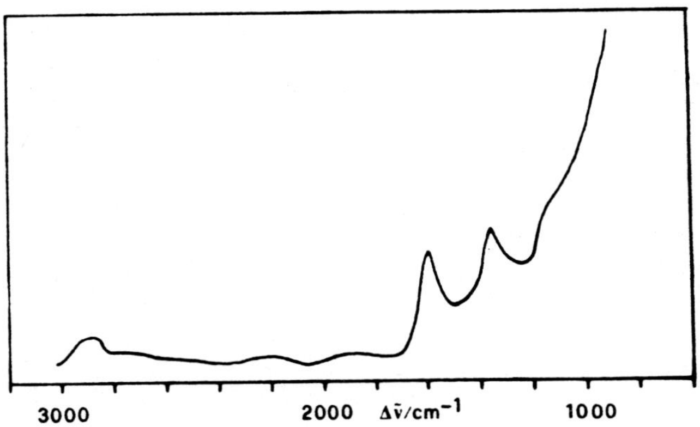

Fig. 11. Raman spectrum of a carbon prosthesis.

In Fig. 11, the Raman spectrum of a carbon prosthesis is shown. The band at ~1580 cm^{-1} is typical of crystalline graphite, while that at ~1350 is due to less-organized carbon. In this context, we can deduce for the carbon prosthesis the presence of graphitized carbon (1580 cm^{-1} band) and of less organized carbon (1350 cm^{-1} band).

REFERENCES.

1 A. Bertoluzza, P. Monti, J.V. Garcia-Ramos, R. Simoni, R. Caramazza and A. Calzavara, Applications of Raman spectroscopy to the ophthalmological field: Raman spectra of soft contact lenses made of poly-2-hydroxyethyl-methacrylate (PHEMA), J. Mol. Struct., 143 (1986) 469-472.
2 Results not yet published.
3 A. Bertoluzza, C. Fagnano, M.A. Morelli, V. Gottardi and M. Guglielmi, Raman defect peaks in the spectra of Na_2O silica gels evolving toward glass, J. Non-Cryst. Solids 82 (1986) 127-136.
4 A. Krajewski, A. Ravaglioli, A. Bertoluzza, P. Monti, M.A. Battaglia, A. Pizzoferrato, R. Olmi and A. Moroni, Structural modifications and biological compatibility of doped bioactive glasses, in press.
5 A. Bertoluzza, M.A. Battaglia, R. Simoni and D.A. Long, Vibrational spectroscopic studies of a new class of oligophosphate glasses of biological interest - Part 2, J. Raman Spectr. 14(3) (1983) 178-183.
6 S.P.S. Porto and R.S. Krishnan, Raman effect of corundum, J. Chem. Phys. 47(3) (1967) 1009-1012.
7 P. Colomban, R. Mercier and G. Lucazeau, Vibrational study of and conduction mechanism in β alumina. II. Non stoichiometric β alumina, J. Chem. Phys. 75(3) (1981) 1388-1399.
8 D.T. Cromer and K. Herrington, The structure of anatase and rutile, J. Am. Chem. Soc. 77 (1955) 4708-4709.
9 V.G. Keramidas and W.B. White, Raman scattering study of the crystallization and phase transformations of ZrO_2, J. Am. Ceram. Soc. 57(1) (1974) 22-24.
10 P.A. Chen, Raman effect in sintered ceramics, J. Am. Ceram. Soc. 57(6) (1974) 275-276.

Author Index

SUBJECT INDEX